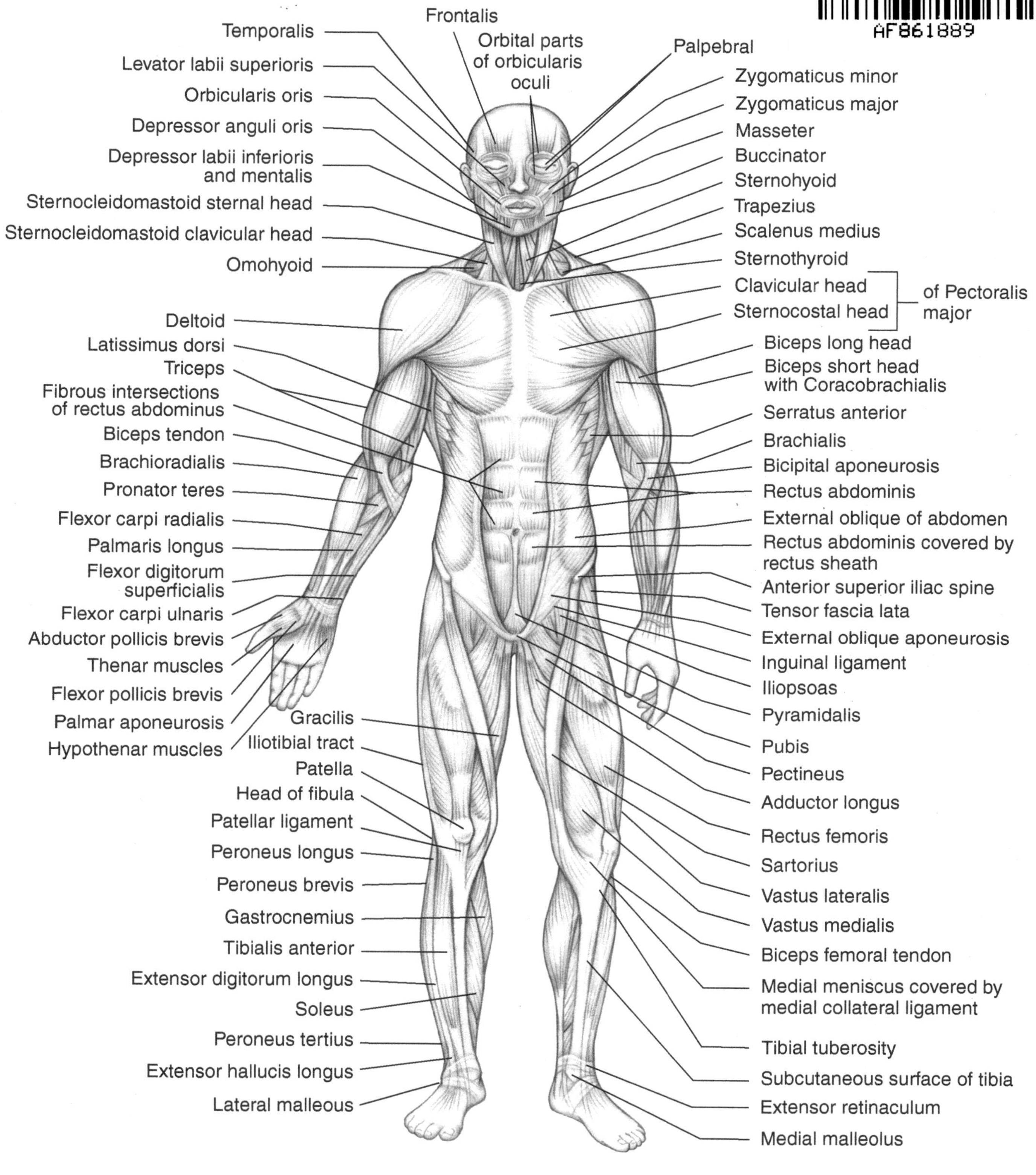
Temporalis
Frontalis
Orbital parts of orbicularis oculi
Palpebral
Levator labii superioris
Orbicularis oris
Depressor anguli oris
Depressor labii inferioris and mentalis
Sternocleidomastoid sternal head
Sternocleidomastoid clavicular head
Omohyoid
Zygomaticus minor
Zygomaticus major
Masseter
Buccinator
Sternohyoid
Trapezius
Scalenus medius
Sternothyroid
Clavicular head
Sternocostal head
of Pectoralis major
Deltoid
Latissimus dorsi
Triceps
Fibrous intersections of rectus abdominus
Biceps tendon
Brachioradialis
Pronator teres
Flexor carpi radialis
Palmaris longus
Flexor digitorum superficialis
Flexor carpi ulnaris
Abductor pollicis brevis
Thenar muscles
Flexor pollicis brevis
Palmar aponeurosis
Hypothenar muscles
Biceps long head
Biceps short head with Coracobrachialis
Serratus anterior
Brachialis
Bicipital aponeurosis
Rectus abdominis
External oblique of abdomen
Rectus abdominis covered by rectus sheath
Anterior superior iliac spine
Tensor fascia lata
External oblique aponeurosis
Inguinal ligament
Iliopsoas
Pyramidalis
Pubis
Pectineus
Adductor longus
Rectus femoris
Sartorius
Vastus lateralis
Vastus medialis
Biceps femoral tendon
Medial meniscus covered by medial collateral ligament
Tibial tuberosity
Subcutaneous surface of tibia
Extensor retinaculum
Medial malleolus
Gracilis
Iliotibial tract
Patella
Head of fibula
Patellar ligament
Peroneus longus
Peroneus brevis
Gastrocnemius
Tibialis anterior
Extensor digitorum longus
Soleus
Peroneus tertius
Extensor hallucis longus
Lateral malleous

Massage Foundations

Taken from:

Tappan's Handbook of Healing Massage Techniques: Classic, Holistic, and Emerging Methods, Fourth Edition
by Patricia J. Benjamin and Frances M. Tappan

Health, The Basics, Sixth Edition
by Rebecca Donatelle and Lorraine Davis

HERITAGE®

PEARSON
Custom Publishing

Taken from:

Tappan s Handbook of Healing Massage Techniques: Classic, Holistic, and Emerging Methods, Fourth Edition
by Patricia J. Benjamin and Frances M. Tappan
Copyright © 2005 by Pearson Education
Published by Prentice Hall
Upper Saddle River, New Jersey 07458

Health, The Basics, Sixth Edition
by Rebecca Donatelle and Lorraine Davis
Copyright © 2004 by Pearson Education
Published by Benjamin Cummings
San Francisco, California 94111

Printed in the United States of America

26 27 V0CR 16 15 14 13 12

ISBN 0-536-08850-0

2007520148

SB

Please visit our web site at *www.pearsoncustom.com*

PEARSON
Custom Publishing

PEARSON CUSTOM PUBLISHING
501 Boylston Street, Suite 900, Boston, MA 02116
A Pearson Education Company

Frances M. Tappan Remembered

1917–1999

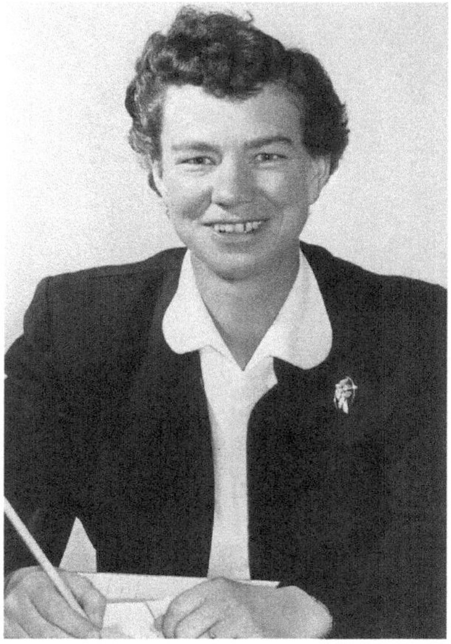

Frances M. Tappan at the University of Connecticut c. 1960.

Frances M. Tappan passed away on August 17, 1999. Her spirit endures in the memories of the many people she touched throughout her full life. Fran was an adventurous soul with a big heart. She was an inspiration to her family, friends, and colleagues—and to two professions dear to her heart, physical therapy and massage therapy.

Dr. Tappan organized the physical therapy program at the University of Connecticut in Storrs in 1950, and served as its leader for the next 25 years. She was active in the American Physical Therapy Association. After she officially retired, Fran continued her work, helping the founders of the Connecticut Center for Massage Therapy in Newington in the early 1980s. She received the American Massage Therapy Association, Council of Schools Award for Excellence in Education in 1989.

Although her other professional accomplishments are many, she will be remembered here for love of massage therapy. Fran believed in massage and its healing capabilities. In the 1940s, she began her study of the different massage techniques used at the time in the developing field of physical therapy. Her first book on massage was called *Massage Techniques: A Case Method Approach* (1961).

Fran traveled to Germany to study Bindegewebsmassage at the Elizabeth Dicke School in Überlingen. In 1975, she went to Taiwan to learn about Chinese medicine and how finger pressure to acupoints can be used to enhance healing. The first edition of *Tappan's Handbook of Healing Massage Techniques* was published in 1980 and reflected her interest in massage techniques practiced worldwide. It was called *Healing Massage Techniques: A Study of Eastern and Western Methods*.

Chapter 26, "The Art of Healing Touch," appeared as "Creating Positive Attitudes towards Healing" in that first edition. It is recommended reading for anyone wanting a sense of Dr. Tappan's personal belief in the healing power of touch.

The next editions of *Tappan's Handbook of Healing Massage Techniques* included even more forms of massage and bodywork, some with alternative ways of understanding human health, disease, and healing. The book's subtitle changed to *Classic, Holistic, and Emerging Methods*.

Tappan's Handbook of Healing Massage Techniques, including this latest edition, is a product of Dr. Tappan's vision. She set the scope, the tone, and the basic philosophy that continues in the work that she began so many years ago. It is a tribute to her dedication and love of hands-on healing.

May Frances M. Tappan be remembered as the curious, open, and kind-hearted spirit that she truly was.

Patricia J. Benjamin

Brief Contents

PART I FOUNDATIONS OF MASSAGE

1 Healing Massage—A Wellness Perspective 1
2 History of Massage 16
3 Effects and Benefits of Massage 34
4 Clinical Applications of Massage 55
5 Endangerment Sites, Contraindications, and Cautions 66
6 Guidelines for Giving Massage 75

PART II WESTERN MASSAGE

7 Western Massage Techniques 105
8 Joint Movements 129
9 Full-Body Western Massage 149
10 Regional Applications 165
11 Hydrotherapy/Thermal Therapies 196
12 Mother and Child 207
13 Healthy Aging 220
14 Terminally Ill and Dying 228
15 Seated Massage in the Workplace 233
16 Infectious and Noninfectious Conditions 241

PART III STUDY GUIDE

Appendix A: 25 Forms of Therapeutic Massage and Bodywork 343
Glossary 361

Contents

Frances M. Tappan–Remembered iii
Introduction to Massage Foundations xv

PART I FOUNDATIONS OF MASSAGE

1 Healing Massage—A Wellness Perspective 3

Learning Outcomes 3
Key Terms/Concepts 4
Introduction 4
Natural Healing Art 4
Massage Definition 5
Massage and Bodywork Traditions 5
Massage and Western Medicine 7
Wellness Perspective 9
Wellness Massage Pyramid 10
Wellness and the Health Professions 12
Clarifying Terminology 12
Summary 13
References 15

2 History of Massage 16

Learning Outcomes 16
Key Historical People 17
Key Terms/Concepts 17
Ancient and Global Heritage 17
Native and Folk Traditions 17
  South Sea Islands 18
  Curanderas 18
Ancient Civilizations 18
  Sumer 18
  China and Japan 19
  India 20
  Greece 20

Rome 20
Turkey 21
Middle Ages and Renaissance Europe 21
Western Massage 22
Ling 22
Mezger 23
Swedish Movement Cure in the United States 23
Conventional and Natural Healing 24
Massage in Conventional Medicine 24
Natural Healing 26
Swedish Massage 26
Sports and Fitness 27
Sports Massage 27
Fitness 28
Decline and Revival in the 20th Century 28
Esalen Massage in the 1970s 28
Milestones at the Turn of the 21st Century 30
Public Policy 30
Standards and Credentials 30
Consumers 31
Summary 31
References 32

3 Effects and Benefits of Massage 34

Learning Outcomes 34
Key Terms/Concepts 34
Effects of Massage 35
Tissue Level Effects 35
Tissue Repair 35
Connective Tissue 37
Organ System Level Effects 38
Integumentary System 38
Skeletal System 38
Muscular System 38
Nervous and Endocrine Systems 40
Cardiovascular System 41
Lymphatic System and Immunity 42
Respiratory System 43
Digestive System 43
Urinary System 43
Reproductive System 43
Organism Level Effects 44
Growth and Development 44
Pain Reduction 44
Stress Reduction 45
Psychological Effects 46
Mental Clarity 46
Reduced Anxiety 46
Emotional Release 47
Feelings of General Wellbeing 47
Mechanisms of Massage 47
Mechanical Effects 48
Physiological Effects 48
Reflex Effects 48

Body–Mind Effects 49
Energetic Effects 49
A Holistic View 49
The Indivisible Body and Mind 49
Limbic System 50
Character Armor 50
Body-Centered Therapy 50
Benefits of Massage for Everyone 51
Benefits for Special Populations 51
Summary 52
References 53

4 Clinical Applications of Massage 55

Learning Outcomes 55
Key Terms/Concepts 55
Clinical Massage Therapy 56
Value of Research 56
Clinical Approach 57
Musculo-Skeletal Pathologies 58
Fibromyalgia 58
Cardiovascular and Lymphatic Pathologies 58
Edema and Lymphedema 58
Immune Function 59
Respiratory Pathologies 59
Anxiety Reduction in Hospitalized Patients 59
Massage for Cancer Patients 60
Pediatric Care 60
Preterm Infants 60
Pediatric Applications 61
Psychological Aspects of Treatment 61
Therapeutic Touch 62
Complement to Chiropractic 62
Summary 63
References 64

5 Endangerment Sites, Contraindications, and Cautions 66

Learning Outcomes 66
Key Terms/Concepts 66
Do No Harm 67
Endangerment Sites 67
General Principles for Safety around Endangerment Sites 69
Contraindications 69
Principles for Contraindications and Cautions 70
Medications 72
Person-Centered Massage 73
Resources 73
Summary 73
References 74

6 Guidelines for Giving Massage 75

Learning Outcomes 75
Key Terms/Concepts 76

The Therapeutic Relationship 76
Dual Relationships 76
Transference and Counter-Transference 77
Professional Demeanor 77
Touching Another Person 77
More Basic than Technique 77
Touch and the Therapeutic Relationship 78
Permission to Touch 78
Informed Consent 78
Gender Considerations 79
Intervention Model 80
Talking and Feedback 80
Confidentiality 81
HIPAA Privacy Rule 81
The Physical Environment 82
Massage Tables and Chairs 82
The Massage Space 83
Topical Substances 84
Positioning and Draping 85
Positioning 85
Draping 86
Physical Self-Care for the Practitioner 91
Hand and Wrist Care 91
Good Body Mechanics 92
Avoiding Strain 94
Emotional Self-Care 97
Performance Elements 98
Length of the Session 98
Amount of Lubricant 99
Sequence of Techniques and Routines 100
Specificity and Direction 100
Pressure, Rhythm and Pacing 100
Summary 101
References 102

PART II WESTERN MASSAGE

7 Western Massage Techniques 105

Learning Outcomes 105
Key Terms/Concepts 105
Western Massage 106
Western Massage Techniques 106
Effleurage 106
Variations of Effleurage 107
Petrissage 112
Variations of Petrissage 112
Friction 115
Variations of Friction 116
Friction Used in Rehabilitation 118
Tapotement 119
Variations of Tapotement 120
Vibration 122
Variations of Vibration 123
Touch without Movement 125
Passive Touch 125
Direct Pressure 125

Summary 127
References 128

8 Joint Movements 129

Learning Outcomes 129
Key Terms/Concepts 129
Joint Movement Techniques 130
Overview of Joint Movements 131
Categories of Joint Movements 131
Uses of Joint Movements 131
General Principles of Joint Movements 131
Joint Movement Techniques 132
Neck 132
Shoulder Girdle 134
Elbow 136
Wrist 138
Hand 138
Chest 140
Hip 140
Knee 142
Ankle 144
Foot 145
Summary 147
References 148

9 Full-Body Western Massage 149

Learning Outcomes 149
Key Terms/Concepts 149
Overview 150
Guidelines for Full-Body Western Massage 151
Draping 151
Sequence of Body Regions 151
Order of Techniques 151
Continuity and Flow 152
Rhythm, Pacing, and Specificity 152
Full-Body Western Massage Routine 152
Prone Position 153
Turning Over 156
Supine Position 156
Summary 164

10 Regional Applications 165

Learning Outcomes 165
Key Terms/Concepts 165
Wholeness and Meaning 166
Head and Face 166
Applications of Massage 166
Anatomy 167
Techniques 167
Neck 170
Applications of Massage 171
Anatomy 171
Techniques 172
Back 174

Applications of Massage 174
Anatomy 175
Techniques 175
Therapeutic Sequence for the Lower Back 175
Back Massage for Relaxation 177
Sedating Effleurage of the Back 177
Buttocks 178
Applications of Massage 178
Anatomy 178
Techniques 179
Lower Extremities 180
Applications of Massage 180
Anatomy 180
Techniques 181
Upper Extremities 185
Applications of Massage 186
Anatomy 186
Techniques 187
Chest and Abdomen 190
Applications of Massage 190
Anatomy 191
Techniques 191
Summary 194
References 195

11 Hydrotherapy / Thermal Therapies 196

Learning Outcomes 196
Historical People and Developments 196
Key Terms/Concepts 197
History of Hydrotherapy 197
Water-Based Therapies 197
Hydrotherapy in Medicine 198
Physical Therapy 199
Healing Properties of Water 199
Whirlpool Baths, Showers, Steam Room, Sauna 200
Hot Applications—Thermo-Therapy 203
Healing Effects of Heat 203
Hot Packs and Massage 203
Cold Applications—Cryotherapy 204
Healing Effects of Cold 204
Cold Packs, Ice, Ice Massage 205
Summary 206
References 206

12 Mother and Child 207

Learning Outcomes 207
Key Terms/Concepts 207
Benefits of Pregnancy Massage 208
Contraindications and Cautions 208
Setting the Environment 208
Positioning Options 209
Pregnancy Massage Session 211
Labor, Delivery, and Recovery 212

Women with Infants and Toddlers 212
Infant Massage 213
  Benefits 213
  Infant Massage Techniques 213
Summary 218
References 218

13 Healthy Aging 220

Learning Outcomes 220
Key Terms/Concepts 220
Effects of Aging and Benefits of Massage 221
Benefits for Elders 221
Working with the Elderly 223
Massage for Elders in Chairs 224
Massage Session for Healthy Aging 225
Cautions 225
Summary 226
References 226

14 Terminally Ill and Dying 228

Learning Outcomes 228
Key Terms/Concepts 228
Caring Touch of Massage 229
Hospice and Palliative Care 229
Massage for the Dying 229
Knowledge and Skills 230
Self-Care 230
Summary 231
References 231

15 Seated Massage in the Workplace 233

Learning Outcomes 233
Key Terms/Concepts 233
History of Workplace Massage 234
Benefits of Massage in the Workplace 234
Seated Massage for Office Workers 236
Popularity of Workplace Massage 237
Summary 239
References 239

16 Infectious and Noninfectious Conditions 241

Objectives 241
Assessing Your Disease Risks 242
  Risk Factors You Can't Control 242
  Risk Factors You Can Control 242
  Types of Pathogens and Routes of Transmission 243
  Bacteria 244
  Viruses 246
  Other Pathogens 249
Your Body's Defenses: Keeping You Well 249
  Physical and Chemical Defense 249
  The Immune System: Your Body Fights Back 250

Fever 251
Pain 251
Vaccines: Bolstering Your Immunity 251
Emerging and Resurgent Diseases 251
Tiny Microbes: Lethal Threats 252
Sexually Transmitted Infections 255
Possible Causes: Why Me? 256
Modes of Transmission 256
Chlamydia 256
Pelvic Inflammatory Disease 257
Gonorrhea 257
Syphilis 260
Pubic Lice 261
Genital HPV 261
Candidiasis (Moniliasis) 261
Trichomoniasis 262
General Urinary Tract Infections 262
Herpes 262
HIV/AIDS 263
A Shifting Epidemic 263
Women and AIDS 264
How HIV Is Transmitted 266
Symptoms of HIV Disease 266
Testing for HIV Antibodies 267
New Hope and Treatments 267
Preventing HIV Infection 268
Noninfectious Diseases 268
Chronic Lung Disease 268
Allergy-Induced Respiratory Problems 268
Hay Fever 270
Asthma 270
Emphysema 272
Bronchitis 272
Sleep Apnea 272
Neurological Disorders 273
Headaches 273
Seizure Disorders 274
Other Neurological Disorders 274
Gender-Related Disorders 275
Menstrual Problems 275
Endometriosis 275
Digestion-Related Disorders 275
Diabetes 275
Lactose Intolerance 277
Colitis and Irritable Bowel Syndrome 277
Peptic Ulcers 277
Musculoskeletal Diseases 278
Arthritis 278
Fibromyalgia 278
Systemic Lupus Erythematosus 278
Low Back Pain 279
Other Maladies 279
Chronic Fatigue Syndrome 279
Repetitive Stress Injuries 280

Taking Charge *280*
Make It Happen! *280*
Summary *281*
Questions for Discussion and Reflection *282*
Accessing Your Health on the Internet *282*
Further Reading *283*

PART III STUDY GUIDE 287

Appendix A: 25 Forms of Therapeutic Massage and Bodywork 343

Glossary 351

Index 360

Introduction to Massage Foundations

Massage is one of the oldest healing techniques in the world. Ancient documents from all over the word record healers using massage as a means to promote and restore health. Today, massage is one of the fastest growing fields of healing. More and more people use massage for relaxation, health, and healing.

Massage Foundations represents a great introduction to therapeutic massage. It explores the history, the effects, and many applications of massage. The focus of this book is to help you build an effective foundation of knowledge which will assist you in your career. It is this foundation that transforms a soothing back rub into therapeutic massage. This book is designed to help you develop this foundation which will help you provide effective therapeutic applications of massage.

TIPS TO LEARNING MASSAGE THERAPY

- **Practice, practice, practice.** Books can only provide a theoretical understanding of massage practices. Great massage therapists have practiced their art over and over again. Each technique you read about in the book will need to be practiced many times to achieve mastery.
- **Learn to feel.** The hands are the most important tool in massage therapy. Learning how to use your hands as tools requires that you learn to feel through your hands in a different way. They both assess conditions as well as help to resolve the conditions. In many cases, your hands become your eyes; they feel what the eyes cannot see. In this way, they become the most important connection between you and the client.
- **Be open-minded.** Massage therapy uses a wide variety of traditions in its modalities. Some of these traditions may seem strange or foreign to you. In some cases, they may even seem counterintuitive to the Western practices of medicine that we are most familiar with. One of massage therapy's greatest strengths is in its willingness to adopt new strategies and modalities. The greatest massage therapists are the ones who are most willing to explore new ideas. Open your mind to the wonderful possibilities that massage therapy can provide.
- **Be patient.** Few great lessons are learned in short periods of time. Massage is no different. It may take a few classes to really grasp some of the more complex concepts in massage. This is okay. It simply takes practice, patience, and perseverance to overcome most obstacles. If you commit

yourself to improving your theoretical and practical knowledge each day, you will succeed in your study of massage therapy.

- **Take care of yourself.** Massage can be a physically demanding professtion. Good body mechanics will help in remediating much of the pressures upon your body. It is important to remember body mechanics and hand care throughout your schooling and your career. Additionally, many traditions of massage believe that energy is transferred between the therapists and the clients. This energy, both positive and negative, travels though you to your client and visa versa. As such, how you care for yourself can have a great impact on the success of your treatment. Maximizing your effectiveness with a client will require that you also take care of yourself.
- **Continue to learn.** Massage therapy is too large of a field to be contained in a single book. In fact, thousands of books have been written about massage therapy. Part of the reason for this is that there are hundreds of massage modalities and thousands of ways to combine these into countless applications. It is important to take this foundation of knowledge and expand it through life long learning. Make it a part of your career to learn new methods and pass this knowledge along to other therapists.

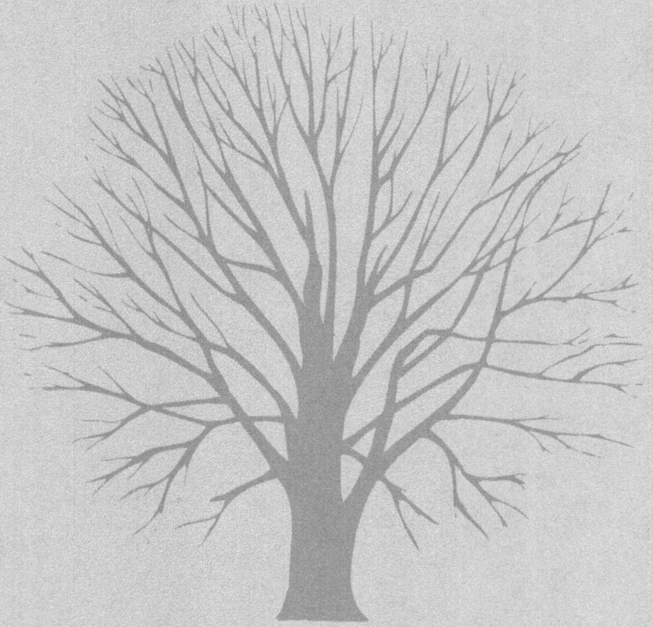

I

Foundations of Massage

CHAPTER ONE

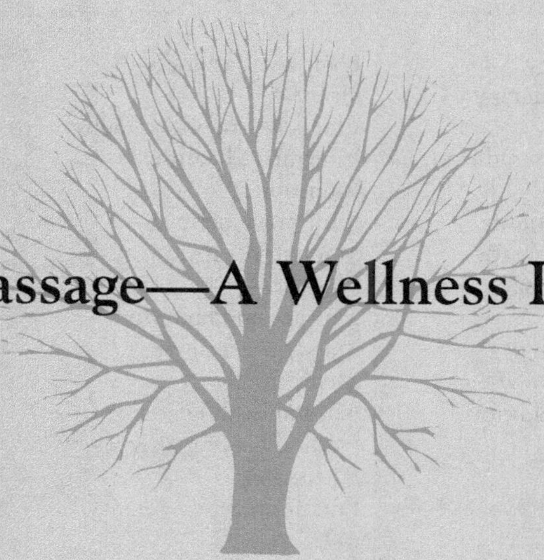

Healing Massage—A Wellness Perspective

LEARNING OUTCOMES

After studying this chapter, the student will have information to:

1. Explain massage as a natural healing art, and as manual therapy.
2. Identify important tenets of the natural healing philosophy.
3. Define the meaning of healing, and contrast it to curing.
4. Define holistic, and discuss the idea of the whole person.
5. Define massage, and analyze the nature of massage techniques, including action and intention.
6. Describe four major world traditions of massage and bodywork.
7. Identify the seven major categories of Western massage techniques.
8. Analyze the relationship of massage to Western medicine as a CAM therapy, and within a system of integrative health care.
9. Use Travis' Illness/Wellness Continuum to compare the wellness and treatment models.
10. Use the Wellness Massage Pyramid to describe the broad scope of massage, and its contributions to achieving high level wellness.
11. Discuss the scope of different health professions using the Wellness Massage Pyramid.
12. Use the language of wellness and treatment appropriately.

LINK LIBRARY TERMS

Massage Therapy • *Massage Business* • *Human Anatomy and Physiology* • *Sports Massage* • *Massage Regulations*

MEDIALINK

A companion CD-ROM, included free with each new copy of this book, supplements the techniques presented in this chapter. Insert the CD-ROM to watch video clips of massage techniques being demonstrated. This multimedia feature is designed to help you add a new dimension to your learning.

KEY TERMS/CONCEPTS

Alternative therapy
Asian bodywork therapy tradition
Ayurvedic massage tradition
CAM therapy
Clients, guests, patients
Complementary therapy
Contemporary massage and bodywork
Eclectic practitioner
Effleurage
Folk and native traditions
Friction
Giver
Healing
High level wellness
Holistic
Illness/wellness continuum
Integrative healthcare
Intention
Joint movements
Manual therapy
Massage
Massage and bodywork
Massage technique
Medical spa
Natural healing arts
Natural healing philosophy
Petrissage
Practitioner
Receiver, recipient
Session
Tapotement
Therapist
Touch without movement
Traditions of massage and bodywork
Treatment model
Treatment, procedure
Vibration
Wellness Massage Pyramid
Wellness model
Western massage technique categories
Western massage tradition

INTRODUCTION

In this first decade of the 21st century, massage is available around the globe—on the streets of China, in the spas of Europe, in the temples of Thailand, in tribal villages in Africa and Australia, and in health clubs and day spas in the United States. Soft tissue manipulation is used by traditional healers such as Hispanic curanderas, and is an integral part of medical systems such as Traditional Chinese Medicine, and Ayurveda in India. It is also being reclaimed as a valuable therapy within modern Western medicine. Its many benefits for preventing illness, healing, and optimizing well-being are being rediscovered by a growing number of people worldwide.

NATURAL HEALING ART

Massage is one of the traditional **natural healing arts.** It has been used for centuries to promote and restore health along with other gifts of nature such as nutritious food, herbs, healing waters, exercise, relaxation, fresh air and sunshine. Massage is a **manual therapy,** i.e., performed by hand. Simple hand tools and electric devices are sometimes used in conjunction with massage by hand. But it is the person-to-person touch that defines massage, and gives massage its unique healing potential.

Many of the tenets of the **natural healing philosophy** formalized in late 19th century are still adhered to by many massage practitioners. These include preference for natural methods of healing, a belief in the existence of an innate healing force, and a holistic view of human life. The wellness perspective described later in this chapter is a modern adaptation of the natural healing philosophy.

The term **healing** has many shades of meaning. Healing in its broader sense means to make healthy, whole, or sound. The word healing also means enhancing health and well-being, as well as the process of regaining health or optimal functioning after an injury, disease, or other debilitating condition. Modern science is confirming the efficacy of massage and other natural methods for maintaining health and for healing.

Healing, especially natural healing, may be contrasted to the concept of *curing.* The connotation of the term *cure* is of something coming from the outside, and given to a passive recipient. Healing, on the other hand, implies the existence of a force at work from within, with the recipient as an active participant in their own recovery. In this text, massage is presented as a method for enhancing the innate healing force already at work as living beings continuously repair themselves and try to maintain an integrated wholeness.

Holistic refers to those approaches to health and healing that take into account the wholeness of human beings, including body, mind, emotions, and spirit. In the holistic paradigm, massage is applied to the physical body, yet it affects all other aspects of the whole person. Although the term holistic is relatively new in the health professions, the concept is of ancient origin and is a basic tenet of the natural healing philosophy. It is also a fundamental principle of the wellness perspective discussed later in the chapter.

MASSAGE DEFINITION

Massage is the intentional and systematic manipulation of the soft tissues of the body to enhance health and healing. Joint movements and stretching are commonly performed as part of massage. The primary characteristics of massage are touch and movement.

The actions and intentions of the practitioner constitute the **massage technique.** Massage techniques are generally described in active terms such as gliding or sliding, percussion, compression, broadening, kneading, friction, vibrating, stretching, and holding. Through the medium of touch, the massage practitioner's actions cause movement in the soft tissues of the recipient. Different massage techniques have different effects. Techniques are chosen by the practitioner and applied in such a way to accomplish the goals of each massage session.

Intention is the aim that guides the action, that is, what the practitioner hopes to accomplish. The intent might be to enhance a biophysical process such as relaxation or circulation, or to balance energy, or to evoke a positive emotional state. It might also be expressed in a more functional way, such as to recover from an athletic competition, to improve posture, or to diminish pain. Intention helps determine choice of techniques and guides the action in subtle ways. Intention is an essential part of the effective application of massage.

Massage falls into the more general category of **massage and bodywork.** The term *bodywork* was coined in the latter 20th century to encompass a wide variety of manual therapies including systems of soft tissue manipulation, movement integration, structural integration, energy balancing, and other approaches to health and healing that involve touch and movement. The terms *massage* and *bodywork* are often used together to describe the broad scope of the occupational field of massage therapy, for example, as in National Certification for Therapeutic Massage and Bodywork. The types of massage described in this text fall into the broad category of massage and bodywork. Some of the more popular systems of massage and bodywork are described in Appendix A. (The book to read for a survey of massage and bodywork systems is *Discovering the Body's Wisdom*, by Mirka Knaster.)

MASSAGE AND BODYWORK TRADITIONS

A *tradition* implies some element of culture that is passed down from generation to generation within a group of people. A tradition is typically defined as originating from an ethnic group, geographic location, or civilization.

Occasionally a tradition of one group is adopted by other groups of people. This has happened time and again throughout history, for example in music, art, games, writing, and health and healing practices. Tradition is not an immutable concept; some say that a tradition is established after only two generations. However, tradition is a useful concept for identifying the origin, and categorizing the many different systems of massage and bodywork.

There are four traditions that encompass most of the systems of massage and bodywork used widely today. These are folk and native traditions, Ayurvedic massage, Asian bodywork therapies (ABT), and Western massage and bodywork. The map in Figure 1–1 shows the origin of these world traditions of massage. Information about the history of these traditions may be found in Chapter 2 in Part IV.

Folk and native traditions of massage and bodywork are characterized by being specific to a small or narrowly defined group of people, and passed down by apprenticeship either through families, or from tribal or village healers. They include both general health and healing goals. Folk and native healing practices are based on how things have been done in the past, and on experience about what brings are about the desired results. These practices are most often performed in a larger context that includes herbal remedies, rituals, and religious beliefs. These traditions often served as the foundations for the more formal and larger traditions that evolved over time. Examples are rubbing techniques of

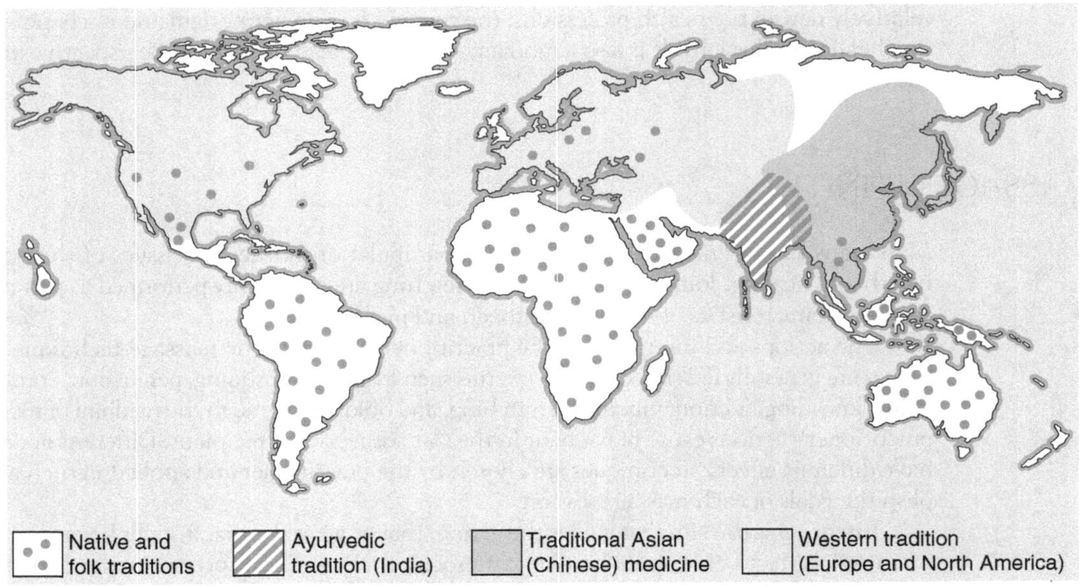

FIGURE 1–1. Map of World Traditions of Massage and Bodywork.

the tribal healers in Africa; lomi-lomi of the Hawaiians; and soft tissue techniques of traditional Hispanic healers, called curanderas.

The **Ayurvedic massage tradition** originated in India, and is based on a comprehensive system of beliefs about health and disease. Its theory can be traced to an ancient text called the Vedas written in the 5th century BCE. Massage is considered essential in Ayurvedic practices to circulate "vayu" (or wind) in vessels called "siras" to promote healthy body functioning. The oil used in massage is chosen carefully according to the recipient's body type, the atmosphere, and the season. Different types of bodywork are also used to balance energy in centers called chakras. Related practices include hatha yoga, breathing exercises, cleansing and vegetarianism. (The book to read is *Ayurvedic Massage*, by Harish Johari.)

The **Asian bodywork therapy (ABT) tradition** includes systems of massage and bodywork with roots in Chinese medicine. These are characterized by reference to energy (chi, ki) channels or meridians, and points along the channels called acupoints. Pressing and rubbing techniques stimulate the movement of energy through the channels to promote balance and harmony. Examples of ABT are tuina or medical massage from China, amma and shiatsu from Japan, and a contemporary system called Jin Shin Do®. Related practices include tai chi, qigong, and acupuncture.

The **Western massage tradition** can be traced to ancient Greek and Roman practices as developed over the centuries in Europe and North America. The Western tradition encompasses massage as a heath practice, for beauty and pleasure, as well as for healing. Its foundation is Western science including anatomy, physiology, and pathology. Scientific research about the efficacy of massage for healing has increased dramatically in the past few decades, and is providing a solid grounding for the use of massage in treatment of certain pathologies, as defined by Western medicine.

Modern Western massage is a system of soft tissue manipulation that evolved out of the work of Pehr Ling and Johann Mezger at the end of the 19th century. Five classic massage technique categories are *effleurage*, *petrissage*, *friction*, *tapotement*, and *vibration*. The classic terminology is common to Swedish massage, and massage as taught in most physical therapy programs. Some schools today use their English equivalents, i.e., sliding/gliding, kneading/compression, friction, percussion, vibration. Touch without movement and joint movements are also incorporated into Western massage. These seven **Western massage technique categories** are simple, adaptable, and useful for describing a variety of healing massage techniques.

Effleurage techniques slide or glide over the skin with a smooth continuous motion. **Petrissage** techniques lift, wring, or squeeze soft tissues in a kneading motion, or press or roll tissues under the hands. **Friction** is performed by rubbing one surface over another repeatedly. **Tapotement** consists of rapid percussive movements performed in a rhythmic manner. **Vibration** may be described as an oscillating, quivering, or trembling motion, or movement back and forth or up and down performed quickly and repeatedly. **Touch without movement** includes passive touch, holding, or laying the hands on the body. **Joint movements** within the scope of Western massage include mobilizing techniques within normal range of motion, and stretching. Figure 1–2 illustrates the basic Western massage techniques.

Contemporary massage and bodywork systems that go beyond the basic Western techniques were developed in the 20th century. Some—like lymphatic massage, trigger points, and myofascial massage—are based in Western anatomy, while others—like polarity therapy and reflexology—rely on alternative health perspectives. In recent years there has been an explosion of interest in many different forms of massage and bodywork as consumers have rediscovered their many benefits for promoting optimal health and healing. Part III describes five systems of contemporary massage and bodywork.

Many practitioners grounded in Western massage incorporate elements of theory and technique from other systems or traditions for an eclectic approach. For example, an **eclectic practitioner** might combine basic Western techniques with contemporary approaches like myofascial or trigger point techniques, and perhaps some reflexology or shiatsu. Part of the art of massage is in choosing the appropriate techniques to accomplish the goals of a session.

MASSAGE AND WESTERN MEDICINE

Massage and bodywork therapies are sometimes called alternative or complementary in relation to Western medicine. This is a curious concept, since massage has been used in Western medicine since ancient Greek times. The reason for this contradiction can be traced to the mid-20th century when massage lost favor within regular medicine, and was largely dropped from mainstream health care. Renewed interest in massage in the late 20th century happened largely within the natural healing tradition during the counterculture of the 1960–1970s. Since the revival occurred outside of what was considered conventional medicine at the time, and included approaches to healing at the fringes or outside of Western science, massage therapy was then considered to be alternative.

This attitude has gradually changed as more scientific research about massage is conducted within mainstream medical institutions. For example, research studies about massage are conducted by the Touch Research Institute at the University of Miami (www.miami.edu/touch-research), and can be found in the AMTA Foundation database (www.amtafoundation.org).

When massage is called an **alternative therapy,** it is generally meant as an *either/or* option outside of mainstream medicine. When it is seen as a **complementary therapy,** it is considered secondary to the treatments of mainstream medicine, but contributing to the patient's recovery.

CAM is an acronym for Complementary and Alternative Medicine. CAM is a broad concept that includes therapies like biofeedback, herbal remedies, homeopathic remedies, acupuncture, Ayurveda, naturopathic medicine, environmental medicine, and various forms of massage and bodywork. Wide use of CAM therapies by consumers prompted the establishment of the National Center for Complementary and Alternative Medicine (NCCAM) within the National Institutes of Health (NIH) in 1998. (www.nccam.nih.gov).

The White House Commission on CAM Policy (2002) cites therapeutic massage, bodywork, and somatic movement therapies as a major CAM domain. Other domains include alternative healthcare systems (e.g., Traditional Chinese Medicine, Ayurveda, chiropractic and naturopathic medicine), mind-body interventions (e.g., meditation and hypnosis), biological-based therapies (e.g., herbal remedies and special diets), energy therapies (e.g., qigong and Reiki), and bioelectromagnetics (e.g., magnet therapy). (www.whccamp.hhs.gov).

A more progressive viewpoint considers massage and bodywork as a choice within an **integrative health care** system offering many options for healing. In integrative health care systems, different therapies exist on equal status, and are chosen for a particular case based on the greatest benefit for the patient. Manual therapies like massage are being integrated into an increasing number of medical settings today.

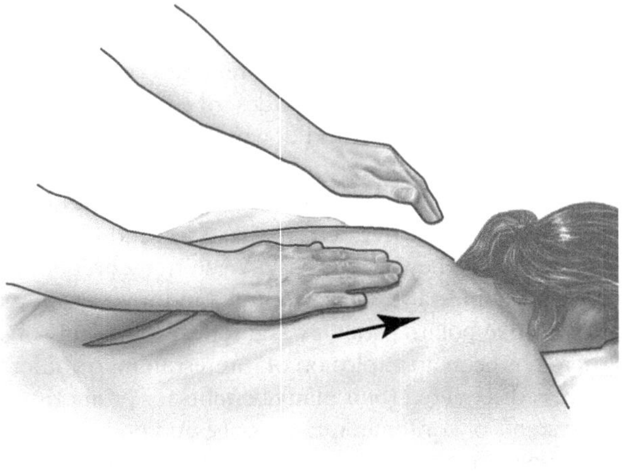

Effleurage—sliding and gliding techniques.

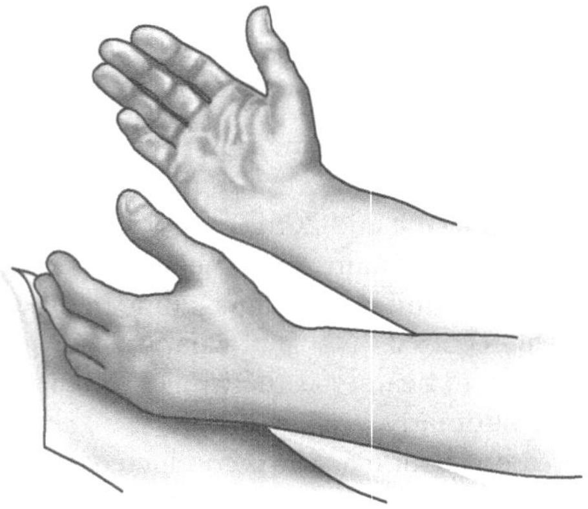

Tapotement—percussion techniques.

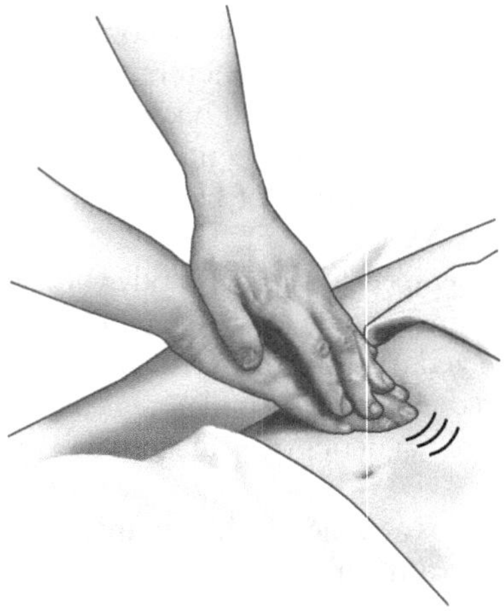

Vibration—oscillating techniques.

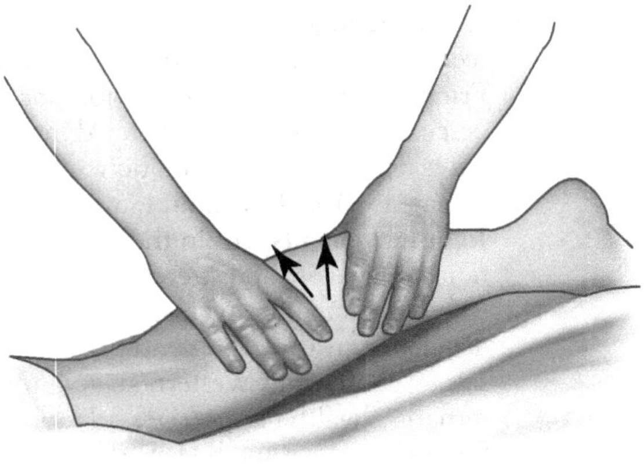

Petrissage—kneading and compression techniques.

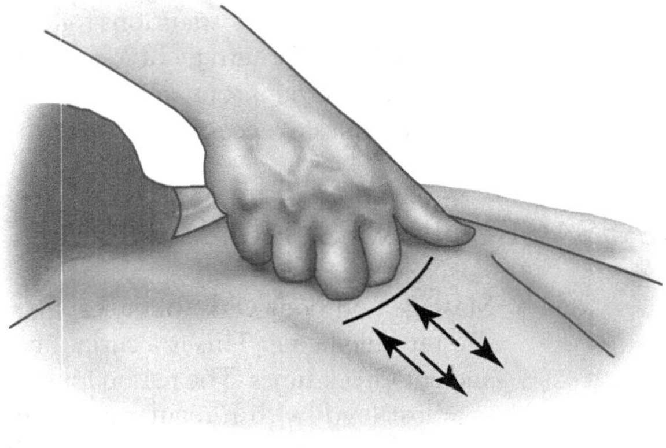

Friction—rubbing techniques.

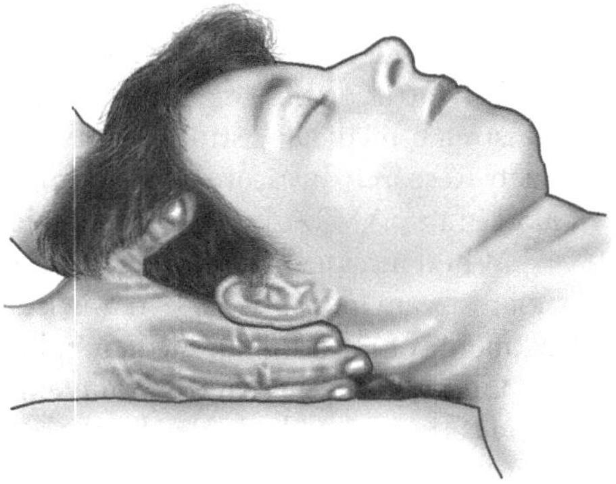

Touch without movement—holding and touching techniques.

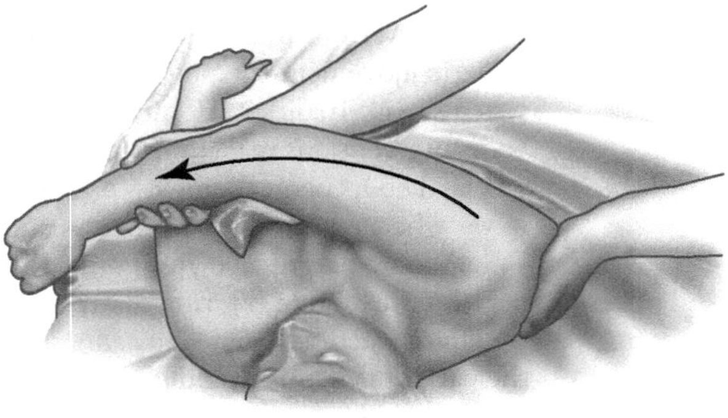

Joint movements—mobilizing and stretching techniques.

FIGURE 1–2. Seven Basic Western Massage Techniques.

In a parallel trend, some North American spas are providing conventional as well as complimentary therapies to patrons who come to them for health and healing services. An integrative approach has been common in European spas for years. The International Spa Association (ISPA) includes "medical spa" as one of the seven categories of spas. A **medical spa** is one that provides "comprehensive medical and wellness care in an environment which integrates spa services, as well as conventional and complementary therapies and treatments" (www.experienceispa.com).

WELLNESS PERSPECTIVE

A wellness perspective goes beyond the old idea of health as the mere absence of disease to the goal of achieving a vibrant, meaningful life. In this paradigm, the individual takes personal responsibility for forming life habits to achieve optimal wellbeing in many areas of their lives. "Wellness" is a concept that took form in the 1970s United States and has been adopted in professions devoted to physical education and fitness, health, recreation and leisure, and health care.

Illness/Wellness Continuum

The diagram of the **illness/wellness continuum**, shown in Figure 1–3, is a useful illustration of the concept of wellness, and of the wellness and treatment models. It was developed by John Travis, MD, a pioneer of the wellness movement, who founded the Wellness Resource Center in Mill Valley, California in 1975. Wellness Associates, a nonprofit educational foundation, continues Travis' work today (www.thewellspring.com).

Travis's **wellness model** spans the entire illness/wellness continuum, from premature death to high level wellness. It includes treatment for disability and the signs and symptoms of disease, as well as movement towards greater awareness, education, and growth to achieve high level wellness. In this diagram the **treatment model** is shown separately and corresponds to the half of the wellness model to the left of "neutral."

High Level Wellness

In its broadest sense, **high level wellness** is a condition of optimal physical, emotional, intellectual, spiritual, social, and vocational wellbeing. It is holistic at its core. The components of wellness and a healthy lifestyle are explained in practical terms in Table 1–1. Achieving optimal wellness in each of these arenas is a lifetime process.

There are many aspects of living that contribute to high level wellness. They include things like good nutrition, adequate exercise, rest, recreation, satisfying and healthy relationships, seeking counsel for handling problems, spending time in nature, and finding meaningful work.

Many have found massage to be an effective method to enhance wellness in a number of ways. Looking at the components of wellness in Figure 1–4, several potential ways come to mind. Massage helps keep soft tissues in healthy condition, improves sleep, and promotes relaxation. It can help one cope with stress, reduce anxiety, and find inner peace. It supports participation in exercise and sports.

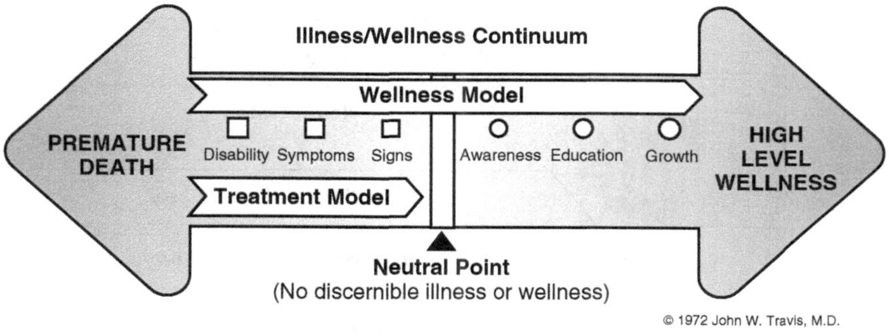

FIGURE 1–3. The illness/wellness continuum. *(Reprinted with permission, Wellness Workbook, Travis & Ryan, Ten Speed Press, Berkeley, CA. © 2000 John W. Travis, MD)*

Table 1–1 COMPONENTS OF WELLNESS AND A HEALTHY LIFESTYLE

Physical wellbeing involves being physically fit; eating nutritiously; being free from chemical dependency and other harmful behaviors; being aware of early signs of illness; getting adequate sleep and rest; preventing accidents.
Emotional wellbeing involves balance in emotions; expressing emotions appropriately and comfortably; showing respect and affection for others; coping successfully with stress and personal problems; seeking counsel when needed.
Intellectual wellbeing includes clear thinking and problem solving; processing information; questioning and evaluating; learning from life experiences; being flexible, creative, and open to new ideas.
Social wellbeing means having satisfying relationships and interacting well with others; having a network of family, friends, and others who can help you in time of need; establishing a sense of belonging within your community.
Spiritual wellbeing is whatever brings meaning and purpose in your life; knowing your purpose in life and being more comfortable expressing love, joy, peace, and fulfillment; feeling connected to your inner self, significant others, and the universe; having hope after setbacks; appreciating nature.
Vocational wellbeing includes school and job satisfaction; working in harmony with others to accomplish something worthwhile.

Source: Seiger, L., Vanderpool, K., & Barnes, D. (1995). *Fitness and wellness strategies.* Madison, WI: Brown & Benchmark (pp. 5–6).

It can provide an avenue for learning more about the body, mind and emotions. It helps develop body awareness and sense of connectedness to the inner self. It can relieve isolation, and help establish a sense of connectedness to others. It offers caring touch in a safe environment. Because each person is an interconnected whole, improving any one of these aspects can help improve others. Each person benefits from massage for their own unique reasons.

WELLNESS MASSAGE PYRAMID

While the illness/wellness continuum is useful, it leaves the impression of a dichotomy between the wellness and treatment models. This is problematic when trying to express one broad scope for massage therapy. This dichotomy in thinking is evident in how the terms are commonly used, that is, with the word

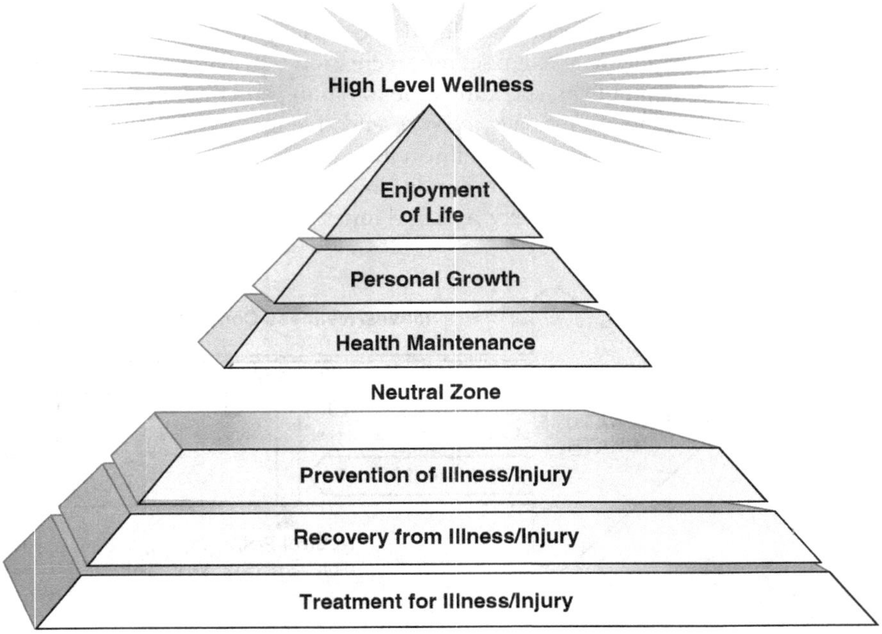

FIGURE 1–4. Wellness massage pyramid.

treatment reserved for massage therapy left of the neutral point (i.e., disability, symptoms, signs), and *wellness* practices reserved for the neutral point to high level wellness (i.e., awareness, education, growth). A different illustration is needed to capture a concept of wellness that includes the entire range of wellness related to massage therapy.

The **Wellness Massage Pyramid** (WMP) in Figure 1–4 tries to capture the inclusive nature of a wellness perspective for massage therapy. The WMP uses some concepts from the illness/wellness continuum, but adds others specific to the potential contributions of massage to high level wellness.

Each level on the WMP represents a major contribution massage can make on a journey to high level wellness, and each level serves as the platform for the next level. The pyramid includes from the base to the top: treatment and recovery from illness and injury, prevention of illness and injury, a neutral zone (absence from illness and injury), and on to health maintenance, personal growth and the enjoyment of life. A three-dimensional view of the pyramid would reveal each of these levels for body, mind, emotions, and spirit.

Using a pyramid to depict a hierarchy of levels for achieving a specific goal is borrowed from Maslow's Hierarchy of Needs in psychology. At the base of the pyramid in Maslow's theory of human motivation are *deficiency needs* that have to be satisfied before *growth needs* may be addressed. Maslow's deficiency needs are physiological, safety, love, and esteem. Once these are met, then growth needs, such as understanding and aesthetic needs, may be addressed, finally allowing for self-actualization and transcendence (Huitt 2002). Maslow's theory is meant to explain human motivation, but the general idea of a pyramid also works well to illustrate needs to be met on the road to high level wellness.

At the base of the WMP is treatment for, recovery from, and prevention of illness or injury. If successful at these levels, i.e., eliminating deficiencies, one gets to a neutral point. Beyond the neutral point, growth toward high level wellness proceeds to the maintenance of good health. This provides a base for physical, psycho-emotional, and spiritual growth, and enjoyment of life. Theoretically, the foundation would be laid on each level to enable a person to proceed to the next level, but it is important not to take this hierarchy too literally.

There is significant gray area between levels. Throughout a lifetime, levels would be revisited periodically to repair any weaknesses from the wear and tear of living, and to address challenges faced in different life stages. And given the multidimensional nature of wellness, you could be addressing different levels simultaneously. For example, from a wellness perspective, people with chronic illnesses might always be in treatment, but may also be maintaining health in other areas, working on personal growth (e.g., spiritual development), and progressing to high level wellness in other dimensions of their lives. The pyramid is simply a tool for understanding the possible contributions of massage therapy on the journey to high level wellness.

The pyramid can be used to explain the many different reasons people seek massage. The treatment and recovery level is perhaps the easiest to understand. A client comes in with a complaint of pain or dysfunction, and massage is used to diminish pain and help in the healing process. Once an acute phase is past, the slow rebuilding of a healthy state begins. It is in the recovery phase that massage is often used to complement a primary treatment.

At the level of prevention, a client may be aware that their stress level is getting too high and may use massage as a strategy to reduce their stress and prevent illness. Or a client may feel their muscles tightening up from repetitive motion and seek massage to prevent damaging strain. These are subclinical situations that would eventually lead to illness or injury if left to progress.

The neutral zone indicates the absence of deficiencies, i.e., signs and symptoms of disease and injury. It is characterized by absence of pain, tolerable stress level, and function for daily living activities. This was the goal in old theories of health. In the WMP, it is a plateau on the way to high level wellness.

At the level of health maintenance, a client might receive regular massage as part of a healthful lifestyle. At this point they are moving past the neutral zone on their way to high level wellness. Massage can help keep the body and mind functioning well both as a kind of pre-prevention strategy, as well as a foundation for being able to participate in personal growth activities and to enjoy life to its fullest.

Beyond health maintenance are the reasons people seek massage as a life enhancement. These might include the healthful pleasure of caring touch, developing greater awareness of our inner selves, feeling integrated in body and mind, or improving physical condition for recreation activities.

The wellness massage pyramid can be used to describe the goals of a massage session. The goals might fall within one or more levels, depending on the client/patient needs at the time and the setting.

A session may be focused primarily at the base of the pyramid in the treatment arena, or on treatment and prevention, or on health maintenance and personal growth, or at several levels simultaneously. Any one massage session could be described as having a certain percentage of time or focus at a particular level of the pyramid.

WELLNESS AND THE HEALTH PROFESSIONS

Several health professions include massage in their scope of practice, e.g., massage therapists, physical therapists, nurses, athletic trainers, chiropractors, and naturopaths. Depending on the profession, massage may be called massage therapy, bodywork, manual therapy, physiotherapy, or simply a modality.

In the context of a profession that utilizes several different modalities, or methods of treating pathology, massage may play a minor role overall. It may be in the same category of modalities as ice packs, hot packs, ultrasound, or whirlpool baths. This is true of most health professions listed above.

In the massage therapy profession, massage and bodywork is the main "modality." Massage therapists are specialists in soft tissue applications, and are called upon to perform massage within the full range of the wellness massage pyramid. Massage therapists themselves sometimes call different systems of massage and bodywork "modalities." This is discouraged, since it does not reflect the complexity of these approaches to healing. *Systems, approaches,* and *forms* are suggested instead of the term modality.

Massage practitioners commonly specialize in one or two aspects of the wellness massage pyramid. For example, most physical therapists concentrate on treatment, recovery and prevention, while many massage therapists focus on health maintenance and personal growth. However, some physical therapists help clients reach personal goals such as improving athletic performance, and a growing number of massage therapists specialize in rehabilitation and in treatment of patients with pathology. Nurses may include massage as part of palliative care for patients in hospitals or nursing homes. Most health professions include at least some aspects of the broad scope of wellness, although individual practitioners may choose to practice within a narrower range of client goals.

Health practitioners in states with occupational licensing generally have their scope of practice defined by law, although that scope may change over time. For example, many jurisdictions now include treatment in the scope of practice of massage therapists, although they are legally prohibited from diagnosing medical conditions in most states.

Massage is used somewhat differently in different health professions according to their scope and theoretical bases, but these professions share a common bond, that is, the massage techniques themselves. The heart of this book is the description of massage techniques and their applications for enhancing health and healing.

CLARIFYING TERMINOLOGY

Terminology used within different health professions and in different settings varies. For example, some health professionals will say they have **clients** or **guests,** while others use the term **patients.** Some call themselves technicians or **practitioners,** while others prefer **therapists.** Some refer to what they do as **treatments** or **procedures,** while others use the term **sessions.**

The word *treatment* has become particularly problematic for massage therapists in their interface with mainstream medicine. Historically, the term *treatment* has been used for a number of different services in settings like spas. For example, a facial, mud bath, or massage might be called a treatment even though its aim is health, beauty, or pleasure.

This becomes confusing for practitioners in health care professions where *treatment* specifically means a method of healing a medical condition. Because many massage therapists are working in mainstream medical settings, and it is important to be clear about scope of practice, it may be time to limit the use of the term *treatment.* It should be reserved for when massage and bodywork is used for treatment of or recovery from a specific medical condition.

The chart in Table 1–2 contains suggestions for terminology to distinguish more clearly when massage is being used in the medical model. The column on the left lists terms more appropriate for more general wellness situations, and the column on the right is more treatment oriented language. Using

Table 1–2 *WELLNESS/TREATMENT TERMINOLOGY CHART*

The terminology listed below can be used to distinguish more clearly between the broad scope of wellness, and specific treatment applications of massage. Wellness terminology is appropriate in a wide variety of settings, while the treatment terminology is used more in clinical or medical settings.

Note: The intent of massage from a wellness perspective is high level wellness in many dimensions of life, and in treatment applications is the alleviation of a specific diagnosed medical condition.

Wellness Terminology	Treatment Terminology
• Client	• Patient, case
• Client history, health history	• Medical history, case history
• Session, appointment	• Treatment
• Assessment, evaluation	• Assessment, diagnosis
• Benefit	• Indication
• Contraindication	• Contraindication
• Problem solving skills, session organizing skills	• Clinical reasoning skills
• Client management	• Case management
• Session plan, session strategy	• Treatment plan, protocol
• Therapeutic approach	• Intervention
• Therapeutic	• Therapy, rehabilitation
• Health profession	• Health care profession
• Practice environment	• Medical environment, health care environment
• Practitioner, massage therapist, bodyworker	• Therapist

the word *treatment* and related terms only in the context of addressing a medical condition would help clarify the intention of a specific massage application.

The terminology used throughout this text is deliberately more inclusive. The one who performs massage will be called the **giver** or practitioner, while the one receiving massage will be called the **receiver** or **recipient.** The word *practitioner* specifically refers to someone trained in massage techniques, and who uses massage in the practice of his or her profession. Session will refer to the period of time in which massage is performed. The term treatment will be reserved for descriptions of medical applications.

SUMMARY

Massage is one of the traditional natural healing arts. It is a manual therapy, i.e., performed by hand, and it is the person-to-person touch that defines massage and gives it a unique healing potential. Many massage practitioners adhere to the tenets of a natural healing philosophy, including a preference for natural methods of healing, the belief in an innate healing force, and a holistic view of human life.

Healing means to make healthy, whole, or sound. It also means to enhance health and wellbeing, and the process of regaining health or optimal functioning after an illness or injury. Healing comes from the inside, and recipients are active participants in their own recovery. In contrast, the connotation of the word *curing* is something coming from the outside, and given to a passive recipient. Massage is presented in this text as a method for enhancing the innate healing force already at work as living beings continuously repair themselves and try to maintain an integrated wholeness.

Holistic refers to approaches to health and healing that take into account the wholeness of human beings including body, mind, emotions, and spirit. In the holistic paradigm, massage is applied to the physical body, yet it affects all other aspects of the whole person.

Massage is the intentional and systematic manipulation of the soft tissues of the body to enhance health and healing. Its primary characteristics are touch and movement. The actions and intentions of the practitioner constitute the massage technique. Through the medium of touch, the practitioner's actions (e.g., sliding, kneading, or stretching) cause movement in the soft tissues. Intention is the aim that guides the action, and is an essential part of the effective application of massage. Massage falls into the general category of massage and bodywork.

Traditions are elements of culture passed down from generation to generation. There are four traditions that encompass most of the systems of massage and bodywork used widely today. These are folk and native traditions, the Ayurvedic massage tradition of India, Asian bodywork tradition based in Chinese medicine, and the Western massage tradition from Europe and North America.

Modern Western massage is a system of soft tissue manipulation first developed in 19th century Europe. The seven Western massage technique categories are effleurage (sliding and gliding), petrissage (kneading and compression), tapotement (percussion), friction, vibration, touch without movement (holding and touching), and joint movements (mobilizing and stretching techniques). Contemporary massage and bodywork systems developed in the 20th century include lymphatic massage, trigger points, myofascial massage, polarity therapy, and reflexology. Eclectic practitioners combine Western massage techniques with techniques from other systems or traditions to accomplish the goals of a massage session.

Massage and bodywork are sometimes called alternative or complementary to Western medicine. Although renewed interest in massage occurred outside of conventional Western medicine in the late 20th century, a growing number of scientific studies are currently conducted within mainstream medical institutions. When massage is referred to as alternative, it is looked upon as an either-or option outside of mainstream medicine. When it is called complementary, it is considered secondary to a conventional treatment but as contributing to a patient's recovery. CAM is the acronym for complementary and alternative medicine. The United States government considers therapeutic massage, bodywork, and somatic movement therapies a major CAM domain.

In an integrative health care system, massage is considered of status equal to other conventional and CAM therapies. Massage is being integrated into many medical settings today, as well as in spas that offer comprehensive medical and wellness care.

The illness/wellness continuum extends from premature death to high level wellness. The wellness model spans the entire length of the continuum with the aim of high level wellness, while the treatment model spans the continuum to the neutral point. High level wellness is a condition of optimal physical, emotional, intellectual, spiritual, social, and vocational wellbeing. Massage can help individuals achieve high level wellness in a number of ways.

The wellness massage pyramid (WMP) combines concepts from the illness/wellness continuum and Maslow's hierarchy of needs to illustrate the many contributions massage can make toward achieving high level wellness. Moving up from the base of the WMP, levels of contribution are treatment of, recovery from, and prevention of illness and injury, the neutral zone, and then health maintenance, personal growth, and enjoyment of life. The WMP can be used to explain reasons people seek massage, as well as describe the goals of a massage session.

Several health professions include massage in their scope of practice. In many health professions, massage is just one modality among others for treatment of a medical condition. For massage therapists, massage is their specialty and is used for the full range of the wellness goals. Although massage is used somewhat differently in different professions, they share a common bond, that is, the massage techniques themselves.

Various health professions use terminology related to massage differently. The terminology used in this text is deliberately inclusive. The one who performs massage will be called the *giver* or *practitioner*, while the one receiving massage will be called the *receiver* or *recipient*. *Session* will refer to the time period in which massage is performed. *Treatment* will be reserved for medical applications.

A look ahead . . .

Our current understanding and practice of massage therapy has evolved over many centuries. In Chapter 2 we will take a closer look at the history of massage to get a sense of its ancient origin, and its development into a valued health and healing practice for the 21st century.

REFERENCES

Huitt, W. G. (2002) Maslow's hierarchy of needs. Retrieved: March 2003 (*http://chiron.valdosta.edu/whuitt/col/regsys/maslow.html*).

Johari, H. (1996) *Ayurvedic massage: Traditional Indian techniques for balancing body and mind*. Rochester, VT: Healing Arts Press.

Knaster, M. (1996) *Discovering the body's wisdom: A comprehensive guide to more than fifty mind-body practices*. New York: Bantam Books.

Seiger, L., Vanderpool, K., & Barnes, D. (1995). *Fitness and wellness strategies*. Madison, WI: Brown & Benchmark.

Travis, J. W., & Ryan, R. S. (2000). *Wellness Workbook*. 2nd edition. Berkeley, CA: Ten Speed Press.

White House Commission on Complementary and Alternative Medicine Policy (2002). *Final Report*. Department of Health and Human Services. (*www.whccamp.hhs.gov*).

WEB SITES

www.amtafoundation.org AMTA Foundation—Research Database

www.experienceispa.com International Spa Association

www.miami.edu/touch-research Touch Research Institute at the University of Miami

www.nccam.nih.gov National Center of Complementary and Alternative Medicine at the National Institutes of Health, Washington, DC.

www.thewellspring.com Wellness Associates

www.whccamp.hhs.gov White House Commission on CAM Policy Report

CHAPTER TWO

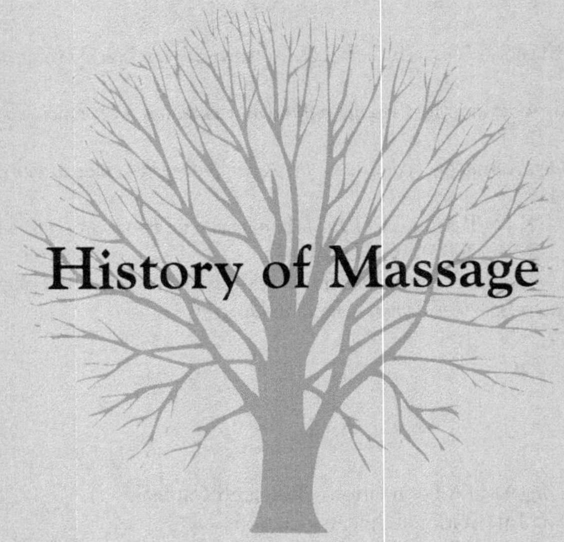

History of Massage

LEARNING OUTCOMES

After studying this chapter, the student will have information to:

1. Appreciate massage as an ancient and global practice.
2. Discuss massage as part of daily life in different native and folk cultures.
3. Describe evidence of massage in the ancient civilizations of Sumer, China and Japan, India, Greece and Rome.
4. Explain how the practice of massage was preserved during Medieval and Renaissance Europe.
5. Describe the beginning of modern Western massage, including the roles of P. H. Ling and J. Mezger.
6. Discuss the uses of massage within conventional medicine from simple medical rubbing to its use in nursing and physical therapy.
7. Discuss the natural healing movement of the early 20th century, including the contributions of J. Harvey Kellogg and Bernarr Macfadden.
8. Describe Swedish massage in its heyday from 1920 to 1950.
9. Trace the development of massage for sports and fitness.
10. Explain the significance of Esalen massage in the 1970s.
11. Identify milestones in the advancement of massage therapy at the turn of the 21st century.

LINK LIBRARY TERMS

Massage Therapy • *Neuromuscular Massage* • *Massage Business* • *Myofascial Release* • *Massage Regulations*

MEDIALINK

A companion CD-ROM, included free with each new copy of this book, supplements the techniques presented in this chapter. Insert the CD-ROM to watch video clips of massage techniques being demonstrated. This multimedia feature is designed to help you add a new dimension to your learning.

KEY HISTORICAL PEOPLE

Avicenna
Celsus
Curanderas
Galen
Graham, Douglas
Hippocrates
Kellogg, J. Harvey
Ling, Pehr Henrik
Lucas-Championnière, Marie Marcellin
Macfadden, Bernarr
McMillan, Mary
Mennell, James
Mezger, Johann Georg
Namikoshi, Torujiro
Pare, Ambrose
Reconstruction Aides
Roth, M.
Taylor, George

KEY TERMS/CONCEPTS

Amma
AMTA Foundation
Anatriptic art
Ayurveda
Commission on Massage Therapy Accreditation
Counterculture
Esalen massage
Greek gymnasium
Hawaiian lomi-lomi
Human potential movement
Massage parlor
Medical rubbing
National Certification Examination for Therapeutic Massage and Bodywork
National Center for Complementary and Alternative Medicine
Natural Healing Movement
Roman Baths
Royal Institute of Gymnastics
Rubdown
Shiatsu
Swedish massage
Swedish movement cure
Touch Research Institute
Traditional Chinese Medicine
Turkish bath
Wellness movement
Yellow Emperor's Classic of Internal Medicine

ANCIENT AND GLOBAL HERITAGE

The history of massage is both ancient and global. Its origin is before recorded history, and it is found in some form in every known culture in the world. Isolated peoples developed their own unique forms of massage and bodywork, which were transformed when their cultures came into contact with each other. Travel, war, trade, immigration, international study, and modern forms of communication have all facilitated the exchange of ideas, and the evolution of the practice of massage on a global scale. Access to the Internet with its vast potential as a reservoir of information is a major advancement for sharing knowledge and transforming the practice of massage today.

The Western massage tradition currently forms the foundation of massage therapy in North America. However, Asian bodywork therapies and Ayurvedic massage are also gaining popularity here. Diverse ethnic populations bring their traditions to the mix.

Knowing about the history of these various traditions helps massage practitioners develop a sense of the vast heritage of which they are a part. (The book to read is *The History of Massage* by Robert N. Calvert, 2002.) Some interesting facts about the uses of massage at various times and in a variety of places will be presented in this chapter. Some of the major forces that shaped massage therapy in North America in the latter part of the 20th century will also be identified.

It will become evident that forms of massage from different time periods, and from all over the world, span the broad scope of the wellness perspective. You will find massage for medical applications, health and fitness, sports massage, and for personal and spiritual development. Some of these forms of massage and bodywork are both historical *and* contemporary to the extent that they continue to be performed in their traditional ways.

As is the custom in many history texts, the more universal designation of dates will be used. The abbreviation "BCE" will be used to denote *before the common era,* often referred to as "BC." The abbreviation "CE" is used to mean *in the common era,* referred to as AD in the Roman calendar.

NATIVE AND FOLK TRADITIONS

In cultures without written records, historical evidence of health practices like massage is difficult to find. The knowledge and skills were handed down in families and in communities through the generations from person to person, and many of these oral traditions have been lost. However, we can learn some things from explorers who first came in contact with indigenous peoples of the world and who described their daily lives in written records. In addition, some ancient forms are still performed by groups who continue to practice their honored traditions. Massage by the South Sea Islanders before their contact with Western civilization and by the curanderas of the southwest United States are examples of native and folk traditions for which we have some reliable information.

South Sea Islands

Descriptions from European and American adventurers offer glimpses of massage as practiced in the South Sea Islands in the 1800s. It was reported that the Maoris of New Zealand called their version of massage *romi-romi,* and the natives of Tonga Island performed *toogi-toogi* for relief of sleeplessness and fatigue. "Melee denotes rubbing with the palm, and fota kneading with the thumb and fingers" (Kellogg, 1923, p. 12). In 1874, Nordhoff described a wellness massage called **Hawaiian lomi-lomi** performed by the natives of the Sandwich Islands:

> To be lomi-lomied you lie down upon a mat, or undress for the night, if you prefer. The less clothing you have on the more perfectly the operation can be performed. To you thereupon comes a stout native with soft fleshy hands, but a strong grip, and beginning with your head and working down slowly over the whole body, seizes and squeezes with indefatigable patience, until in half an hour, whereas you were weary and worn out, you find yourself fresh, all soreness and weariness absolutely and entirely gone, and mind and body soothed to a healthful and refreshing sleep (Murrell, 1890, p. 10).

The Maori of New Zealand are reported to have treated clubfoot in infants with massage. In his study of the genetics of clubfoot, Beals tells of the practice of continuous massage of the clubfoot by the older women of the family, which he said had surprisingly good results. It was a practice passed down from generation to generation, but which virtually disappeared with the advent of European medicine in New Zealand (Beals, 1978).

Curanderas

Today in the Southwestern United States, Hispanic healers called **curanderas** continue folk traditions from Spain and Mexico that are combined with Native American remedies. Their roots can be traced to the Moors of 8th century Spain, then to the Spaniards who came to the Americas in the 15th century, and also to Native Americans, particularly the Aztecs of ancient Mexico (Torres).

Curanderas are female healers called upon when a family's chief caregiver needs assistance. Curanderas totals are those who practice all the various healing specialties, including herbs, midwifery, massage, and ritual. Curanderas totals have a strong spiritual dimension to their methods and are described as using "ritualism and symbolism in their art and are able to move in and out of dimensions not bound to earth." It is believed that curanderas inherit their power to heal, although some families with no heritage of healing may be given the *don,* translated as "gift," or more loosely as the "heart."

Sobardoras are curanderas who specialize in massage and may also use herbal remedies in their work. They perform soft tissue manipulations as well as "bonesetting" types of joint manipulations. Sobardoras learn their art by apprenticeship (Perrone, Stockel, & Krueger, 1989).

ANCIENT CIVILIZATIONS

Written and pictorial records from the ancient civilizations of Sumer, China and Japan, India, Greece, and Rome contain descriptions of massage and exercise. Many of the forms of massage and bodywork found today trace their roots to these ancient practices.

Sumer

A clay tablet from Sumer dating from 2100 BCE describes a remedy that uses an herbal mixture and "rubbing" and "frictions."

> Pass through a sieve and then knead together turtle shells, naga-si plant, salt, and mustard. Then wash the diseased part with beer of good quality and hot water, and rub with the mixture. Then friction and rub again with oil, and put on a poultice of pounded pine (Time-Life Books, 1987, p. 41).

China and Japan

The **Yellow Emperor's Classic of Internal Medicine** (c. 500 BCE), is often cited as the first book on Chinese medicine. It became the foundation for **traditional medicine** practiced in the Asian countries of China, Japan, and Korea (Monte, 1993, p. 20). Essential concepts in Chinese medicine include yin and yang, life energy called *qi* or *chi,* which moves in patterns defined by energy channels, and the five element (fire, wood, water, metal, earth) theory. Ancient health practices and therapies from China include acupuncture with needles, acupressure using finger pressure on acupunture points, a form of massage called tuina, and forms of exercise called chi kung and tai chi.

Massage and bodywork was not confined to medicine in China. In the 1700s, Chinese barbers offered a form of massage to seated patrons in addition to other personal services like cutting hair and cleaning ears. Figure 2–1 is a drawing from an actual street scene in China in the 1790s. It appears to be a form of percussion (Benjamin 2002).

Anma, or **amma,** is a form of Japanese massage that was brought from China via the Korean peninsula in the sixth century CE. At that time, the Japanese assimilated the Chinese medical philosophies that came to Japan as kampo, i.e., "the Chinese way." Amma became an accepted Japanese healing practice.

Shiatsu is a modern form of Japanese bodywork developed in the 1940s by **Torujiro Namikoshi.** Shiatsu incorporates many of the ideas from Western science with traditional Japanese amma. Shiatsu was introduced into the United States in the 1950s by Torujiro's son, Toru Namikoshi.

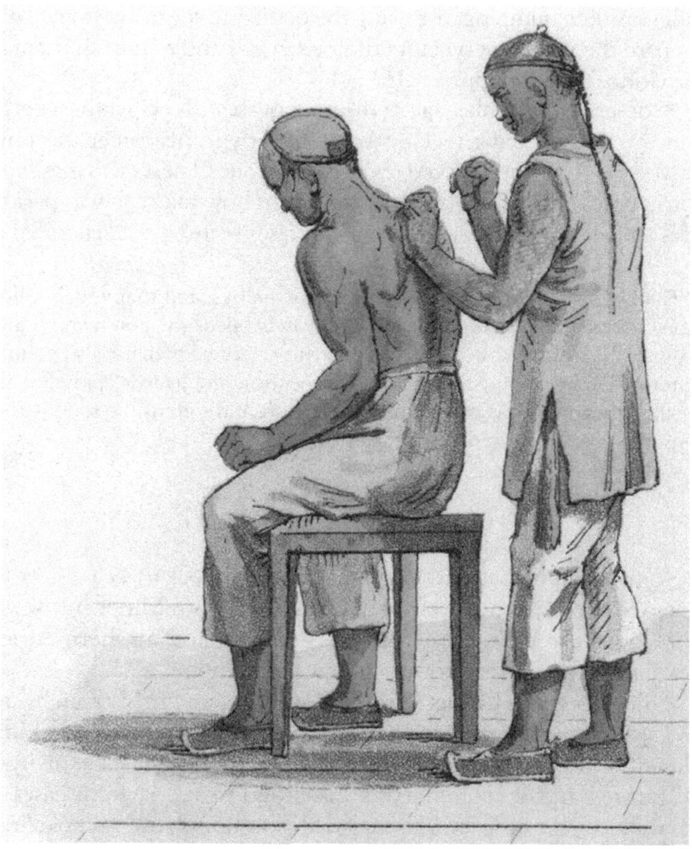

FIGURE 2–1. Chinese barber performing a form of percussion on a seated patron in China in the 1790s. From *Picturesque Representations of the Dress and Manners of the Chinese* by Thomas M'Lean, published 1814.

India

Ayurveda, "knowledge of long life" and the traditional medicine of India, is said to have been given to a Hindu seer by the god Indra. The Ayurvedic system goes back to at least the fifth century BCE and is based on the Vedas, the ancient philosophical and spiritual writings of India (Monte, 1993, p. 30).

Ayurvedic health practices include guidelines for vegetarian eating, forms of cleansing, movements and postures (hatha yoga), breathing exercises, meditation, and massage. Essential concepts in Ayurvedic theory include a life force called *prana,* energy centers called *chakras,* the five great elements (earth, water, fire, air, ether), and the three *doshas (vata, pita, kapha).* The ancient wisdom of Ayurveda continues to be practiced today and has been popularized in the West in the writings of Deepak Chopra (Chopra, 1991).

The recent revival of infant massage in the United States has been patterned in part on the ancient practice of baby massage in India. Leboyer's popular book, *Loving Hands: The Traditional Indian Art of Baby Massage* (1982), shows Shantala, an Indian woman, massaging her baby as she learned from her mother, who learned from her mother, and so on back in time.

Greece

In ancient Greece, the uses of massage for healing, health, and sports were well advanced. **Hippocrates** (450–377 BCE) wrote of the utility of friction after sprains and reduced dislocations and recommended abdominal kneading and chest clapping (Kleen, 1921, p. 2). Aristotle (384–322 BCE), a Greek philosopher and tutor of Alexander the Great, is said to have recommended rubbing with oil and water as a remedy against weariness. Alexander the Great (356–323 BCE), who conquered a vast empire from Egypt to India, reportedly had a personal *triptai* (massage specialist) named Athenophanes, "whose business it was to rub the great emperor and to prepare his bath" (Kleen, 1921, p. 2).

The **Greek gymnasia** in ancient Athens and Sparta were centers run by the state for free men and youths, which contained facilities for exercises, frictions, and baths. The exercises included wrestling, boxing, running, jumping, throwing the quoit and spear, and some ball games. Massage with oil was used to prepare the young men before their exercises and to refresh them after their exercises and after their baths (Johnson, 1866, pp. 15–16).

A description of massage performed in the Greek gymnasia is offered by **Galen** (c. 130–200 CE). Galen was a respected Greek doctor who early in his career was physician to the gladiators, and who later went to Rome and served several emperors. Galen's writings preserve knowledge of the Greek traditions and contain valuable descriptions of how massage was performed in ancient times. Galen describes the effects of massage before exercises (*tripsis paraskeuastike*) and after exercises (*apotherapeia*):

> Rubbing which prepares for gymnastic exercises, and that which follows the same, is subservient to the exercises. The former heats and moderately opens the pores, and liquifies the excretions retained in the flesh, and softens the solid parts, and this is termed preparatory or paraskeuastic rubbing. But the other is termed after-administering (apotherapeutic); and as it is applied with a larger amount of oil, it at the same time moistens by means of the grease, and softens the solid parts, and carries off what is contained in the pores (Johnson, 1866, pp. 19–20).

Rome

The Roman Empire dates from approximately 27 BCE to 476 CE. At the height of its power, the Roman Empire extended from present-day Turkey and Asia Minor in the east to the British Isles in the west and included the territories of southern Europe and northern Africa. The Romans adopted much of Greek culture and spread it throughout their empire.

Aulus Cornelius **Celsus** (25 BCE–50 CE), a Roman physician, is credited with compiling a text called *De Medicina,* a series of eight books covering all of the medical knowledge of his time. In the text, he describes the use of exercises, frictions, inunctions (i.e., applying oil or ointment), rubbing, brushing, ligatures, and dry cupping to prevent and treat certain diseases. Active movements prescribed include walking, running, swimming, riding on horseback, and playing at ball (Georgii, 1880, p. 3).

The Romans borrowed many of the features of the Greek gymnasia to create the **Roman Baths.** The ruins of a famous Roman Bath may still be toured in the former Roman city of Aquae Sulis, now the city of Bath, England. Also at this site is a temple to the Roman goddess of wisdom, Minerva. The Aquae Sulis baths were in operation from approximately 60 to 410 CE. The baths themselves consisted of a space for undressing (*apodyterium*), an exercise court, a warm room (*tepidarium*), a type of steamroom (*caldarium*), and a cold pool (*frigidarium*). At Aquae Sulis, there was also a great swimming pool and immersion baths where one could sit up to the neck in hot curative waters. Both men and women came to these baths.

The Roman writer Seneca (4 BCE–65 CE) left a vivid description of the noise of the Roman bath above which he was trying to study. The passage included complaints about the noise of people exercising and the following passage about massage:

> Or perhaps I notice some lazy fellow, content with a cheap rub-down, and hear the crack of the pummelling hand on his shoulder varying in sound according as the hand is laid on flat or hollow (Cunliffe, 1978, p. 16).

Turkey

After the fall of the Roman Empire in 476 CE, the idea of the Roman Bath was preserved in Turkey and brought back into Western civilization as the **Turkish bath** during the Renaissance. In Turkey it was customary for women, as well as men, to go to the baths as part of their health regimen. The Turkish bath became very popular in the big cities of Europe and the United States in the 19th century.

After partaking of the various forms of hot and cold waters at the *hammam* or Turkish baths, a patron would receive a rather rigorous form of bodywork. The following is a description of a bodywork session given at the *hammam* in Constantinople in the mid-19th century:

> The tellack (two, if the operation is properly performed) kneels at your side, and bending over, grips and presses your chest, arms, legs, passing from part to part like a bird shifting its place on a perch. He brings his whole weight on you with a jerk; follows the line of muscle with an anatomical thumb . . . draws the open hand strongly over the surface, particularly round the shoulder, turning you half up in doing so . . . You are now turned on your face; and . . . he works his elbow round the edges of your shoulder-blades, and with the heel, hard, the ankle of the neck . . . You are then raised for a moment to a sitting posture, and a contortion given to the small of the back with the knee, and a jerk to the neck by the two hands holding the temples (Johnson, 1866, pp. 29–30).

Turkish baths can still be found in some of the major cities of the world. It is noteworthy that the tradition of the Greek gymnasia, the Roman baths, and the Turkish baths is still with us in the form of the modern health club. The basic format of exercise space, swimming pool, showers, steamroom, sauna, whirlpool, and massage room, continue this ancient tradition.

MIDDLE AGES AND RENAISSANCE EUROPE

The Middle Ages in Europe extended roughly from 500 to 1300 CE. This is often considered a period of backwardness in Europe, where the Roman Empire collapsed with the invasion of "barbarian" tribes like the Celts and Saxons. The classical Greek and Roman medical writings, including those about the medical use of friction and rubbing, were lost for a time, and not brought back to Europe until the Renaissance (1300–1600 CE). The Arabs in Turkey and the Near East, as well the monks in Ireland, preserved the writings of Hippocrates, Galen, and others. Some of the information concerning rubbing and frictions was also preserved at this time in the folk healing traditions in Europe.

The Middle Ages were not all darkness, however. A book translated from Arabic into Latin in the 11th century called the *Tacuinum Sanitatis* expounded on the six things that are necessary for everyone in the daily preservation of health. These were listed as the treatment of air, right use of foods and drink, correct use of movements and rest, proper sleep, correct use of elimination and retention of humors, and the regulating of the person by moderating joy, anger, fear, and distress. It notes that "the secret of the preservation of health, in fact, will be in the proper balance of all these elements, since it is the disturbance of this balance that causes illnesses" (Arano, 1976, p. 6).

The *Tacuinum Sanitatis* is evidence of the rich knowledge about healthy living that was known in the Middle Ages and of an early holistic philosophy of health and disease in Europe. It contains the seeds of the philosophy and practices of natural health and healing, which were in full swing by the late 19th century. Natural healing is one of the major traditions of which massage is a significant part.

It should be noted that the Arabic physician **Avicenna** (980–1037 CE) wrote about massage in his famed medical texts. Avicenna said: "the object of massage is to disperse the effete matters formed in the muscles and not expelled by exercise. It causes the effete matter to disperse and so remove fatigue" (Wood & Becker, 1981).

The classical writings of the Greeks and Romans were reintroduced into Europe during the Renaissance. These included writings about the use of frictions and rubbing in the treatment of disease and injuries. This no doubt renewed interest in massage as a medical treatment in the great learning centers of Europe, particularly in France, England, Germany, Russia, and Sweden.

One of the founders of modern surgery, **Ambrose Pare** (1517–1590) of France, wrote about the use of frictions for joint stiffness and wound healing. Pare described different types of frictions simply as gentle, medium, and vigorous.

WESTERN MASSAGE

Two figures loom large in the history of massage in the 19th and early 20th centuries: Pehr Henrik Ling of Sweden and Johann Georg Mezger of Amsterdam. Their pupils have taken their systems of active and passive movements, combined and expanded upon them, and spread them throughout the world. Western massage is a synthesis of techniques developed by these two men.

Ling

Pehr Henrik Ling (1776–1839) was a fencing master, poet, playwright, and educator. He believed that movements of the body had the power to protect, educate, express, and heal. Ling developed four different systems of movement: military, educational, aesthetic, and medical. He described them in his treatise *The General Principles of Gymnastics*, published one year after his death in 1840 (Ling, 1840a). In the late 19th and early 20th centuries, Ling's educational gymnastics were taught in the public schools of the United States as Swedish gymnastics, and his system of medical gymnastics was known popularly as the **Swedish movement cure.** The movement cure consisted of passive and active movements used to treat chronic disease conditions.

Ling is eulogized as having put medical gymnastics on scientific ground. However, a reading of his treatise in the original Swedish reveals the more metaphorical thinking of a poet. He believed that human beings are made up of mechanical, chemical, and dynamic forces. The mechanical force is roughly equivalent to movements of the muscles, and the chemical force has to do with processes like digestion, elimination, and the secretions of glands. The dynamic force is an interesting mix of mental, emotional, and spiritual aspects. Balance in these three forces is necessary to maintain health, while imbalance results in disease. The mechanical force, the realm of passive and active movements, is sometimes used to reestablish balance and, therefore, health, in the human organism (Roth, 1851, pp. 25–32).

Ling's medical gymnastics included both active and passive movements. In his *Notations to the General Principles*, Ling identified the passive movements with descriptive terms like shaking, hacking, pressing, stroking, pinching and squeezing, kneading, clapping, vibrations, and rolling. He instructed that oil may be used to decrease skin friction, but that "this hinders the manipulation of the inner abdominal organs" (Ling, 1840b).

The types of diseases treated by medical gymnastics in the 19th century included a variety of ailments such as congestion of the head, humming in the ears, asthma, emphysema, gastritis, constipation, incontinence, and hernia. Nervous conditions such as epilepsy, neuralgic pain, and paralysis were also treated. Explorations into the treatment of mental diseases by movements were also conducted (Roth, 1851).

Ling believed that practitioners of his work need a thorough grounding in anatomy and physiology. However, in the *Means or Vehicles of Gymnastics*, he cautioned his pupils against a mechanistic view of the human body with these words:

> May anatomy—that holy genesis, which reveals the great work of the Creator to the eye of man, and teaches him at one and the same time how small and yet how great he is—be the gymnast's most treasured fundamental principle; but let him contemplate these forms—not as if they were lifeless ones—but . . . as though they were living, not as constituting an inert mass, but the instrument of the soul, animated with the latter throughout (Ling, 1840c).

Ling established the **Royal Institute of Gymnastics** in Stockholm in 1813 to teach his systems of gymnastics. His pupils took educational and medical gymnastics to major cities all over the world, and by the late 19th century, people interested in natural health and healing were traveling to the Royal Institute to learn Ling's systems from those who carried on his work.

Ling's major legacy to the practice of massage lies in his belief that active and passive movements skillfully applied can help maintain and restore health and balance in the human organism. His holistic view of human beings has persisted, and his work was part of the evolution of the modern concepts of holistic health and wellness. The exercises of Ling's educational gymnastics were the forerunners of modern forms of calisthenics and physical fitness. In addition, the Swedish movements were carried on in the early practice of physical therapy.

Mezger

Johann Georg Mezger (1838–1909), a physician in Amsterdam, also believed that passive movements had the power to heal. Although he never published a detailed description of his work, his pupils von Mosengeil and Helleday did write articles about Mezger's massage. Mezger categorized the methods of soft tissue manipulation into four broad technique categories using the French terms *effleurage* (stroking), *petrissage* (kneading), *friction* (rubbing), and *tapotement* (tapping).

The popularity of Mezger's work was instrumental in reviving the interest in massage in medical settings (Nissen, 1920, pp. 7–8). The general categories of movements he defined have proved very useful and form the basis of Western massage. Vibration was added later as a fifth category as it gained popularity in the late 1800s.

Swedish Movement Cure in the United States

Ling's medical gymnastics, or movement cure as it was known in English-speaking countries, was well established in England and in the United States by the late 1800s. **Dr. M. Roth** studied at the Royal Institute and wrote the first book in English on Ling's system in 1851, *The Prevention and Cure of Many Chronic Diseases by Movements*. Figure 2–2 shows two drawings from Roth's book. One drawing depicts superficial friction being performed for respiratory congestion, and the other shows passive rotation of the foot used to increase circulation in the lower limbs to affect circulation in the head and chest. Note that the patient (recipient) and the operator (practitioner) are in various positions to best facilitate the

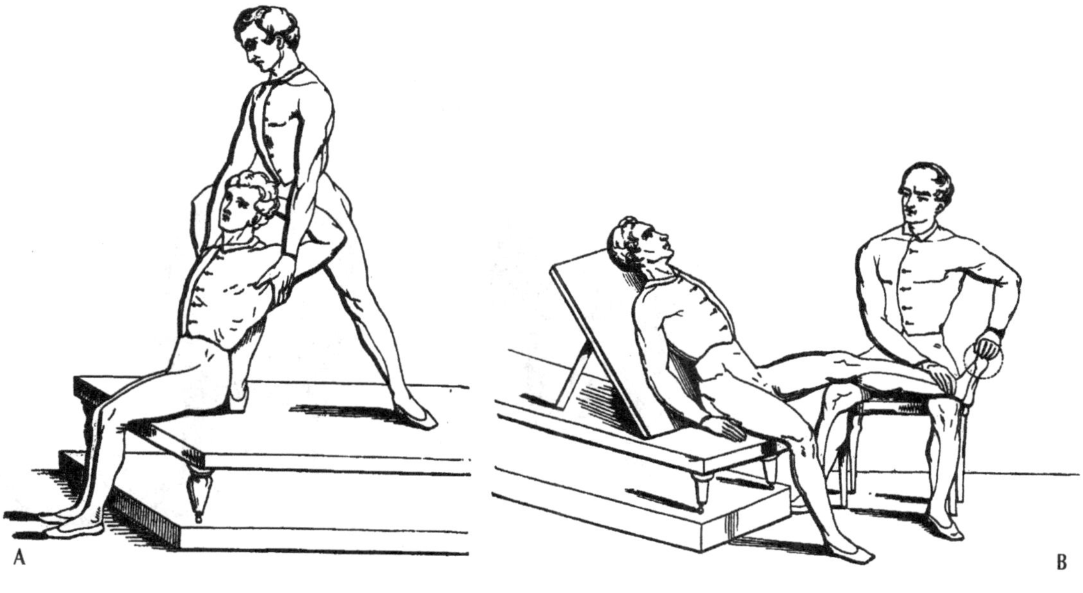

FIGURE 2–2. Drawings from Dr. Roth's book, *The Prevention and Cure of Many Chronic Diseases by Movements*, published in 1851. A. Superficial friction on the sides of the chest for respiratory congestion. B. Passive rotation of the foot to increase circulation.

movements being performed. The convention of lying on a table during the entire session was a later development adopted after the popularization of full-body massage.

The Swedish movement cure was first brought to the United States in 1854 by **Dr. George Taylor** of New York. Other prominent names in the early history of the movement cure in the United States are Hartvig Nissen in Washington, DC (1889), Baron Nils Posse in Boston (1894), Kurre Ostrom in Philadelphia (1905), and Axel Grafstrom in New York (1904).

By the early 20th century, Mezger's massage was adopted by practitioners of the Swedish movement cure, and you begin to see the two terms used together. For example, they are both used in the title of Ostrom's book, *Massage and the Original Swedish Movements* (1905). Figure 2–3 shows drawings of massage of the the neck and shoulders from Ostrom's book.

CONVENTIONAL AND NATURAL HEALING

Various forms of soft tissue manipulation and passive movements continued to be developed as methods for promoting health and healing into the 1900s. The most popular forms continued to be massage and the Swedish movements, later combined into what was called Swedish massage.

Massage in Conventional Medicine

The use of massage in conventional medicine (as opposed to folk remedies, natural healing, and other "alternative" practices) can be found in the medical literature of Europe and the United States dating from the 1700s. It was generally called frictions, rubbing, or **medical rubbing.** In 1866 Walter Johnson wrote a history of medical massage with the lengthy title, *The* ***Anatripic Art:*** *A history of the art termed anatripsis by Hypocrates, tripsis by Galen, friction by Celsus, manipulation by Beveridge, and medical rubbing in ordinary language, from the earliest times to the present day.*

Marie Marcellin Lucas-Championnière (circa 1880) claimed that in fractures, the soft tissue union as well as the bony union should be considered from the start. Sir William Bennett of England was impressed with Lucas-Championnière's idea and started a revolutionary treatment with the use of massage at St. George's Hospital in circa 1899. Albert J. Hoffa published his book, *Technik der Massage*, in Germany in 1900. This book is still a good basic text on massage, giving clear descriptions of how to execute the techniques and advocating the procedures that underlie all modern techniques. The book by Max Bohm, *Massage: Its Principles and Techniques*, written in 1913, includes interpretations of Hoffa's techniques. In 1902, **Douglas Graham** published *A Treatise on Massage, Its History, Mode of Application and Effects*. This text finally aroused the interest of the medical profession in the United States in massage and its therapeutic effects.

Sir Robert Jones, a leading orthopedic surgeon in England, was an enthusiast of the Lucas-Championnière treatment of fractures. Jones was to have an influence on two of the great figures of

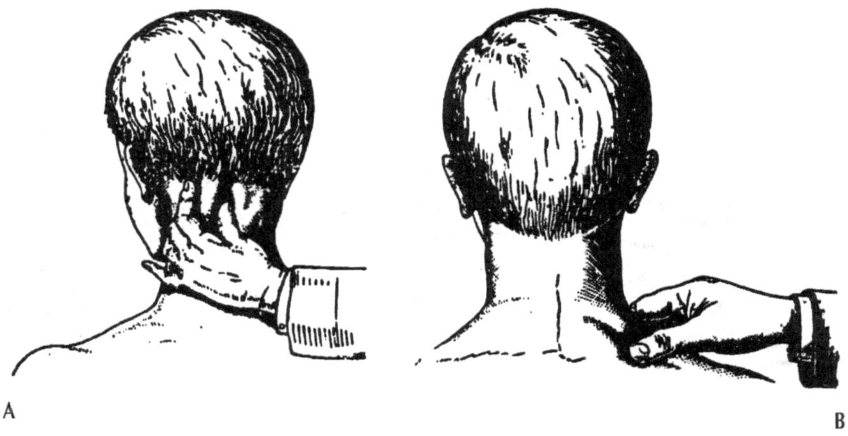

FIGURE 2–3. Drawings of kneading the neck muscles from Ostrom's book, *Massage and the Original Swedish Movements*, published in 1905. A. Kneading the posterior neck muscles. B. Kneading the upper trapezius.

physical therapy in the United States. Mary McMillan was associated with Jones's clinic at Southern Hospital in Liverpool, England, from 1911 to 1915, and **James B. Mennell** worked with Jones at the Special Military Surgical Hospital, Shepherd's Bush, England. Mennell (1880–1957) wrote his text, *Physical Treatment by Movement, Manipulation and Massage,* in 1917 during World War I. Mennell's text was a compilation of the manual therapeutics that he saw in various European countries, and he considered his book to be a rationale of massage treatment. He endeavored to show the importance of care and gentleness in giving massage. Mennell was a medical officer and lecturer on massage at the Training School of St. Thomas' Hospital in London, England, from 1912 to 1935. He was very influential in shaping the practice of physical therapy in its early years.

During World War I, E. G. Bracket and Joel Goldthwait became interested in the reconstruction (i.e., rehabilitation) work that was being done among the Allied nations. They initiated the Reconstruction Department of the United States Army in 1918. The department consisted of physiotherapy, occupational therapy, and curative workshop divisions. Short intensive courses were arranged in recognized schools of physical education throughout the country to train women, called **Reconstruction Aides,** to perform physiotherapy, including massage, on wounded soldiers (McMillan, 1925, p. 10).

In his book, *A Practice of Physiotherapy* (1926), C. M. Sampson, MD describes the types of modalities used in the developing field of physiotherapy, including massage. Figure 2–4 is a photograph of a corner of the general massage section of an army hospital. It shows four operators, as practitioners were then called, working with soldiers who are seated in chairs, and lying or sitting on tables. Massage was applied to assist in rehabilitation.

Mary McMillan, who figured prominently in the development of the profession of physical therapy, received her special training in London at the National Hospital for Nervous Diseases, at St. Bartholomew's Hospital, and at St. George's Hospital with William Bennett. At the Southern Hospital in Liverpool, McMillan was in charge of massage and therapeutic exercises at Greenbank Cripples' Home. She came to the United States as Director of Massage and Medical Gymnastics at Children's Hospital in Portland, Maine. She later served as chief aide at Walter Reed Hospital and instructor of the special war emergency course at the Reed College Clinic for training reconstruction aides during World War I. McMillan was director of physiotherapy at Harvard Medical School while she was writing her book, *Massage and Therapeutic Exercise,* from 1921 to 1925.

Physical therapists trained for rehabilitation work during and after World Wars I and II continued to expand the field of physical therapy for treating a number of orthopedic conditions. They were called upon in the 1930–50s to treat victims of the polio epidemics of that time. But as Gertrude Beard

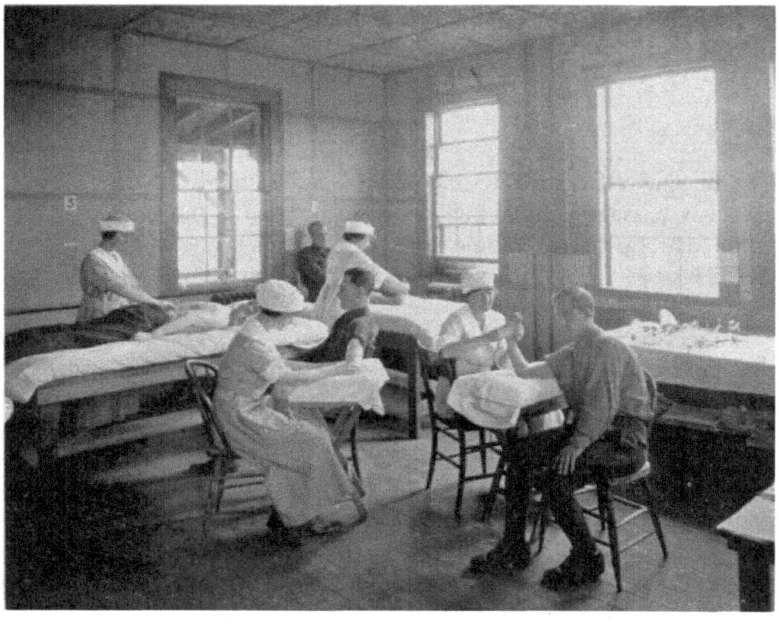

FIGURE 2–4. A corner of the general massage section of an army hospital from Sampson's book, *A Practice of Physiotherapy,* published in 1926.

noted, the amount of massage being prescribed by physicians in the United States declined in the decades following World War II. She speculates that this was due to the fact that massage is time consuming, sometimes strenuous, demands real skill, and the basis for prescribing it was largely empiric rather than scientific (Beard, 1964, p. 1). (For more information, read *Healing the Generations: A history of physical therapy and the American Physical Therapy Association*, edited by W. Murphy, 1995.)

Natural Healing

Massage and the Swedish movements were also practiced by proponents of natural healing, which was considered non-conventional therapy in the early 1900s. These practitioners used various natural remedies to treat different ailments and generally rejected the allopathic methods of drugs and surgery. The philosophy of natural healing includes the belief that humans are created with innate healing powers that can be facilitated by various natural methods such as rest, sunshine, heat and cold applied by water (hydrotherapy), exercise, massage, proper nutrition, laughter, and herbal remedies. Natural healing in the late 1800s and early 1900s also included magnetic healing, a form of energy work (Bilz, 1898).

The Battle Creek Sanitarium in Battle Creek, Michigan, run by **John Harvey Kellogg** (1852–1943), was a natural healing resort of the early twentieth century. Kellogg advocated a host of natural health practices he called "biologic living," including vegetarianism, physical exercise, sunshine, fresh air, colonic irrigation, various forms of bathing, and massage. There was no alcohol, no coffee, no tea, and no smoking. Kellogg and his brother invented the first cold cereal and started the breakfast cereal industry (Armstrong & Armstrong, 1991, pp. 107–111). Kellogg's book, *The Art of Massage*, was first published in 1895.

C. W. Post (1854–1914), of Post brand cereal fame, opened a competing sanitarium on the outskirts of Battle Creek called La Vita Inn. Post featured what he called "mental healing." In 1895 in a self-published book called *I Am Well*, Post offers this advice, which sounds much like relaxation techniques used today:

> Seek an easy position where you will not be disturbed. Relax every muscle, close your eyes and go into silence where mind is plastic to the breathings of Spirit, where God talks to son (Armstrong & Armstrong, 1991, p. 111).

Bernarr Macfadden (1868–1955) was a popular proponent of natural health practices, which he called *physical culture*. In the early 1900s, he opened a string of physical culture resorts in the East and Midwest. His *Physical Culture* magazine was launched in 1898 and was popular well into the 1930s. Macfadden's Physical Culture Training School in Chicago graduated "doctors" of hydropathy, kinesitherapy, and physcultopathy. His health regimen consisted of proper breathing, relaxation, diet, fasting, bathing, singing, exercise, and massage. He was considered a huckster by some, but was successful in bringing the tradition of natural health to the general public (Armstrong & Armstrong, 1991, pp. 203–213).

Swedish Massage

The heyday of Swedish massage was from about 1920 to 1950. During this time, the genre called **Swedish massage** came to include massage, Swedish movements, various forms of hydrotherapy, heat lamps, diathermy, and colonic irrigation. The focus was on health. "Reducing massage" was popular in the 1930–1940s, since massage was believed at that time to be a beauty aid that helped reduce fat on the thighs and waistline.

Practitioners were trained in private vocational schools called colleges, such as the College of Swedish Massage in Chicago. A typical women's class in "scientific massage technique" in the 1940s is shown in Figure 2–5. At this time, women and men were separated, and there was very little cross-gender legitimate massage outside of medical facilities (Benjamin, 1993).

Graduates of these colleges of Swedish massage often opened their own establishments, called **massage parlors** or health centers. In the 1920–1930s, the word *parlor* was simply a term for a functional room like a funeral parlor or beauty parlor. A *masseuse* was a female massage therapist, and a *masseur* was a male. Graduate masseuses worked in upscale beauty parlors such as Helena Rubenstein and Elizabeth Arden. Sometimes exercise classes were offered along with Swedish massage services. Graduates of colleges of Swedish massage could also find jobs at the YMCA, private health clubs, resorts, hospitals, and with professional sports teams. Many practitioners of Swedish massage were proponents of the tradition of natural healing and worked with alternative medical practitioners, especially chiropractors and naturopaths.

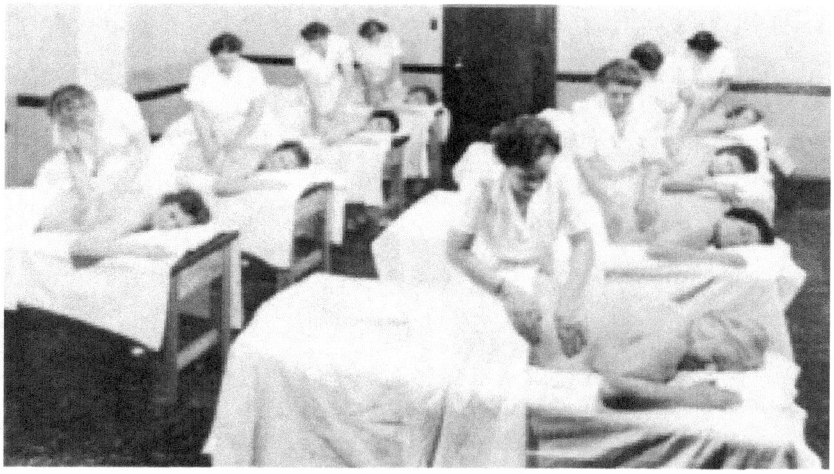

FIGURE 2–5. A women's class in "scientific massage techniques" from a catalog of the College of Swedish Massage in Chicago, circa 1940s.

SPORTS AND FITNESS

Sports Massage

Massage has been part of the sports and fitness scene since ancient Greek times. The **rubdown** was a well established practice by athletes in the United States and England in the late 1800s. A rubdown consisted of superficial skin friction with the hand, a brush, a coarse towel, or a horsehair glove. It was said that "Oxford athletes are never allowed to do cross country running without first rubbing their legs with horsehair gloves or with hands" (Pollard, 1902, p. 21).

H. Joseph Fay wrote about the use of massage in sports in 1916. In his book, *Scientific Massage for Athletes*, he describes massage as being used for ridding the muscles of wastes, which bring about fatigue and stiffness, and to produce additional growth of bone and muscle. He says that the practical trainer "works the meat, or muscle, between the hide and the bone so that it's in its highest state for exercise" (Fay, 1916, p. 20).

Harry Andrews, another trainer-masseur from that era, is shown in Figure 2–6 massaging an athlete's lower leg. Andrews believed that the "rubbing, stroking, pinching, and slapping . . . arouse the latent energy and reinvigorate the limbs, nerve centres, and muscular system generally" (Andrews, 1910, p. 22).

Massage performed by trainers was a familiar sight at college and amateur athletic events in the first part of the 20th century. Albert Baumgartner, a former trainer at the State University of Iowa, wrote *Massage in Athletics* in 1947. He describes massage as being used in preparation for a workout or competition, during rest periods between activities, for reconditioning or recuperation to revitalize the body, and in the treatment of minor injuries. Baumgartner also recognized the psychological benefits of massage to the athlete.

By the 1950s, massage had largely disappeared from the American sports scene. The profession of athletic training was growing, and trainers specialized in the prevention and treatment of athletic injuries using many of the methods of physical therapy. As physical therapists decreased their use of massage in the 1950s, so did athletic trainers.

In the 1970s, the tradition of massage for athletes was revived within the growing profession of massage therapy. Impressed by the success of European athletes who used massage in their training regimens, athletes in the United States began seeking massage to enhance performance and to complement other restorative methods. The American Massage Therapy Association launched a National Sports Massage Team in 1986 to promote massage for athletes. Sports massage was included as part of the official medical team at the centennial Olympics in Atlanta in 1996, and has been a presence at the Olympics ever since. Sports massage has become a specialty among massage therapists, and is popular for both amateur and professional athletes.

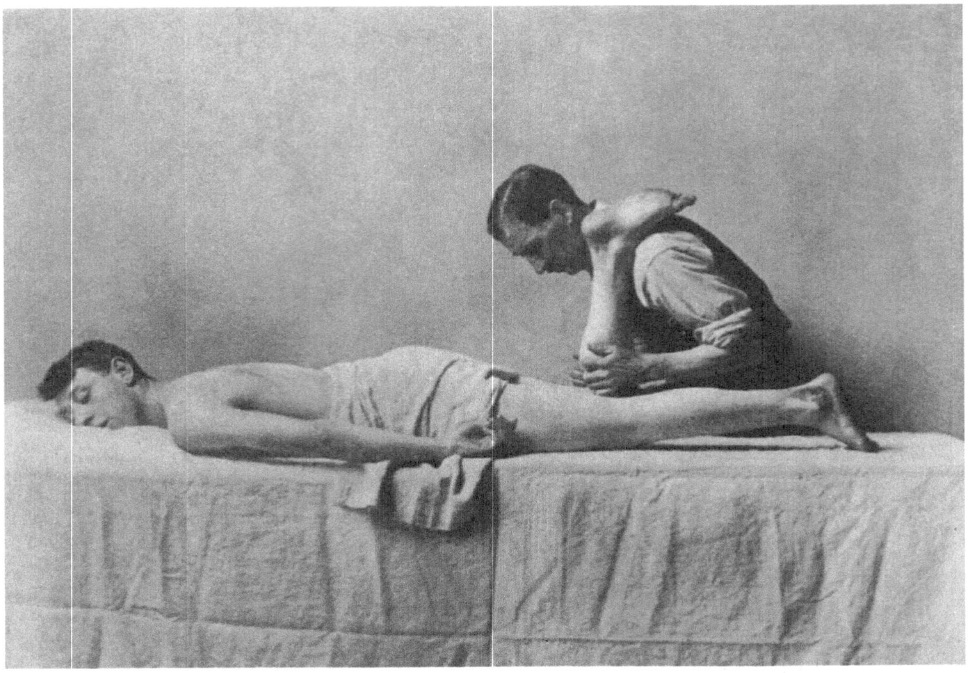

FIGURE 2–6. Harry Andrews, trainer and masseur, massaging the leg of an athlete circa 1910. From *Massage & Training* by Harry Andrews, published in 1910.

Fitness

Just as the ancient Greek gymnasia were not solely for elite athletes, YMCAs and health clubs offer various physical fitness activities for the general population. The YMCA tradition of exercise and massage was well established by 1915 when R. Tait McKenzie described the workouts at the "Y" as consisting of a mixture of Swedish gymnastics, German gymnastics, and games, ending with a bath and a rubdown (McKenzie, 1915, p. 70). By 1953, the health services at the YMCA offered massage and related services for general wellness. The scope of services offered was described by Frierwood:

> The technician uses massage, baths (shower, steam, electricity cabinet), ultraviolet irradiation (artificial and natural sunlight), infrared (heat), instruction in relaxation and in some cases directed exercise. The adult members secure a relief from tensions, gain a sense of well-being, give attention to the personal fitness and develop habits designed to build and maintain optimum health and physical efficiency throughout the lifespan. (1953, p. 21)

DECLINE AND REVIVAL IN THE 20TH CENTURY

In the 1950s, the practice of massage went into a period of decline. "Massage parlors" were used as cover for prostitution, ruining the image of legitimate practitioners. Other modalities were taking precedence in physical therapy, and the therapeutic value of massage was being questioned in professional publications. In the sports arena, trainers were specializing in injuries and the tradition of massage as a training aid was largely forgotten. It was a time of social conservatism, and the undressing and touching that happen in a massage session were uncomfortable for many in the general public. Most private massage schools closed down.

Esalen Massage in the 1970s

Two things happened in the 1960s to help revive the practice of massage: the **counterculture** and the **human potential movement.** Young people in the 1960s rejected the conservative, conformist, "untouchable" values of the 1950s, and began a search for a deeper meaning in life. Many became "hippies" and a culture counter to the mainstream was born. These were the post World War II baby boomers reaching young adulthood.

At the same time, a group of accomplished professionals started meeting at the Esalen Institute in Big Sur, California, in search of the limits of human potential. In the seminars at the Esalen Institute established in 1962, people explored their feelings in encounter groups, tried meditation, delved into various spiritual practices, learned physical exercises from Asia such as tai chi, and various forms of massage and bodywork. TV, movies, and popular magazines such as *Look* and *Life* brought knowledge of the Esalen experience to the American public. Americans were breaking out of the confines of the 1950s and exploring their potential in new ways (Leonard, 1988). (For more about the history of Esalen, go to *www.esalen.org*.)

A form of massage was developed at the Esalen Institute that was to affect the field of massage therapy dramatically. **Esalen massage** was not about technique, although it was loosely based on a simple form of Western massage that emphasized long flowing strokes, scented oils and incense. It was about making connection with the inner self, and with each other. It was not about professional massage at first, but about people connecting with each other on a deep level. As George Downing explained in his *Massage Book* (1972):

> The core of massage lies in its unique way of communicating without words . . . When receiving a good massage a person usually falls into a mental-physical state difficult to describe. It is like entering a special room until now locked and hidden away; a room the very existence of which is likely to be familiar only to those who practice some form of daily meditation . . . Trust, empathy and respect, to say nothing of a sheer sense of mutual physical existence, for this moment can be expressed with a fullness never matched by words (p. 1).

Many of those who embraced the ideals of the counterculture and the human potential movement tried Esalen massage as part of that experience. Others, searching for drugless spiritual or mystical experiences, studied Eastern philosophy and cultures. Many joined ashrams where they learned health practices of India, which include vegetarianism, meditation, yoga, and massage. Some studied Taoism, and tried health practices from China and Japan, including tai chi, chi kung, and shiatsu. China opened its doors to Western trade in 1972, and the ancient art of acupuncture was reintroduced to Western medicine.

Many of the values, as well as the practices, of the tradition of natural health and healing from earlier in the century were revived in the 1970s. Some of those who learned massage in ashrams, growth centers, or out of books wanted to try making a living doing massage professionally. Many still hold onto the values of the counterculture and resist efforts to "professionalize" the field of massage therapy. Others join professional associations and are active in legislative efforts, and in promoting research related to massage therapy.

The opening up to massage that happened in the 1960–1970s had a tremendous impact on the emerging profession of massage therapy. There was a significant growth in the number of practitioners and potential receivers of massage. The number of massage and bodywork training programs increased dramatically, and there was an infusion of youthful energy, spirit, and hope. The concepts of holistic health and healing were revived and expanded. There was openness to new ideas and diversity, and an expansion of thinking beyond Western science and medicine. The values of caring, heart, and connection became defining qualities of the work (Benjamin, 1996).

The cultural revolution of the 1960–1970s has affected health professions other than massage therapy. The **wellness movement,** undoubtedly influenced by the human potential movement, gained ground in the 1970s within the traditional fields of health, physical education, and recreation. The concept of wellness was promoted by people like John Travis, MD, who developed the illness/wellness continuum mentioned in Chapter 1.

Many hospitals today have picked up the concept, and offer "wellness programs" designed to teach good health habits and illness prevention. In the spirit of the wellness movement, they emphasize self-responsibility for health, and address holistic health, i.e., body, mind, emotions, and spirit.

In addition, methods that "touch" patients in a human way are being re-examined for their therapeutic value. For example, the American Nurses Association has recognized massage therapy as an official nursing subspecialty. The National Association of Nurse Massage Therapists (*www.nanmt.org*) is a member of the Nursing Organization Alliance (NOA). Many nurses have also adopted Therapeutic Touch, a form of energy work that has become a respected healing practice (*www.therapeutic-touch.org*).

MILESTONES AT THE TURN OF THE 21ST CENTURY

There were several noteworthy milestones for massage therapy in the 1990s and early 2000s. Most significant were an increase in research about massage therapy, a growing interest in CAM therapies by the U.S. government, the advent of a National Certification Examination for Therapeutic Massage and Bodywork, upgrading of curriculum standards for massage therapy programs, and a growing number of states in the United States licensing massage therapists.

The number of published research studies regarding massage therapy skyrocketed during the last decade of the 20th century. The **AMTA Foundation** was incorporated in 1992. A major part of their mission is to fund research about the efficacy of massage therapy. A database of massage therapy research was made available on their Web site in 2001 (*www.amtafoundation.org*).

The **Touch Research Institute** (TRI) was also created in 1992 at the University of Miami School of Medicine, with Tiffany Field as director. It was the first center in the world devoted to basic and applied research in the use of touch in human health and development. Information about the many studies sponsored by TRI can be accessed through their Web site (*www.miami.edu/touch-research*).

In addition, the first International Symposium on the Science of Touch was held in May 2002 in Montreal, Quebec, Canada. It was sponsored by the Canadian Touch Research Center. Presenters from all over the world participated in the event. Summaries of their presentations are available on line (*www.ccrt-ctrc.org*).

This increase in research and its availability to massage practitioners will help improve the quality of care given to clients and patients, and expand our understanding of the benefits of massage for different populations. It will also bolster the acceptance of massage therapy in an integrative health care system. Chapters 3 and 4 will review some of these study findings in more detail.

Public Policy

The Office of Alternative Medicine (OAM) was established within the U.S. National Institutes of Health (NIH) in 1992. Its charge was to explore "unconventional medical practices," and to recommend further research on the subject. *Alternative Medicine—Expanding Medical Horizons: A Report to the National Institutes of Health on Alternative Medical Systems and Practices in the United States* (1994) was published to summarize their findings.

The OAM was designated a Collaborating Center in Traditional Medicine by the United Nations World Health Organization in 1996. The status of the OAM was elevated to "center" in 1998, when it became the **National Center for Complementary and Alternative Medicine** (NCCAM). The NIH has subsequently awarded several grants for research projects on manual healing methods, including massage therapy (*www.nccam.nih.gov*).

The White House Commission on Complementary and Alternative Medicine issued its final report in March 2002. It made recommendations about coordination of CAM research, education of CAM practitioners, dissemination of information about CAM, and access to and delivery of CAM therapies. It urged the U.S. government to support research to determine which CAM therapies were effective for particular pathologies. The report also recognized the contribution of CAM approaches to wellness and health promotion (*www.whccamp.hhs.gov*).

Standards and Credentials

The **National Certification Examination for Therapeutic Massage and Bodywork** was first given in June 1992. Thus began the process of establishing valid credentials for massage therapists. Over 50,000 massage practitioners have become nationally certified since that time. The NCBTMB has developed massage therapy and specialty exams, and promoted the study of ethics via their recertification process, and Code of Ethics and Standards of Practice documents (*www.ncbtmb.org*).

In addition, in the United States an increasing number of states have passed occupational licensing laws for massage therapists. To date, 31 out of the 50 states have licensing laws. A list of states with massage licensing can be found in Appendix C. Check the American Massage Therapy Association Web site for the most up-to-date information about state licensing laws (*www.amtamassage.org*).

The **Commission on Massage Therapy Accreditation** (COMTA) received approval by the U.S. Department of Education in 2002, and the number of accredited massage therapy programs is growing. COMTA has initiated competency-based curriculum standards more clearly defining basic knowledge and skills for massage therapists (*www.comta.org*).

Consumers

Most importantly, consumers continue to receive massage for the whole range of goals outlined in the wellness massage pyramid. An article appeared in the *New England Journal of Medicine* in January 1993 titled "Unconventional Medicine in the United States." It was a report of a national survey that looked at the prevalence of the use of what was called "unconventional medicine," which included therapies such as chiropractic, acupuncture, relaxation techniques, herbal remedies, energy healing, hypnosis, spiritual healing, and massage therapy. Massage ranked third in alternative therapies used by the general public, with only relaxation techniques and chiropractic reported more frequently. The article concluded that the frequency of use of unconventional therapy in the United States is much higher than previously reported (Eisenberg et al., 1993, pp. 246–252). In a follow-up study of trends in alternative healthcare conducted in 1997, massage therapy was cited as one of the fastest growing CAM therapies in the United States (Eisenberg et al., 1998, pp. 1569–1575).

The American Massage Therapy Association reports increasing acceptance and use of massage therapy by consumers of all ages. In a 2002 Opinion Research study, 28% of adults reported having had a massage in the past 5 years, up from 17% in 1997. And a survey of medical practitioners ranked massage therapy highest (74%) among CAM approaches in terms of being perceived as always or usually effective. An increasing number of workplaces are offering massage as an employee benefit (AMTA 2002 "Demand for Massage Therapy"). The upcoming period in the history of massage therapy looks promising indeed.

SUMMARY

The history of massage is both ancient and global. It is used for health and healing in native and folk cultures all over the world. In the writings of the ancient civilizations of Sumer, China, India, Greece, and Rome we find descriptions of highly developed forms of massage. During the Middle Ages, classical Greco-Roman culture was preserved by Arabs in Turkey and the Near East, and monks in Ireland, and reintroduced into Europe during the Renaissance. The Turkish bath, which included a form of bodywork, was an evolution of the Greek gymnasium and Roman baths. Today's health clubs, with their workout facilities, swimming pools, steam rooms, whirlpools, and massage rooms, are part of this legacy.

Two men influential in the development of modern Western massage were Pehr H. Ling (1776–1839) of Sweden, and Johann G. Mezger of Amsterdam (1838–1909). Ling developed a system of active and passive movements to treat medical conditions and strengthen the body that in the late 1800s was called the Swedish Movement Cure in the United States. Mezger popularized the use of the familiar French terms for the Western massage technique categories of effleurage, petrissage, tapotement, and friction. In the 1900s the work of Ling and Mezger was further developed by their pupils, and found its way into conventional medicine, used both by nurses and physical therapists. Western massage was also an important part of the non-conventional healing methods of proponents of natural healing.

Swedish massage was very popular in the 1920–1940s. In its heyday Swedish massage was a set of therapies that included massage, Swedish movements, hydrotherapy, heat lamps, diathermy, and colonic irrigation. Swedish massage was offered at places like health clubs, the YMCA, resorts, reducing salons, and private establishments called massage parlors. Women massage therapists were called masseuses, and men were called masseurs.

Massage went through a period of decline in the 1950s. It was being used as a cover for prostitution, and its popularity in the United States as a health practice for the general public waned in the conservative climate of that decade. Massage was also losing credibility as a therapeutic modality within medical professions at that time.

Massage was revived as a valuable health and healing practice in the 1970s. The counterculture and human potential movement helped bring to light the benefits of massage as a holistic health practice. Esalen massage and sports massage raised public awareness, and helped invigorate the practice of massage. In addition, forms of massage from China and India came to the United States during this period.

In the 1990s and early 2000s, there were several noteworthy milestones in the history of massage therapy. There was an increase in scientific research about massage, and the creation of institutions to fund research and make results widely available via the Internet. The U.S. government began to develop public policy related to CAM therapies, and provide support for further study. Standards for massage therapists were raised with advent of national certification and USDE-recognized accreditation of training programs. The use and acceptance of massage continued to grow among consumers and other health professionals.

A look ahead . . .

Our understanding of the effects and benefits of massage continue to evolve. Chapter 3 presents some of the current theories about how massage enhances health, and reviews recent research on its efficacy.

REFERENCES

Alternative Medicine—Expanding Medical Horizons: A Report to the National Institutes of Health on Alternative Medicine Systems and Practices in the United States (1994). Available from the Office of Alternative Medicine, National Institutes of Health, 6120 Executive Blvd. #450, Rockville, MD 20892-9904.

AMTA (2002) *Demand for massage therapy use and acceptance increasing*. Retrieved: March 2003 (*http://amtamassage.org*).

Andrews, H. (1910). *Massage & training*. London: Health & Strength, Ltd.

Arano, L. C. (1976). *The medieval health handbook: Tacuinum sanitatis*. New York: George Braziller.

Armstrong, D., & Armstrong, E. M. (1991). *The great American medicine show: Being an illustrated history of hucksters, healers, health evangelists, and heroes from Plymouth Rock to the present*. New York: Prentice-Hall.

Baumgartner, A. J. (1947). *Massage in athletics*. Minneapolis, MN: Burgess.

Beals, K. R. (1978). Clubfoot in the Maori: A genetic study of 50 kindreds. *New Zealand Medical Journal, 88*, 144–146.

Beard, G., & Wood, E. C. (1964). *Massage principles and techniques*. Philadelphia: W. B. Saunders.

Benjamin, P. J. (1993). Massage therapy in the 1940's and the College of Swedish Massage in Chicago. *Massage Therapy Journal, 32*(4), 56–62.

Benjamin, P. J. (1996). The California revival: Massage therapy in the 1970–80's. Presentation at the AMTA National Education Conference in Los Angeles, CA, June 1996.

Benjamin, P. J. (2002). Shampooing—A journey to the East. *Massage Therapy Journal,* 41(2), 140–144.

Bilz, F. E. (1898). *The natural method of healing: A new and complete guide to health*. Translated from the latest German edition. Leipiz: F. E. Bilz.

Bohm, M. (1913). *Massage: Its principles and techniques*. Translated by Elizabeth Gould. Philadelphia: Lippincott.

Calvert, R. N. (2002). *The history of massage: An illustrated survey from around the world*. Rochester, VT: Healing Arts Press.

Chopra, D. (1991). *Perfect health: The complete mind/body guide*. New York: Harmony Books.

Cunliffe, B. (1978). *The Roman baths: A guide to the baths and Roman museum*. City of Bath: Bath Archeological Trust.

Downing, G. (1972). *The massage book*. New York: Random House.

Eisenberg, D. M., Kessler, R. C., Foster, C., Norlock, F. E., Calkins, D. R., & Delblanco, T. L. (1993). Unconventional medicine in the United States. *New England Journal of Medicine, 328*(4), 246–252.

Eisenberg, D. M., Davis, R. B., Ettner, S. L. et al. (1998). Trends in alternative medicine use in the United States, 1990–1997. *Journal of the American Medical Association*, 280 (18), 1569–1575.

Fay, H. J. (1916). *Scientific massage for athletes*. London: Ewart, Seymour & Co.

Frierwood, H. T. (1953). The place of the health service in the total YMCA program. *Journal of Physical Education*, 21.

Georgii, A. (1880). *Kinetic jottings*. London: Henry Renshaw.

Grafstrom, A. (1904). *A text-book of mechano-therapy (massage and medical gymnastics), prepared for the use of medical students, trained nurses, and medical gymnasts*. Philadelphia: W. B. Saunders.

Graham, D. (1902). *A treatise on massage, its history, mode of application and effects*. Philadelphia: Lippincott.

Hoffa, A. (1978). *Technik der massage* (13th ed). Stuttgart, Germany: Ferdinand Enke. Translated for Fran Tappan by Ruth Friedlander.

Johnson, W. (1866). *The anatriptic art*. London: Simpkin, Marshall & Co.
Kellogg, J. H. (1923). *The art of massage*. Battle Creek, MI: Modern Medicine Publishing Co.
Kleen, E. A. (1921). *Massage and medical gymnastics*. New York: William Wood & Company.
Leboyer, F. (1982). *Loving hands: The traditional art of baby massage*. New York: Alfred A. Knopf.
Leonard, G. (1988). *Walking on the edge of the world: A memoir of the sixties and beyond*. Boston: Houghton Mifflin.
Ling, P. H. (1840a). The general principles of gymnastics. In *The collected works of P. H. Ling*. (1866). Stockholm, Sweden. Translated by Lars Agren and Patricia J. Benjamin. Unpublished.
Ling, P. H. (1840b). Notations to the general principles. In *The collected works of P. H. Ling*. (1866). Stockholm, Sweden. Translated by Lars Agren and Patricia J. Benjamin and published in *Massage Therapy Journal*, Winter 1987.
Ling, P. H. (1840c). The means or vehicle of gymnastics. Translated by R. J. Cyriax. In *American Physical Education Review*, *19*(4), April 1914.
McKenzie, R. T. (1915). *Exercise in education and medicine*, 2nd ed. Philadelphia: W. B. Saunders.
McMillan, M. (1925). *Massage and therapeutic exercise*, 2nd ed. Philadelphia: W. B. Saunders.
Mennell, J. B. (1945). *Physical treatment*, 5th ed. Philadelphia: Blakiston.
M'Lean, T. (1814) *Picturesque representations of the dress and manners of the Chinese*. London: Howlett and Brimmer.
Monte, T., & the Editors of East West Natural Health (1993). *World medicine: The East West guide to healing your body*. New York: Putnam.
Murphy, W. (Ed.) (1995) *Healing the generations: A history of physical therapy and the American Physical Therapy Association*. Lyme, CT: Greenwich Publishing Group.
Murrell, W. (1890). *Massotherapeutics or massage as a mode of treatment*. Philadelphia: Blakiston.
Nissen, H. (1889). *A manual of instruction for giving Swedish movement and massage treatment*. Philadelphia: F. A. Davis.
Nissen, H. (1920). *Practical massage and corrective exercises with applied anatomy*. Philadelphia: F. A. Davis.
Ostrom, K. W. (1905). *Massage and the original Swedish movements*. Philadelphia: Blakiston.
Perrone, B., Stockel, H. H., & Krueger, V. (1989). *Medicine women, curanderas, and women doctors*. Norman, OK: University of Oklahoma Press.
Pollard, D. W. (1902). Massage in training. An unpublished thesis, International Young Men's Christian Association Training School, Springfield, MA.
Posse, N. (1895). *The special kinesiology of educational gymnastics*. Boston: Lothrop, Lee & Shepard.
Roth, M. (1851). *The prevention and cure of many chronic diseases by movements*. London: John Churchill.
Sampson, C. W. (1926). *A practice of physiotherapy*. St. Louis: C. V. Mosby.
Time-Life Books. (1987). *The age of god-kings: Timeframe 3000–1500* B.C. Alexandria, VA: Time-Life Books.
Torres (no date). *The folk healer: The Mexican-American tradition of curanderismo*. Kingsville, TX: Nieves Press.
Wood, E. C., & Becker, P. D. (1981). *Beard's massage*, 3rd ed. Philadelphia: W. B. Saunders.

WEB SITES

www.amtafoundation.org American Massage Therapy Association Foundation
www.amtamassage.org American Massage Therapy Association
www.ccrt-ctrc.org Canadian Touch Research Center
www.comta.org Commission on Massage Therapy Accreditation
www.esalen.org Esalen Institute
www.nanmt.org National Association of Nurse Massage Therapists
www.ncbtmb.org National Certification Board for Therapeutic Massage and Bodywork
www.therapeutic-touch.org Nurse Healers-Professional Associates International
www.miami.edu/touch-research Touch Research Institute
www.nccam.nih.gov National Center of Complementary and Alternative Medicine
www.worldofmassagemuseum.org World of Massage Museum
www.whccamp.hhs.gov White House Commission on Complementary and Alternative Medicine

ADDITIONAL REFERENCES

Videos

"Esalen massage." (1999). Big Sur, CA: Esalen Institute. (*www.esalen.org*)
"Hawaiian lomi-lomi: Level 1" Venture, CA: Hawaiian Healing Arts. (*www.lomi-lomi.com*)

CHAPTER THREE

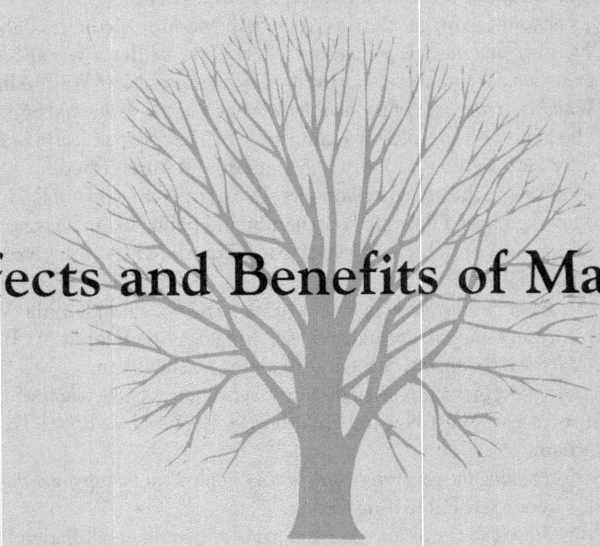

Effects and Benefits of Massage

LEARNING OUTCOMES

After studying this chapter, the student will have information to:

1. Explain the effects of massage at the tissue and organ system levels.
2. Explain the effects of massage at the organism level.
3. Describe the psychological effects of massage.
4. Explain various mechanisms for the effects of massage.
5. Describe how different massage techniques are applied for different effects.
6. Appreciate the holistic view of the effects of massage.
7. Discuss the beneficial effects of massage for everyone.
8. Discuss the beneficial effects of massage for special populations.

KEY TERMS/CONCEPTS

Adhesions
Analgesia
Anxiety reduction
Benefits of massage
Body alignment
Body awareness
Body-centered therapy
Character armor
Effects of massage
Emotional release
Endorphins
Energetic effects
Flexibility
Holistic
Hyperemia
Hypertonic
Immunity
Ischemia
Limbic system
Mechanical effects
Mental clarity

LINK LIBRARY TERMS

Complementary and Alternative Medicine • *Massage Therapy* • *Neuromuscular Massage* • *Massage Business* • *Natural Healing* • *Massage Regulations*

MEDIALINK

A companion CD-ROM, included free with each new copy of this book, supplements the techniques presented in this chapter. Insert the CD-ROM to watch video clips of massage techniques being demonstrated. This multimedia feature is designed to help you add a new dimension to your learning.

Week 3

Mind-body effects
Muscle relaxation
Neural-gating mechanism
Pain-spasm-pain cycle
Posture
Psychological effects
Reflex effects
Relaxation response
Sensory input
Thixotropy
Tissue repair
Venostasis
Wellness massage

Massage is valued for its ability to promote optimal body function, enhance overall health and well-being, and for its specific therapeutic effects. Through the years many theories have been proposed for how and why massage works. In this chapter we will explore some of those theories, and review research that examines the effects of massage and its many benefits.

EFFECTS OF MASSAGE

Effects of massage refer to changes that occur in the body, mind, and emotions of the recipient during a massage session. They are the outcomes of a session, for example, muscle relaxation, increased alertness, or reduced anxiety. Massage practitioners keep these effects in mind as they apply soft tissue techniques to accomplish therapeutic goals.

Different massage techniques are chosen for their specific effects, and are applied to elicit the desired response in the receiver. For example, tapotement has a stimulating effect if received for a short time and may have a sedating effect if received for a longer period of time. Effleurage applied slowly, rhythmically, and with light to moderate pressure usually has a relaxing effect, but applied briskly may feel invigorating.

Practitioners who know how to apply massage techniques to obtain specific effects will be more successful in achieving session or treatment goals. (Refer to *Outcomes-Based Massage* by Andrade & Clifford, 2001.) Information about Western massage techniques and how to apply them for specific effects is found in Part II, Western Massage.

The remainder of this chapter takes a systematic look at the effects of massage as understood in Western anatomy and physiology. The levels of organization found in standard anatomy and physiology textbooks provides a useful framework for studying the effects of massage, i.e., tissue level, organ system level, organism level. Psychological effects are discussed at the whole organism level. Effects that have practical implications from the wellness perspective will be highlighted. The potential effects of massage are summarized in Table 3–1.

TISSUE LEVEL EFFECTS

Massage improves the overall health of cells and tissues of the body, primarily by increasing blood and lymph circulation. The "milking" action of petrissage techniques and the sliding movements of effleurage are very effective in moving body fluids to facilitate natural processes. Increased fluid circulation improves delivery of oxygen and nutrients to tissue cells, and helps in removal of metabolic wastes and byproducts of the inflammatory process (Yates 1990).

Tissue Repair

Healing from tissue injuries such as burns, bruises, sprains, and wounds has three physiological phases. This **tissue repair** process consists of *inflammation* to stabilize the injured area, *regeneration* to restore the tissue structure, and *remodeling* for healthy scar formation. Massage can play an important role in the tissue repair process.

The initial reaction to injury, called inflammation, is designed to stabilize the situation and prepare damaged tissues for repair. Inflammation results in increased blood flow to the area causing redness, warmth, swelling, pain, and decreased function. The lymphatic system plays an important role in

Table 3–1 SUMMARY OF THE EFFECTS OF MASSAGE[a]

Physical Effects	
Tissue Level	
	Enhance tissue repair and scar formation
	Improve connective tissue health
	Improve pliability of fascia
	Break adhesions and separate tissues
Organ System Level	
Integumentary system	Stimulate sensory receptors in skin
	Increase superficial circulation
	Remove dead skin
	Add moisture with oil or lotion
	Increase sebaceous gland secretions
	Facilitate healthy scar formation
Skeletal System	Promote good joint function
	Promote optimal joint flexibility and range of motion
	Promote proper skeletal alignment
Muscular System	"Milk" metabolic wastes into venous and lymph flow
	Promote specific and general muscle relaxation
	Promote optimal body flexibility
	Relieve myofascial trigger points
	Release myofascial adhesions
Nervous System	Stimulate parasympathetic nervous system (i.e. relaxation response)
	Reduce pain (e.g. neural-gating mechanism)
	Sharpen body awareness
Endocrine System	Release of endorphins (with nervous system)
Cardiovascular System	Increase general and local circulation
	Enhance venous return
	Reduce blood pressure and heart rate
	Increase red blood cells in circulation
Lymphatic System and Immunity	Increase lymph fluid movement
	Improve immune function via stress reduction
Respiratory System	Encourage diaphragmatic breathing
	Relax muscles of respiration
	Promotes good structural alignment and rib cage expansion
Digestive System	Digestion improved with relaxation
	Facilitate bowel movement
Urinary System	Enhances circulation to kidneys
	Increased urinary production and bladder tension
Reproductive System	Reproductive function improved with relaxation
	Promote general breast health
Organism Level	
Growth and Development	Improve growth and development in infants
Pain Reduction	Relieve muscle pain from tension and poor circulation
	Deactivate myofascial trigger points
	Activate neural-gating mechanism
	Induce release of endorphins and enkephalins
Stress Reduction	Trigger relaxation response
Psychological Effects	
	Increase mental clarity
	Reduce anxiety
	Facilitate emotional release
	Promote feelings of general well-being

[a]These effects do not occur during every massage session. The massage techniques used and the qualities of movement (e.g., rhythm, pacing, pressure, direction, duration) help determine which effects are likely to occur. The physical, mental, and emotional condition of recipients and their openness to massage might also have impact on which effects occur.

the resolution of inflammation by removing fluid that creates swelling and surveying that fluid for harmful microorganisms. The length of the inflammatory phase will vary depending on the severity of the initial trauma, and the strength of the individual's immune system. Massage is contraindicated in the immediate location of an injury during the inflammatory phase, especially in the presence of infection. Once the signs of inflammation subside, massage can be applied safely around the injury site.

In the regeneration phase, the tissue structure is rebuilt and restored. New tissue replaces damaged tissue of the same type. This involves removing damaged cells, excess fluids, and other byproducts of inflammation, as well as delivering the building blocks for new tissue formation. By improving general and local circulation, massage facilitates this transportation process.

Massage can also play a role in the remodeling phase of tissue repair by encouraging healthy scar formation. Deep transverse friction is used in rehabilitation to help form strong mobile scar tissue. Deep friction helps break interfiber adhesions by forcibly broadening the tissues. This in turn helps produce more parallel fiber arrangement and fewer transverse connections in the tissue that may inhibit movement (Cyriax & Cyriax, 1993). Subcutaneous scar tissue may be loosened by careful and persistent friction; however, further research is needed to establish whether deeper scarring in connective tissue can be realigned once it is formed.

A less understood role for massage in tissue repair is related to its promotion of stress reduction. A study reported in *Lancet*, a British medical journal, showed that wounds healed more slowing in people suffering from chronic stress. Researchers found that the stressed group had lower levels of interleukin-1 beta, an immune system substance known to play a role in wound repair (Greene, 1996, p.16). To the extent that massage reduces stress, it may help wounds heal faster.

Connective Tissue

Connective tissue is the most pervasive tissue in the body. It fills internal spaces, provides structural support, and is a vehicle for fluid transportation and energy storage. Three classifications of connective tissue are fluid (e.g., blood and lymph); supporting connective tissue (e.g., cartilage and bone); and connective tissue proper (e.g., ligaments, tendons, fascia). Some general connective tissue considerations and the nature of fascia will be discussed briefly in the following paragraphs.

Connective tissue has a property called **thixotropy,** which means that it becomes more fluid and pliable when it is mobile, and firmer when it is immobile. Pressing, friction, stretching, and other movements of massage raise the temperature and the energy level of the tissue slightly and create a "greater degree of sol (fluidity) in organic systems that are already there but are behaving sluggishly." (Juhan, 1987, pp. 69–70).

In addition to promoting healthy function, massage helps to *prevent* some connective tissue abnormalities and dysfunction. For example, massage techniques such as kneading and deep friction have been found to help prevent the formation of abnormal collagenous connective tissue called *fibrosis* (Yates, 1990).

Fascia is a connective tissue that surrounds all muscles, bones, and organs and helps to give them shape. Fascia literally holds the body together and can be thought of as continuous sheets of supportive tissue, which envelop the entire body and its parts. (For more detail about fascia read *The Endless Web: Fascial Anatomy and Physical Reality* by Schultz & Feitis, 1996.)

In healthy bodies, fascial tissues are pliable and move freely. With chronic stress, chronic immobility, trauma, or disease, this connective tissue may become thickened, rigid or may stick to other tissues forming adhesions. Adhesions result in restricted movement and impair the ability of the affected tissues to conduct exchanges of nutrients and cellular wastes. Massage can improve tissue function by helping to restore tissue pliability and break adhesions.

Certain massage techniques break **adhesions** formed when fascial tissues stick to each other or to other tissues. The simple mechanical action of some massage techniques separates tissues, for example, lifting, broadening, and applying a shearing force across the parallel organization of fibers. Kneading, skin rolling, deep transverse friction, broadening techniques, and myofascial techniques are examples of effective methods for separating and "unsticking" adhering tissues.

Chapter 12 provides more detailed information about massage for healthy fascia. The discussion of increased joint mobility and flexibility in the Muscular System section of this chapter has further information on connective tissue and massage.

ORGAN SYSTEM LEVEL EFFECTS

Massage has specific effects on the different organ systems of the body. In addition to keeping the organ tissues healthy and enhancing healing, massage can also improve the function of the system as a whole. And since organ systems interact in myriad ways, the effects of massage on any system impacts others as well. Overlapping function is especially obvious in certain system pairings such as muscular-skeletal, circulatory-lymphatic, nervous-endocrine, and respiratory-circulatory-muscular.

Integumentary System

The integumentary system includes the skin and its accessory structures such as hair, nails, and sebaceous and sweat glands. Sensory receptors in the skin detect touch, pressure, pain, and temperature and relay that information to the nervous system.

The skin is the primary point of contact between the giver and receiver of massage. One of the major effects of pressure to the skin is stimulation of the sensory receptors found here. This stimulation may have beneficial effects such as general relaxation, pain reduction, and body awareness. Good **body awareness** enhances a person's sense of integrity and wholeness, and is important for good mental and emotional health.

In order for the exocrine glands in the skin (i.e., sebaceous and sweat glands) to work properly, skin pores must be free from blockage. Pores may become blocked with substances like dirt, makeup, dried oils and sweat, or the accumulation of dead skin cells. Bathing with soap and water, and hydrotherapy such as whirlpool, steam room, and sauna, help open pores. Exfoliating, or removing dead skin cells by scraping or frictioning (i.e., with loofa, brush, or coarse towels) is an old health and beauty practice.

The friction of massage also increases the temperature of skin, which promotes perspiration and increases sebaceous oil secretions. Oil and lotion applied to the skin during massage add moisture needed to prevent further drying or cracking. This is especially beneficial in dry climates, on aging skin, and with certain dry skin conditions.

Massage can facilitate the formation of healthy scar tissue on the skin surface following lacerations, surgery incisions, or burns. Applying cross-fiber and with-fiber friction techniques to scars during the remodeling or scar maturation phase helps form strong mobile scars, break adhesions to underlying tissues, and reduce scar thickness.

Skeletal System

The skeletal system includes the bones of the skeleton, associated cartilage, ligaments, and other stabilizing connective tissue structures. In addition to general tissue health promoted by good circulation, massage and related joint movements help maintain good joint function and range of motion. Movement of the joints stimulates production of synovial fluid that keeps joints moving smoothly.

Optimal range of motion is achieved when the bones are in proper alignment and the tissues surrounding the joints are healthy, pliable, and relaxed. Joint flexibility (i.e., flex-ability) is enhanced with massage and stretching movements. Flexibility is discussed in greater depth in the Muscular System section of this chapter.

Proper body alignment is necessary for optimal functioning of the skeletal system. Maintaining alignment or body posture is discussed below as a function of the combined muscular and skeletal systems.

Muscular System

The muscular system includes skeletal muscles, associated connective tissue (i.e., fascia and tendons), and motor and sensory neurons related to movement. Proprioceptors, important sensory neurons that monitor the movement and position of the body in space, are located in the skeletal muscles and associated connective tissue.

The importance of muscular system health for overall wellbeing cannot be overestimated. It is through the musculature and the movement it produces that so many other health benefits derive: for example, good circulation, body heat, metabolism, kinesthetic awareness, and even emotional balance. Problems in the musculature cause untold pain, and reduced quality of life. It is not surprising that massage therapy is valued so highly for its role in maintaining good health and function of the muscular system.

Cellular Level Activity. Muscles maintain normal cellular level activity and balance through movement. Muscle contraction puts mechanical pressure on the veins and lymphatic vessels, thereby pushing fluids along and carrying away metabolic byproducts. As the muscles relax, fresh blood flows into them, bringing nutrients to the area. This balancing action is disturbed through under-activity or over-activity.

Under-activity disturbs balance, since the muscle contractions that provide the "milking" effect are less than needed for good fluid circulation. Waste products then accumulate in the muscle tissue, and the arrival of nutrients is slowed. When illness or injury results in muscular inactivity, massage can mimic the action of muscle contraction, thereby improving fluid circulation.

Over-activity, for example, from strenuous exercise or work, also disturbs balance at the cellular level. Insufficient time between contractions decreases the inflow of nutritive products and oxygen to muscle tissues. In addition, metabolic waste products are formed faster than they can be eliminated. Muscle tension increases and muscles shorten due to reduced cellular nutrition. Muscle tension worsens the situation by further limiting fluid circulation.

Massage given immediately after strenuous activity reduces muscle stiffness and soreness. A combination of effleurage (i.e., sliding) and petrissage (e.g., kneading, compression) flushes metabolic wastes, brings oxygen and nutrients to the area, and enhances tissue repair. These are important benefits of post-event, inter-event, and recovery sports massage (see Figure 3–1). (For further information on massage for athletes refer to *Understanding Sports Massage* by Benjamin & Lamp, 1996.) Also see the discussion on increased blood circulation in the Cardiovascular System section.

Muscle Relaxation. Massage is often used to relax **hypertonic** or tense muscles. There are several ways that **muscle relaxation** may be effected. Reduction of general muscle tension may be due in part to stimulation of the parasympathetic nervous system via relaxation massage. There may also be a conscious letting go of muscle tension by the higher brain centers as the recipient assumes a passive state during a massage session.

General muscle relaxation may also be traced to increased sensory stimulation that accompanies the application of massage techniques. Yates (1990) reasons that massage causes a massive increase in the **sensory input** to the spinal cord, which results in readjustments in reflex pathways, which leads to spontaneous normalization of imbalances of tonic activity between individual muscles and muscle groups. Residual muscle tension left over from past activity or emotional stress is released as the system balances itself (pp. 11–12). Thus, muscular relaxation results from the general application of a variety of basic massage techniques such as effleurage, petrissage, friction, tapotement, and vibration.

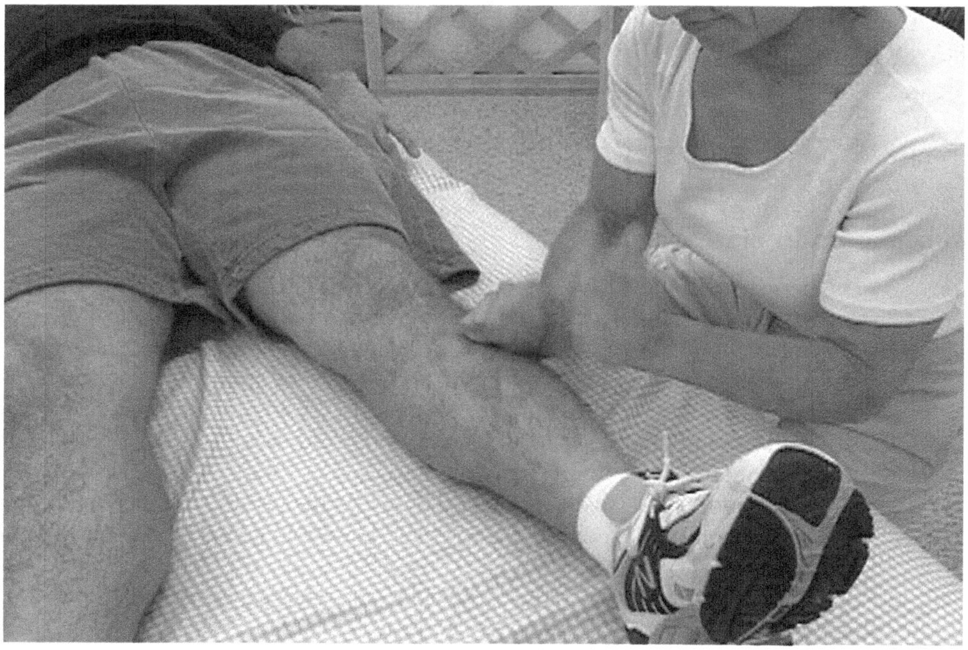

FIGURE 3–1. Massage for athletes improves performance.

Manual techniques may be applied to relax specific muscles. For example, in a technique called *muscle approximation*, the combined action of the muscular and nervous systems is utilized to reduce muscle tone. In this technique, the practitioner slowly and forcibly draws the attachments of the muscle closer together. This decreases stretch of the muscle spindles, which are composed of nerve filaments coiled around specialized muscle fibers. Muscle spindles cause contraction when muscles are suddenly elongated, i.e., stretch reflex. Approximation causes slack in the muscle, and is held until the muscle spindles stop firing and the muscle fibers relax. Approximation is useful for treating muscle spasms.

Another muscle relaxation method called the *origin and insertion technique* by Rattray is useful when direct work on the muscle belly is too painful. In the origin and insertion technique, cross-fiber and with-fiber friction is performed on the attachments of the targeted muscle in small segments until the muscle fibers relax. Eventually overall muscle tone is reduced. This works by stimulating sensory receptors called Golgi tendon organs located in tendons near muscle attachments. When Golgi tendon organs fire, they inhibit contraction of the associated muscle (Rattray 1994, pp. 43-44).Since muscular relaxation is one of the fundamental effects of massage, there are many other manual techniques for promoting muscle relaxation discussed throughout the text.

Increased Joint Mobility and Flexibility. **Flexibility** refers to the degree of range of motion in a joint. It is a function of the combined muscular and skeletal systems with some nervous system involvement. Hypertonic muscles, scarring in muscle and connective tissues, myofascial adhesions, trigger points, and general connective tissue thickening and rigidity may all restrict movement at joints. Massage and passive joint movements can be used effectively to help maintain joint mobility and normal range of motion by addressing any abnormal conditions found in the soft tissues surrounding the joint.

In a study conducted by sport physical therapists and a massage therapist, massage was found to significantly increase range of motion in the hamstrings. The massage techniques used in the study were light and deep effleurage, stretching effleurage, petrissage (kneading), and friction (deep circular and deep transverse). Increased flexibility lasted for at least seven days after the massage (Crosman, Chateauvert, & Weisburg, 1985). Additional information on improving flexibility through joint movements may be found in Chapter 8.

Posture. Proper **body alignment** or good posture is the combined function of the muscular, skeletal, and nervous systems. Poor posture usually results from a combination of factors such as ergonomically inadequate workstations or tools, injuries, or poor postural habits. Poor posture often leads to imbalances between muscle groups, hypertonic and shortened muscles, fascial adhesions, trigger points, and other problem conditions. Or vice versa: Muscle imbalances or pathologies may result in poor body alignment.

Some forms of massage and bodywork specifically focus on helping clients improve their body alignment. After analyzing the client's posture and identifying the probable cause of misalignment, massage and related joint movements are applied with the goal of proper alignment. This might involve strategies such as relaxing and elongating muscles with massage, lengthening muscle groups with stretching, or breaking fascial adhesions with myofascial techniques.

Nervous and Endocrine Systems

The nervous and endocrine systems work together, to coordinate organ system functions and respond to environmental stimuli. The nervous system controls relatively swift responses like those related to movement, while the endocrine system regulates slower responses such as metabolic rate. Nervous system anatomy consists of the central nervous system (i.e., brain and spinal cord), and peripheral nervous system (i.e., sensory receptors and motor neurons). A division of the nervous system that regulates the activity of smooth muscle, cardiac muscle, and glands is called the autonomic nervous system, which plays an important role in relaxation massage.

The endocrine system is composed of endocrine glands that secrete hormones that regulate important body processes such as cell growth and division, general metabolism, water loss and blood calcium levels.

Some of the effects of massage related to the nervous system have already been discussed. For example, stimulation of sensory receptors in the skin enhances body awareness, and plays an important role in muscle relaxation and pain reduction. The effects of massage on growth and development in infants are directly related to stimulation of the nervous system via the skin and through body movement.

Some massage and movement techniques use the nervous system to affect desired results. For example, some assisted stretching techniques deliberately activate proprioceptors in muscles to effect relaxation and elongation.

One of the most important effects of massage is its ability to elicit the relaxation response. This combined autonomic nervous system and endocrine system response is discussed below in more detail under the Organism Level, since it involves many organ systems as well as mental and emotional states.

Cardiovascular System

Cardiovascular system anatomy includes the heart, blood vessels (i.e., arteries and veins), and blood, which is considered a fluid connective tissue. The cardiovascular system is essentially a fluid transportation system for things like nutrients, waste products, dissolved gases, hormones, and cells and molecules for body defense.

The cardiovascular and lymphatic systems are transportation systems that rely specifically on the movement of fluids to carry out their functions. Good fluid circulation in these important body systems is a key to health at the cellular level.

The benefits of increased circulation include improved nutrient delivery and increased metabolic waste removal via the blood. It is also important for tissue repair, as building blocks for new tissues are brought to an area and damaged cells are removed. When pathogens enter the body, fluids deliver macrophages to attack the invaders and help prevent disease. The team action of these two body systems is succinctly described by Yates (1990):

> Increases in blood and lymph circulation are the most widely recognized and frequently described of the physiological effects of massage therapy. Changes in blood and lymph circulation are appropriately discussed together because they have effects in common on the clearance of metabolic wastes, and the byproducts of tissue damage and inflammation, the absorption of excess of inflammatory exudate, and on the delivery of oxygen and nutrients to tissue cells (p. 20).

Blood Circulation. Massage improves both general and local blood circulation. Several studies have shown that capillary vessel dilation and increased blood flow in an area occur with massage. Even light pressure was shown to have an effect (Wood & Becker, 1981, pp. 25–26).

Superficial friction produces **hyperemia** or increased local circulation in the skin and underlying connective tissue. As a result the skin appears red and feels warm. This effect is the result of the release of a chemical called *histamine* that causes dilation of capillaries in the area.

Deep effleurage and petrissage have specifically been shown to increase blood volume in an area. This increased flow is thought to last for some time after massage. For example, Bell (1964) reported that after a 10-minute massage of the calf, blood flow to the area doubled. This effect lasted 40 minutes. The benefits of increased circulation include improved nutrient delivery, and increased metabolic waste removal via the blood.

Venous Return. The mechanical action of deep effleurage enhances venous flow in the limbs. This technique physically pushes blood through venous circulation.

The structure of veins dictates the direction of the application of deep stroking on the limbs. A dictum in classic Western massage states that deep stroking should always be "toward the heart," or moving distal to proximal.

Veins are low-pressure tubes. Movement of blood through them is aided by muscle contraction and by valves that prevent pooling due to the effects of gravity. Deep effleurage in the direction of the natural movement of blood enhances the flow. Applying massage in the opposite direction puts pressure on the valves and could possibly damage them.

Damage to valves results in a condition known as varicose veins. In varicose veins we find static, pooled blood. The constant pressure of pooled blood weakens the vein walls even further, causing a vicious cycle of pooling and weakening. Over time the veins become fragile. Under these conditions, massage could cause the vein to rupture, or release clots formed in the pools, into general circulation. Therefore, massage is locally contraindicated over superficial varicose veins, and generally contraindicated for someone with a history of blood clots.

The mechanical action of kneading and other forms of petrissage also assist in venous return, much the same way muscle contraction does during exercise. Compression of the tissues increases local circulation and blood in the capillaries is moved along toward the larger veins.

Venostasis is a condition in which the normal flow of blood through a vein is slowed or halted. Muscular inactivity can bring about venostasis, particularly in inactive or paralyzed limbs. Other causes for venostasis include varicose veins and pressure on the vessels from edema of the surrounding tissues. Massage given for this condition should first address the proximal aspects of an inactive limb before massage of the distal area. This ensures that the circulatory pathways are open enough to carry the venous flow from the distal area back toward the heart.

Blood Pressure. Researchers Barr and Taslitz (1970) found that blood pressure is temporarily decreased for about 40 minutes after a massage session. The decrease in pressure is thought to result from a greater capacity for blood in the capillaries due to local vasodilation, and greater permeability of capillary walls. The more blood in the capillaries, the less in other vessels to cause pressure on vessel walls. Reduction in both systolic and diastolic pressure was duplicated in research by Cady and Jones (1997).

Also, as mentioned above, one of the long-term effects of eliciting the relaxation response regularly and learning to control stress is decreased blood pressure in individuals with hypertension. This saves wear and tear on the circulatory system and improves circulation overall.

Red Blood Cells. Massage increases the number of circulating red blood cells, thereby increasing the oxygen carrying capacity of the blood. Red blood cells stored in the liver and spleen are thought to be discharged during massage, as well as RBC in stagnant capillary beds returned to circulation (Mitchell 1894; Pemberton 1939).

Lymphatic System and Immunity

The lymphatic system is made up of a network of lymphatic vessels, a fluid called lymph, and organs (i.e., lymph nodes) that contain a large number of lymphocytes. The lymphatic system functions to return fluids from body tissues to the blood; transport hormones, nutrients, and waste products from tissues into general circulation; and defend the body from infection and disease via white blood cells or lymphocytes.

Lymph Fluid Movement. Lymph is a viscous fluid that moves slowly through the lymphatic vessels. These vessels are, for the most part, non-contractile. Lymphatic pressure is naturally lower, and lymph fluid movement slower than venous blood flow.

The movement of lymph through the capillaries, ducts, and nodes of the lymphatic system depends on outside sources such as the contraction of muscles, action of the diaphragm, and pressure generated by filtration of fluid from the capillaries. Lack of mobility due to a sedentary lifestyle, confinement to bed or a wheelchair, pain, or paralysis seriously interferes with flow of lymph fluid. It has been known for some time that massage techniques, especially effleurage and petrissage, mechanically assist general lymphatic flow (Drinker et al., 1941; Elkins et al., 1953; Mortimer et al., 1990). Special lymphatic massage techniques have been developed to maximize the effects of moving lymph through superficial capillaries. (For more detailed information on the lymph system related to massage, read *A Primer on Lymphedema* by Deborah G. Kelly, 2002; and *Compendium of Dr. Vodder's Manual Lymph Drainage* by Renato Kasseroller, 1998). Lymphatic massage is described in more detail in Chapter 14.

Immunity. **Immunity** is defined as "the resistance to injuries and disease caused by specific foreign chemical compounds and pathogens" (Martini & Bartholomew 1999, p. 269). It is a complex phenomenon in which the lymphatic system plays an important part.

Massage affects immunity by enhancing the immune response, which is designed to destroy or inactivate pathogens, abnormal cells, and foreign molecules such as toxins. By improving lymphatic flow as described above, massage facilitates the transport of lymphocytes that participate in the immune response. This is a direct mechanical result of massage techniques like effleurage and petrissage that help move body fluids.

Massage also appears to improve immunity through a number of other mechanisms. Recent studies show massage to be associated with increased natural killer (NK) cells and increased CD4 cells, as well as decreased anxiety and cortisol levels. High cortisol levels inflict wear and tear on the body over time by inhibiting the production and release of white blood cells, blocking T and B cell function, and interfering with the production of interleukins, which are important for communication among white cells (Ironson, 1996; Zeitlin, 2000).

Respiratory System

The respiratory system includes the lungs and the passageways leading to the lungs (i.e., nose, nasal cavity and sinuses, trachea, bronchial tubes). It acts with the circulatory system to effect an exchange of gases between the body and the environment. The respiratory system relies on the diaphragm and other skeletal muscles to produce breathing.

Massage enhances respiratory function by improving general blood circulation, and encouraging relaxed diaphragmatic breathing. Massage can also address tension and shortening in skeletal muscles involved in respiration. To the extent that massage facilitates good posture, it helps achieve the structural alignment and rib cage expansion necessary for optimal vital capacity, i.e., the amount of air moved into or out of the lungs during a single respiratory cycle.

Digestive System

The digestive system consists of a muscular tube called the digestive tract (i.e., oral cavity, pharynx, esophagus, stomach, small intestine, large intestine, rectum and anus), and accessory organs including the salivary glands, gall bladder, liver and pancreas. Functions of the digestive system include ingestion, mechanical processing and chemical breakdown of food and drink, secretion, absorption of water and nutrients, and excretion of waste products.

Massage enhances digestion through eliciting the relaxation response, in which digestive activity is increased. One of the negative effects of stress accumulated over a long period of time is disruption of the normal digestive processes, which can cause indigestion. Relaxation massage as part of a stress reduction program helps prevent digestive maladies.

Abdominal massage has been used for decades to facilitate bowel movement in people suffering from constipation. The direct mechanical effects of massage move the contents of the large intestine, and initiate reflex effects that stimulate peristaltic movement (DeDomenico & Wood, 1997). Abdominal techniques of infant massage assist bowel and gas movement and help relieve distress. Abdominal massage for adults is described in Chapter 10, and for infants in Chapter 22.

Urinary System

The structures of the urinary system include the kidneys, ureters, urinary bladder, and the urethra. The primary function of the urinary system is removal of waste products from the blood, and their excretion out of the body. It also helps regulate blood volume and pressure, as well as blood composition.

Because massage enhances function of the cardiovascular system, it indirectly affects the urinary system, which filters the blood. Better circulation to the kidneys leads to improved blood filtration overall. In addition, one of the results of activation of the parasympathetic nervous system via relaxation massage is increased urinary production and bladder tension. It is not uncommon to have to go to the bathroom after receiving a relaxing massage.

Reproductive System

The male and female reproductive organs are not appropriate targets for therapeutic massage, although they do benefit from improved general cardiovascular function, as do all body systems. There is evidence that chronic stress can impair sexual function, so to the extent massage promotes relaxation it could be said to benefit the reproductive function.

There are specialized approaches to massage for pregnant women, and some massage therapists are trained to work with midwives and health care practitioners during delivery. They often combine Western massage techniques with others such as shiatsu or, in some cases, folk healing traditions. Chapter 22 describes preganancy massage. (Refer to *Mother-Massage: A Handbook for Relieving the Discomforts of Pregnancy* by E. Stillerman, 1992.)

Women's breasts contain mammary glands and lymphatic vessels surrounded by pectoral fat pads and other connective tissues. A layer of loose connective tissue separates the mammary complex from underlying muscle. Breast massage is a specialized skill that helps promote well-breast health, and is a complementary therapy for women undergoing treatment for breast cancer. (Refer to *Breast Massage* by Debra Curties, 1999.) Breast massage requires informed consent from the client, and may be beyond the legal scope of practice for some practitioners.

Occasionally in males, increased circulation to the groin area results in erection of the penis. This does not necessarily indicate sexual arousal. With no sexual arousal, the erection will subside naturally. This is the situation in the vast majority of cases.

However, if there is sexual arousal, it is advised to stop the session immediately, state your perception, and ask the client if your perception is correct. If you still believe that there is sexual arousal regardless of what the client says, or if you are uncomfortable, inform the client that the massage is over, and leave the massage room to allow the client to get dressed. The ethical issues with the client should be dealt with outside of the immediate massage environment.

ORGANISM LEVEL EFFECTS

The effects of massage at the organism level include phenomena that impact the person beyond the effects on any one or two organ systems. Important phenomena affected by massage include growth and development in infants, stress reduction, pain reduction, and certain psychological effects.

Growth and Development

Touch has been found to be essential for the proper growth and development of infants and children. Holding, cuddling, rocking, stroking, and other forms of touching are all necessary for infants to thrive. There is also evidence that adequate pleasurable tactile experience in early life can influence the development of personality traits such as calmness, gentleness, and non-aggressiveness (Brown, 1984, pp. 41–120; Juhan, 1987, pp. 43–55; Montagu, 1978, pp. 76–157).

The importance of stimulation to the skin for proper growth and development cannot be overestimated. The skin develops from the same primitive cells as the brain and is a prime sensory organ. Stimulation of the tactile nerve endings in the skin provides information about the outside world and helps the brain organize its circuitry for proper development. This is also true for movement and information received through the kinesthetic sense. Thus "the use of touch and sensation to modify our experience of peripheral conditions exerts an active influence upon the organization of reflexes and body image deep within the central nervous system" (Juhan, 1987, p. 40).

As infants learn about the world around them through touch and movement, they also learn about themselves and their own bodies. Juhan expresses this idea, "by rubbing up against the world, I define myself to myself" (Juhan, 1987, p. 34).

Massage is an excellent way to provide systematic and regular touching to growing infants (see Figure 3–2). The massage of infants has been practiced widely all over the world, and has been increasing in use in the United States as more caregivers become aware of its benefits. Chapter 22 describes infant massage in more detail.

Pain Reduction

Pain is defined in Taber's as "a sensation in which a person experiences discomfort, distress, or suffering due to irritation of or stimulation of sensory nerves, esp. pain sensors" (Thomas, 1985). **Analgesia,** or pain reduction, is one of the benefits of massage that follows from its ability to elicit the relaxation response, relieve muscle tension, and improve circulation.

Massage may be used effectively to reduce pain caused by certain conditions. For example, muscle relaxation and improved local circulation can help relieve pain associated with tense muscles and the accompanying **ischemia** or lack of blood supply. Massage may also be used to help interrupt a **pain–spasm–pain cycle** induced by hypertonic or tense muscles. By relaxing the muscle and relieving the pain of the spasm, the cycle is broken and healing can take place. The use of specific techniques such as approximation as described above can be very effective for this purpose (Kresge, 1983; Rattray, 1994; Yates, 1990).

It is also thought that massage reduces pain by activating the **neural-gating mechanism** in the spinal cord through increase in sensory stimulation. The theory is that by activating fast, large nerve

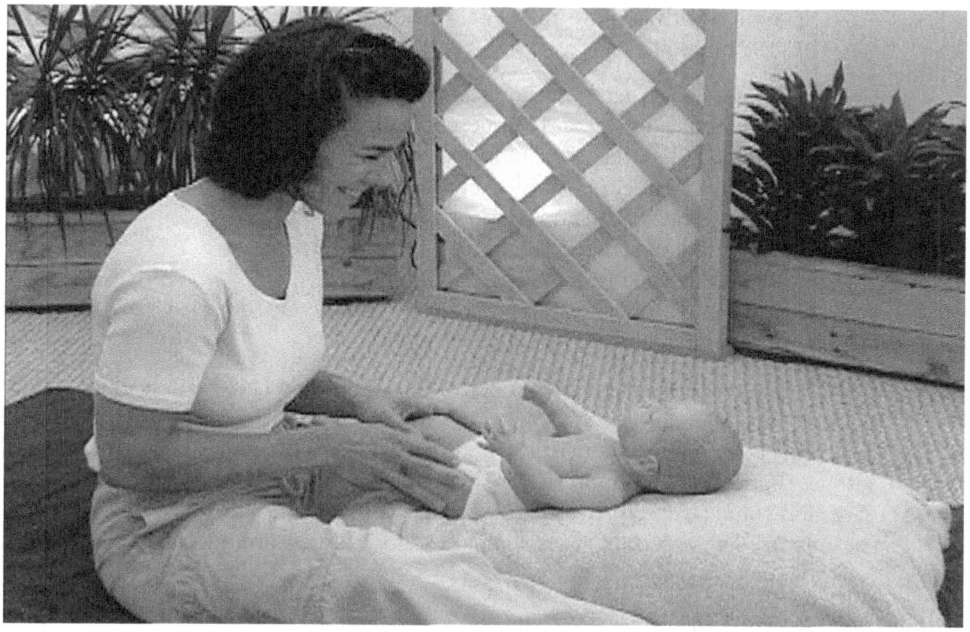

FIGURE 3–2. Massage for infants promotes growth and development.

fibers that carry tactile information, transmission from slower, smaller pain-transmitting nerve fibers is blocked. The perception of pain may be reduced for minutes or hours through the additional sensory input created by massage techniques. Activation of the neural-gating mechanism has been suggested as an explanation for the temporary analgesia associated with deep friction massage in the treatment of tendinous and ligamentous injuries (Yates, 1990).

Research by de Bruijn (1984) noted that the high degree of analgesia resulting from deep transverse friction is preceded by painful irritation of the affected tissues. De Bruijn concluded that friction massage was a promising treatment for soft tissue injuries since the eventual pain-reduction effect allowed the patient to use the affected tissue for better healing.

Myofascial trigger points (TP) are known to cause pain at the site of the TP, at satellite trigger points, and in muscles that lie within the reference zone of the TP. Massage (e.g., ischemic compression and muscle stripping) and stretching are therapies often used in deactivating trigger points (Travell & Simons, 1983, 1992). See Chapter 13 for further discussion of neuromuscular massage and the relief of trigger points.

There is also evidence that massage induces the release of neurochemicals called **endorphins** and enkephalins. These substances modulate pain-impulse transmission in the central nervous system and induce relaxation and feelings of general wellbeing. They are the body's natural painkillers. The mechanism involved in not clearly understood and may be a combination of psychological, as well as physical, reactions to massage (Yates, 1990).

Stress Reduction

Soothing massage is commonly recognized as an effective relaxation technique. It is one of several stress-management methods known to trigger the relaxation response. Other popular methods include meditation, guided imagery, progressive relaxation, abdominal breathing, hatha yoga, and biofeedback.

Back massage is especially effective for stress management, and its application for relaxation is described in more detail in Chapter 10. Several studies have confirmed the benefits of back massage for reducing stress in hospitalized patients (Bauer and Dracup 1987; Fakouri and Jones 1987; Fraser and Kerr 1993). The value of back massage for stress reduction is directly related to its ability to activate the parasympathetic nervous system, and elicit the physiological phenomenon called the **relaxation response.** Inducing the relaxation response counters the damaging effects of a chronic stress response by bringing balance to the body's systems.

Specific health benefits of the relaxation response cited by Robbins, Powers, and Burgess (1994, pp. 191–192) include:

- Decreased oxygen consumption and metabolic rate, less strain on energy resources
- Increased intensity and frequency of alpha brain waves associated with deep relaxation
- Reduced blood lactates, blood substances associated with anxiety
- Significantly decreased blood pressure in individuals with hypertension
- Reduced heart rate and slower respiration
- Decreased muscle tension
- Increased blood flow to internal organs
- Decreased anxiety, fear, and phobias, and increased positive mental health
- Improved quality of sleep

During the relaxation response, a person feels totally relaxed and is in a pleasant semi-awake state of consciousness.

Full-body massage consisting predominantly of effleurage and petrissage, with fewer specific techniques that cause discomfort, is very effective in eliciting the relaxation response. The qualities of such a session could be described as light, smooth, and flowing. The relaxing effects of this type of session may be enhanced with certain types of music, soft lighting, warm room temperatures, and minimum talking.

PSYCHOLOGICAL EFFECTS

The psychological effects of massage (i.e., on the mind and emotions) are less well understood than the physical effects, although they are related to the physical effects in many ways. The most well studied mental and emotional effects of massage include increased mental clarity, reduced anxiety, and feelings of general wellbeing. A phenomenon called *emotional release*, which is an interesting interface of body, mind, and emotions, may also occur during massage.

Mental Clarity

Two studies performed at the Touch Research Institute in Miami suggest that massage helps improve **mental clarity,** i.e., sharpening cognitive skills like solving problems, remembering information, or paying focused attention. In one study, 15-minute massage sessions were given to hospital personnel over a five-week period during their lunch hour. People reported feeling more relaxed, in better moods, and more alert after receiving massage. Similarly, students who received massage during finals week reported being more relaxed and less anxious and said that they remembered information better after an 8-minute massage session (Field 2000).

In a job stress study conducted in 1993, subjects received a 20-minute massage in a chair twice weekly for a month (see Figure 3–3). They reported less fatigue and demonstrated greater clarity of thought, improved cognitive skills, and lower anxiety levels. EEG, alpha, beta, and theta waves were also altered in ways consistent with enhanced alertness (Field, Fox, Pickens, Ironsong, & Scafidi, 1993).

Massage is used with athletes in pre-event situations to help spark the alertness necessary for competition. For pre-event readiness, sports massage sessions are 15–20 minutes in duration, have an upbeat tempo, and use techniques to increase circulation and joint mobility. Tapotement is frequently employed for stimulation (Benjamin & Lamp, 1996, pp. 67–68).

In each of the cases mentioned above, the massage sessions were relatively short—between 8 and 20 minutes. Increased mental alertness is most likely related to sensory stimulation and enhanced circulation to the brain. Improved mental clarity may also be the result of a calmer mind.

Reduced Anxiety

A consistent finding of research on massage is that it **reduces anxiety** significantly. This is true for the general public as well as for those with chronic diseases, and those hospitalized for different reasons. Anxiety is measured through subjective self-reporting instruments, as well as the more objective measure of cortisol levels in saliva and urine. Anxiety reduction would be an expected result of the relaxation response and action of the parasympathetic nervous system. It may also be related to the release of endorphins (Field 2000; Kaard & Tostinbo 1989; Rich 2002).

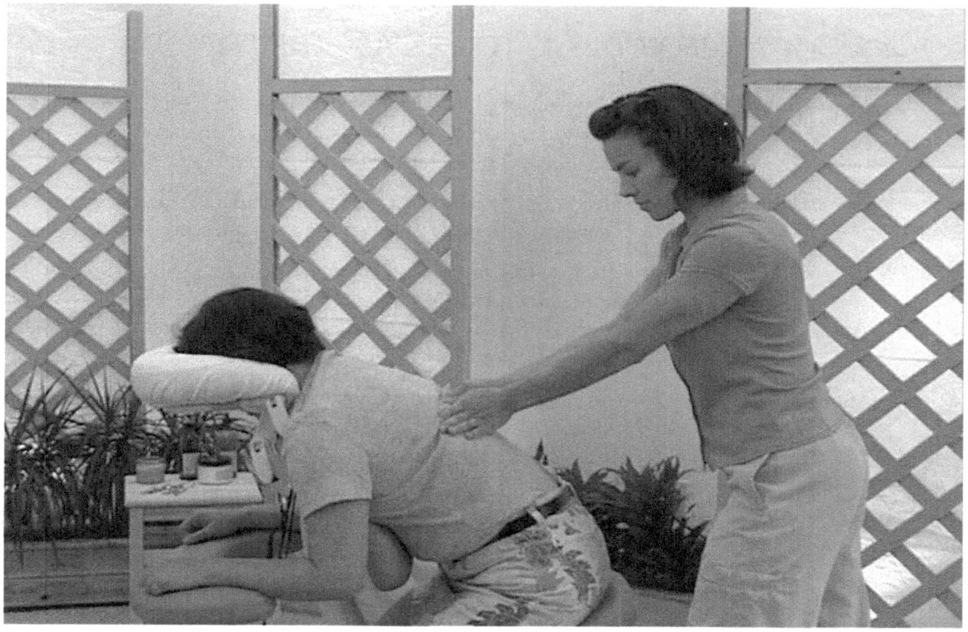

FIGURE 3–3. Seated massage increases mental clarity and alertness.

Emotional Release

A phenomenon called **emotional release** sometimes occurs during a massage session. Unexpressed emotions that are held in the receiver's body may come to the surface in various forms such as being tearful, feeling anger, fear, or grief. Although emotional release is a phenomenon familiar to many massage practitioners, relatively little is known about the mechanisms involved. It is possible that during deep relaxation, a person's natural psychological defenses are lowered, allowing them to feel or express emotions held inside.

Some forms of massage and bodywork specifically address the emotions, and practitioners are trained to deal with issues brought up during emotional release. Releasing unexpressed emotions can be an important step in a physical or psychological healing process. (Refer to *Where Healing Waters Meet: Touching Mind & Emotion Through the Body* (1989) and *Compassionate Touch: The Role of Human Touch in Healing and Recovery* (1993) by Clyde Ford, D.C.)

Massage practitioners should be considerate of their clients during an emotional release, and be good listeners, but be mindful of their own scope of practice. Clients should be referred to other health professionals as needed to resolve deep emotional problems.

Feelings of General Wellbeing

Stated in positive terms, massage is shown to increase feelings of general wellbeing. This likely involves the same mechanisms as anxiety reduction, that is, relaxation response and release of endorphins. Tactile pleasure associated with relaxation massage and simple caring touch may also contribute to feelings of wellbeing.

It is interesting to note that prolonged exposure to pain and other stressors has been shown to deplete the stores of endorphins, leading to an increased perception of pain and despair. To the extent that massage helps to manage pain and stress, and to release endorphins, it may contribute to a more positive outlook.

MECHANISMS OF MASSAGE

Several mechanisms have been identified to explain how the effects of massage are produced. Some of these theories are recognized within the Western biomedical model, while others are on the cutting edge of alternative and body–mind studies. The mechanisms presented here include mechanical, physiological, reflex, body–mind, and energetic. Table 3–2 outlines the mechanisms used to explain the effects of massage.

Table 3–2 MECHANISMS TO EXPLAIN THE EFFECTS OF MASSAGE

Mechanical Effects	The result of physical forces such as compression, stretching, shearing, broadening, and vibration of tissues. Occurs on the gross level of physical structure. *Examples:* venous return, lymph flow, breaking adhesions
Physiological Effects	Organic processes of the body on cellular, tissue, or organ system levels. *Examples:* activation of parasympathetic nervous system; release of endorphins
Reflex Effects	The result of pressure or movement in one part of the body having an effect in another part; or effects mediated through the nervous system. *Examples:* muscle relaxation, increased mental clarity, pain reduction, normalizing system function
Mind–Body Effects	The result of the interplay of body, mind, and emotions in health and disease processes. *Examples:* relaxation response, anxiety reduction
Energetic Effects	The result of balancing or improving the flow of energy within and around the body. *Examples:* Therapeutic Touch, Polarity Therapy, Asian Bodywork Therapy

Some effects are produced by more than one mechanism. For example, changes in local blood circulation during and after massage are thought to occur through direct physical and mechanical effects on vessels; circulatory changes mediated by the local release of vasodilator chemicals (e.g., histamine); or circulatory changes elicited by reflex responses of the autonomic nervous system to tissue stimulation. (Yates 1990).

Furthermore, a specific massage technique may produce a number of different effects. This is a further example of the holistic nature of human beings, and the complexity of effects produced by something seemingly simple like massage.

Mechanical Effects

Mechanical effects are the result of physical forces such as compression, stretching, shearing, broadening, and vibration of body tissues. These effects occur on the more gross level of physical structure. Examples of mechanical effects include enhanced venous return from deep effleurage; elongation of muscles by stretching; increased lymph flow from kneading and deep effleurage; and breaking tissue adhesions with deep transverse friction or myofascial massage.

Physiological Effects

Physiological effects refer to organic processes of the body. These effects involve biochemical processes at the cellular level, but may also occur at the tissue and organ system levels. Examples of physiologic effects include the various results of the relaxation response produced by activating the parasympathetic nervous system; decrease in anxiety by facilitating the release of endorphins; and proper development and growth in infants assisted by the tactile stimulation that occurs during massage.

Reflex Effects

Andrade and Clifford (2001) explain **reflex effects** as functional change mediated by the nervous system (p. 12). Sensory receptors in the skin and proprioceptors in muscles are stimulated by massage and joint movements, thereby eliciting reflex effects. Some examples of reflex effects are muscle relaxation, enhanced mental clarity, and pain reduction.

A different type of reflex effect forms the theoretical basis for a type of bodywork called *reflexology*. In this largely unexplained phenomenon, pressing or massaging one part of the body (e.g., ears, hands, or feet) is believed to have a normalizing effect on an entirely different part of the body. It is not clear if the apparent effects occur through the nervous system or some other mechanism. Chapter 15 explains more about reflexology.

Body–Mind Effects

Body–mind effects acknowledge the interplay of body, mind, and emotions in health and disease. This concept has a long tradition in natural healing, in most native cultures, and in healing traditions of China and India. Western medical science is beginning to confirm demonstrable links between our physical bodies and our mental and emotional states. The new science of psychoneuro-immunology has grown out of these studies.

The body–mind connection can be easily seen in the relaxation response, a physiological process involving the parasympathetic nervous system. The relaxation response is elicited by practices such as meditation, which quiets the mind, or by the tactile stimulation of massage. Other examples of body–mind effects of massage include reduction in anxiety and release of unexpressed emotions held in the body. The discussion of body–mind effects is continued below.

Energetic Effects

Massage and bodywork have been described as balancing, or improving the flow, of energy. What this energy is, and how it relates to the body, are yet to be determined in terms of Western science. However, there are ancient traditions of massage and bodywork, primarily from China and India, based on concepts of energy flow. Therapeutic Touch is a form of energy work adopted by many nurses that addresses the energy field of the recipient. Other popular forms of energy bodywork include polarity therapy and reiki (Claire, 1995).

There are many theories about how energy flows in and around the body, and many practitioners and receivers alike report "feeling" energy. Energy work is currently outside of the understanding and general acceptance of Western biomedicine, but it has persisted over time and is found to be useful by many people.

A HOLISTIC VIEW

Theoretically dividing the human organism into body, mind, and emotions is a useful exercise for discussing the effects of massage. Perhaps it is a product of Western thought and science to think of human beings as divided in this way. However, it should always be remembered that we live as whole or **holistic** persons, and that these effects interact with each other in complex ways to produce an overall effect that may be greater than the sum of its parts. Western medicine is just beginning to explore the holistic nature of human beings.

The Indivisible Body and Mind

The body and mind function as a single unit, i.e., in a holistic way. For example, emotions are felt in and expressed through the body. Love is felt deeply in the physical self, as is hate. Facial expressions are a window to our emotions. Mental and physical pain can be indistinguishable.

Physical manifestations of emotions include the blush of embarrassment, sweaty palms in nervousness, the clenched fist of anger, wide-eyed fear, and the quickened heartbeat of those in love. Some believe that body posture may be read for its emotional sources. For example, raised shoulders indicating fear; rounded shoulders carrying the weight of the world; or forward, hunched shoulders for self-protection and fear of being hurt (Dychtwald, 1977).

The connectedness of body and mind can be traced to our beginnings as an embryo. In the third week of life, there are three layers of cells. The outer layer, or ectoderm, eventually develops into the skin, brain, and nervous system. Thus the physical structures that allow us to feel physical sensations are from the same source as those through which we experience emotions. Juhan observes that "depending on how you look at it, the skin is the outer surface of the brain, or the brain is the deepest layer of the skin" (Juhan, 1987, p. 35).

This connection between the skin and the nervous system has profound implications when studying the effects of massage on the mind and emotions. In touching the outermost part of the physical body, we are able to touch the innermost parts of our patients and clients.

Research on touch has borne out this connection. For example, babies deprived of touch fail to develop properly and suffer retarded bone growth, failure to gain weight, poor muscular coordination, immunological weakness, and general apathy (Montagu, 1978). Massage, as a form of structured touch, has been used successfully to help premature infants gain weight and thrive (Field 2000).

Limbic System

The concept of the **limbic system** helps shed light on how the physical and emotional components of a person are related and how body memories are created. From a physiological perspective, the lymbic system is defined as follows:

> Limbic system—a group of structures within the rhinencephalon of the brain that are associated with various emotions and feelings such as anger, fear, sexual arousal, pleasure and sadness. The structures of the limbic system are the cingulate gyrus, the isthmus, the hippocampal gyrus, the uncus, and the hippocampus. The structures connect with various other parts of the brain (Anderson & Anderson, 1990).

Memory researchers have been able to trace the flow of information from touch receptors in the skin through the spinal cord and brain stem into different parts of the brain. This activates the limbic system to experience emotions related to the touch and to create memories or images of tactile experiences (Knaster, 1996, pp. 123–124).

There is the possibility, therefore, that memories are activated, as well as created, by touch. This has a variety of important implications for practitioners. For example, if the recipient of massage has experienced caring touch primarily in a sexual context, the touch of the practitioner might bring up feelings and memories that would be confusing and inappropriate during a session. Or a recipient who has been physically or sexually abused may have difficulty accepting healing touch without hardening against it. Touch may similarly be used to help in the healing and recovery process.

Character Armor

Wilhelm Reich (1897–1957) introduced the concept of **character armor,** or muscular tension caused by suppression of emotions. For example, unexpressed anger often causes tension in the muscles of the back and arms that would have been used to strike out. Or unexpressed grief may result in shallow breathing and stiffening of muscles used in crying. In the process of relaxing the affected muscles, the suppressed emotions may be felt by the recipient. Massage practitioners sometimes encounter such armoring and should be prepared to help the patient or client understand the release of emotions that sometimes happens.

The above discussion merely touches lightly on the complexity of the body, mind, and emotion relationship. Many of the concepts are in the theoretical stages of development. Research into the holistic nature of human beings is continuing to confirm and clarify ideas that have been little understood before in the context of Western medicine. In her book *Discovering the Body's Wisdom,* Mirka Knaster explores these ideas in more detail and offers a comprehensive introduction to the subject (1996).

Body-Centered Therapy

Massage has been called a **body-centered therapy,** since it works primarily through touch and movement of the body to enhance the overall wellbeing of the recipient. This concept includes the energetic aspect of the person as well, as, for example, in polarity therapy and Asian forms of bodywork.

Explained in Western scientific terms, massage produces effects on the parasympathetic nervous system, releases endorphins, stimulates sensory receptors, relaxes muscles, or gives pleasure. Any of these effects may, in turn, enhance the mental and emotional wellbeing of the recipient.

Practitioners experience the interconnectedness of human beings in many ways. For example, a practitioner may be focused on some physical aspect such as relaxing hypertonic muscles, and the recipient's experience might also have an emotional component such as painful memories of an accident that caused trauma to the area. A psychotherapist may witness the physical effects of stress, such as tension headaches, in their clients. Awareness of how the body, mind, and emotions interact will enable practitioners to better serve their clients.

BENEFITS OF MASSAGE FOR EVERYONE

When the effects of massage support general health and wellbeing or the ongoing healing process, there are **benefits** by definition. A general wellness or health massage aims to normalize body tissues and to optimize function. Everyone can benefit from the health-promoting effects of wellness massage.

The main intention in a general **wellness massage** is to elicit the relaxation response, promote muscular relaxation, and to enhance circulation of fluids, digestion, and elimination. The effects of general relaxation alone have an impact on many physiological and psychological aspects of health and wellbeing. Massage also provides healthy touch, which is a basic human need.

BENEFITS FOR SPECIAL POPULATIONS

The effects of massage may be especially beneficial for people with special needs. These benefits are the natural effects of a wellness massage tailored for a unique individual. For example, pregnant women who tend to have back and leg strain may find special benefit in the effects of massage related to muscle relaxation and improved circulation. Infants benefit from the extra tactile stimulation provided by regular massage for their normal growth and development. Chapter 22 discusses massage for mother and child. The elderly may find massage beneficial for mitigating the normal effects of the aging process and providing healthy caring touch (see Figure 3–4). Massage for healthy aging is discussed in Chapter 23.

Some practitioners are going to workplaces and providing wellness massage for people who sit at desks or similar workstations all day. Massage chairs are commonly used in this environment. The special chairs offer a convenient delivery model and give access to the upper body, which is stressed in office workers. Workplace wellness massage is described more fully in Chapter 25.

For centuries, athletes have benefited from massage as part of their training regimen. The intent of sports massage is to help athletes stay in top condition during strenuous training, prepare for competition, recover after competition, and recover from injury. See Chapter 21 for more information about sports massage.

People going through stressful life situations may benefit from the relaxing effects of massage. Massage may be used in psychotherapy treatment to help reduce anxiety as emotional issues are dealt with. Massage for mental and emotional wellness is also described in Chapter 4.

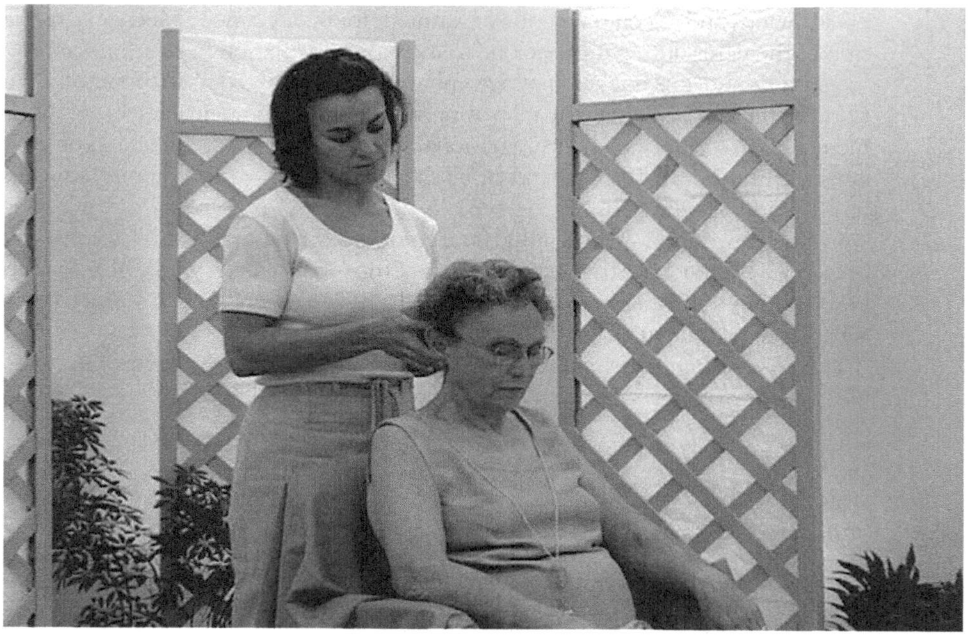

FIGURE 3–4. Massage promotes healthy aging.

People with life-threatening illnesses, those in hospices, and their caregivers may benefit from the psychological benefits of massage. Even those for whom treatment of a condition is not an option may improve the quality of their lives with massage, as explained in Chapter 24.

SUMMARY

Effects of massage refer to changes that occur in the body, mind, and emotions of the recipient during a massage session. Practitioners who know how to apply massage techniques to obtain specific results will be more successful in achieving session or treatment goals.

Massage improves the overall health of cells and tissues of the body. It assists the tissue repair process, especially in the regeneration and remodeling phases. Massage is contraindicated in the inflammation phase of tissue repair. To the extent that massage lowers stress it may help wounds heal faster.

Massage causes connective tissues to become more fluid and pliable, and prevents some connective tissue abnormalities and dysfunction. Certain massage techniques can "unstick" adhering fascial tissues.

Massage improves the overall functions of organ systems. Oil applied during massage moisturizes the skin, and massage stimulates sensory receptors, as well as exocrine glands. Cross-fiber massage techniques assist in healthy scar formation.

Massage promotes good joint mobility and flexibility, and proper alignment of the skeletal system. By improving local circulation, massage alleviates some of the negative effects of under-activity and over-activity of the muscular system. It can reduce muscle stiffness and soreness after strenuous activity, and relax hypertonic or tense muscles. Massage works through the nervous system to increase body awareness, relax muscles, and reduce pain.

Massage improves the function of the circulatory and lymphatic systems by helping to move fluids through the systems. It produces hyperemia locally, and increases blood volume in an area. Mechanical action of deep effleurage enhances venous flow in the limbs, and so deep stroking should always be towards the heart to prevent damage to valves in the veins. Massage can also play a part in decreasing blood pressure, and increasing the number of circulating red blood cells. Massage assists in movement of lymph fluid through the lymphatic system, and enhances immunity.

Massage improves respiratory system function by enhancing general circulation, relaxing muscles of respiration, and encouraging deep diaphragmatic breathing. Relaxation massage improves digestive system function, and abdominal massage is used to treat constipation.

Massage can address the needs of pregnant women, and breast massage is a specialty used for well-breast health and as complementary treatment for breast cancer. Men can experience non-sexual erection of the penis during massage due to increased circulation in the groin area.

On the organism level, massage enhances growth and development of infants. It has pain reduction effects, and can elicit the relaxation response. Psychological effects of massage include increased mental clarity, reduced anxiety, emotional release, and increased feelings of general wellbeing. Mechanisms through which the effects of massage are produced include mechanical, physiological, reflex, body-mind, and energetic.

The connection of body, mind, and emotions has profound implications when studying the effects of massage. In touching the outermost part of the physical body we are able to touch the innermost parts of our patients and clients. Massage is called a body-centered therapy, since it works primarily through touch and movement to create its effects.

Everyone can benefit from the general health promoting effects of massage. Special populations also benefit from massage planned to address their special needs.

A look ahead . . .

Practitioners in several health professions use massage and related bodywork approaches to treat specific medical conditions. Chapter 4 looks at the clinical applications of massage, and some of the research that supports its use in treatment.

REFERENCES

Anderson, K. N. & Anderson, L. E. (1990). *Mosby's pocket dictionary of medicine, nursing & allied health*. St. Louis: C.V. Mosby Company.

Andrade, C., & P. Clifford. (2001) *Outcomes-based massage*. Philadelphia: Lippincott Williams & Wilkins.

Barr, J. S., & N. Taslitz. (1970) Influence of back massage on autonomic functions. *Physical Therapy*, 50.

Bauer, W. C., & Dracup, K. A. (1987). Physiological effects of back massage in patients with acute myocardial infarction. *Focus on Critical Care, 14*(6), 42–46.

Bell, A. J. (1964). Massage and the physiotherapist. *Physiotherapy, 50*, 406–408.

Benjamin, P. J., & Lamp, S. P. (1996). *Understanding sports massage*. Champaign, IL: Human Kinetics.

Brown, C. C., ed. (1984). *The many facets of touch*. Johnson & Johnson Baby Products Company.

de Bruijn, R. (1984). Deep transverse friction: Its analgesic effect. *International Journal of Sports Medicine*, *5*(suppl.), 35–36.

Cady, S. H., and G. E. Jones. (1997) Massage therapy as a workplace intervention for reduction of stress. *Perceptual and Motor Skills*, 84(1), 157–158.

Claire, T. (1995). *Bodywork: What type of massage to get, and how to make the most of it*. New York: William Morrow.

Crosman, L. J., Chateauvert, S. R., & Weisburg, J. (1985). The effects of massage to the hamstring muscle group on range of motion. *Massage Journal*, 59–62.

Curties, D. (1999). Breast massage. Toronto: Curties-Overzet Publications.

Cyriax, J. H., & Cyriax, P. J. (1993). *Illustrated manual of orthopedic medicine*, 2nd ed. Boston: Butterworth & Heinemann.

DeDomenico, G., & Wood, E.C. (1997) *Beard's Massage*, 4th ed. Philadelphia: W.B. Saunders.

Drinker, C. K., & Yoffey, J. M. (1941). *Lymphatics, lymph and lymphoid tissue: Their physiological and clinical significance*. Cambridge: Harvard University Press.

Dychtwald, K. (1977). *Body-mind*. New York: Jove Publications.

Elkins, E. C., Herrick, J. F., Grindlay, J. H., et al. (1953). Effects of various procedures on the flow of lymph. *Archives of Physical Medicine*, 34, 31.

Fakouri, C., & Jones, P. (1987). Relaxation ℞: Slow stroke back rub. *Journal of Gerontological Nursing, 13*(2), 32–35.

Field, T. (2000). *Touch therapy*. London: Churchill Livingstone.

Field, T. M., Fox, N., Pickens, J., Ironsong, G., & Scafidi, F. (1993). Job stress survey. Unpublished manuscript. Touch Research Institute, University of Miami School of Medicine. Reported in *Touchpoints: Touch Research Abstracts, 1*(1).

Ford, C. W. (1989). *Where healing waters meet: Touching mind & emotion through the body*. Barrytown, NY: Station Hill Press.

Ford, C. W. (1993). *Compassionate touch: The role of human touch in healing and recovery*. New York: A Fireside/Parkside book.

Fraser, J., & Kerr, J. R. (1993). Psychophysiological effects of back massage on elderly institutionalized patients. *Journal of Advanced Nursing, 18*, 238–245.

Greene, E. (1996). Study links stress reduction with faster healing. *Massage Therapy Journal, 35*(1), 16.

Ironson, G., Field, T. et al. (1996). Massage therapy is associated with enhancement of the immune system's cytotoxic capacity. *International Journal of Neuroscience*, 84: 205–217.

Juhan, D. (1987). *Job's body: A handbook for bodywork*. Barrytown, NY: Station Hill Press.

Kaard, B., & Tostinbo, O. (1989). Increase of plasma beta endorphins in a connective tissue massage. *General Pharmacology, 20*(4), 487–489.

Kasseroller, R. (1998). *Compendium of Dr. Vodder's Manual Lymph Drainage*. Heidelberg: Karl F. Haug Verlag.

Kelly, D. G. (2002) *A primer on lymphedema*. Upper Saddle River, NJ: Prentice Hall.

Knaster, M. (1996). *Discovering the body's wisdom*. New York: Bantam.

Kresge, C. A. (1983). Massage and sports. In O. Appenzeller & R. Atkinson (eds.), *Sports medicine: Fitness, training, injuries* (pp. 367–380). Baltimore: Urban & Schwarzenberg.

MacKenzie, J. (1923) *Angina pectoris*. London: Henry Frowde and Hodder and Stoughton.

Martini, F. H. & Bartholomew, M. S. (1999). *Structure & Function of the Human Body*. Upper Saddle River, N.J.: Prentice-Hall.

Mitchell, J. K. (1894). The effect of massage on the number and haemoglobin value of the red blood cells. American Journal of Medical Science, *107*, pp. 502–515.

Montageu, A. (1978). *Touching: The human significance of the skin*, 2nd ed. New York: Harper & Row.

Mortimer, P. S., Simmonds, R., Rezvani, M., et al. (1990). The measurement of skin lymph flow by isotope clearance: Reliability, reproducibility, injection dynamics, and the effects of massage. *Journal of Investigative Dermatology*, 95, 666–682.

Pemberton, R. (1939). Physiology of Massage. In *American Medical Association Handbook of Physical Therapy*, 3rd ed. Chicago: Council of Physical Therapy.

Rattray, F. S. (1994). *Massage therapy: An approach to treatments*. Toronto, Ontario: Massage Therapy Texts and MA Verick Consultants.

Rttray, F., & L. Ludwig (2000). *Clinical massage therapy: Understanding, assessing and treating over 700 conditions*. Toronto, Canada: Talus Incorporated.

Rich, G. J. (2002) *Massage therapy: The evidence for practice*. New York: Mosby.

Robbins, G., Powers, D., & Burgess, S. (1994). *A wellness way of life*, 2nd ed. Madison, WI: Brown & Benchmark.

Schultz, R. L., & R. Feitis (1996). *The endless web: Fascial anatomy and physical reality*. Berkeley, CA: North Atlantic Books.

Stillerman. E. (1992). *Mother-Massage*. New York: Delta/Delcorte.

Thomas, C. L. (ed.) (1985). *Taber's cyclopedic medical dictionary*. Philadelphia: F. A. Davis.

Travell, J. G., & Simons, D. G. (1983). *Myofascial pain and dysfunction: The trigger point manual*. Baltimore: Williams & Wilkins.

Travell, J. G., & Simons, D. G. (1992). *Myofascial pain and dysfunction: The lower extremities*. Vol. 2. Baltimore: Williams & Wilkins.

Wood, E. C., & Becker, P. D. (1981). *Beard's massage*, 3rd ed. Philadelphia: W. B. Saunders.

Yates, J. (1990). *A physician's guide to therapeutic massage: Its physiologic effects and their application to treatment*. Massage Therapists Association of British Columbia, Vancouver, BC, Canada.

Zeitlin, D., et al. (2000). Immunological effects of massage therapy during academic stress. *Psychosomatic Medicine*, 62, 83–87.

ADDITIONAL REFERENCES

Videos

"Anatomy and Pathology for Bodyworkers." Santa Barbara, CA: Real Bodywork. (*www.deeptissue.com*)

CHAPTER FOUR

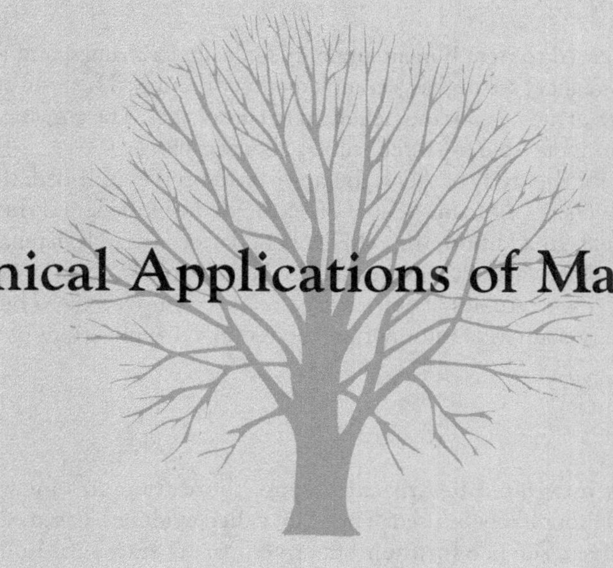

Clinical Applications of Massage

LEARNING OUTCOMES

After studying this chapter, the student will have information to:

1. Define clinical massage therapy.
2. Locate research about clinical massage therapy.
3. Explain Yates' principle-based theory of massage treatment.
4. Discuss three major clinical approaches to massage.
5. Describe the benefits of massage in treating specific pathologies.
6. Discuss the benefits of massage for hospitalized patients.
7. Discuss the benefits of massage for cancer patients.
8. Explain how massage improves development of preterm infants.
9. List applications of massage in pediatric care.
10. Explain how massage benefits people with conditions worsened by stress.
11. Discuss the benefits of massage for people with psychiatric disorders.
12. Describe therapeutic touch and its potential as a clinical approach.
13. Explain how massage is used to complement chiropractic care.

KEY TERMS/CONCEPTS

Clinical massage therapy
Complementary
Contraindicated
Direct therapeutic effects
Evidence-based
Indicated
Integrated health care
Palliative care
Principle-based therapy
Research literacy

LINK LIBRARY TERMS

Massage Therapy • *Neuromuscular Massage* • *Massage Business* • *Polarity Therapy* • *Massage Regulations*

MEDIALINK

A companion CD-ROM, included free with each new copy of this book, supplements the techniques presented in this chapter. Insert the CD-ROM to watch video clips of massage techniques being demonstrated. This multimedia feature is designed to help you add a new dimension to your learning.

CLINICAL MASSAGE THERAPY

Massage has been used to treat human ailments since ancient times, and is currently being integrated into a number of medical settings as a complementary therapy. The term **clinical massage therapy** describes applications of massage for the treatment of pathologies. The growing interest in massage for treatment has led to an increase in research studies about its efficacy.

Two centers for the study of touch therapies have been established: the Touch Research Institute (TRI) at the University of Miami School of Medicine in Florida, and the Canadian Touch Research Center in Montreal. In addition, the AMTA Foundation research database lists thousands of studies about the benefits of massage and its clinical uses. The National Library of Medicine search service called PubMed offers access to studies about massage reported in over 4,000 health-related journals. Table 4–1 lists some major sources of information about clinical applications of massage.

VALUE OF RESEARCH

In the emerging **integrated health care** scene, those therapies for which there is more scientific research will more likely be used. These are called **evidence-based,** since research provides some verifiable objective evidence for their effectiveness. As stated in the Forward to Touch Therapy (Field 2000):

> One of the principal requirements of modern health care provision can be summed up by the term, "evidence-based." It is no longer sufficient for any therapeutic approach to simply rely on a long history of use, or popularity, or widespread availability, to justify its continued acceptance (especially if insurance reimbursement is anticipated) (pp. vii).

Evidence from scientific studies can more clearly substantiate the benefits of massage in treating certain diseases, as well as identify contraindications. Applications of clinical massage therapy will become safer and more effective as the result of research.

Table 4–1 SOURCES OF INFORMATION ABOUT CLINICAL APPLICATIONS OF MASSAGE

Institution Web sites	Touch Research Institutes (TRI) at the University of Miami School of Medicine www.miami.edu/touch-research Canadian Touch Research Centre (CTRC) www.ccrt-ctrc.org National Center for Complementary and Alternative Medicine (NCCAM) at the National Institutes of Health, Washington, DC www.nccam.nih.gov
Massage research database Web sites	Massage Therapy Research Database AMTA Foundation www.amtamassage.org/foundation/dbase.htm National Library of Medicine www.ncbi.nlm.nih.gov/PubMed
Books	***Clinical Massage Therapy*** by Fiona Rattray and Linda Ludwig (Toronto, Canada: Talus Incorporated, 2000) **A Massage Therapist's Guide to Pathology,** 2nd ed., by Ruth Werner (Philadelphia: Lippincott, Williams & Wilkins, 2002) **A Physician's Guide to Therapeutic Massage** by John Yates (Toronto, Canada: Curties-Overzet, 2004) ***Making Sense of Research: A Guide to Research Literacy for Complementary Practitioners*** by Martha Brown Menard (Toronto, Canada: Curties-Overzet Publications, 2003) ***Massage Therapy: The Evidence for Practice*** by Grant Jewell Rich (Philadelphia: Mosby, 2002) ***Pathology A to Z—A Handbook for Massage Therapists,*** 2nd ed., by Premkumar (Calgary, Canada: VanPub Books, 2000) ***Touch Therapy*** by Tiffany Field (Philadelphia: Churchhill Livingston, 2000)

It has been argued that the nature of massage as a holistic therapy makes it unsuited for scientific inquiry. For example, many practitioners distrust the formula approach to massage used in research to minimize variables in treatment. They understand the importance of varying the approach for the unique individual receiving the massage. Nevertheless, there are certain aspects of massage and its effects that can be measured objectively and provide valuable information to practitioners.

Knowledge gained from research is essential to an approach to treatment that Yates calls **principle-based therapy.** Principle-based massage is in contrast to recipe-based or formula massage, in which each client receives exactly the same treatment (i.e., same techniques applied in same way) for a particular condition. Yates describes the foundation of principle-based therapy as the creation of an overall treatment plan directed toward the achievement of specific treatment goals. Such a plan takes into consideration the condition being treated, tissue involvement, and most importantly in terms of research, the therapeutic potential of different treatment methods. Principle-based therapy also allows for variation:

> Appropriate treatment techniques and modalities are selected, integrated and adapted as necessary to achieve specific effects and are modified according to the changing physiological and psychological state of the patient as treatment proceeds. Treatment is therefore patient-centered rather than technique-centered (Yates 1999, pp. 3–4).

Research takes on practical importance for the selection of techniques based on their healing potential. It can help sort out which massage techniques or approaches are most effective for particular pathologies. Research is most useful for adding to our understanding of the applications of massage, not as a means for developing recipes for treatment. A deeper level of knowledge complements those aspects of massage therapy practice that are intuitive and artful.

Research literacy is important for all massage therapists, especially those in clinical settings. Research literacy includes understanding the scientific method, locating research articles, and reading, analyzing, and evaluating specific studies. (The book to study is *Making Sense of Research: A Guide to Research Literacy for Complementary Practitioners* by Martha Brown Menard, 2003.)

CLINICAL APPROACH

Massage is **indicated** for treating a particular injury or illness if it contributes to the alleviation of the diagnosed condition, or helps ease its symptoms. Massage may be **contraindicated,** or not advisable, if its use as a form of treatment would be detrimental to the client. The word *patient* is most often used to describe a person being treated. However, the word *client* is gaining ground in clinical settings to infer a degree of empowerment on the part of the person receiving treatment. Rattray and Ludwig define client "as a person who is able to make choices about health care" (2000, p. ix).

There are three useful ways of thinking about the clinical benefits of massage therapy, i.e., for its complementary, palliative, or direct therapeutic effects. For example, massage is sometimes indicated as **complementary** to a primary treatment method to enhance its effectiveness and create a more favorable environment for healing. This is especially true for massage designed to help clients relax and reduce anxiety, thereby improving the body's own healing process.

Massage may also be used as **palliative care** to reduce symptoms and discomfort associated with certain diseases or with their treatment. For example, massage has been successful in reducing some of the negative side effects of cancer treatment. By helping to make patients more comfortable, massage is indirectly involved in the healing process. Massage may also be indicated for its more **direct therapeutic effects** such as for relieving constipation, relaxing hypertonic muscles, or for healthy scar formation.

Clinical massage therapy includes Western massage as well as specialized soft tissue manipulation techniques developed to address specific body structures or organ systems. These specialized approaches include neuromuscular massage (i.e., trigger point therapy), deep transverse friction, myofascial massage, lymphatic massage, breast massage, and an energy approach called Therapeutic Touch.

The remainder of this chapter will discuss some of uses of massage in medical settings and some of the promising research that has been done on its clinical applications. It is just a sampling of the growing amount of information available, and points to areas where the study of the clinical applications of massage has been strong.

MUSCULO-SKELETAL PATHOLOGIES

Massage is routinely incorporated into the rehabilitation of musculo-skeletal injuries by physical therapists, athletic trainers, and massage therapists. It is also frequently used as a complement to chiropractic.

Massage is particularly effective in relieving muscle tension, increasing flexibility and range of motion, promoting healthy scar tissue, and reducing muscular pain. These direct therapeutic effects on the muscular system were discussed in Chapter 3.

Deep transverse friction has been especially effective in the treatment of repetitive strain injuries (RSI) such as tendinitis/tenosynovitis, (i.e., inflammation of tendons and tendon sheaths), and bursitis (i.e., inflammation of the fluid sacs around joints). Deep friction techniques increase local circulation, help separate adhesions, and have an analgesic or pain reducing effect (de Bruijin, 1984; Hammer, 1993).

Pain caused by hypertonic muscles can be relieved with massage. For example, tension headaches resulting from tense and shortened cervical muscles have been successfully treated with massage (Puustjarvi, K. et al., 1990). Massage has also been effective in treating subacute chronic low back pain (Cherkin et al, 2001; Preyde, 2000). These findings are particularly encouraging since tension headaches and low back pain afflict so many people in the modern world.

Neuromuscular and myofascial massage are specialized techniques that relieve myofascial pain and dysfunction. Chapters 12 and 13 discuss these techniques in more detail.

Fibromyalgia

Fibromyalgia syndrome (FMS) is a chronic condition characterized by widespread muscle pain and stiffness, and tenderness at specific body sites. The pain and fatigue associated with FMS can be debilitating. Other common symptoms of this syndrome are disturbed sleep, severe headaches, and osteoarthritis. Mental and emotional problems such as anxiety and depression often accompany FMS. Although there is no known cure for FMS, massage can address many of its symptoms. The general effects of massage that offer relief are reduction of stress and anxiety, more restful sleep, more positive outlook, improved circulation, and relief for sore and stiff muscles (Sunshine et al, 1996; Field, 2000).

CARDIOVASCULAR AND LYMPHATIC PATHOLOGIES

Relaxation massage may be beneficial in treating some cardiovascular pathologies such as hypertension (high blood pressure), and cardiac arrhythmia (Curtis, 1994; Longworth 1982). It not only reduces heart rate and blood pressure, but also reduces anxiety which helps give the patient a more positive outlook and improved feelings of wellbeing.

A study by nurses Bauer and Dracup (1987) found that back massage consisting of effleurage had a positive effect on the perception of relaxation and comfort reported by patients with acute myocardial infarction. Although they could not confirm improvement in the pathology, the massage had no apparent detrimental effects.

In another study, patients hospitalized in a cardiovascular unit of a large medical center in New York City who received Therapeutic Touch had a significantly greater reduction in anxiety scores than those who received casual touch or no touch (Heidt, 1981). A fuller discussion of Therapeutic Touch can be found later in this chapter.

Edema and Lymphedema

Edema, or excess interstitial fluid in the tissues, is not a disease, but rather a condition of fluid buildup or swelling. The edema itself can cause pain from increased fluid pressure, and from the buildup of toxins due to decreased circulation (Premkumar 1999).

Edema may occur with minor muscular injuries such as strains and sprains, or with conditions that cause venostasis such as varicose veins or prolonged standing (e.g., swollen feet or ankles). Petrissage and effleurage applied with light to moderate pressure distal to proximal can help reduce these types of edema in the limbs.

Lymphedema is a specific type of edema caused by poor lymph circulation, for example, after removal of lymph nodes during cancer surgery. Massage in general, and lymphatic massage in particular, are useful methods of reducing edema in the extremities. The beneficial effects of manual lymph drainage for patients with chronic and postmastectomy lymphedema continues to be confirmed. It has been noted that permanent and regular treatment is necessary for these conditions (Badger, 1986; Bunce et al., 1994; Kurz et al., 1978; Zanolla et al., 1984). Lymphatic massage is discussed further in Chapter 14.

A note of caution: Massage is contraindicated in cases of edema due to chronic cardiac, kidney, or liver problems.

IMMUNE FUNCTION

One of the basic positive effects of massage is improvement in immune function, as noted in Chapter 3. One of the first major studies to link massage and improved immunity was conducted by the Touch Research Institute in 1996. In a group of HIV-positive men who received daily massage for a month, the majority had significant increase in the number and activity of NK cells. The men showed reduced anxiety and stress, lower cortisol levels, as well as increased serotonin levels during the month of massage.

> Given that elevated stress hormones (catecholamines and cortisol) negatively affect immune function, the increase in NK activity probably derived from the decrease in these stress hormones following massage therapy (Field 2000, pp. 201–205).

To the extent that massage helps reduce stress and thus improves immune function, it can be considered an important disease prevention measure. Health problems caused by compromised immunity include frequent infections, autoimmune disorders, and possibly, cancer (Corwin, 1996; Field, 2000).

RESPIRATORY PATHOLOGIES

Massage is used as a complementary therapy for people with respiratory conditions such as chronic bronchitis, emphysema, and asthma. The benefits of massage for these patients include anxiety reduction and relaxation that deepens breathing patterns, relaxation and lengthening of muscles tense from labored breathing, and reduced fatigue overall. Passive movement of the rib cage, as well as percussion on the back and chest, can help loosen mucus for more productive coughs.

Children with asthma have been the subjects of several recent research projects. In one study, children with asthma were found to have lower anxiety, improved attitude towards the asthma condition, and increased peak airflow after regular massage by their parents. Over a one-month period, these children had fewer asthma attacks. The study suggested that daily massage may lead to improved airway tone, decreased airway irritability, and better control of asthma in children (Field, 2000, pp.179–186).

In another study, asthma, bronchitis, and emphysema patients received a form of bodywork called Trager Psychophysical Integration®, which consists of gentle painless, passive movements. Focus was on the neck, abdomen and chest wall. After treatment, improvement was found in forced vital capacity, respiratory rate, and chest expansion. Patients reported general relaxation and decrease in anxiety and tension (Witt & MacKinnon, 1986).

An increase in thoracic gas volume, peak flow and forced vital capacity was found in 4 out of 5 COPD patients receiving a combination of massage and myofascial trigger point therapy, i.e., neuromuscular massage. The neuromuscular techniques were specifically directed to improve the function of chronically hypertonic muscles involved in breathing (Beeken et al., 1998).

Note that the studies cited above used different massage therapy approaches to achieve their positive results. The overall objectives were to reduce stress, improve diaphragmatic breathing, relax and lengthen the muscles of respiration. Studies help identify specific techniques that are effective for these goals.

ANXIETY REDUCTION IN HOSPITALIZED PATIENTS

The ability of massage to elicit the relaxation response and reduce anxiety accounts for much of its value as a complement to standard medical treatment. Nurses in particular have found massage useful in caring for patients hospitalized for a variety of conditions.

For example, back massage was found to be an effective, noninvasive technique for promoting relaxation and improving communication with elderly, institutionalized patients. The nurses who conducted the study noted the potential of massage for reducing the common dehumanizing effects of institutional care (Frazer and Kerr, 1993). Those results were confirmed by another study of slow stroke back rub for the elderly by two other nurses, Fakouri and Jones (1987).

Another study by nurses examined the effects of therapeutic massage on hospitalized cancer patients. Primary techniques used were effleurage, petrissage, and trigger point therapy. They found that massage therapy significantly reduced the patients' perceived level of pain and anxiety, while enhancing their feelings of relaxation. Objective physiologic measures, i.e., heart rate, respiratory rate, and blood pressure, tended to decrease, providing further indication of relaxation (Ferrell-Torry and Glick, 1993).

MASSAGE FOR CANCER PATIENTS

Massage was once listed as a general contraindication for cancer patients. It is now recognized as a valuable complementary therapy, and cancer patients who receive massage are reporting relief from a number of physical, mental and emotional discomforts related to the disease and its treatment.

General benefits of massage especially important to cancer patients include reduced stress and anxiety, improved sleep, improved immune system function, pain relief, and the comfort of caring touch (Rhiner et al 1993; Sims 1986; Weinrich & Weinrich 1990).

Cancer patients who undergo surgery may benefit from the effects of massage related to faster recovery from anesthesia, faster wound healing, separation of adhesions around incisions, healthy scar formation, and reduction of edema and lymphedema. Massage has also been linked to reduced pain and less need for pain medication. Hospitalized patients find relief from muscle soreness caused by prolonged bed rest. Improved circulation from massage helps prevent pressure and bed sores.

Massage has also been found to reduce some of the negative side effects of radiation and chemotherapy such as fatigue, nausea, diarrhea, loss of appetite, and insomnia (MacDonald, 1995). However, the timing of massage in relation to treatment can be important; for example, the patient may be overtaxed and negative side effects worsened if massage is received too soon after a bout of chemotherapy.

The benefits of massage on the emotional level can be significant. Massage can help a cancer patient deal with depression, and offer pleasant social interaction providing relief from isolation. It can help reestablish a positive body image, and reclaim the body as an ally. It empowers patients to participate in their healing process, and helps rebuild hope (Chamness, 1996; Rattray 2000).

Breast massage is increasing in use as a clinical application for women who have experienced breast cancer. It is especially useful for post-mastectomy patients, including for general wound healing, healthy scar formation, and treating lymphedema. (Refer to *Breast Massage* by Debra Curties, 1999).

The concern about metastasis, or that massage may spread cancer, is still real in some cases. For example, massage should be avoided completely around the site of a tumor, or where a tumor has recently been removed. Massage practitioners should consult the patient's physician to assess the potential for harm from massage, and to get advice on how to proceed safely. (Refer to *Massage Therapy & Cancer* by Debra Curties (1999); and *Medicine Hands: Massage Therapy for People with Cancer* by Gayle Macdonald (1999)).

PEDIATRIC CARE

Massage is being used increasingly in the care of hospitalized children, from infants to adolescents. Many of the uses of massage in pediatric care are similar to uses for adults, e.g., rehabilitation and anxiety reduction. A unique benefit for infants is the tactile stimulation provided by massage, which is essential for proper growth and development.

Much of the recent interest in massage for children has been generated by the work of Tiffany Field, PhD, who in 1991 founded the Touch Research Institute (TRI) at the University of Miami School of Medicine, Department of Pediatrics. The research being performed at TRI on a variety of pediatric conditions can be reviewed on their Web site.

Preterm Infants

Building on research done in the 1970s, Field found that preterm infants who received tactile stimulation during their stay in the transitional care nursery setting experienced greater weight gain, increased motor activity, more alertness, and improved performance on the Brazelton Neonatal Behavioral Assessment Scale. Tactile stimulation was applied by gentle stroking of the head and neck, across the shoulders, from upper back to the waist, from the thighs to the feet, and from the shoulders to the hands. Additional stimulation was provided by passive flexion/extension movements of the arms and legs (Field et al., 1986).

Subsequent research has shown that massage also benefits cocaine-exposed preterm infants. In addition to better weight gain, massaged infants showed significantly fewer postnatal complications and stress behaviors than the control infants did (Wheeden et al., 1993).

Pediatric Applications

A review of some of the research being done at TRI demonstrates the broad range of situations in which massage is found to be a useful treatment for children. Descriptions of the research for the results below, and for many other studies, can be found in the book *Touch Therapy* by Tiffany Field (2000) and on the TRI Web site (www.miami.edu/touch-research.)

- **Asthmatic children:** 20-minute massages given to asthmatic children by their mothers for one month resulted in decreased anxiety levels and improved mood for both children and parents; the children's cortisol levels decreased; and they had fewer asthma attacks and were able to breathe better.
- **Autistic children:** After one month of massage therapy, the autistic children were less touch sensitive, less distracted by sounds, more attentive in class, related more to their teachers, and received better scores on the Autism Behavior Checklist and on the Early Social Communications Scales.
- **Diabetic children:** A pilot study showed that as a result of massage given to diabetic children by their parents, both children and parents showed lower anxiety and less depressed mood levels; the children's insulin and food regulation scores improved, and blood glucose levels decreased to the normal range.
- **Depressed adolescent mothers:** After 10 massage sessions over a five-week period, depressed adolescent mothers reported lower anxiety; showed behavioral and stress hormone changes, including decreases in anxious behavior and in pulse and salivary cortisol levels; and a decrease in urine cortisol levels, suggesting lower stress levels.
- **Infants of depressed adolescent mothers:** Full-term infants born to depressed adolescent mothers were given 15 minutes of massage two times a week for six weeks. These infants gained more weight, showed greater improvement on emotionality, sociability, and soothability temperament dimensions and on face-to-face interaction ratings, and had greater decreases in urinary stress catecholamines/hormones (norepinephrine, epinephrine, cortisol) than the controls who were simply rocked.
- **Children with posttraumatic stress disorder:** Children traumatized by Hurricane Andrew were massaged at their schools two times a week for one month. The massaged children had less depression, lower anxiety levels, and lower cortisol (stress hormone) levels than children in the control group.

Although further research is needed to substantiate much of what has been found to date, massage appears to be a promising adjunct to treatment of children with a variety of disorders.

PSYCHOLOGICAL ASPECTS OF TREATMENT

Massage is used to address the psychological and emotional problems of patients receiving medical treatment. For example, several of the studies mentioned in this chapter found massage to be beneficial in the reduction of the anxiety of patients hospitalized for serious medical conditions.

Massage may also help in the treatment of patients with medical conditions significantly worsened by stress. For example, in a study by Joachim (1983), patients with chronic inflammatory bowel disease, ulcerative colitis, or Crohn's disease (ileitis) who received massage for relaxation had fewer episodes of pain and disability from the disease.

Massage may also help patients hospitalized for psychiatric reasons. In a study by Field et al. (1992), hospitalized depressed and adjustment-disorder children and adolescents who received massage were less depressed and anxious and had lower saliva cortisol levels (an indication of less depression) than patients who watched relaxation videotapes.

Psychotherapy patients not hospitalized may also benefit from the effects of massage related to stress and anxiety reduction, improved body awareness, and the ability to receive pleasurable nonsexual touch. For example, some massage therapists work with psychotherapists in the treatment of survivors of sexual and physical abuse. Massage has been found to be beneficial in helping these patients reconnect with their bodies, develop a more compassionate relationship with their physical being, and experience their bodies as a "source of groundedness and eventually of strength and even pleasure—good things instead of a bad thing" (Benjamin, 1995, p. 28).

THERAPEUTIC TOUCH

Therapeutic Touch is a form of manual therapy in which the energy field of the recipient is rebalanced, thus promoting health and healing. Although it does not fall directly into the category of soft tissue massage, it is performed by many massage practitioners and integrated into their work. It has found special acceptance by nurses, who find it effective in caring for patients.

Therapeutic Touch was developed by Dolores Krieger, PhD, RN, in the 1970s. She explains the technique as one of centering; then placing the hands in the recipient's energy field to detect a break in energy flow, pressure, or dysrhythmias; then rebalancing or repatterning the energy field by sweeping hand movements a few inches above the skin. She explains what happens as a profound relaxation response that has a positive effect on the immune system, which allows self-healing to reassert itself (Karpen, 1995).

Kreiger explains that Therapeutic Touch has been found to have more effect on some conditions than others. For example, it seems to have a positive effect in working with fluid and electrolyte imbalances, dysfunctions of the autonomic nervous system, lymphatic and circulatory dysfunctions, and musculoskeletal problems. She further explains that:

> Some collagen dysfunctions respond, such as rheumatoid arthritis, but lupus is resistant. Within the endocrine system, the thyroid, adrenals, and ovaries respond, but there is little success with the pituitary and variable success with the pancreas in treating diabetes. In psychiatric disorders, manic depressives and catatonics respond, but there has been little success with schizophrenics. (Karpen, 1995)

Therapeutic Touch was found to have potential in the treatment of tension headache pain (Keller & Bzdek, 1986). Therapeutic Touch has also been used successfully to help reduce the stress of hospitalized children (Kramer, 1990). Research and articles about Therapeutic Touch can be found in nursing journals such as the *American Journal of Nursing* and *Nursing Research*. Further information about Therapeutic Touch research is available from Nurse Healers–Professional Associates, which was established in 1977 under the leadership of Dolores Kreiger (see Appendix A). The NH-PA is a voluntary, nonprofit cooperative whose international exchange network facilitates the exchange of research findings, teaching strategies, and developments in the clinical practice of Therapeutic Touch (www.therapeutic-touch.org).

COMPLEMENT TO CHIROPRACTIC

Chiropractic care is gaining increasing recognition as an effective treatment for certain conditions. Massage is often given as a complement to chiropractic care to help prepare the body for chiropractic adjustments, to relieve tension and pain in muscles and related soft tissues, and to prevent future musculoskeletal misalignment.

The term *chiropractic adjustment* is used here to mean a technique in which bones and joints are manipulated to return the body to proper alignment. This often involves a forceful thrusting movement or manipulation. Such adjustments are performed on *subluxations*, a condition of misalignment in a joint, which often results in structural, nervous system, and chemical dysfunctions.

Local massage is sometimes used in preparation for an adjustment. Massage relieves muscle tension and warms up the soft tissues in the area, making joints more pliable and more easily adjusted. Massage may be given along with heat and ultrasound in this preparatory routine.

A general massage (1 half to 1 hour long) may also be good preparation for an adjustment. In addition to preparing the immediate area of concern, it helps induce general relaxation and accustoms the recipient to touch. The recipient may be more receptive to other hands-on treatment in such a relaxed state. Massage after an adjustment may help the muscles remain relaxed and prevent a tightening reaction to the treatment. Regular massage may help adjustments last longer by keeping muscles relaxed and lengthened.

Therapeutic massage may also be used to address some of the muscular problems that bring patients for adjustments. These include nerve constriction due to tight muscles, poor circulation, trigger points, damaged tissues, and the pain–spasm–pain cycle. Massage used with ice can help relieve muscles in spasm. Recent research shows massage to be an effective treatment for low back pain (Cherkin et al., 2001; Preyde, 2000).

SUMMARY

The term *clinical massage therapy* refers to applications of massage for the treatment of pathologies. In an integrated health care system, therapies that are evidenced-based, i.e., supported by scientific research, are more likely to be used. Research on clinical applications of massage is available through centers for the study of touch, and on the Internet in research databases. Research literacy is important for massage practitioners in clinical settings.

Knowledge gained from research is essential to a principle-based approach to massage therapy. In the principle-based approach, massage techniques are chosen, applied, and adapted to reach treatment goals. This is in contrast to a recipe-based approach, where the same techniques are applied in every case.

Massage is indicated for injuries and illness if it contributes to their alleviation, or helps ease symptoms. Three useful ways of thinking about the clinical benefits of massage are for its complementary, palliative, or direct therapeutic effects.

Massage has been found effective in relieving musculo-skeletal conditions such as repetitive strain injuries, tension headaches, and low back pain. It relieves symptoms of fibromyalgia. Massage is used in treatment of cardiovascular and lymphatic disorders such as hypertension, edema, and lymphedema. It improves immune function, which is important in the treatment of many diseases.

Massage is a useful complementary therapy for people with respiratory conditions such as chronic bronchitis, emphysema, and asthma. Several different massage therapy approaches have been studied for their effects on people suffering from COPD.

Massage has been used effectively as a palliative measure to reduce anxiety in hospitalized patients, as well as reduce pain and improve communication. Benefits of massage for cancer patients include reduced stress and anxiety, faster recovery from surgery, and reduction of the side effects from cancer treatment. Emotional benefits for cancer patients include help in dealing with depression, reestablishing a positive body image, and rebuilding hope.

Massage has been used successfully in pediatric care for children with asthma, autism, diabetes, depression, and posttraumatic stress disorder. It helps preterm infants gain weight and develop more normally.

Massage is an effective complement to treatment of conditions worsened by stress. It relieves the anxiety and stress of psychiatric patients.

Therapeutic Touch is a form of manual therapy that rebalances the energy field of the patient. It has been found effective in treatment of fluid and electrolyte imbalances, dysfunction in the autonomic nervous system, and lymphatic and circulatory disorders. Nurses have been particularly involved in the development of Therapeutic Touch and its use with patients.

Massage is an effective complement to chiropractic care. It helps prepare the body for adjustment, and addresses some of the muscular problems of chiropractic patients.

A look ahead . . .

While massage has many beneficial effects, there are certain circumstances in which it should be modified or avoided altogether for the health and safety of the recipient. Chapter 5 presents guidelines for endangerment sites, contraindications, and cautions for giving massage.

REFERENCES

Badger, C. (1986). The swollen limb. *Nursing Times* (England), *82*(31), 40–41.

Bauer, W. C., & Dracup, K. A. (1987). Physiological effects of back massage in patients with acute myocardial infarction. *Focus on Critical Care, 14*(6), 42–46.

Beeken, J., et al. (1998). Effectiveness of neuromuscular release massage therapy on chronic obstructive lung disease. *Clinical Nursing Research, 7*(3), 309–325.

Benjamin, B. E. (1995). Massage and body work with survivors of abuse: Part I. *Massage Therapy Journal, 34*(3), 23–32.

Bunce, I. H., Mirolo, B. R., Hennessy, J. M., et al. (1994). Post-mastectomy lymphedema treatment and measurement. *Medical Journal* Australia, *161*, 125–128.

Chamness, A. (1996). Breast cancer and massage therapy. *Massage Therapy Journal, 35*(1, Winter).

Cherkin, D. C., Eisenberg, D. et al. (2001). Randomized trial comparing traditonal Chinese medical acupuncture, therapeutic massage, and self-care education for chronic low back pain. *Archives of Internal Medicine 161*(8), 1081–1088.

Corwin, E. J. (1996). *Handbook of pathophysiology*. Philadelphia: Lippincot.

Curties, D. (1999). *Breast Massage*. Toronto, Canada: Curties-Overzet Publications.

Curties, D. (1999). *Massage Therapy and Cancer*. Toronto, Canada: Curties-Overzet Publications.

Curtis, M. (1994). The use of massage in restoring cardiac rhythm. *Nursing Times* (England), 90(38), 36–37.

de Bruijn, R. (1984). Deep transverse friction; its analgesic effect. *International Journal of Sports Medicine, 5*, 35–36.

Fakouri, C., & Jones, P. (1987). Relaxation ℞: Slow stroke back rub. *Journal of Gerontological Nursing, 13*(2), 32–35.

Ferrell-Torry, A. T., & Glick, O. J. (1993). The use of therapeutic massage as a nursing intervention to modify anxiety and the perception of cancer pain. *Cancer Nursing, 16*(2), 93–101.

Field, T. (2000). *Touch Therapy*. London: Churchill Livingston.

Field, T. M., Morrow, C., Valdeon, C., et al. (1992). Massage reduces anxiety in child and adolescent psychiatric patients. *Journal of the American Academy of Child and Adolescent Psychiatry, 31*(1), 125–131.

Field, T. M., Schanberg, S. M., Scafidi, F., et al. (1986). Tactile/kinesthetic stimulation effects on preterm neonates. *Pediatrics, 77*(5), 654–658.

Frazer, J., & Kerr, J. R. (1993). Psychophysiological effects of back massage on elderly institutionalized patients. *Journal of Advanced Nursing, 18*, 238–245.

Hammer, W. I. (1993) The use of transverse friction massage in the management of chronic bursitis of the hip and shoulder. *Journal of Manipulation and Physical Therapy, 16*(2), 107–111.

Heidt, P. (1981). Effect of therapeutic touch on anxiety level of hospitalized patients. *Nursing Research, 30*(1), 32–37.

Joachim, G. (1983). The effects of two stress management techniques on feelings of well-being in patients with inflammatory bowel disease. *Nursing Papers, 15*(5), 18.

Karpen, M. (1995). Dolores Kreiger, PhD, RN: Tireless teacher of Therapeutic Touch. *Alternative & Complementary Therapies*, April/May, 142–146.

Keller, E., & Bzdek, V. M. (1986). Effects of therapeutic touch on tension headache pain. *Nursing Research, 35*(2), 101–106.

Kramer, N. A. (1990). Comparison of therapeutic touch and casual touch in stress reduction of hospitalized children. *Pediatric Nursing, 16*(5), 483–485.

Kurz, W., Wittlinger, G., Litmanovitch, Y. I., et al. (1978). Effect of manual lymph drainage massage on urinary excretion of neurohormones and minerals in chronic lyphedema. *Angiology, 29*, 64–72.

Longworth, J. D. (1982). Psychophysiological effects of slow stroke back massage in normotensive females. *Advances in Nursing Science 4*, 44–61.

Macdonald, G.(1999). *Medicine Hands: Massage Therapy for People with Cancer*. Tallahassee, FL: Findhorn Press.

MacDonald, G. (1995). Massage for cancer patients: A review of nursing research. *Massage Therapy Journal*, Summer, 53–56.

Menard, M. B. (2003). *Making sense of research: A guide to research literacy for complementary practitioners*. Toronto: Curties-Overzet Publications.

Premkumar, K. (1999). Pathology A to Z: A handbook for massage therapists. 2nd Ed. Calgary, Canada: Van Pub Books.

Preyde, M. (2000). Effectiveness of massage therapy for subacute low-back pain: A randomized controlled trail. *CMAJ, 162*(13), 1815–1820.

Puustjarvi, K., Airaksinen, O., & P.J. Pontinen (1990). The effects of massage in patients with chronic tension headache. *Acupuncture Electrotherapy Research, 15*(2), 159–162.

Rattray, F. and L. Ludwig (2000). *Clinical massage therapy: Understanding, assessing and treating over 700 conditions*. Toronto, Canada: Talus Incorporated.

Rhiner, M., Ferrell, B. R., Ferrell, B. A., & Grant, M. M. (1993). A structured non-drug intervention program for cancer pain. *Cancer Practice, 1*, 137–143.

Sims, S. (1986). Slow stroke back massage for cancer patients. *Nursing Times, 82*, 47–50.

Sunshine, W., Field, T., et al. (1996) Fibromyalgia benefits from massage therapy and transcutaneous electrical stimulation. *Journal of Clinical Rheum*. *2*(1), 18–22.

Weinrich, S. P., & Weinrich, M. C. (1990). The effect of massage on pain in cancer patients. *Applied Nursing Research, 3*, 140–145.

Wheeden, A., Scafidi, F., Field, T., et al. (1993). Massage effects on cocaine-exposed preterm neonates. *Developmental and Behavioral Pediatrics, 14*(5), 318–322.

Witt, P. L., MacKinnon, J. (1986). Trager psychosocial integration: A method to improve chest mobility of patients with chronic lung disease. *Physical Therapy*, *66*(2), 214–217.

Yates, J. (1999). *A physician's guide to therapeutic massage: Its physiological effects and treatment applications*, 2nd edition. Vancouver, BC: Massage Therapists' Association of British Columbia.

Zanolla, R., Monzeglio, C., Balzarini, A., & Martino, G. (1984). Evaluation of the results of three different methods of postmastectomy lymphedema treatment. *Journal of Surgical Oncology, 26*, 210–213.

WEB SITES

AMTA Foundation *(www.amtafoundation.org)*
Canadian Touch Research Center *(ccrt-ctrc.org)*
National Library of Medicine *(ncbi.nlm.nih.gov/PubMed)*
Nurse-Healers–Professional Associates International *(www.therapeutic-touch.org)*
Touch Research Institute *(www.miami.edu/touch-research)*

ADDITIONAL REFERENCES

Videos

"Cancer massage video." Canada Institute of Palliative Massage. Nelson, British Columbia, Canada: Sutherland Massage Productions. (*www.sutherlandmassageproductions.com*)

"AIDS massage video." Canada Institute of Palliative Massage. Nelson, British Columbia, Canada: Sutherland Massage Productions. (*www.sutherlandmassageproductions.com*)

"Massage for children with Down Syndrome." Canada Institute of Palliative Massage. Nelson, British Columbia, Canada: Sutherland Massage Productions. (*www.sutherlandmassageproductions.com*)

CHAPTER FIVE

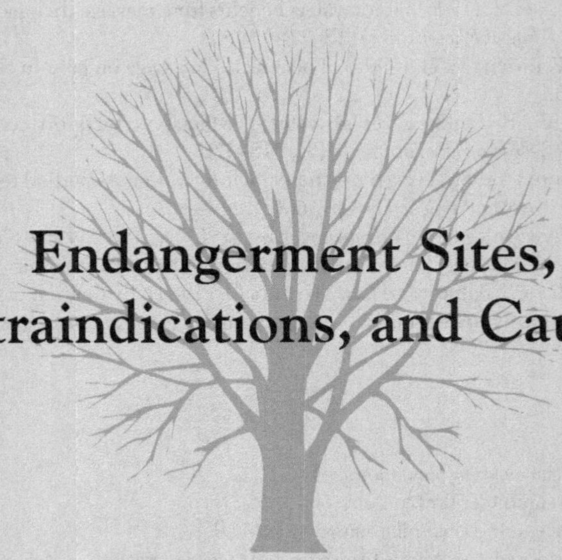

Endangerment Sites, Contraindications, and Cautions

LEARNING OUTCOMES

After studying this chapter, the student will have information to:

1. Locate major endangerment sites.
2. Discuss the general principles of safety around endangerment sites.
3. Distinguish between general and regional contraindications for massage.
4. List and explain the general principles for contraindications and cautions for massage.
5. Discuss considerations related to medications.
6. Explain the concept of person-centered massage.
7. Identify sources of information about endangerment sites and contraindications for massage.

KEY TERMS/CONCEPTS

Caution
Contraindications
Do no harm
Endangerment site
General contraindications
Health history
Local contraindications
Medications
Person-centered massage
Professional library
Regional contraindication

LINK LIBRARY TERMS

Massage Business • *Massage Regulations*

MEDIALINK

A companion CD-ROM, included free with each new copy of this book, supplements the techniques presented in this chapter. Insert the CD-ROM to watch video clips of massage techniques being demonstrated. This multimedia feature is designed to help you add a new dimension to your learning.

DO NO HARM

One of most basic rules of giving therapeutic massage is to **do no harm.** Guidelines for helping you make decisions about what to do and what to avoid, to protect the health and safety of your clients will be presented in this chapter. Topics addressed will include endangerment sites, contraindications, cautions, and resources for further information.

The variety of massage approaches used today complicates the issue somewhat. These forms vary from deep tissue structural massage of the physical body to light work affecting the energy within and around the physical body. An endangerment site or a contraindication in one form of bodywork may be considered perfectly safe for a different form.

This chapter will focus on endangerment sites, contraindications, and cautions that are important when giving Western massage and forms that use similar techniques. This includes all techniques applied to the physical body that involve pressing, stroking, friction, kneading, tapping, and vibrating. Chapters devoted to other types of massage and bodywork will address contraindications and cautions for that particular type of work.

Knowledge of Western anatomy and physiology is essential to ensure the safety of the person receiving massage and bodywork. It is particularly important to know the location of major nerves and blood vessels, glands, and visceral organs. Endangerment sites, contraindications, and cautions will be discussed in this chapter in terms of Western science and pathologies.

ENDANGERMENT SITES

Endangerment sites are areas of the body where delicate structures are less protected and, therefore, may be more easily damaged when receiving massage. Caution is required when performing massage on or around endangerment sites. The following paragraphs identify the location of endangerment sites, and describe cautions when working in those areas. Figure 5–1 shows the general location of endangerment sites on the anterior and posterior body.

Anterior Neck. The anterior neck is the triangular area on the front of the neck defined by the sternocleidomastoid (SCM) and includes the sternal notch, which is the depression found on the superior aspect of the sternum. Delicate structures located in the anterior neck region are the carotid artery, jugular vein, vagus nerve, larynx, and thyroid gland. Deep pressure on any of these structures is dangerous.

Pressure within the anterior triangle of the neck, including the depression formed by the sternal notch, should be avoided entirely in most forms of massage. Some advanced techniques address cervical muscles from the anterior neck, but they should be performed only by experienced therapists with special training. The gentle superficial stroking during lymphatic massage and non-contact forms of energy work are possible exceptions to the no-touch rule.

Great care should be taken when performing neck massage on the elderly due to the likelihood of atherosclerosis and the potential for dislodging a thrombus that could lead to stroke. Too much pressure from massage could also cause further damage to blood vessels in the area. Only light pressure should be used on the neck, if massage is applied to the neck at all.

Vertebral Column. The vertebral column protects spinal cord of the central nervous system. The spinous processes of the cervical, thoracic and lumbar vertebrae can be felt along the middle of the neck and back. Massage techniques that apply heavy pressure or that involve thrusting or percussion movements should not be performed directly over the spinous processes.

Thoracic Cage. The thoracic cage consists of the ribs and sternum. The thoracic cage is relatively flexible to allow for breathing, and ribs 1–10 attach to the sternum with cartilage. The lower tip of the sternum called the xiphoid process is a slender piece of bone that can break under pressure and be driven into the liver, causing severe damage. Avoid strong pressure or impact over the sternum overall, and especially the xiphoid process. Heavy pressure over the anterior and lateral surfaces of the rib cage should also be avoided, especially in the elderly.

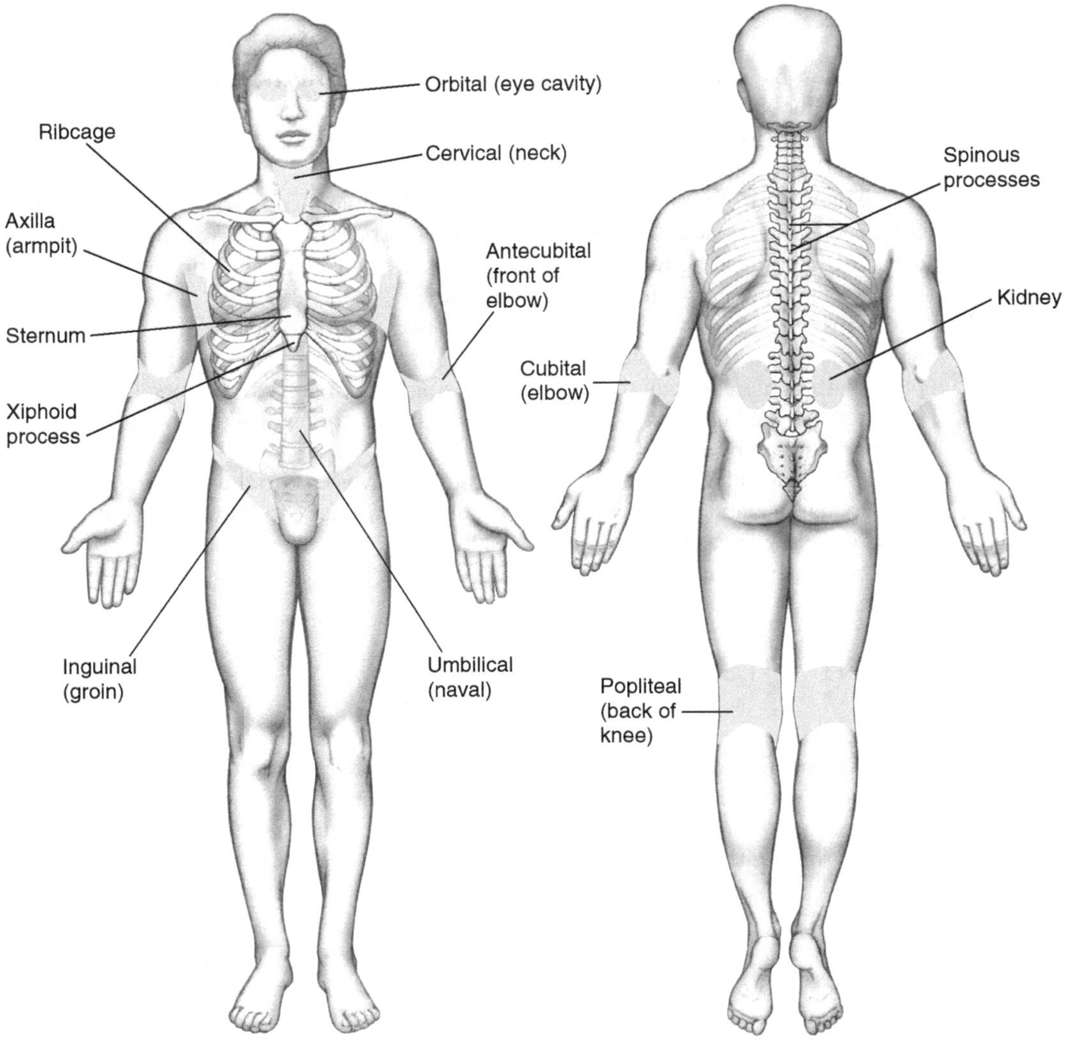

FIGURE 5–1. Endangerment sites—anterior and posterior views.

Axilla. Delicate circulatory and nervous structures are relatively exposed in the axilla or armpit area. These include the brachial artery, axillary artery and vein, cephalic vein, and the nerve complex of the brachial plexus. Deep pressure in this area should be approached with caution.

Elbow. Two places around the elbow area require caution. One is the space just medial to the olecranon process where the ulnar nerve is relatively exposed. This is the "funny bone" area that causes sharp pain when hit. The second area is the anterior surface, or fold, of the elbow. This area is similar to the popliteal fossa found posterior to the knee as described later on. Vulnerable structures found in this area include the brachial vein and artery, median cubital vein, and median nerve. These structures are all close to the surface and unprotected by muscle. Moderate broad pressure may be applied to the area, but deep specific pressure should be restricted to the surrounding muscles and their attachments.

Umbilicus. The umbilicus or "belly button" is a sensitive area superficial to the descending aorta and abdominal aorta. Avoid direct heavy pressure to the umbilicus.

Kidney Area. The kidneys are located on either side of the spine generally at the level between the 3rd lumbar and 12th thoracic vertebrae. They are positioned behind the parietal peritoneum and against the deep muscles of the back. Superficial or deep stroking and pressing techniques may be applied carefully to the muscles of the back located in the kidney area. However, only very light pressure should be used when performing percussion techniques over this area.

Inguinal Area. The inguinal or groin area is located roughly where the thigh and the trunk meet on the anterior side of the body. The femoral nerve and major blood vessels to the lower extremities cross there, i.e., femoral artery, great saphenous and femoral veins. When the thigh is flexed, a depression is created in the area exposing the more delicate structures. Great care should be taken when applying deep pressure into this area, for example, when reaching for the iliopsoas. This should be attempted only by students under supervision and by practitioners with advanced training.

Popliteal Fossa. The muscles of the posterior lower extremity cross the knee laterally and medially, leaving the center space relatively unprotected. This is the popliteal fossa. The popliteal artery and vein and the tibial nerve are located there. Avoid heavy specific pressure over this area. Follow the muscles around the popliteal fossa when massaging them.

Eyes. Take great care when working around the eyes. Be careful not to slip and hit the eyeball by accident. Only the very lightest pressure is used when stroking the eyelid.

Major Veins in Extremities. Major veins in the extremities are being included under endangerment sites because structural damage can occur to the valves within the veins if deep effleurage is applied improperly. Always apply deep flushing effleurage to the arms and legs from distal to proximal, that is, toward the heart, and with the flow that opens the valves.

GENERAL PRINCIPLES FOR SAFETY AROUND ENDANGERMENT SITES

Here are some general principles to keep in mind to protect the receiver's body from structural damage during massage. Remember, your first responsibility is to do no harm.

1. Always adjust the pressure you use to match the part of the body, the condition of the tissues, and the person you are working on. Any part of the body can be damaged if too much pressure is used.
2. Avoid heavy pressure anyplace where nerves, blood vessels, or lymph vessels are close to the surface or are unprotected by muscle or bone.
3. Be careful around joints where delicate structures are less protected by skeletal muscle.
4. If you feel a pulse, it means that you are on a major artery. Move to a different place immediately.
5. If the receiver feels searing, burning, shooting, electrical sensations, "pins and needles," or numbness, you may be pressing on a nerve. Move to a different place immediately.
6. Any abnormal structure is a potential endangerment site. Get information about structural abnormalities, and proceed with caution when you are sure it is safe to do so.
7. Always work with awareness, and when in doubt, do not take a chance that might lead to injury.

CONTRAINDICATIONS

Contraindications are conditions or situations that make the receiving of massage inadvisable because of the harm it might do. In the treatment model, a contraindication is "any symptom or circumstance indicating the inappropriateness of a form of treatment otherwise advisable" (Thomas, 1985). For **general contraindications,** avoid massage altogether. For **regional** or **local contraindications,** avoid only the specific area of the body affected.

Cautions are areas of potential danger that require thoughtful consideration and possible modifications of technique application. Cautions may or may not involve a pathology.

Practitioners should be alert to possible contraindications and cautions for every client. A **health history** taken during the initial visit will provide information about previous conditions or situations to be aware of and current health status. Appendix E contains health history forms for general wellness massage, as well as treatment-oriented sessions. Practitioners should check with regular clients at every session to see if their health status has changed in significant ways, especially if they are known to have a condition that is a contraindication or for which special cautions apply.

Knowledge of normal anatomy and physiology, as well as the nature of common pathologies, is important for the massage practitioner. Such knowledge may help prevent a well-meaning practitioner from causing harm. Those performing clinical applications need to be especially well versed in the pathologies that they are treating.

Be sure you fully understand the origin of any symptom of disease reported by a client. This will help in the selection of appropriate techniques and of positioning to best support the health of the massage recipient. If a client reports having a condition or disease that you are not familiar with, use your professional resources (see below) to get more information before proceeding with the massage.

Some general principles can be used to help determine whether receiving massage might be harmful. Some of the more common conditions and situations encountered in a massage practice are listed below.

PRINCIPLES FOR CONTRAINDICATIONS AND CAUTIONS

1. **Severe Distress.** *Do not perform massage when the recipient is experiencing severe distress.*
   For example:
   - Feels physically ill or nauseated
   - Is in severe pain
   - Has a fever
   - Has been seriously injured recently
2. **Acute Inflammation.** *Do not perform massage in the presence of acute inflammation.* Signs of inflammation are redness, heat, swelling, and pain. Any diagnosed condition that ends in "itis" is either a general or local contraindication.
   For example:
   - **Appendicitis.** Massage will spread inflammation throughout abdomen; avoid massage entirely.
   - **Rheumatoid arthritis.** Avoid massage over acutely inflamed joints (local contraindication); use caution even when not acute. Avoid traction of joints and spine.
   - **Phlebitis.** Inflammation of a vein; completely avoid site of disease, usually the legs.
   - **Locally inflamed tissues.** Signs are redness, heat, swelling, and pain. Avoid the surrounding area. On limbs, work proximal to the affected area.
3. **Loss of Structural Integrity.** *Understand the physician's recommendations and the relevant anatomy and physiology in cases where there is a loss of integrity in an area.*
   For example:
   - **Over recent surgery.** Only those specifically trained to work with scar tissue should attempt this work.
   - **Around burns.**
   - **Recent fractures.** Wait for physician's approval before performing massage in the area of recent fracture.
   - **Artificial joint replacements.** Check recommended restrictions in range of motion in replaced joints.
4. **Skin Conditions.** *Do not touch areas of the skin where there is a pathologic condition that is contagious or that may be worsened or spread by applying pressure or rubbing.*
   For example:
   - **Rashes**
   - **Boils**
   - **Athlete's foot**
   - **Herpes simplex (e.g., cold sores)**
   - **Impetigo.** A skin infection usually caused by staph or strep.
   - **Allergies.** Clients with skin allergies, may react negatively to certain oils or lotions used during massage. Check with recipient for substances to avoid, and be alert to skin reactions during the session.
5. **Decreased Sensation.** *Use extreme care in amount of pressure used when the client has decreased sensation.* Recipients cannot give accurate feedback regarding pressure and may also have

abnormal vasomotor response to the massage. May be due to stroke, diabetes, spinal cord injury, or medication.

6. **Increased Sensitivity to Touch.** *Massage only to recipient's tolerance or comfort when there is increased sensitivity to touch.* Clients who are ticklish or who have ticklish areas (e.g., feet) generally find light superficial stroking unpleasant and annoying. They may respond well to deeper, slower pressure, or to percussion techniques on the ticklish area.
7. **Cardiovascular Disorders.** *For clients with cardiovascular system disorders, research the condition carefully, including getting a physician's recommendation if serious.* Be aware of medications the client is taking and their potential as contraindications for massage.
   For example:
   - **High blood pressure.** If high, even with treatment, avoid circulatory massage.
   - **Low blood pressure.** Someone with low blood pressure may be more susceptible to fainting after receiving massage either on a table or on a massage chair. Be sure that such a client gets up slowly from a horizontal position.
   - **Cardiac arrhythmias or carotid bruit.** Avoid lateral and anterior neck.
   - **Severe atherosclerosis.** Massage only with the physician's permission, and then only very superficially.
   - **Severe varicose veins.** Tissues easily damaged and tendency to clotting; avoid massage of the area.
   - **Stroke.** Avoid circulatory massage, especially massage of neck. Blood thinners are usually prescribed after stroke, so use light pressure with all soft tissue manipulation.
8. **Spreading Disease by Circulation.** *Do not perform circulatory massage when there is a pathologic condition that might be spread through the lymph or cardiovascular systems.*
   For example:
   - Blood poisoning (lymphangitis). Inflammation of the lymphatic vessels; appears as steaks of red on the skin.
   - Malignant melanoma. A cancerous mole or tumor that metastasizes or spreads easily through the bloodstream or lymph system.
   - Swollen glands (i.e., lymph nodes). The immune system may be attempting to filter out bacteria or other pathogens, and draining them may cause an infection to spread.
9. **Bleeding and Bruising.** *Do not perform massage near an area where there is bleeding or bruising.*
   For example:
   - A bruise; avoid pressure to immediate area.
   - Whiplash or other acute trauma. Any situation in which there is tearing of tissue and where there may be bleeding into the tissue during the first 24 to 48 hours after the trauma; avoid massage in area, and if severe trauma avoid massage totally (see principle 1 above).
10. **Edema.** *Be sure of cause of edema before proceeding with massage.* Acute edema resulting from trauma, edema from inflammation due to bacterial or viral infection, pitted edema indicating tissue fragility, lymphatic obstruction due to parasites, and edema due to deep vein thrombosis are all contraindications for massage (Rattray, 2000). In cases of general edema caused by cardiac, liver, or kidney disease, avoid massage altogether.
11. **Compromised Immunity.** Be especially careful with personal and environmental hygiene when a client's immune function is depressed, e.g., after organ transplant when immune system is depressed with medication, with AIDS/HIV, or chronic fatigue syndrome.
12. **Osteoporosis.** Osteoporosis is a disease in which bones become fragile, brittle, and fracture easily. Avoid deep pressure and vigorous joint movements with a client with diagnosed osteoporosis, someone whom you suspect to have the disease, or those in a high-risk category (e.g., small, sedentary postmenopausal women; frail elderly; or someone with hyperkyphosis or "dowager's hump."
13. **Personal Appliances**
    - **Contact Lenses.** If a client is wearing contact lenses, take special care when working around the eyes to avoid pressure on the lenses and to avoid dislodging or moving the lenses. If using a face cradle when the recipient is prone, make sure that no pressure is put on the recipient's eyes. Taking the contact lenses out during massage is preferable.
    - **Hearing Aid.** If a client wears a hearing aid, be careful not to dislodge it while massaging around the ears. If it is turned on, massage on the head or around the ears may make a lot

of noise and be annoying. Remember that a client with severe hearing loss will not be able to hear you ask for feedback, or give directions. Be sure they can see you if you talk to them.

MEDICATIONS

Medications are used by an increasing number of people for a variety of ailments. This includes prescription, as well as over-the-counter, drugs. This also includes medications for short-term use, for example, common cold medications and pain-killers (analgesics) like aspirin; and longer term use, for example, heart medications or antidepressants. Massage practitioners need to be more aware of what their clients are taking, and understand the implications for massage therapy. Table 5–1 lists some of the most common considerations for massage and medications.

A client's medication may affect the scheduling of massage sessions, the length of sessions, techniques used and their application, or client behavior. Types of medications that require caution include, but are not limited to, those that alter sensation (e.g., numbing); affect the blood and circulation (e.g., prevent clotting, regulate blood sugar level); compromise tissue integrity (e.g., corticosteroids), or alter mood (e.g., depressants, antidepressants). Check with the health care provider who prescribed the medication if in doubt. (For more detailed guidelines on massage and medications, refer to *Massage Therapy & Medications: General Treatment Principles* by Randal S. Persad, 2001.)

Persons under the influence of alcohol or recreational drugs should not receive massage. These drugs alter sensation, affect mood, and in many cases, reduce good judgment.

Table 5–1 GUIDELINES FOR MASSAGE AND MEDICATIONS

The following chart summarizes some important points to consider when working with clients taking medication. If in doubt, check with clients and their health care providers about potential for harm and how to avoid it.

Scheduling of Sessions

- Massage after the client's scheduled dosage if the medication is needed for condition stability, i.e., to ensure maximum bioavailability of the medication. For example, with insulin-dependent diabetics, chronic pain clients, epileptic patients.
- Massage before or shortly after the client's scheduled dosage if medication decreases the client's perception of pain and their ability to give accurate feedback. For example, clients taking drugs like non-steroidal anti-inflammatories, narcotic analgesics, and central nervous system depressants.

Session Length

- Shorten the session if the medication significantly depletes the energy level of the client, causing abnormal fatigue. For example, clients taking hypertension medications, anti-anxiety drugs, and many antidepressants.
- Shorten the session if the medication significantly decreases the emotional stability of the client, causing them to feel emotionally volatile or easily overwhelmed. For example, clients taking corticosteroids (long term), or medications that have side effects that cause mood fluctuations, anxiety, or depression.

Selection of Massage Techniques

- **For drugs that alter clotting mechanisms,** e.g., anticoagulants, platelet inhibitors, and aspirin and other non-steroidal anti-inflammatories—Avoid high-pressure techniques like muscle stripping, deep kneading, ischemic compression, and cross-fiber friction.
- **For drugs that alter protective responses,** e.g., centrally acting muscle relaxants, narcotic analgesics, anti-anxiety drugs—Avoid deep massage, tense-relax stretching, and any technique that requires accurate client feedback for safe application.
- **For drugs that compromise tissue integrity,** e.g., corticosteroids, long-term use or injected directly into joints or tissues—Avoid deep pressure techniques, heavy tapotement, forced stretching, skin rolling and wringing.
- **For drugs that mask pain responses,** e.g., anti-inflammatories, analgesics—Rely less on client feedback and more on observation and palpation to determine appropriate pressure and technique applications.
- **For drugs that alter a client's cooperativeness,** or **make them less communicative,** e.g., narcotic analgesics and anti-anxiety medications—Take time to ask questions as needed for accurate health histories and ongoing feedback during massage.

Information from ***Massage Therapy & Medications: General Treatment Principles*** by Randall S. Persad (Toronto, Canada: Curties-Overzet Publications, 2001.)

PERSON-CENTERED MASSAGE

It is easy to lose sight of the person when there is pathology involved. From the wellness perspective, massage can be thought of as person-centered rather than pathology-centered. In other words, practitioners may give massage to people with pathologies, but the people are more than their pathologies. In fact, practitioners often find themselves working around pathologies.

This may be the case when a person has a condition for which deep or vigorous massage is contraindicated. A light massage may be appropriate to add an element of care, comfort, and stress reduction as a complement to standard medical care. For example, there would be few pathologies for which stroking the hand or head of an elderly person is contraindicated.

Most of the contraindications and cautions mentioned above are based on common sense, given some knowledge of anatomy, physiology, and pathology. If the giver of massage is motivated by sincere concern, is gentle in giving, and is receptive and responsive to feedback from the recipient, the experience will most likely be a healthy one for both people. Even in the hands of a child, massage given with love and sensitivity can be supportive and helpful.

RESOURCES

Personal professional libraries should include some basic resources for information about conditions and pathologies commonly encountered in massage practices. This information can provide insights into possible contraindications and cautions, and implications for performing massage. Pathologies may also be researched at a local library, a library at a school of medicine, and on the Internet. See Table 4–1, Sources of Information about Clinical Applications of Massage.

A basic **professional library** for massage practitioners should include a good anatomy and physiology text, an atlas of human anatomy, a general pathology text, and a medical dictionary. Pathology books written especially for massage therapists have been published recently, and are valuable references that include special considerations for massage including contraindications and cautions. (Refer to *Clincal Massage Therapy*, by Fiona Rattray and Linda Ludwig (2000); *Massage Therapist's Guide to Pathology*, by Ruth Werner (2000); *Pathology A to Z—A Handbook for Massage Therapists*, by Kalyani Premkumar (1999.))

Practitioners working with special populations should have applicable references for basic information. There are books available on massage with specific populations (e.g., pregnant women, children, elderly, cancer patients). An up-to-date general reference book for common medications and their effects and side effects would also be useful.

One of the best resources for information may be the recipient himself or herself. Recipients are often very knowledgeable about their own pathologies, especially if they have lived with a chronic condition for some time. The recipient's health care providers may also serve as valuable resources when there is any doubt as to the safety of someone receiving massage.

SUMMARY

One of the most basic rules of giving therapeutic massage is to do no harm. Massage practitioners should be aware of endangerment sites, contraindications and cautions to ensure the health and safety of clients.

Endangerment sites are areas of the body where delicate structures are less protected and therefore more easily damaged when receiving massage. Endangerment sites include the anterior neck, vertebral column, thoracic cage, axilla, elbow, umbilicus, kidney area, inguinal area, popliteal fossa, eyes, and the major veins in the extremities. General principles for performing massage related to endangerment sites include adjusting pressure to avoid damage, care around joints, avoiding pressure directly on major arteries and nerves, care around abnormal structures, and always working with awareness.

Contraindications are conditions that make receiving massage inadvisable because of the harm it might do. For general contraindications, massage should be avoided altogether. For local or regional contraindications, only the specific area of the body affected should be avoided. Cautions are areas of potential danger that require thoughtful consideration and possible modifications of technique application.

Acute distress and acute inflammation are general contraindications for massage. Other contraindications and cautions include loss of structural integrity, skin problems, decreased sensation, increased sensation, cardiovascular disorders, diseases spread by circulation, bleeding and bruising, edema, compromised immunity, osteoporosis. Take caution with clients wearing contact lenses and hearing aids.

Clients may be taking medications including prescription and over-the-counter drugs. A client's medication may affect the scheduling of massage sessions, the length of sessions, techniques used and their application, or their behavior. Types of medications that require caution include those that alter sensation, affect the blood and circulation, compromise tissue integrity, or alter mood. Persons under the influence of alcohol or recreational drugs should not receive massage since they alter sensation, affect mood, and reduce good judgment.

From the wellness perspective, massage can be thought of as person centered. Practitioners may give massage to people with pathologies, but the people are more than their pathologies.

Personal professional libraries should include an anatomy/physiology text, atlas of human anatomy, a pathology book, medical dictionary, and books specific to special populations encountered in practice. Access to the Internet is useful for finding information about specific pathologies. The recipient him- or herself and caregivers are also good sources of information about safety for receiving massage.

A look ahead . . .

Establishing and maintaining a successful massage practice involves many factors, including developing good client relationships and creating a therapeutic environment. Longevity is secured by self-care measures that preserve your own health and wellbeing. Effective application of massage requires an understanding of various performance elements. Chapter 6 describes general principles for giving massage that provide the context for performing healing massage techniques.

REFERENCES

Persad, R. (2001). *Massage Therapy & Medications*. Ontario, Canada: Curties-Overzet Publications.

Premkumar, K. (1999) *Pathology A to Z–A handbook for massage therapists*. Calgary, Canada: VanPub Books.

Rattray, F., and Ludwig, L. (2000). *Clinical massage therapy: Understanding, assessing and treating over 70 conditions*. Toronto, Canada: Talus Incorporated.

Thomas, C. L., ed. (1985). *Taber's cyclopedic medical dictionary*. Philadelphia: F. A. Davis.

Werner, R. (2000). *Massage therapist's guide to pathology*, 2nd ed. Philadelphia: Lippincott Williams & Wilkins.

CHAPTER SIX

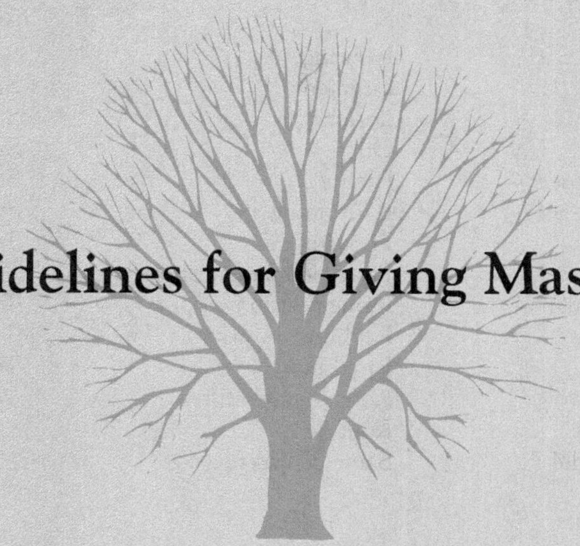

Guidelines for Giving Massage

LEARNING OUTCOMES

After studying this chapter, the student will have information to:

1. Establish good therapeutic relationships.
2. Maintain professional boundaries.
3. Project a professional demeanor.
4. Appreciate the significance of touch in massage.
5. Be aware of gender considerations in a massage practice.
6. Demonstrate the use of informed consent.
7. Apply the seven-step intervention model.
8. Engage in appropriate level of talk during massage.
9. Maintain confidentiality of client information.
10. Comply with HIPAA standards regarding client records.
11. Create an ideal physical environment for massage.
12. Choose topical substances used in massage.
13. Provide for client safety and comfort.
14. Take physical and emotional self-care measures.
15. Analyze the elements of massage performance.

LINK LIBRARY TERMS

Massage Business • *HIPPA* • *Massage Regulations*

MEDIALINK

A companion CD-ROM, included free with each new copy of this book, supplements the techniques presented in this chapter. Insert the CD-ROM to watch video clips of massage techniques being demonstrated. This multimedia feature is designed to help you add a new dimension to your learning.

KEY TERMS/CONCEPTS

Air quality
Boundaries
Cleanliness/neatness
Confidentiality
Counter-transference
Cross-gender massage
Direction
Draping
Dressing arrangements
Dual relationships
Emotional release
Feedback
Informed consent
Intervention Model
Lighting
Liniment
Lotion
Oil
Pacing
Positioning
Pressure
Professional demeanor
Prone position
Reclining position
Rhythm
Room temperature
Routine
Same-gender massage
Self-care
Side-lying position
Sound
Specificity
Standards of practice
Supine position
Tenting
Therapeutic relationship
Topical substances
Touch
Transference
Verbal interaction

Guidelines for providing safe, effective massage and bodywork are presented in this chapter. They take into consideration the nature of the therapeutic relationship, the physical environment, the comfort and safety of the recipient, self-care for the practitioner, and the performance of the massage itself. These guidelines are relevant no matter what specific form, approach, or style of massage and bodywork you practice.

THE THERAPEUTIC RELATIONSHIP

The **therapeutic relationship** involves an implicit agreement regarding the roles of the massage practitioner and the client. The role of the practitioner is to provide massage within the scope of practice of their training and credentials. The role of the client is to receive massage, participate in the therapy, and fulfill financial and appointment obligations within the agreement.

Maintaining clarity about the roles in the therapeutic relationship is achieved by keeping professional **boundaries.** A boundary is defined as "a limit that separates one person from another," and its function is "to protect the integrity of each person." Keeping good boundaries includes practicing within personal limitations, not exploiting the relationship for personal gain, limiting the impact of transference and counter-transference, avoiding dual relationships, not engaging in any sexual activity, and respecting the client's freedom of choice and self-determination (NCBTMB Standards of Practice).

McIntosh (1999) identifies some common mistakes related to boundaries. The first involves going outside of your area of expertise, for example, claiming to provide treatment beyond your training, or advertising expertise in some skill after a weekend workshop, giving advice outside of the scope of practice, or delving into emotional problems without training in psychotherapy. Another mistake is losing the distinction between personal and professional lives; for example, going out socially with clients, or mutual sharing of personal lives.

Boundaries within most health care settings are usually well established. However, boundaries in the context of a private massage practice, or in a spa, health club, or similar non-medical setting need to be carefully maintained by the practitioner.

Dual Relationships

A **dual relationship** is any relationship other than the primary one of practitioner and client. For example, if your client is also your friend, a tenant, an employer, or your stockbroker, there is potential for conflict in the practitioner–client relationship. Dual relationships can end in confusion of roles and weakening professional boundaries. Dual relationships should be avoided if possible, and entered into only with caution.

Transference and Counter-Transference

Transference happens when clients respond to practitioners as they might have responded to an important person from their childhood, e.g., parent, teacher, or other authority figure. They *transfer* those positive or negative feelings onto the practitioner. It is an unconscious, irrational phenomenon.

Counter-transference is similar, except that practitioners transfer feelings from their past onto the client. In both cases, the feelings have little to do with the actual relationship with the massage practitioner and client. The boundaries between the present and the past become blurred.

In a typical case of transference, a client might "fall into the illusion that we are wiser and somehow better than they are," or try too hard to please us as they would a parent. Transference can also manifest as sexual feelings or "crushes." Maintaining good professional boundaries, and awareness of the potential confusion, can help keep clarity in these situations. (For a comprehensive discussion of the practitioner–client relationship refer to *The Educated Heart* by Nina McIntosh, 1999; and *The Ethics of Touch* by Ben Benjamin and Cherie Sohnen-Moe, 2003.)

PROFESSIONAL DEMEANOR

The **professional demeanor,** i.e., appearance and behavior of the practitioner, are important in putting the receiver of massage at ease. Your demeanor should inspire confidence and a sense of safety, and help establish the professional nature of the relationship. This is especially important in a relationship based primarily on touch.

Clothing should be neat, clean, modest, and comfortable, allowing freedom of movement. Avoid clothing that may be sexually suggestive such as tight pants, short shorts, and shirts that expose the chest or midriff. Jewelry should be minimal. Avoid rings that might scratch the client, and dangling bracelets and necklaces.

The practitioner should be free from offensive odors. This includes odors from the body and clothes, and strong perfumes and colognes. Some practitioners bathe or change shirts during the day to stay fresh. After a spicy meal, or just a long day, you may want to consider a breath freshener. Smokers should be particularly aware to eliminate odors on their clothes, hands, and breath.

Language used by the practitioner also sets the tone of the professional relationship. Practitioners should speak in a way that can be clearly understood, avoiding unduly technical and scientific language and jargon. Practitioners should speak to the understanding and educational level of the receiver. However, care should be taken in referring to the body, and sexually suggestive words and expressions avoided.

The physical contact inherent in massage establishes a close relationship between practitioner and receiver. This relationship should be understanding and sympathetic, but never personal.

TOUCHING ANOTHER PERSON

It has been observed that "touch is our most social sense," because it implies interaction with another person. Human beings have an innate touch hunger. Touch is essential for proper growth and development in infants, and for well being at all stages of life. Touch deprivation has been linked to increased stress, physical violence, sleep disturbance, and suppressed immune response. (For further information about the importance of touch read *Touching: The Significance of the Human Skin* by Ashley Montagu, 1978; and *Touch* by Tiffany Field, 2001).

Touch is the primary mode of personal interaction during massage. It is essential that the practitioner be knowledgeable about the psychosocial implications of touch, as well as its physical nature. Practitioners giving massage need to be skilled in touch.

More Basic than Technique

Touch is more basic than technique. To touch means "to come into contact with." In massage, that contact happens on a physical and an energetic level, and is achieved primarily through the hands of the practitioner. From the holistic perspective, you touch the whole person, and what may seem to be only physical touch often has profound effects on the mind, emotions, and spirit of the receiver.

Touch can communicate care and compassion, confidence, calmness, focus, and skillfulness. It can also convey anxiety, apprehension, anger, distractedness, disinterestedness, and lack of confidence. Practitioners should always be aware of their state of being, because whatever it is, it will be communicated through touch to a sensitive receiver. Prepare yourself to give massage by being aware of your intention to be caring and compassionate, and by becoming calm and focused.

A unique feature of touch is that when you touch another person, you are touched yourself. When you are giving touch, you are also receiving touch. This is one reason why giving massage can be such a rewarding experience. However, this can also necessitate some self-care. For example, a practitioner who comes in contact with someone who is experiencing grief, anger, anxiety, or extreme stress can pick up some of the negative effects of these emotions. Self-care techniques like meditation, talking to a colleague, or consciously "washing away" negative energy after a session can limit the degree to which you are affected by the negative "vibes" of your clients. It is important to take care of yourself, while you remain a source of care and compassion for your clients.

Touch and the Therapeutic Relationship

Comfort levels with touch vary for a number of reasons. People from different cultural backgrounds will have different experiences with and attitudes toward touch. For example, studies have shown that people from Great Britain and northern Europe experience touch less in social interaction than those from Mediterranean countries such as Spain, Italy, and Greece (Montagu, 1978).

Appropriate touch in one situation or with one client may be inappropriate in other circumstances. The practitioner must cultivate an awareness of their own, and each client's, comfort with touch. The practitioner's challenge is to create an openness to the touch of massage.

The practitioner should be clear about the difference between friendly, caring, and even affectionate touch and sexual touch. Sexual touch is never appropriate in a professional setting.

Many men and women have been the victims of physical and sexual abuse. Many more have endured the traumatic stress of natural disaster, war, or other disturbing events. These people need special care regarding touch. The practitioner should be aware of each receiver's reaction to touch, and ensure that he or she feels safe and comfortable.

It is possible that the receiver of massage may interpret your touch in a way that was not intended. He or she may project his or her own issues regarding touch onto you. Your touch may be perceived as abusive or sexual when you had no such intention. When that transference happens, clear verbal communication is essential to clear up any misperceptions. Clear professional boundaries are especially important in a therapeutic relationship based on touch.

PERMISSION TO TOUCH

When a person agrees to receive massage from a practitioner, there is an implicit permission to touch. However, when the touch occurs in certain areas, especially those that feel vulnerable, there should be an *explicit* permission to touch that specific area for therapeutic purposes. This is true for areas like the upper or inner thigh, the lower abdomen, and around breast tissue in women.

Informed Consent

In an **informed consent** statement, the practitioner explains what they are going to do (e.g., massage the abdomen), why they are doing it (i.e., therapeutic intention), what the client should expect, and asks permission to touch the area. The client should clearly understand that they have the option of saying "no" either before or at any time during the proposed action. The elements of informed consent are summarized in Table 6–1.

In cases where the recipient has suffered physical or sexual abuse, there may be additional vulnerable areas. For example, if someone has been physically abused with beatings on the back of the legs and buttocks, these may be emotionally sensitive areas to be considerate of and receive permission to work on. You may not know beforehand about these situations, so it is wise to be aware of the client's reactions to touch throughout the session.

Informed consent is a good idea at any time the recipient might be unpleasantly surprised. For example, communicate with the recipient before going deep into the tissues, or pressing into painful

Table 6–1 *ELEMENTS OF INFORMED CONSENT*

Used when the massage practitioner plans to touch a vulnerable body area (e.g., upper or inner thigh, lower abdomen, or breast tissue in women), or plans to apply a technique that may feel strange or cause unusual or increased pain.

1. Explain what you propose to do.
2. Explain your intent.
3. Describe what the client should expect.
4. Give the client the option to say no either before beginning or at any time during the application. Be alert to nonverbal as well as verbal signals.
5. Ask permission to touch the area.

Examples

Intended action: To massage into the muscle attachments on the inner thigh.

1. "I would like to massage your upper thigh thoroughly, including the inner thigh."
2. "This will help relax those tense muscles in your legs. The muscle attachments are at the knee and the pelvis."
3. "I'll secure the drape around the groin so that you will be covered appropriately, and will just massage up to the drape. The inner thigh can be sensitive, so it may feel strange to you."
4. "At any time, if you don't like how it feels, let me know and I'll stop."
5. "Is it OK to go ahead?"

Intended action: To apply pressure to sensitive points on the cervical muscles.

1. "I'd like to press some of the sensitive spots on your neck."
2. "I suspect that they are trigger points causing your tension headaches. Pressing the points helps deactivate and relieve them."
3. "You will feel pain if I press directly on a trigger point, and it may also refer pain into your head. I will ask for feedback on the location of the points, and the amount of pressure I'm using."
4. "If the pressure seems to be too much, let me know and I'll reduce it. And we can stop at any time."
5. "Is it OK to begin?"

trigger points. If you sense that the recipient is uncomfortable physically or emotionally with your touch, it is best to ask permission to continue.

GENDER CONSIDERATIONS

Because of its basis in touch and the interpersonal nature of massage, there are certain considerations related to gender to be aware of. These may be peculiar to a person's cultural background, or to the professional setting. Professional demeanor, good boundaries, and good verbal communication skills will help make the following situations less troublesome. This is true regardless of the gender of the practitioner and the receiver.

Cross-gender massage has become more common. When women give massage to men, or men to women, they need to be especially clear about the non-sexual nature of their work and establish clear professional boundaries. Sexualizing the professional relationship by either party is unacceptable, and if allowed by the practitioner, is unethical.

Same-gender massage may also be an issue for some clients. In some cases, a client or patient may unconsciously transfer their personal aversion to homosexual orientation to the practitioner–client relationship. This presents problems in a same-gender situation, whether the practitioner is homosexual or not. In Western culture, touch is often equated with sexual touch, so that any touch by another person may have sexual overtones. Practitioners need to be mindful of this cultural dilemma. This poses special problems when nurturing and compassion are called for. Practitioners need to meet the needs of their clients in a way that is comfortable and acceptable.

Male practitioners working with women clients should be mindful that most cases of sexual harassment and abuse are committed towards women. Chances are high that some of the women recipients of massage have such histories. It is also possible that the women may not identify this past experience as a problem in the present. Men must approach all women as possible survivors of abuse and must be aware of and especially sensitive to their need for clear boundaries.

Needless to say, any of the considerations mentioned above could apply to either gender. Clear boundaries and professional demeanor are keys to addressing these gender considerations.

INTERVENTION MODEL

During the massage itself, if a client touches you inappropriately, appears to be sexually aroused, makes comments of a sexual nature, or otherwise appears to sexualize the situation, apply an intervention model. Steps in the seven-step **intervention model** include:

1. Stop the session using assertive behavior.
2. Describe the behavior you are concerned about.
3. Ask the client to clarify their behavior.
4. Re-state your intent and professional boundaries.
5. Evaluate the client's response.
6. Continue or discontinue the session as appropriate.
7. Document the situation.

(For further discussion refer to *The Ethics of Touch* by Ben Benjamin and Cherie Sohnen-Moe, 2003.)

It is important not to ignore client misbehavior. A practitioner should never continue the session if they feel that the client is sexualizing the massage. The seven-step intervention model is summarized in Table 6–2.

TALKING AND FEEDBACK

Whether, and how much, **verbal interaction** should go on during a massage session depends on the purpose of the session and the needs of the receiver. The practitioner should be aware of the amount and nature of talking taking place, and structure the session in the best interests of the receiver.

When relaxation is a primary goal, talking should be kept to a minimum. Silence allows receivers to sink further into a relaxed state and be quietly with themselves. They are more likely to be receptive to the relaxing effects of music playing and to the "letting go" that happens during relaxation. A soft voice should be used for necessary communications.

People who are nervous about receiving massage, especially for the first time, may need more verbal interaction. The practitioner may want to give more direction, describe what he or she is doing and ask for frequent feedback to help put the person at ease.

Certain types of techniques require frequent **feedback** on pain level for the safety of the recipient, and for information on the effectiveness of techniques. For example, the receiver may give feedback to

Table 6–2 SEVEN-STEP INTERVENTION MODEL

Used when the client's behavior is inappropriate; for example, if they sexualize the session in any way.

1. Stop the session using assertive behavior.
2. Describe the behavior you are concerned about.
3. Ask the client to clarify their behavior.
4. Re-state your intent and professional boundaries.
5. Evaluate the client's response.
6. Continue or discontinue the session as appropriate.
7. Document the situation.

help pinpoint the precise location of trigger points, or to determine how much to stretch a muscle safely. Feedback can take different forms. A receiver whose face winces in pain, or whose muscles tighten up, or who gives a deep sigh is offering feedback on his or her state of being. The practitioner should be aware of this nonverbal feedback and use it during the flow of the session.

Sometimes a recipient will experience what is called an **emotional release.** Suppressed emotions may be stored in our bodies, and these feelings may be released in a massage session as a person is touched, or as the recipient relaxes and lets down emotional defenses. This may be as simple as a sigh or crying. Practitioners should not attempt to delve into the meaning of such a release of emotions, but should simply be present and supportive.

Practitioners can also give useful feedback to recipients. For example, they may call the receiver's attention to a muscular holding pattern or mention when a formerly tense muscle relaxes. In this way, a person can become more aware of his or her own body.

Talking may also be of a more social nature. This should be kept to a minimum in most cases during a session. An exception may be an elderly person who has little other social contact and wants to talk, or a person who has recently experienced something upsetting and needs to talk about it. Careful judgment is needed in instances like these to prevent crossing professional boundaries.

Practitioners should avoid talking to receivers about their own lives and troubles. A good rule of thumb is to follow the lead of the receiver by listening and responding only to the receiver's questions or comments. This helps you determine whether the interaction is coming from your own or the receiver's needs. You should not get your needs met at the expense of the therapeutic relationship. Practitioners should be especially mindful of their scope of practice and not delve into psychotherapy unless properly trained. It may be useful to keep a referral list for receivers who ask for help finding a psychotherapist.

Practitioners should develop skill in recognizing and establishing the amount and nature of verbal interaction that is best in a given situation. Since the primary mode of communication in massage is touch, usually less talk is better.

CONFIDENTIALITY

In a professional relationship, there is an implicit trust that the practitioner will keep information about the receiver confidential. The ethical principle of **confidentiality** is based on the client's right to privacy. This includes information found on a health history form; information told to the practitioner during a session, or before or after a session; and observations about a client related to physical, mental, or emotional condition. It is a matter of respecting the privacy of the receiver, and in medical settings, confidentiality is a legal matter.

There are exceptions to the general rule of confidentiality, for example, talking to another health professional about a receiver's condition in order to serve him or her better. A practitioner receiving professional supervision may discuss a case with a supervisor. Confidential information may also be divulged if required by law, or in cases of emergency.

In non-medical settings such as health clubs, salons or spas, confidentiality is a matter of professional standards, and respect for the receiver. It is considered unethical to gossip about a client or to give information about him or her without permission.

The National Certification Board for Therapeutic Massage and Bodywork has published a **Standards of Practice** that addresses issues related to professionalism, confidentiality, roles and boundaries, and prevention of sexual misconduct. The standards give more detail about acceptable professional behavior. The standards of practice can be found on the Internet (www.ncbtmb.org).

HIPAA PRIVACY RULE

In 1996, the U.S. Congress passed the Health Insurance Portability and Accountability Act. The HIPAA Privacy Rule is a federal standard designed to protect the medical records of individuals. In general, HIPAA requires a health care provider to inform patients/clients about their privacy rights and how their information can be used. Providers must adopt and implement privacy procedures, and train employees to comply. In an office or clinic, a person must be designated as responsible for seeing that privacy policies are followed.

Patients/clients should be able to see their records, and obtain copies upon request. They may ask for corrections to records if they find mistakes.

Patient/client records must be secured, and kept away from anyone who does not need to see them. For example, records should be kept in locked file cabinets preferably in isolated records rooms, and passwords needed to access client files on the computer. Patients/clients must give written consent for use and disclosure of information for treatment, payment, and health care operations.

HIPAA is administered by the U.S. Department of Health & Human Services (HHS), and enforcement and complaints are handled by the HHS Office of Civil Rights (OCR). Information about HIPAA can be found on the HHS website at (www.hhs.gov/ocr/hipaa).

THE PHYSICAL ENVIRONMENT

Massage Tables and Chairs

Massage tables are specially designed for the needs of the massage practitioner. A massage table should be adjustable in height and have a removable, adjustable face cradle. Tables vary in length, width, and type of padding and covering (e.g., soft or hard vinyl). A typical portable massage table and a face cradle are shown in Figure 6–1a,b.

The type of table you choose depends on the type of work you do, and the setting. For example, if you work in a setting in which tables are rarely moved, you may want a stationary table for its stability. If you carry your table from place to place, you will want a lightweight portable table. If you do sports massage, you may want a narrow table. Some shiatsu practitioners get up on the table for better leverage, and so a wider table is more practical. There are special tables for pregnant clients, and tables with hinges that permit a reclining or partial sitting position.

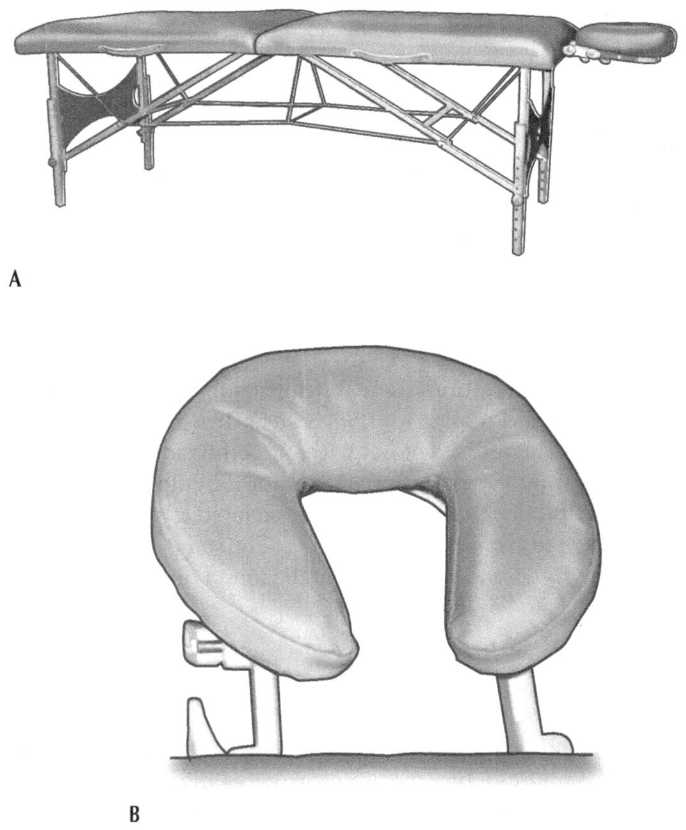

FIGURE 6–1. Massage table and face cradle. **A.** Adjustable massage table. **B.** Adjustable face cradle.

Your table is an important investment. To see a variety of tables, you may want to visit a massage supplies showroom, or a trade show or convention, or check table manufacturers on the Internet. A good quality table is a wise investment.

The massage chair is specially designed to provide maximum comfort while receiving massage in a seated position while fully clothed. Chairs usually have a seat, knee rests, armrest, chest cushion, and face cradle. There should be adjustments for the chest cushion and the face cradle. A typical massage chair is shown in Figure 6–2a,b. This type of massage chair was introduced in the 1980s, and chairs are continually undergoing improvement in design.

Whenever possible, practitioners should use equipment specially designed for massage. However, sometimes practitioners have to improvise in less than ideal situations. For example, massage may be given to people in wheelchairs, to the bedridden elderly or ill, to workers at their desks, or even at poolside at a swim meet. In these circumstances, care should be taken to ensure the safety and comfort of the receiver while providing for good body mechanics for the practitioner.

The Massage Space

Massage is given in a variety of settings, including private offices, chiropractic clinics, health clubs, spas or salons, training rooms, medical clinics and hospitals, nursing homes, and hospices. On-site massage in special massage chairs is given in commercial businesses and other public places. Whatever the location, there are certain factors in the environment that will help maximize the benefits of the session. Important factors to consider include the room temperature, air quality, lighting, sound, dressing arrangements, and overall cleanliness and neatness.

The **room temperature** should be warm enough so that the receiver is comfortable. When the receiver is partially or fully unclothed under a drape, a comfortable room temperature is usually around 75ºF. Receivers often get cold during massage as they relax. Ways to help keep them warm include an electric mattress pad underneath the bottom sheet, a heat lamp overhead, or a blanket on top. Turning up the heat in the room is a less desirable solution, because the practitioner may then get overheated while working.

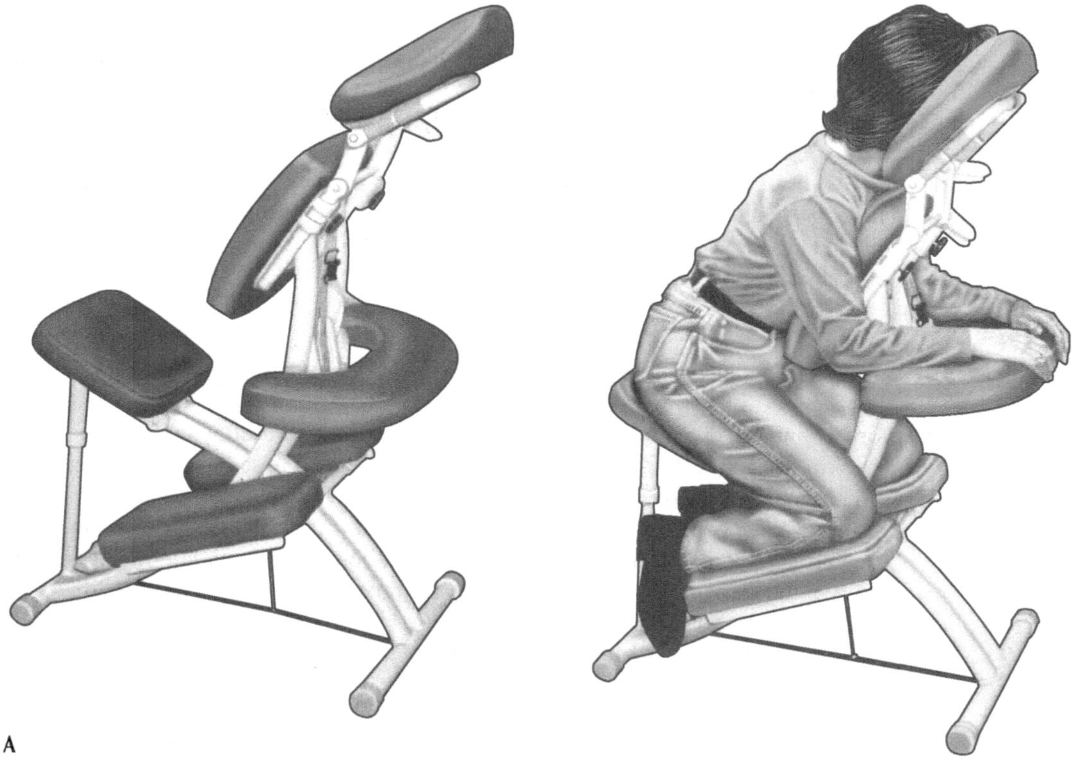

A

B

FIGURE 6–2. Massage chair. **A.** Adjustable massage chair. **B.** Recipient positioned in massage chair.

Air quality should be fresh and pleasant, and rooms well ventilated. This may be a challenge in some places like hospitals or beauty salons where strong odors are present, or in buildings where smoking is allowed. Also consider allergens such as pollen and animal hair. Electric air cleaners may be used, and in the summer, air conditioners can help keep air fresh. However, when using an air conditioner, be mindful of the warmth of the room.

Lighting is an important consideration. Soft and indirect lighting are more restful than harsh and direct lighting. Overhead lighting may shine in the receiver's eyes when he or she is supine on a table, as will the sun if doing massage in an outdoor setting such as at a spa or at an athletic event. In places where overhead lighting cannot be controlled, you may provide the receiver with a light shield for the eyes when he or she is supine.

Sound can help create a peaceful and healing environment, or a stimulating one. Music elicits certain emotions and is often used to create a particular effect. In general, popular and vocal music should be avoided if the intent is to relax. Use of popular music may also confuse the professional relationship, since it is normally heard in social situations. Numerous CDs and tapes are available with music specifically designed for relaxation, and some specifically for massage.

Sometimes it is desirable to have a background of more stimulating music, for example, when the receiver must go back to work immediately, or for an athlete receiving massage just before an event. Music that is stimulating, while not stressful or frenetic, is appropriate in these situations. The receiver's taste in music should be taken into consideration and a variety of choices made available.

For some people, silence, or a fish tank bubbling in the background, is most restful. Fish tanks are known to have a relaxing effect on most people. There are also machines that produce "white noise" to mask annoying outside noises.

Dressing arrangements should be convenient and provide a private space for receivers to disrobe and get onto the table. If there is only one table in a room, then the practitioner may simply leave the room while the recipient is disrobing. In a situation where there is more than one table in the room, such as in a training room or clinic, gowns may be provided for the receivers to use when walking from the dressing area to the massage table. Robes are often provided for this purpose at spas.

It is generally considered a breach of professional boundaries for recipients to be seen naked as they are preparing for massage. Exceptions are in cases where the person receiving massage needs assistance dressing, such as with the elderly or disabled. Even in these cases, care should be taken to preserve the modesty of the recipient as much as possible.

Overall **cleanliness** and **neatness** of the space where massage is given should be maintained. Not only does this provide a sanitary environment for the recipient, it helps create a calm, peaceful, and cheerful atmosphere. Oil bottles should be neatly arranged and wiped clean, and clean linens neatly stacked or stored away. Used sheets and towels should be placed in a closed container and kept out of sight. Floors should be cleaned, carpets vacuumed frequently, and furniture dusted.

There may be local health department regulations concerning sanitation in places where massage is provided. These may include the materials used on the floor, how sheets and towels are stored, and how floors should be cleaned.

TOPICAL SUBSTANCES

Many forms of massage and bodywork use some kind of topical substance to enhance their effects or to minimize skin friction during the application of techniques. These are classified as liniments, oils, lotions, or combinations of these.

Liniments have been used for centuries for sore and stiff muscles and for sprains and bruises. They are particularly popular with athletes. A **liniment** is a liquid or semi-liquid preparation for rubbing on or applying to the skin for therapeutic purposes. Liniments are typically counter-irritating and contain ingredients like camphor, menthol, and turpentine. Herbal preparations might contain rosemary, wild marjoram, or cayenne pepper. Since they contain irritants, rubbing with them too vigorously may cause blistering. If liniments are used, they are usually rubbed onto the skin after massage of an area.

Oils serve as a lubricant to minimize uncomfortable skin friction during sliding and kneading techniques. Certain vegetable oils may also add moisture and nutrients to the skin. Commonly used vegetable oils include almond, olive, and grape seed. Mineral oils are sometimes used, and are generally washed out of sheets more easily than vegetable oils. Vegetable oils trapped in sheets can spoil and turn rancid, causing sheets to have an unpleasant odor. However, some consider vegetable oils healthier for both the giver and the receiver of massage.

Jojoba (pronounced *ho-ho-ba*) is an oil-like substance made from seeds of the jojoba plant found in the North American desert. Native Americans used jojoba for skin and hair care. Many massage practitioners use jojoba either by itself or in combination with lotions, because it is hypoallergenic and healthy for skin, and washes out of sheets easily.

Practitioners choose their oils based on a number of factors. These include properties such as the "feel" of the oil (e.g., thick or thin), inherent nutrients, and scent. Unscented oils are available. Massage oils should be of a high quality and cold pressed. Oils developed specially for massage can be purchased from suppliers.

Lotions are semi-liquid substances containing agents for moisturizing the skin or for therapeutic purposes such as reducing itching or local pain. Lotions are absorbed into the skin, unlike oils, which tend to stay on top of the skin. Lotions are good for situations in which lubrication is desired for a warm-up phase, but more friction is desired later in the session. Those who don't like the feel of oil on their skin may prefer lotions. Lotions also tend to be more water soluble than oils and are, therefore, more easily washed out of sheets.

Practitioners experiment with different topical substances and concoct combinations of substances to get the properties that best enhance their work. They frequently mix different oils, or lotions and oils.

Some substances are more likely to cause allergic reactions. Also, some skin types are more easily irritated. Scent can be an important consideration. People going back to work after massage may desire an unscented substance. Men usually prefer different scents than women. Care should be taken in choosing a topical substance for each unique client or patient.

POSITIONING AND DRAPING

Positioning

Placing the receiver in a comfortable and safe position on the table, called **positioning,** is essential for effective application of massage. The recipient's position can also allow easier access to particular muscles or regions of the body.

The receiver should not have to exert muscular effort to stay in position or to hold draping in place. Various size bolsters, pillows, or rolled towels are used to support body areas and position receivers properly.

In the **supine position** (i.e., face up), a bolster under the knees takes pressure off of the lower back, and a neck roll provides support in the cervical area. In the **prone position** (i.e., face down), support is put under the ankles to ease pressure on them, and small cushions may be placed under the shoulders for women and men with large chests. The face cradle is adjusted for comfort and better access to the cervical area. See Figures 6–3, 6–4, and 6–5.

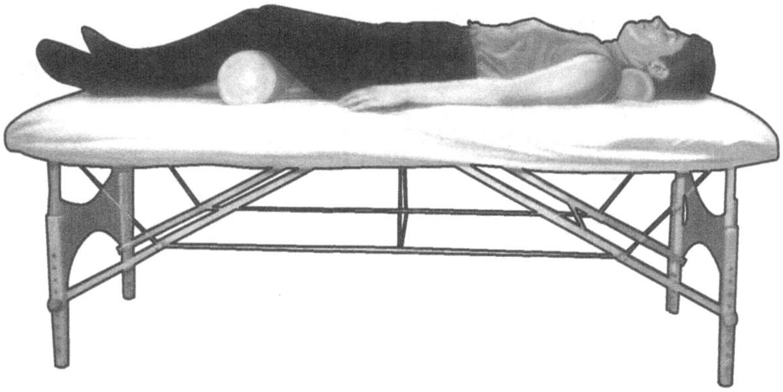

FIGURE 6–3. Supine position. Placement of bolsters under the knees and neck.

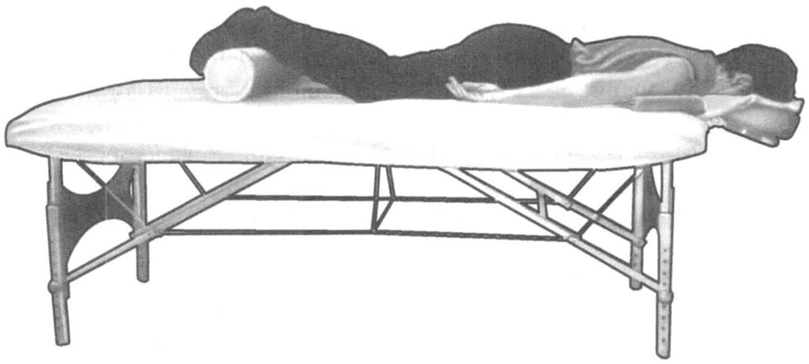

FIGURE 6–4. Prone position. Placement of bolsters under ankles and shoulders, head supported by face cradle.

In the **side-lying position,** support is provided for the superior leg and arm, and under the head. In the **reclining** or semi-supine position, a backrest is created either by adjusting a special hinged table, or by propping the recipient up with bolsters. A bolster is placed under the knees to prevent them from over-extension. See Figures 6–6 and 6–7.

Draping

Covering the body during massage, or **draping,** serves to protect the receiver's modesty, provide clear professional boundaries, and keep the receiver warm. Skill in draping helps the receiver feel safe and allows for maximum relaxation. Draping should be substantial enough to provide a sense of safety and modesty. The use of thin sheets or narrow small towels may leave the recipient feeling exposed and uncomfortable.

When clients remove their clothing and are draped for massage, some general guidelines apply. The genitals and women's breasts should be draped at all times. Mutual consent or familiarity between practitioner and receiver are not good reasons to ignore this guideline. An exception might be during breast massage, but only after special training and with informed consent from the client. Draping can be adjusted to allow access to areas close to the genitals or breasts (e.g., attachments to the adductors or

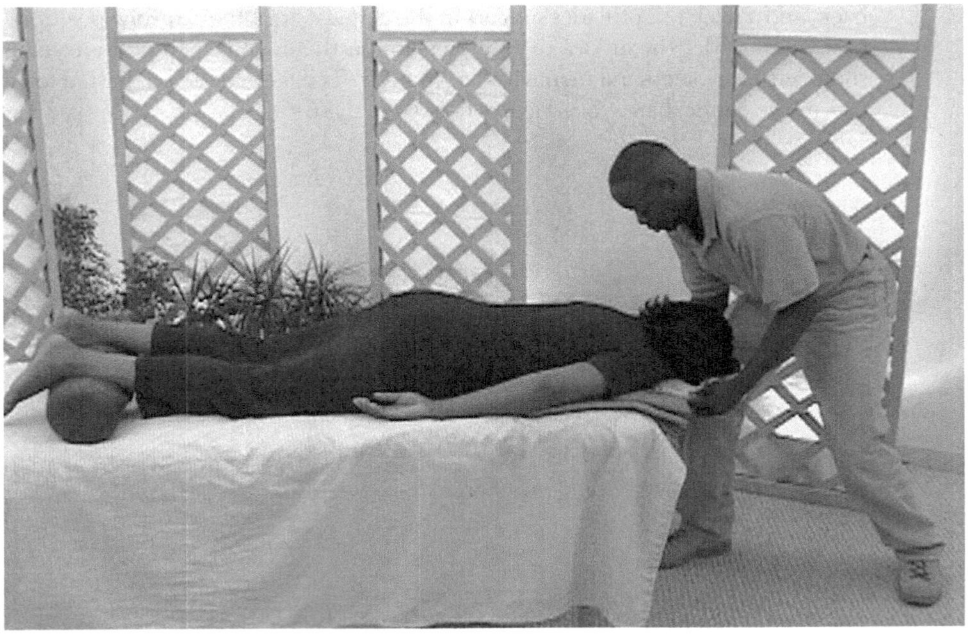

FIGURE 6–5. Face cradle adjustment for comfort of receiver.

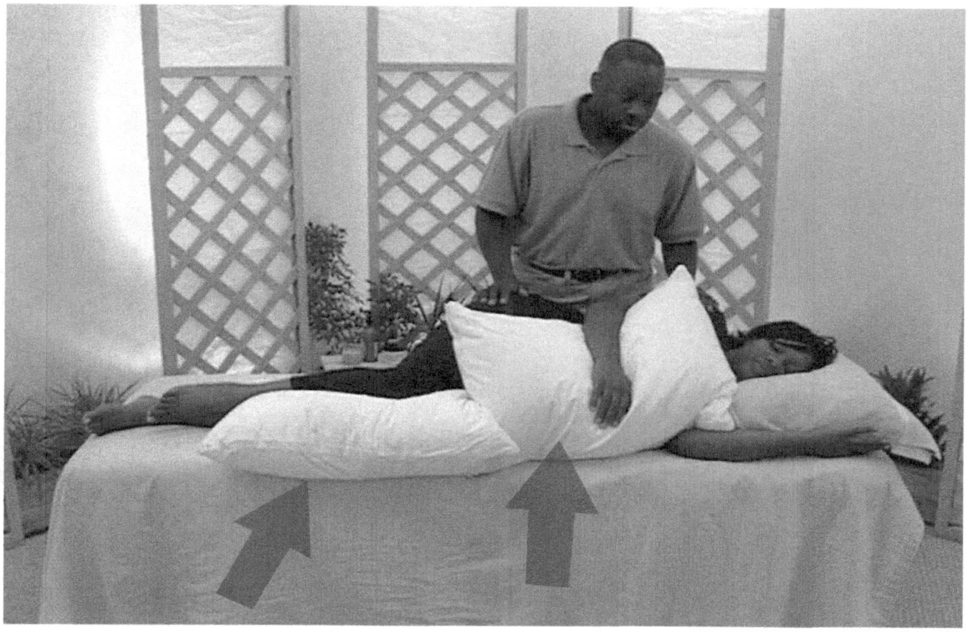

FIGURE 6–6. Side-lying position. Placement of bolsters under the superior leg, arm, and head.

pectoralis major muscle), while maintaining clear professional boundaries. This should be done only with informed consent.

Draping with a sheet provides maximum coverage. The part to be massaged is uncovered and then recovered during the session. Skillful tucking will enhance the security of the drape and prevent inadvertently exposing the receiver. Figure 6–8a–c demonstrates undraping the arm prior to massage.

Preserve the client's modesty when undraping the leg. The leg is lifted at the thigh. The drape is pulled underneath and securely tucked around the hip. Figures 6–9a,b and 6–10a–c demonstrate undraping and securing the drape for the leg.

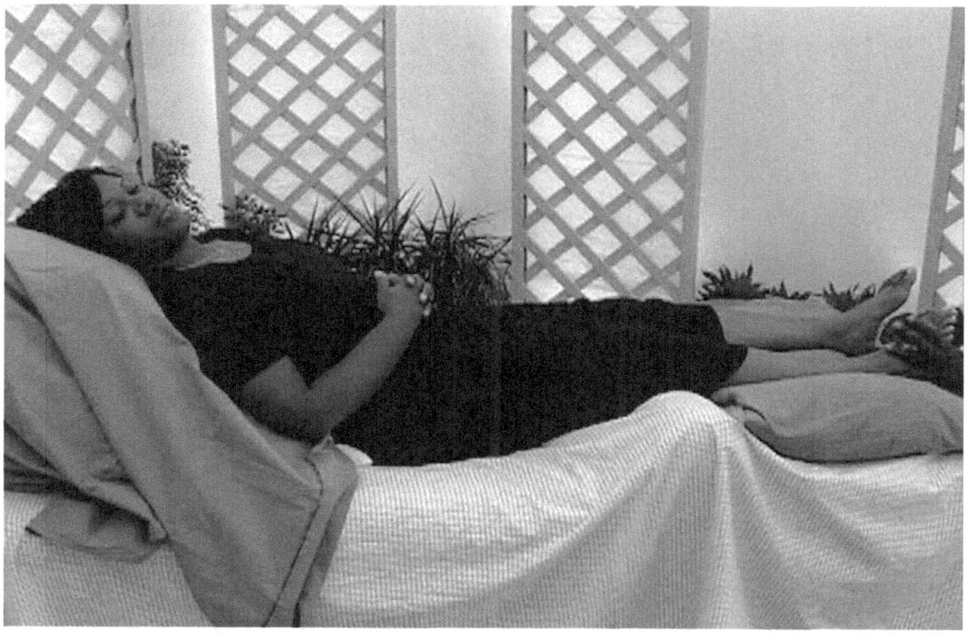

FIGURE 6–7. Reclining position. Back supported and placement of bolster under the knees.

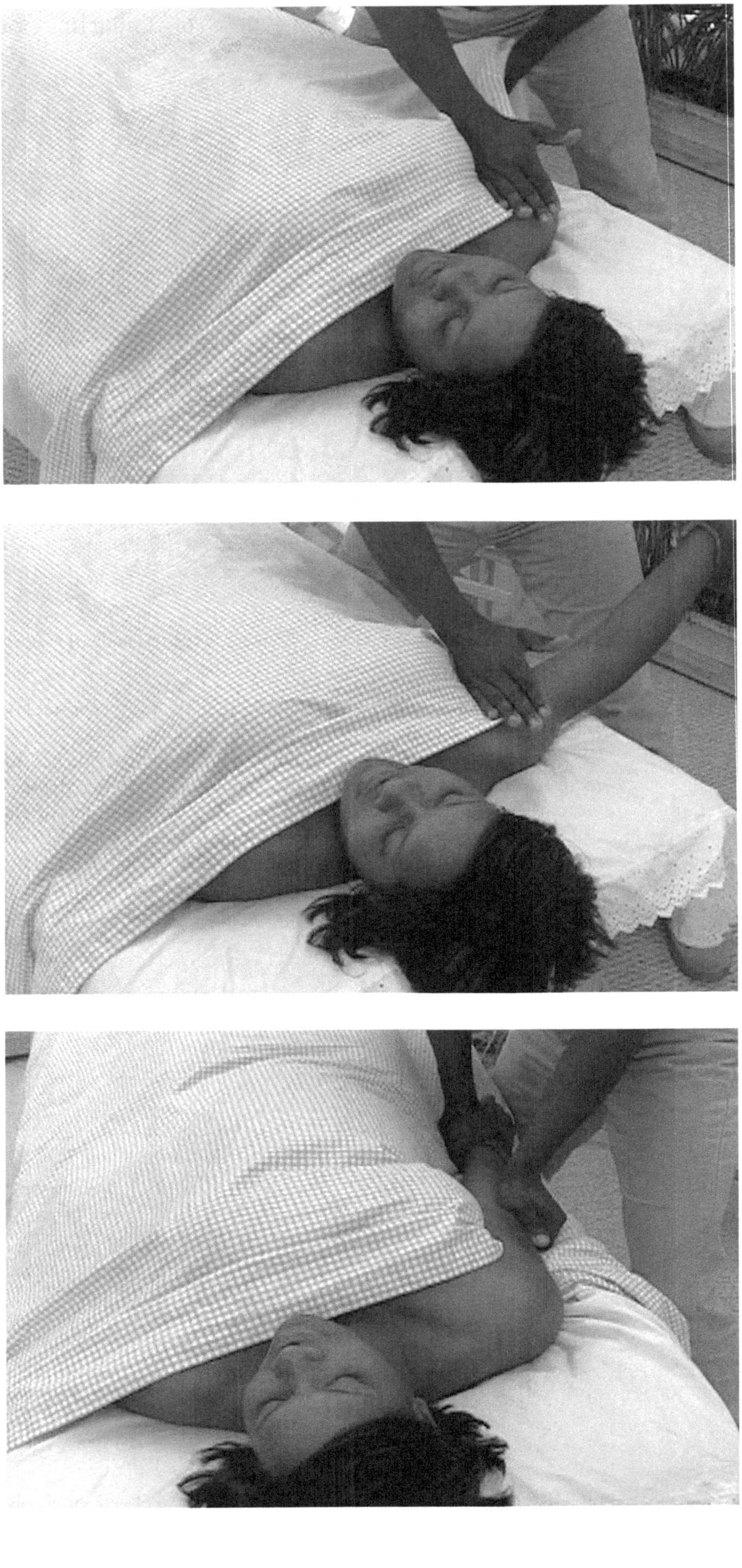

FIGURE 6–8. Draping for massage of arm. **A.** Undraping the arm prior to massage. **B.** Lift arm and tuck sheet underneath. **C.** Arm on table ready for massage.

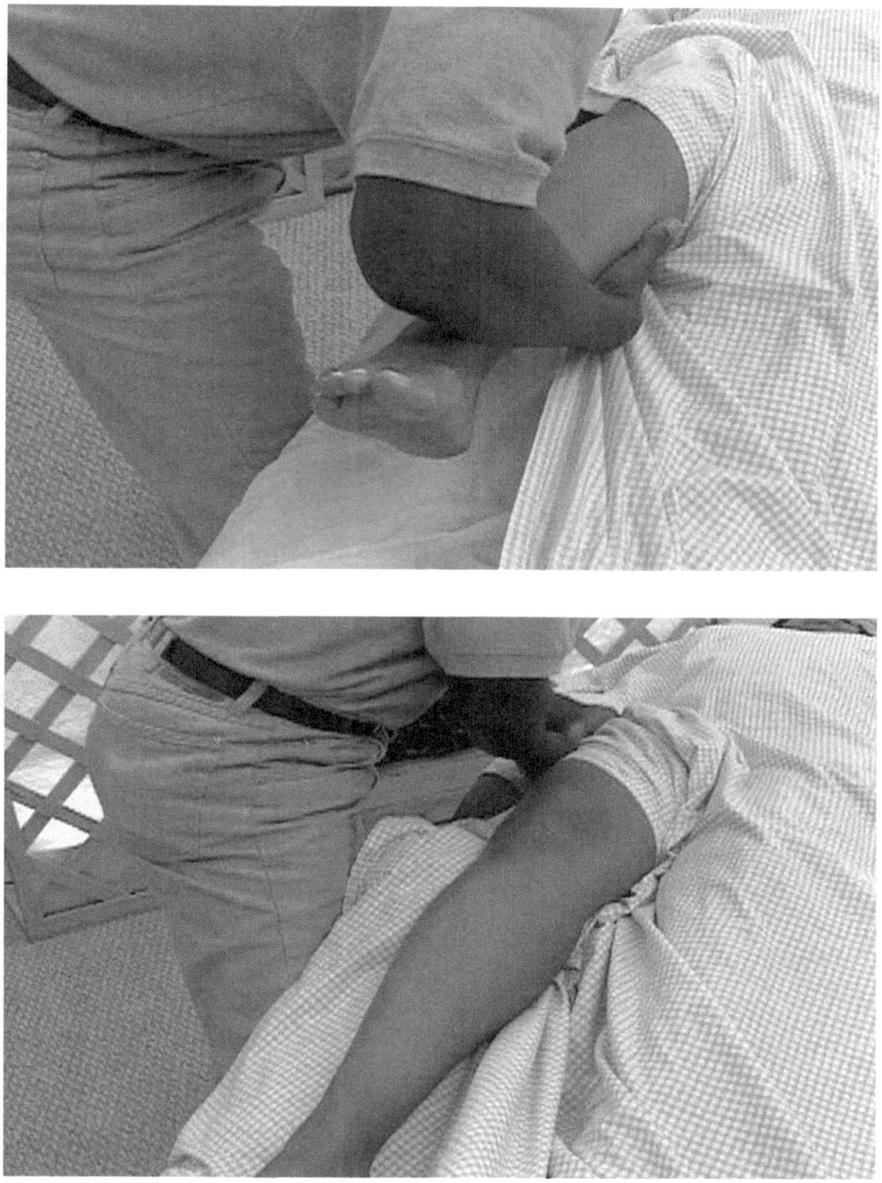

FIGURE 6–9. Draping for massage of leg in supine position. **A.** Lift leg and pull drape underneath. **B.** Secure drape around hip.

Prior to massage of a woman's abdomen or chest area, the breasts are draped with a towel. This is done with informed consent. To begin, a towel is placed over the breasts on top of the sheet. Either you or the client can hold the towel in place as you pull the sheet down to the waist, exposing the upper chest and abdomen. The towel remains covering the breasts. Tuck the sheet around the recipient's hips. Figure 6–11a,b demonstrates proper draping for woman's breasts.

When the receiver is changing from the supine to the prone position, or vice versa, the sheet should be held in place while the person turns over under it. This **tenting** technique allows the receiver to turn over and avoid getting wrapped up in the sheet. Care should be taken not to expose the receiver to the practitioner or to others who might be in the room. See Figure 6–12.

Large towels may also be used for draping. The same general guidelines for modesty apply whatever type of drape is used.

In some situations, receivers do not remove their clothes and draping is unnecessary. For example, receivers usually remain clothed during pre-event and post-event sports massage, chair massage, and some shiatsu and other energy-balancing sessions.

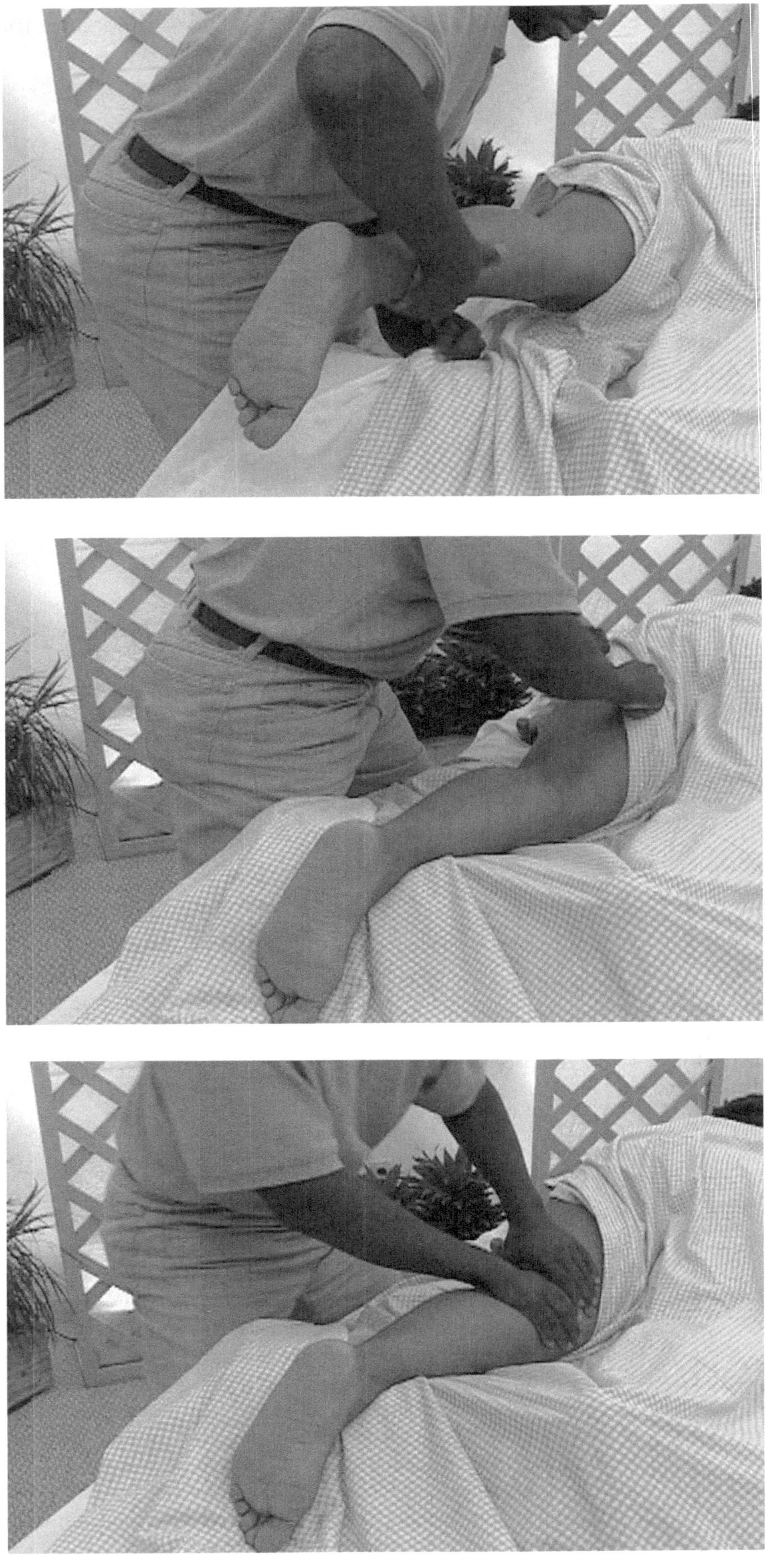

FIGURE 6–10. Draping for massage of leg in prone position. **A.** Lift leg and pull drape underneath. **B.** Secure drape around upper leg and hip. **C.** Massage undraped leg.

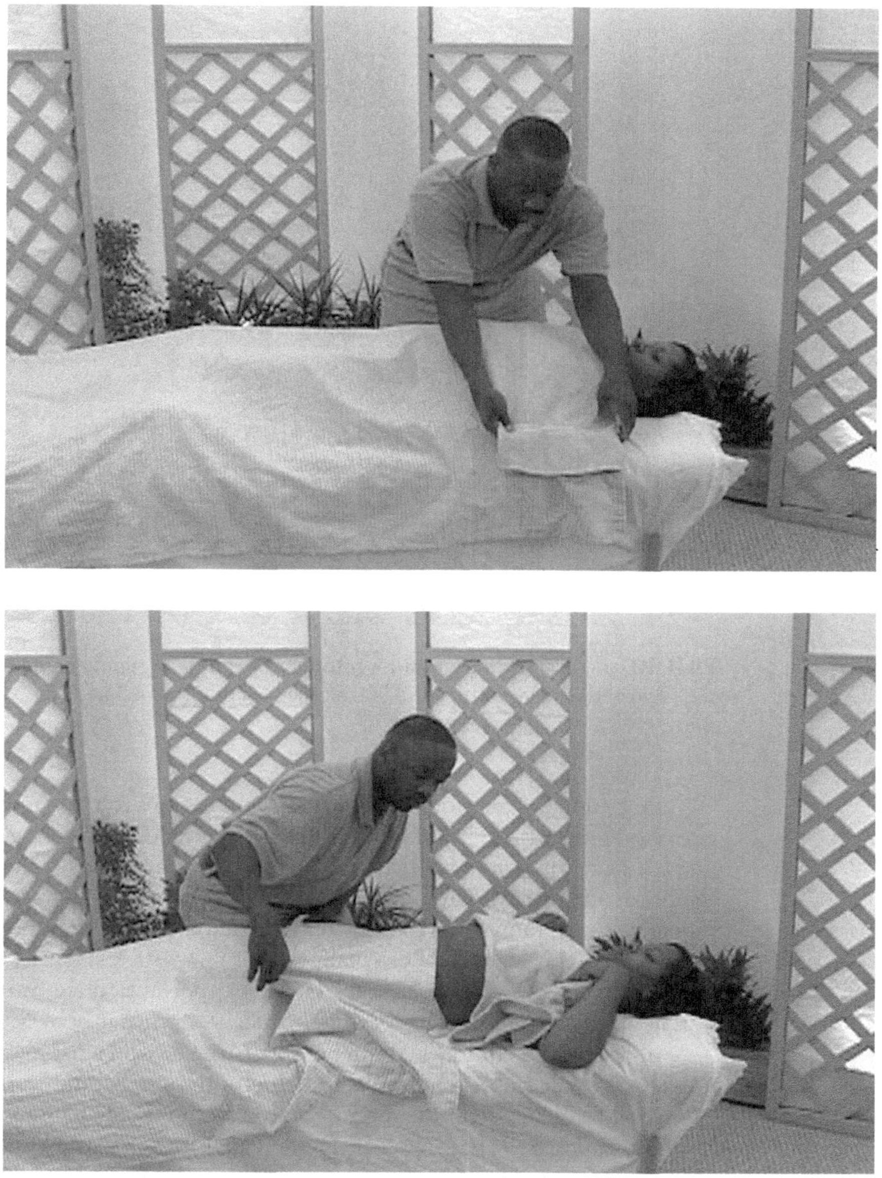

FIGURE 6–11. Draping for a woman's chest. **A.** Place towel over the breasts, and hold the towel in place. **B.** Pull the sheet down to expose the chest and abdomen. Towel remains in place. Tuck the sheet under the hips.

PHYSICAL SELF-CARE FOR THE PRACTITIONER

Physical self-care is essential for the wellbeing and longevity of the massage practitioner. In addition to general health practices, practitioners need to pay special attention to their hands and wrists, posture, and body mechanics. Scheduling of sessions should also be taken into consideration.

Hand and Wrist Care

The hands are the primary means for giving massage. Nails should be clipped so short that they cannot be seen if the hands are held up with the palm toward the face. Rings and bracelets should be avoided, since they might scratch or distract the receiver. Hands should be washed thoroughly before and after every session. This will help protect both the giver and receiver of massage from communicable diseases. Practitioners who smoke should be especially careful to remove odors from their hands. The hands should always be warm and dry before touching the receiver. If necessary, they can be warmed beneath a heat lamp, by hot water, or by rubbing them briskly together. Hands may be dried with a towel or by applying powder to them.

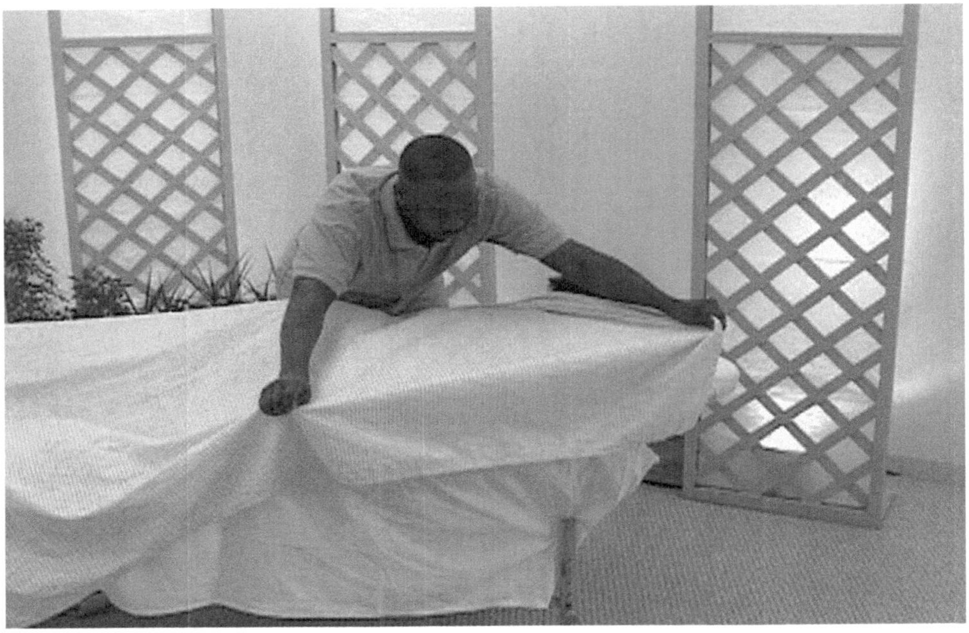

FIGURE 6–12. Creating a tent for turning from prone to supine or vice versa. Pin one side of the sheet against the table with the leg or hip, and lift the sheet so that the recipient can turn over underneath the sheet.

Practitioners can protect themselves from injuries to the hands, arms, and back with conditioning exercises, proper hand position and body mechanics during massage, the use of a variety of techniques, and adequate time for rest between sessions. Common injuries sustained by massage practitioners include tendinitis and tenosynovitis, damage caused by overuse and repetitive strain, and nerve impingement injury (e.g., carpal tunnel and thoracic outlet syndromes). A conditioning program should include exercises to strengthen the upper body, especially the hands, wrists, and arms. Flexibility may be maintained through regular stretching. (The books to read for injury prevention are *Body Mechanics for Manual Therapists* by Barbara Frye, 2000, and *Body Mechanics and Self-Care Manual* by Marian W. Dixon, 2001.)

In applying techniques, strain on finger, thumb, and wrist joints should be minimized. The thumb is especially vulnerable to misuse during high-pressure techniques like trigger point work. Stacking the joints is a protective technique in which pressure is applied along the line of the bones, and through joints, as opposed to being applied at a right angle or across the joint. Figure 6–13a shows correct thumb alignment for applying direct pressure. Avoid applying pressure with the thumb abducted since this puts strain on the joint, as shown in Figure 6–13b.

Wrists should be kept in a neutral position (i.e., neither flexion nor extension) as much as possible when applying techniques (see Figure 6–14). When applying compression techniques, avoid hyperextension at the wrist. If reinforcing one hand with the other during compression techniques, place the top hand directly over the metacarpals, and *not* over the bent wrist. Correct and incorrect positions for compression are demonstrated in Figure 6–15a–c.

Consider the use of the elbow or a special massage tool to apply direct sustained pressure when working in heavily muscled areas. Chapter 13 offers useful suggestions for applying direct pressure safely. The forearm can be used to apply broad effleurage to the thighs or to the back, as demonstrated in Figure 6–16.

Good Body Mechanics

Good body mechanics will minimize shoulder and back problems. First, be sure your table is at the proper height for you. A table too high or too low can cause poor body mechanics and put undue strain on your body. To determine a good table height, stand facing the table with your hands at your sides, as shown in Figure 6–17. Adjust the legs so that your knuckles touch the tabletop. Notice your

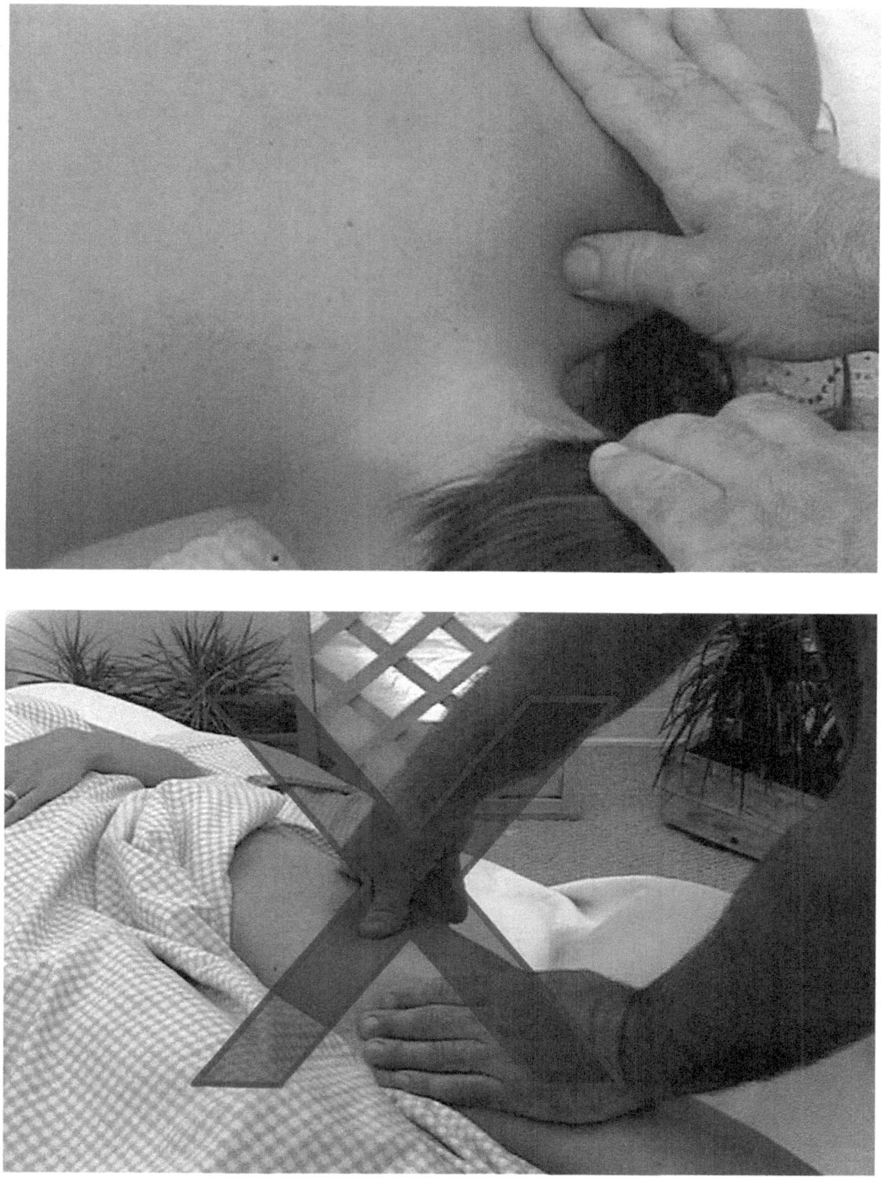

FIGURE 6–13. Correct thumb position when applying pressure. **A.** Correct thumb-wrist alignment for applying direct pressure. **B.** Incorrect position with thumb abducted will cause injury to the joints.

alignment when performing massage at that height. Further adjust the table up or down as needed to keep good alignment of back and neck.

Keep your back and neck in alignment during the session, and bend your knees to lower your body. Avoid bending your back excessively (see Figure 6–18), which puts strain on your back and neck.

Martial arts stances, for example from tai chi, are very effective for keeping good alignment when giving massage. They help take the strain off of your back by using the legs to generate power. These stances not only help keep the back in alignment, but also position you to use body leverage to apply deep pressure.

When facing the head or foot of the table, use a forward leaning stance. Good body alignment and leg position for the forward leaning stance are demonstrated in Figure 6–19a,b. Notice that the front leg is bent more than the rear leg, and pressure is applied as you lean slightly into the technique by shifting the weight from one leg to the other.

When facing the table directly, a side-to-side, or horse, stance is effective. Figure 6–20a,b demonstrates body and foot alignment for the horse stance.

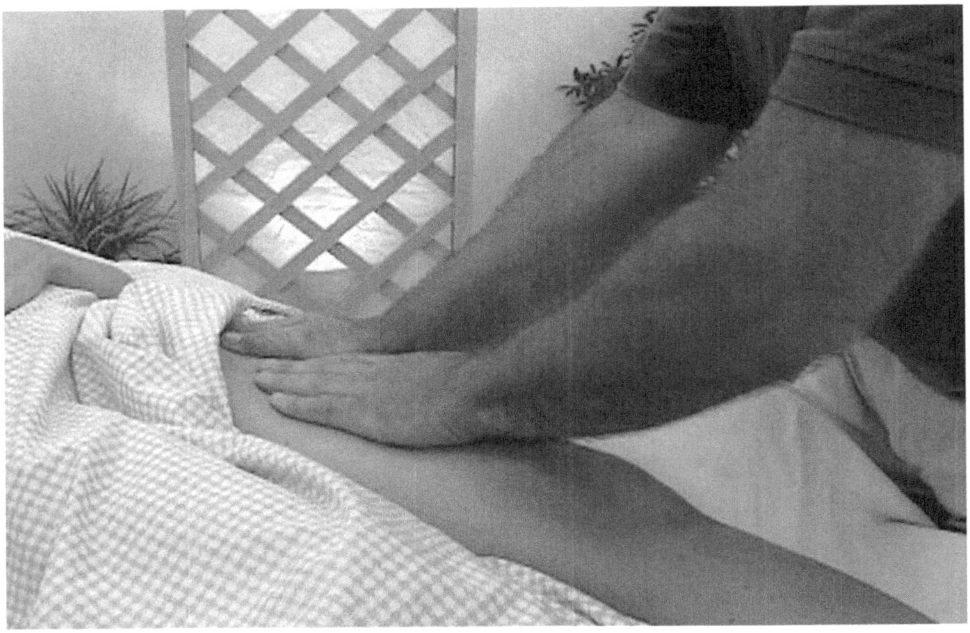

FIGURE 6–14. Wrist in neutral position while performing effleurage.

Sitting on a chair or stool while massaging the receiver's head, hands, and feet also helps minimize strain on the body. Sit near the edge of the seat with your feet flat on the floor and upper body in good alignment. The height of the chair should be adjusted to allow you to keep your wrists in a neutral position. See Figure 6–21a,b.

Avoiding Strain

The warming-up phase of a massage session not only prepares the client for massage, but may also help warm up the practitioner's hands and body. Including a variety of techniques in a session also helps minimize repeated strain on a particular joint or body area of the practitioner.

There are techniques for relaxing tense muscles that cause less strain to the practitioner's body, for example, positional release techniques and some forms of energy work. Techniques that strain the practitioner's body should be alternated with less stressful techniques to provide a resting phase to a session. At the end of a session, the hands are often hot or feel "charged" with energy. Running cold water on the hands after washing them is helpful.

The number of massage sessions any practitioner can perform safely in one day depends on the type of massage performed, his or her strength and fitness, and the quality of his or her body mechanics. Someone just starting out doing massage must build the strength and stamina to perform the work safely. A sudden drastic increase in the number of sessions performed per week may lead to strain, pain, and possible injury.

The following are guidelines for scheduling sessions for a week. They take into account how much work you can expect to perform and maintain your own health and wellbeing. Generally, you should schedule *no more than:*

- Five 1-hour sessions in one day, if you work four days per week
- Four 1-hour sessions in one day, if you work five days per week
- Twenty hours per week total

Furthermore, you should:

- Have 15- to 20-minute breaks between sessions
- Have at least a 30-minute break after three consecutive one-hour sessions
- Do no more than four one-hour sessions in one day, if the type of massage is strenuous

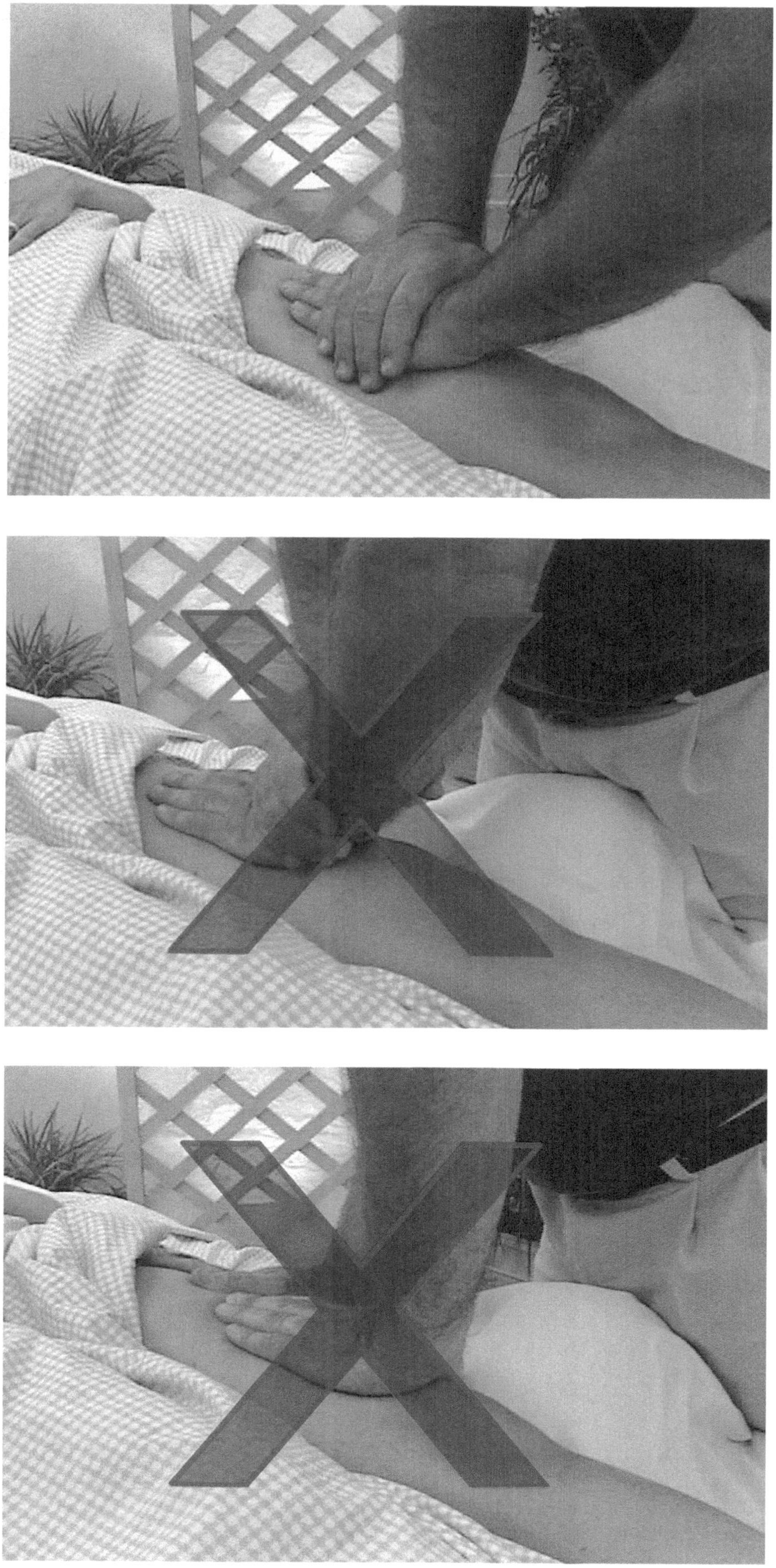

FIGURE 6–15. Correct wrist position while performing compression. **A.** Correct wrist position for compression techniques. **B.** Incorrect position with wrist hyperextended will cause wrist injury. **C.** Incorrect position with pressure directly on the wrist with the other hand will cause wrist injury.

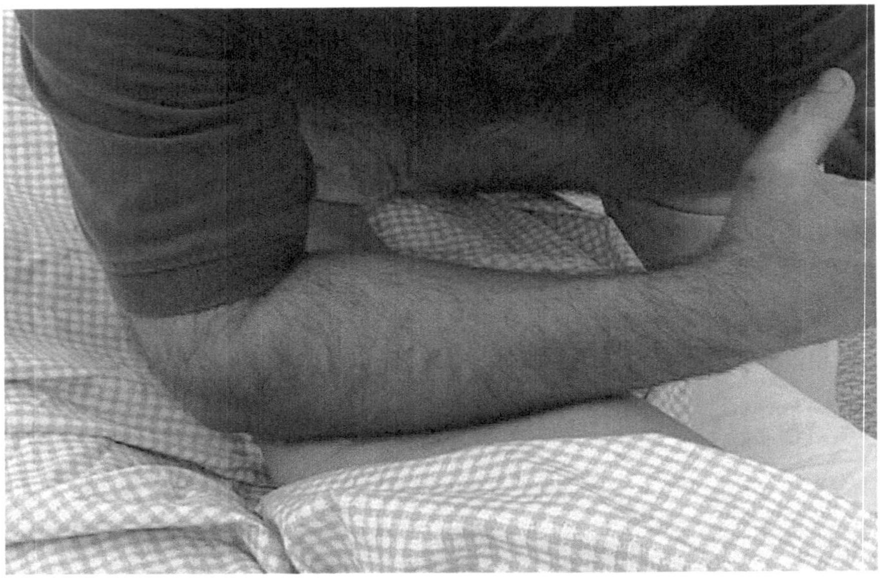

FIGURE 6–16. Use of forearm for performing effleurage on the hamstring muscles.

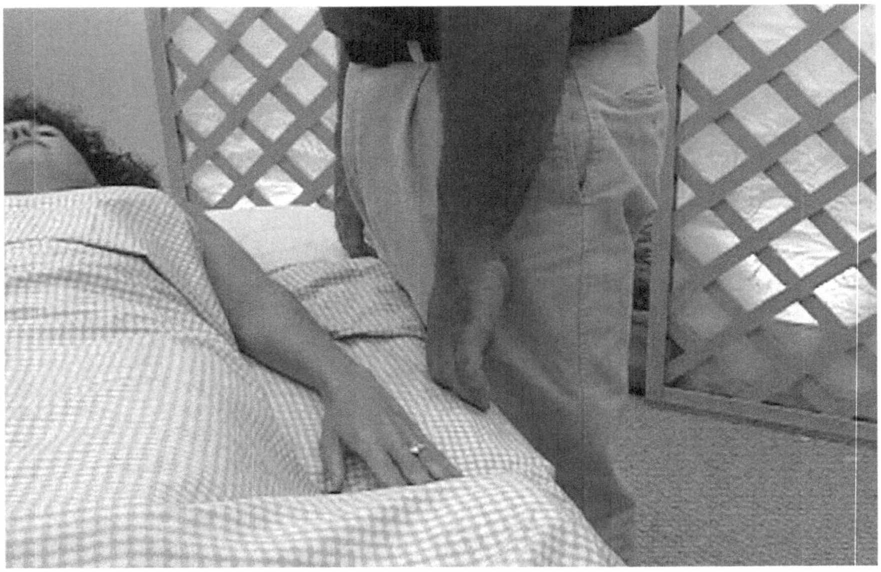

FIGURE 6–17. Determining a good table height. Stand facing the table with your hands at your sides. Adjust the table lags so that your knuckles touch the table top.

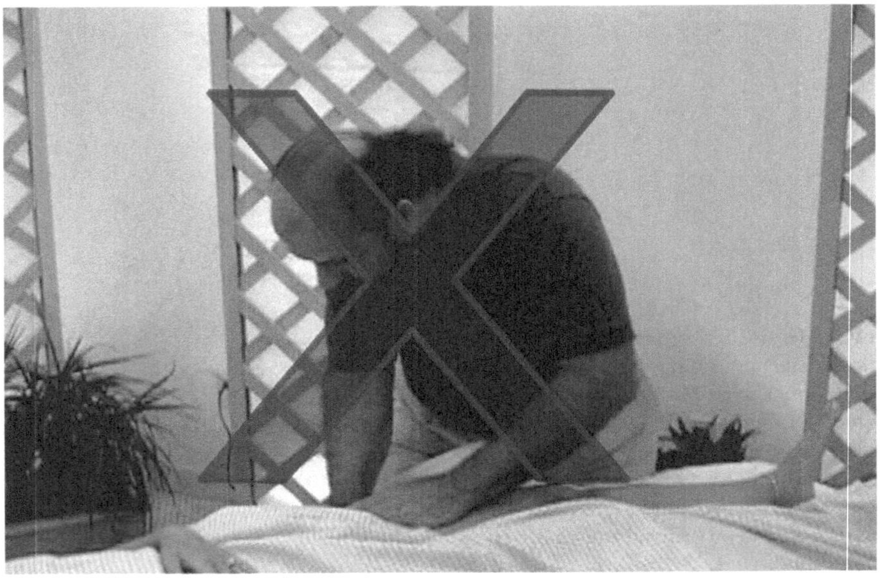

FIGURE 6–18. Incorrect body alignment with back bent and head forward.

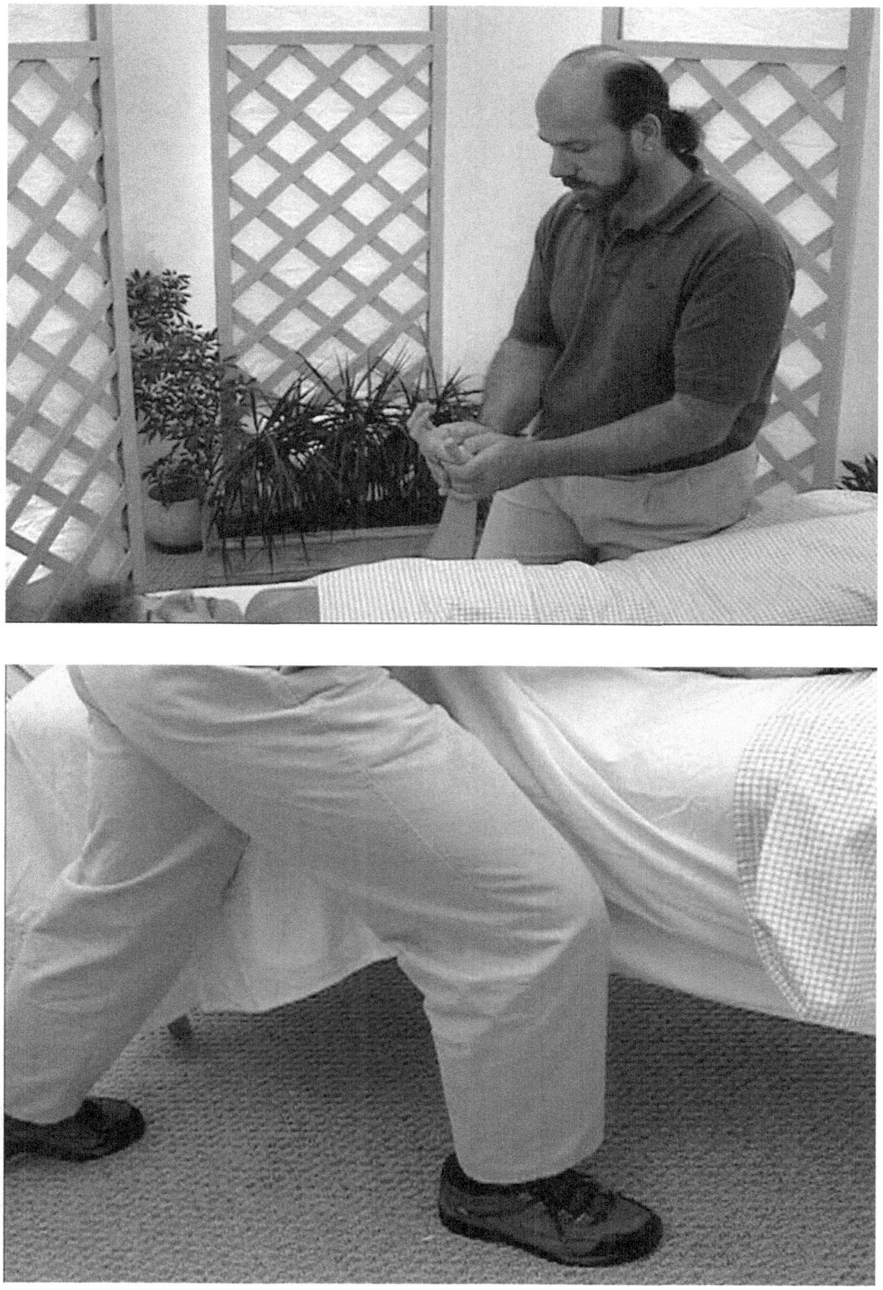

FIGURE 6–19. Good body mechanics when facing the head or foot of the table. **A.** Head and back in alignment. **B.** Legs and feet in forward leaning stance.

If you have a private massage practice, you will also need time to clean linens, keep client or patient records, do financial bookkeeping, and perform other chores related to having your own business.

EMOTIONAL SELF-CARE

Emotional self-care is often overlooked, but it is equally important to prevent stress and burnout. Establish and maintain clear professional boundaries. The practitioner's job is to help patients or clients, not to rescue them from their life's problems. It is useful to have a fellow practitioner with whom to discuss upsetting situations. Peer and professional supervision can help you keep clear boundaries and sort out confusing situations that come up in the practitioner–recipient relationship.

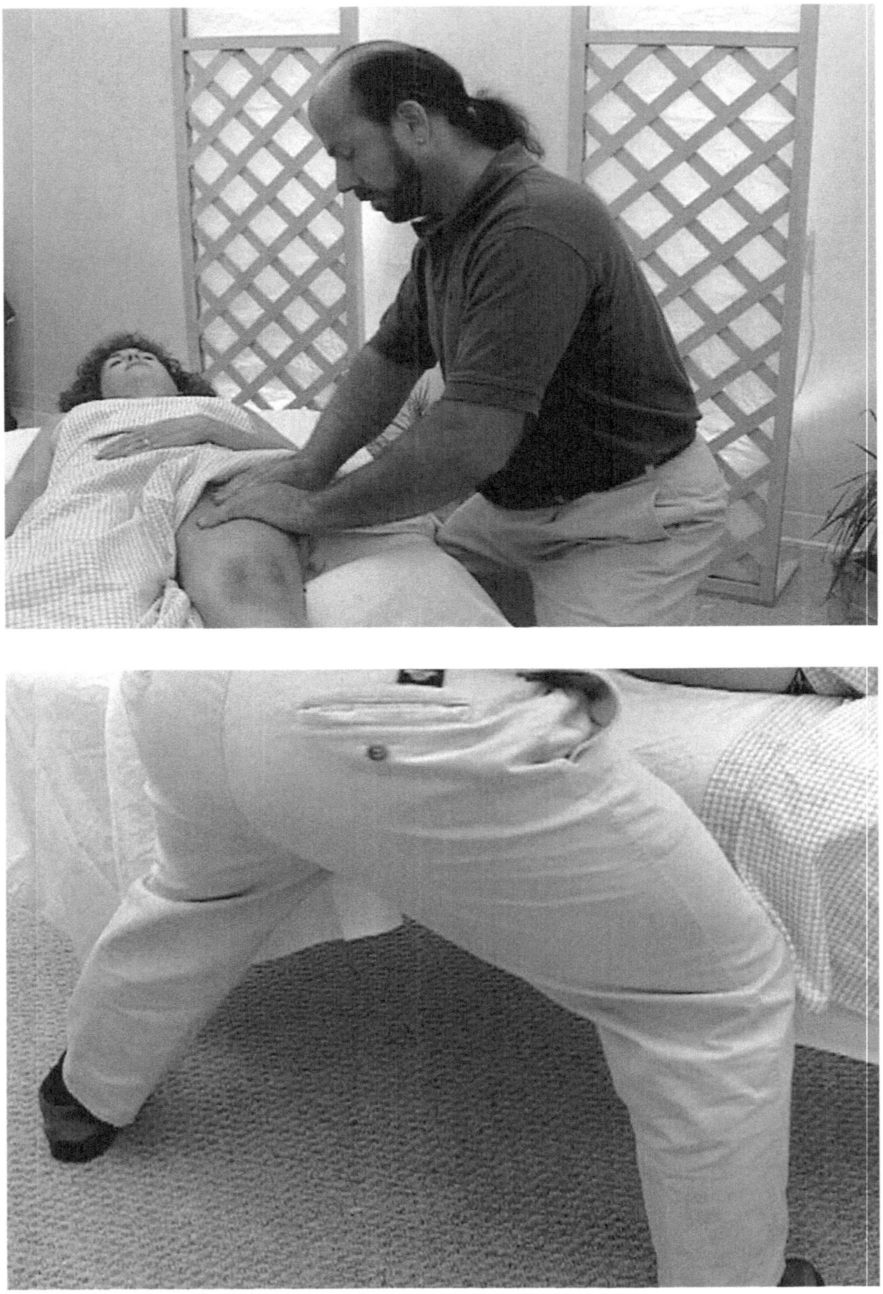

FIGURE 6–20. Good body mechanics when facing table directly. A. Head and back in alignment. B. Legs and feet in horse stance.

PERFORMANCE ELEMENTS

Length of the Session

Session lengths vary depending on the goals and the setting in which it is given. For example, massage sessions for general health purposes last from 30 to 90 minutes, with 60 minutes the most common. This is typical at a health club, spa, or private massage therapy practice. Chair massage given to employees of a business may last 15–20 minutes. Athletes may receive pre-event massage for 15 minutes and general maintenance massage for 30 minutes to 1 hour. Massage that is part of a larger therapy session (e.g., physical therapy) may last as little as 10 minutes. Guidelines for session length will be given for each type of massage described later in this book.

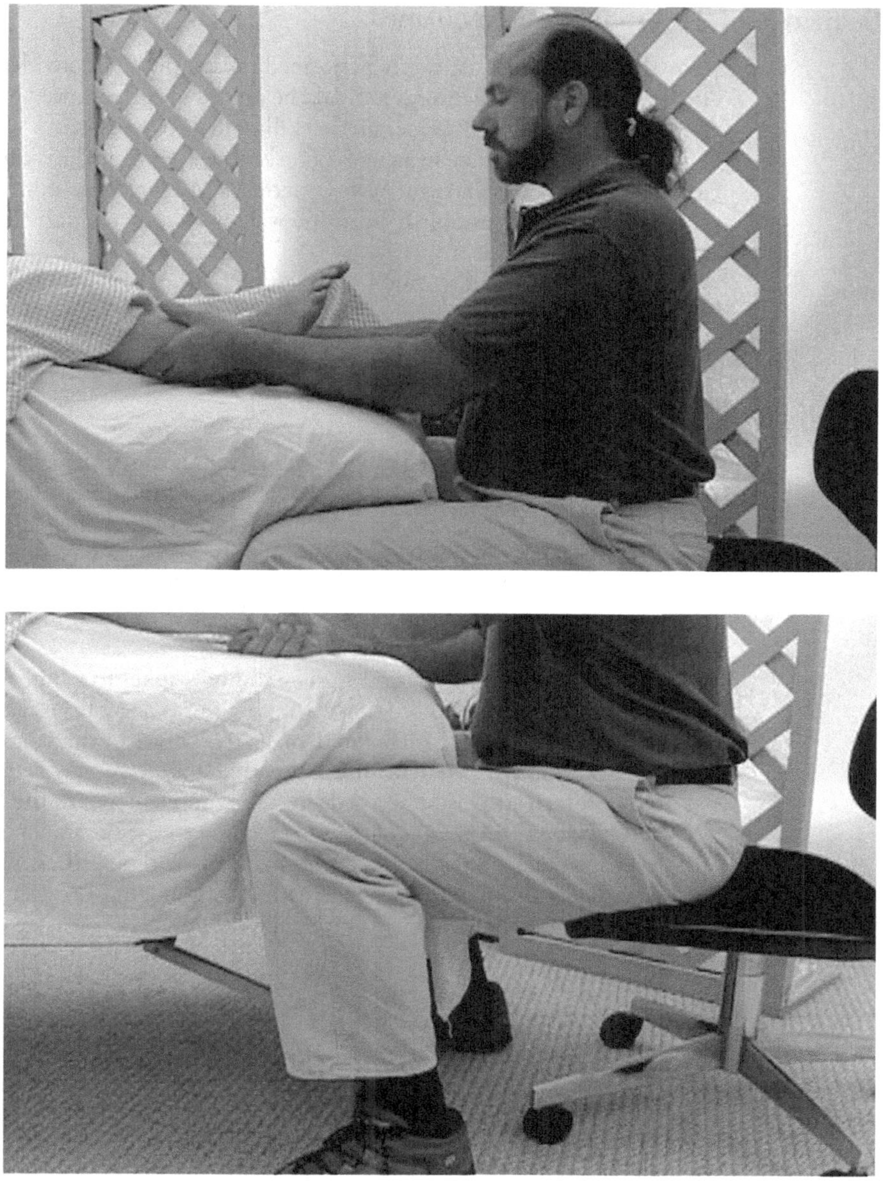

FIGURE 6–21. Good body mechanics for sitting on chair while performing massage. **A.** Sit with back and head in alignment. **B.** Sit near edge of chair with feet flat on floor.

Amount of Lubricant

Generally speaking, you should use the least amount of lubricant needed to get the job done. Too much lubricant prevents firm contact, and the hands will only slip and slide over the surface of the skin. This is especially true when doing more specific work on small areas and when friction is used. Too little lubricant can cause skin irritation, especially in people with thick hair on the arms, legs, or chest, and in people with fair skin. More oil may be used when warming up an area with sliding movements and then wiped off for techniques that are best performed with less lubricant. Recipients of massage may benefit from extra lubricant to relieve dry skin. Additional lotion or oil may be applied after massaging a particular body area as a moisturizer.

The face is an area where little, if any, lubricant should be used. Care should be taken not to get oil or lotion in the hair when working on the neck. Recipients may want to wear surgical or shower caps to keep lubricants out of the hair.

Lubricant should be absorbed into the skin, or wiped off of the skin, before clothes are put back on. Some substances can stain clothes, or certain scents may be difficult to wash out. Rubbing with a dry towel will remove most lotions and oils, and alcohol may be used when more thorough removal is desired.

Sequence of Techniques and Routines

Individual techniques are rarely performed in isolation, but are blended into sequences for the desired effects. Deep specific techniques should be preceded and followed by superficial warming ones. Smooth transitions between techniques give a skillful feel to a session.

Routines are regular sequences of techniques performed in almost the same way each time. A routine may also include a regular sequence of body sections addressed during a session. Experienced practitioners usually establish a routine way of working, which they vary depending on the needs of the receiver.

Routines are useful to establish a smooth pattern of working and are an effective way to learn new massage techniques. Routines will be presented for some of the different approaches discussed later in this book.

Specificity and Direction

Much of massage is performed in a general way and over larger areas of the body. For example, long sliding strokes are often performed over the whole back, and muscle *groups* are kneaded and stretched as opposed to individual muscles. This more general way of applying techniques is appropriate for effects such as warming an area, eliciting the relaxation response (a total body reaction), or relaxing a muscle group.

The **direction** of technique application may be expressed in terms of general anatomical terminology (e.g., proximal, distal, medial, lateral), or in relation to a specific body structure (e.g., toward the muscle attachment).

For example, when performing deep sliding strokes to a limb, always move in the direction of venous flow, that is, distal to proximal. Moving fluids away from the heart, or against venous flow, can cause backflow of blood, which can damage the valves in the veins.

Lighter sliding movements using superficial pressure may be performed proximal to distal. These are used as return strokes between deep sliding movements to the limbs distal to proximal. They may also be used when finishing an area before going to the next area of the body.

Massage practitioners are said to be working with **specificity** if they focus their use of techniques on a specific condition and in a small area (e.g., relieving a trigger point with thumb pressure, or deep transverse friction on a tendon). This requires thorough knowledge of anatomic structures and good palpation skills.

Pressure, Rhythm, and Pacing

Pressure, rhythm, and pacing describe different qualities of applying massage techniques. These qualities will vary with the desired effect of the session, of a sequence of techniques, or of a single technique.

Pressure is related to the force used in applying techniques and to the degree of compaction of tissues as the technique is applied. The amount of pressure used in any one situation will depend on the intended effect and the tolerance or desires of the recipient. Generally speaking, when working an area, pressure should be applied lightly at first then more deeply if desired, then finishing lightly. This allows tissues to be warmed and prepared gradually, and the body to adjust better to the cessation of deep pressure. If too much pressure is used too quickly on a specific area, tissue damage and bruising may result. Too light pressure may cause tickling, and too deep pressure may elicit a tensing response. Both effects are undesirable.

Rhythm refers to a recurring pattern of movement with a specific cadence, beat, or accent. Rhythm may be described as smooth, flowing, or uneven. Rhythm is important when applying techniques generally and in sequence, as with sliding movements and kneading. Working specifically slows or stops the rhythm, as when you slow down to press a trigger point or acupoint. Each massage practitioner has his or her own rhythm for working, which is developed over time. A smooth, flowing, and regular rhythm helps to elicit relaxation in the receiver. An uneven rhythm may be stimulating, or in some cases distracting, to a receiver. Avoid breaking contact with the skin once a session has begun. Abruptly taking the hands off of the body can be unpleasant to the recipient.

Pacing refers to the speed of performing techniques. Generally, a slower pace is more relaxing, while a faster pace more stimulating. Choice of pace depends on the desired effect.

It is the skillful blending of all of these performance elements that comprise the art of massage.

SUMMARY

The therapeutic relationship involves an implicit agreement regarding the roles of the practitioner and the receiver of massage. Professional boundaries help keep those roles clear. Maintaining boundaries involves avoiding dual relationships, being aware of the potential effects of transference and counter-transference, and staying within your scope of practice.

Professional demeanor also helps establish the professional nature of the relationship, and inspires confidence. The practitioner's clothing is neat, clean, and modest, and jewelry minimal. The practitioner and the surrounding space are free of offensive odors. Professional tone is set through appropriate language.

Touch is the primary mode of interaction during massage. From a holistic perspective, what may seem to be only physical touch can have profound effects on the mind, emotions, and spirit. Knowledge of the human need for touch and its cultural implications gives the practitioner insight for better understanding clients and patients. Practitioners prepare to give massage by being aware of intention to be caring and compassionate, and by becoming calm and focused. Self-care techniques can help limit the degree to which practitioners absorb negative "vibes" from receivers.

It is the practitioner's challenge to create openness in the receiver to the touch of massage. Factors like cultural background and history of abuse need to be considered when putting receivers at ease. Practitioners must remain aware of the potential for transference and counter-transference related to touch. Sexual touch is never ethical in a professional setting.

Permission to touch should be sought before massaging vulnerable areas. Informed consent involves describing the proposed action, explaining its intent and what to expect, and asking permission to proceed. The recipient always has the option of saying no, either before or during the application.

Cross-gender situations necessitate special clarity about the non-sexual nature of massage. Clear boundaries and professional demeanor are keys to addressing gender considerations that arise during a massage session. The seven-step intervention model is a procedure for responding to misbehavior by a client.

The appropriate level of verbal interaction during massage depends on the purpose of the session and the needs of the receiver. Getting feedback from the receiver to ensure their health and safety is desirable. Practitioners should remain present and supportive if a receiver experiences an emotional release, and remain clear about the limits of their scope of practice. Since the primary mode of communication in massage is touch, usually less talk is better.

Information about the client or patient is kept confidential. Exceptions include consultation with another health professional, in emergencies or as required by law. The HIPAA Privacy Rule is a federal standard to protect confidentiality of medical records.

A good massage table is adjustable for height and has an adjustable face cradle. Massage chairs are specially made for massage of clothed clients and also have many adjustments. Good massage equipment is a wise investment.

Important factors to consider in setting up the massage space are comfortable room temperature, fresh air quality, indirect lighting, peaceful sounds, private dressing arrangements, and overall cleanliness and neatness. Topical substances used in massage include liniments, oils, and lotions. Practitioners may mix ingredients to get properties that enhance their work. A wide selection of topical substances is available from manufacturers.

Receivers are positioned on the table for comfort, safety, and access to areas to be massaged. Table positions include supine, prone, side-lying, and reclining. The body is draped with a sheet for modesty and warmth. The genitals and women's breasts are draped at all times. Body regions are uncovered before being massaged and recovered afterward. In some situations such as sports events and for chair massage, receivers remain clothed and draping is not used.

The practitioner's hands are clean, nails trimmed, and jewelry that might scratch the receiver removed. Injury to hands is avoided by conditioning exercises, proper technique and adequate rest. Injury to thumbs is minimized by applying pressure through the joints and not while the thumb is abducted. Wrists are held in neutral position, and hyperextension and pressure on wrists avoided.

Good body mechanics involves keeping the back and neck in good alignment, and using the legs to generate power. Martial arts stances, such as the forward-leaning and horse stances, are effective for keeping good body alignment. Table height is adjusted to facilitate healthy body mechanics.

A healthy schedule for massage includes no more than 20 one-hour sessions per week and no more than five in one day. Adequate breaks between sessions helps avoid strain on the body. Emotional self-care helps prevent stress and burnout.

Session lengths vary depending on the goals of the session and the setting, and range from 15 to 90 minutes. One hour is a typical time for full-body table massage. Chair massage given on site generally lasts 15–20 minutes.

The amount of lubricant used for massage depends on the substance used and the techniques performed. Generally speaking, use the least amount needed to get the job done.

Massage techniques are performed in sequences for specific effects. Practitioners develop routine ways of working that are varied to address each client's needs. Elements of technique application include direction, specificity, pressure, rhythm, and pacing. It is the skillful blending of these performance elements that comprise the art of massage.

A look ahead . . .

The guidelines outlined in this chapter support the actual application of techniques. Chapter 7 describes in detail the Western massage technique categories of effleurage, petrissage, tapotement, friction, and vibration.

REFERENCES

Benjamin, B. E., and Sohnen-Moe, C. (2003) *The ethics of touch.* Tucson, AZ: SMA Inc.

Dixon, Marian W. (2001). *Body mechanics and self-care manual.* Upper Saddle River, NJ: Prentice Hall.

Field, T. (2001). *Touch.* Cambridge, MA: The MIT Press.

Frye, B. (2000). *Body mechanics for manual therapists: A functional approach to self-care and injury prevention.* Stanwood, WA: Freytag Publishing.

McIntosh, N. (1999). *The educated heart: Professional guidelines for massage therapists, bodyworkers and movement teachers.* Memphis, TN: Decatur Bainbridge Press.

Montagu, A. (1978). *Touching: The human significance of the skin,* 2nd ed. New York: Harper & Row.

National Certification Board for Therapeutic Massage and Bodywork (2000) *Standards of Practice.* Retrieved March 2003 (*www.ncbtmb.org*).

WEB SITES

HIPAA Privacy Guidelines (www.hhs.gov/ocr/hipaa)

National Certification Board for Therapeutic Massage and Bodywork (www.ncbtmb.org)

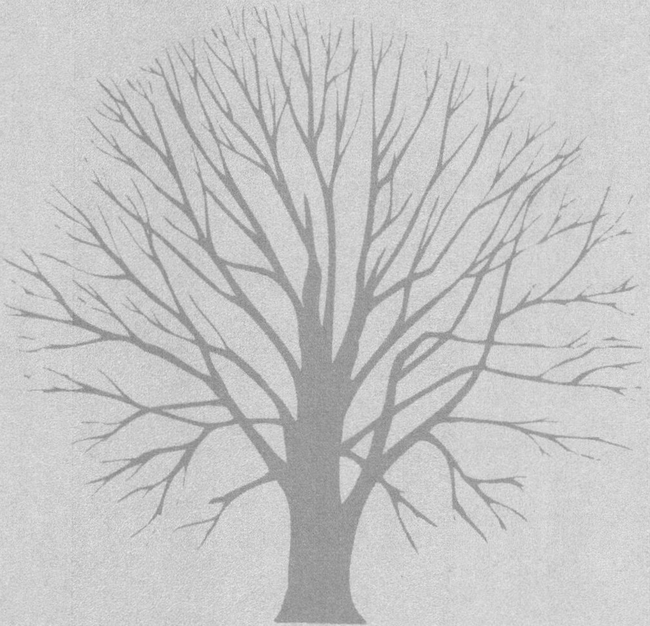

II

Western Massage

CHAPTER SEVEN

Western Massage Techniques

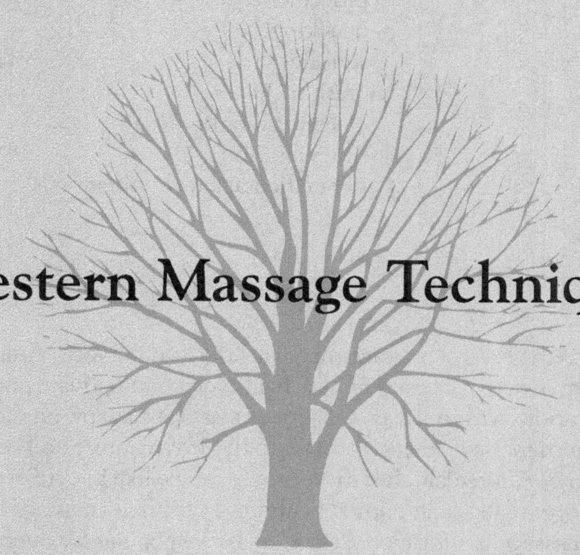

LEARNING OUTCOMES

After studying this chapter, the student will have information to:

1. Describe the Western massage technique categories.
2. Choose different techniques for their effects.
3. Perform variations of basic techniques.
4. Vary rhythm, pacing, and pressure for different effects.

KEY TERMS/CONCEPTS

- Swedish massage
- Western massage
- Western massage techniques
- Effleurage
  - basic sliding effluerage
  - stripping
  - shingles effleurage
  - bilateral tree stroking
  - three-count stroking of trapezius
  - horizontal stroking
  - Mennell's superficial stroking
  - nerve strokes
  - knuckling
- Petrissage
  - basic two-handed kneading
  - one-handed kneading
  - alternating one-handed kneading
  - circular two-handed petrissage
  - alternating fingers-to-thumb petrissage
  - skin rollling
  - compression
  - rolling
- Friction
  - superficial warming friction
  - sawing
  - deep friction
  - deep transverse friction
  - Cyriax friction

LINK LIBRARY TERMS

Swedish Massage • *Massage Business* • *Massage Regulations*

MEDIALINK

A companion CD-ROM, included free with each new copy of this book, supplements the techniques presented in this chapter. Insert the CD-ROM to watch video clips of massage techniques being demonstrated. This multimedia feature is designed to help you add a new dimension to your learning.

Tapotement
- hacking
- rapping
- cupping
- clapping
- slapping
- tapping
- pincement
- quacking
- squishes

Vibration
- electric vibrator
- fine vibration
- light effleurage with vibration
- shaking
- jostling

Touch without movement
- passive touch
- direct pressure
- ischemic compression

WESTERN MASSAGE

Western massage is the basis of massage therapy performed in North America and Europe today. It is the most common form of massage found in spas, health clubs and private practice, and is the foundation for therapeutic applications within the professions of massage therapy, physical therapy, and nursing.

Today's Western massage traces its origin to the 19th century and the work of Pehr Ling of Sweden and Johann Mezger of Amsterdam. It is the legacy of people like Ling (Swedish movements), Mezger (classic massage), Kellogg (massage in natural healing), McMillan (massage in physical therapy), and many others. **Swedish massage** is a form of Western massage popular for over 100 years. See Chapter 2 for a more detailed view of the history of Western massage in conventional medicine and natural healing.

The effects, benefits, and indications for Western massage are understood in terms of Western concepts of anatomy and physiology and Western notions of health and disease. This is in contrast to Chinese medicine and Ayurveda (India). The techniques of Western massage are recognized as valuable for improving circulation of blood and lymph, relaxing muscles, improving joint mobility, inducing general relaxation, and promoting healthy skin. See Chapters 3 and 4 for a more thorough discussion of massage and Western science.

WESTERN MASSAGE TECHNIQUES

Western massage techniques fall into seven categories: effleurage, petrissage, friction, tapotement, vibration, touch without movement, and joint movements. The first five techniques are the classic massage categories, and the last two complete the picture of massage therapy as practiced today. These are the same categories used by J. Harvey Kellogg in the early 20th century to describe the "procedures of massage" (Kellogg 1929). The categories of Western massage are useful for thinking about how techniques are performed, their physiological effects, and common uses.

This chapter will describe the techniques of soft tissue manipulation, while joint movements will be described in Chapter 8. Keep in mind that there is an endless number of variations of massage techniques, and that the ones presented in this text are merely representative of many possibilities. Always perform techniques taking into consideration endangerment sites, contraindications and cautions, as described in Chapter 5, and using good hand and body mechanics, as presented in Chapter 6.

EFFLEURAGE

Effleurage techniques slide or glide over the skin with a smooth, continuous motion. Pressure may be light to moderate, as when applying oil or warming an area, or may be deep, as when facilitating venous return in heavily muscled areas. Experienced practitioners can perform effleurage in many different ways to suit the body area and to evoke specific effects.

Effleurage is perhaps the most versatile of the Western techniques and is used most frequently. For example, effleurage is usually used to begin a session, especially when oil or lotion is applied. It accustoms the receiver to the touch of the practitioner. It is used as a connecting or transition technique. It is often performed as a break from more specific techniques, to move gracefully from one area to another, to conclude work on an area, or to end the session.

While performing effleurage, a practitioner skilled in palpation can assess the general condition of the soft tissues and the firmness and shape of the musculature. Sensitive fingers may find areas of tension or holding. In some cases where there is pain, effleurage may be the only technique employed.

Effleurage can affect the recipient's body and mind in a variety of ways. The qualities of pressure, pacing, and rhythm may be varied for different effects. For example, when effleurage is performed with moderate pressure, slowly and smoothly on the back, it may stimulate the parasympathetic nervous system and evoke the relaxation response. It enhances venous return in the limbs when performed with moderate to deep pressure moving distal to proximal. Deep effleurage may also provide a passive stretch to a muscle group.

Variations of Effleurage

Basic sliding effleurage is performed with the palms and fingers of the hands, the thumbs, fists, or forearms. When using the palms and fingers, mold the hands to the surface of the body. This provides full contact, as shown in basic effleurage of the leg in Figure 7–1. The thumbs may be used in small places like between the metatarsals of the foot, as in Figure 7–2. More pressure may be applied using the forearms or fists in broad places like the back and hamstrings, as seen in Figure 7–3.

Stripping is a type of basic sliding effleurage performed with deep pressure along the length of the muscle fibers, typically done with the thumb. See Figure 7–4. It is commonly performed on the long muscles in the arms and legs, and on the cervical muscles. Stripping is specific to a particular muscle and usually follows the muscle to its site of attachment. If the muscle is wider than the thumb, stripping is performed in parallel lines to cover the entire muscle. Stripping separates and helps lengthen muscle fibers. It is a useful technique to follow direct pressure to trigger points.

Shingles effleurage refers to alternate stroking, first one hand then the other in continuous motion, with the strokes overlaying each other like shingles on a roof. One hand always remains in contact with the receiver as the other hand is lifted. This gives the feeling of unbroken contact. Shingles effleurage is commonly applied to the back with hands parallel to the spine and to the direction of movement as shown in Figure 7–5. It may also be performed with hands perpendicular to the spine and to the direction of movement.

Bilateral tree stroking traces a pattern reminiscent of branches growing out from both sides of the trunk of a tree. It is usually performed on the back starting with the hands on either side of the spine, and moving laterally across the shoulders or around the sides as far as you can reach. This movement is repeated as you progress to cover the entire back. It may be performed standing at the head and progressing from the shoulders toward the hips as shown in Figure 7–6. It may also be done standing at the side moving from hips to shoulders.

Three-count stroking of the trapezius is performed in three strokes, alternating hands with each movement. Count one begins at the origin of the lower trapezius and moves toward its insertion in the shoulder. Count two begins just as the first stroke concludes, moving from the origin of the middle trapezius toward the insertion. As soon as the first hand has completed its slide over the lower trapezius, it lifts and crosses over to the origin of the upper trapezius to begin count three. Count three moves

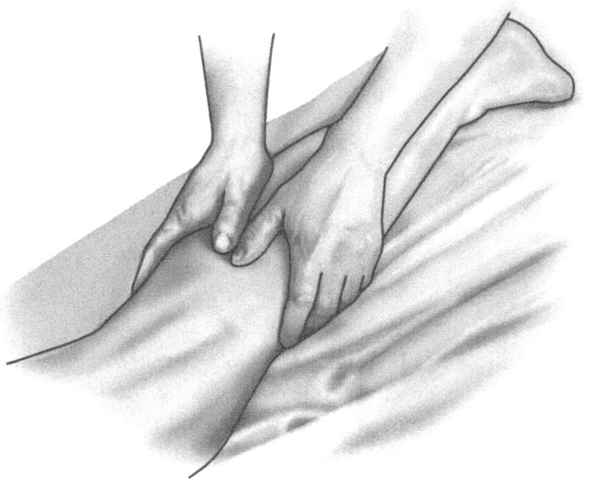

FIGURE 7–1. Basic sliding effleurage using the palms of the hands provides full contact with the leg.

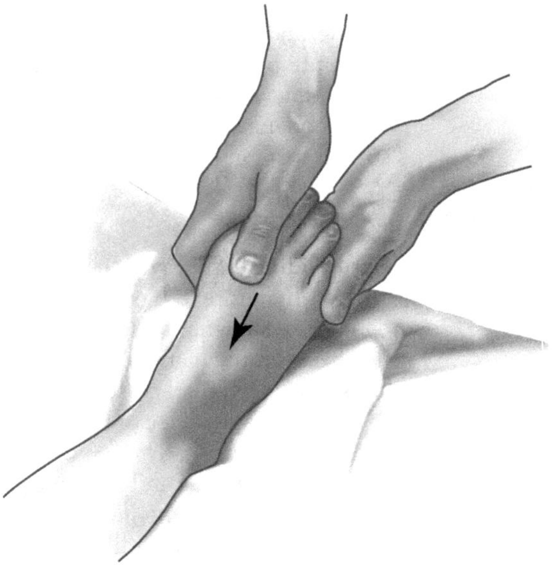

FIGURE 7–2. Basic sliding effleurage using the thumb gets into the small spaces between the metatarsals of the foot.

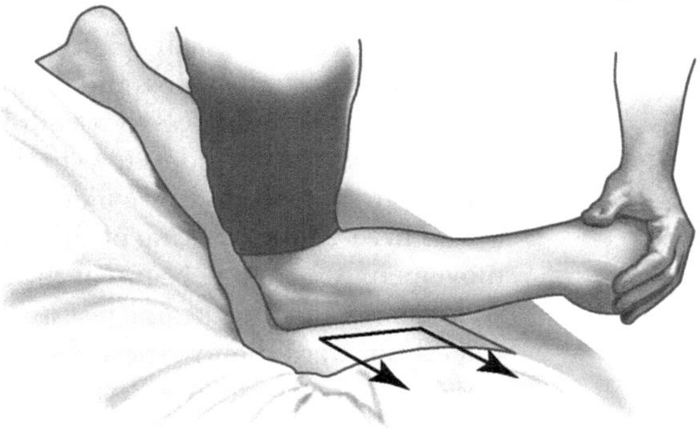

FIGURE 7–3. Basic sliding effleurage using the forearm applies broad, deep pressure to an area.

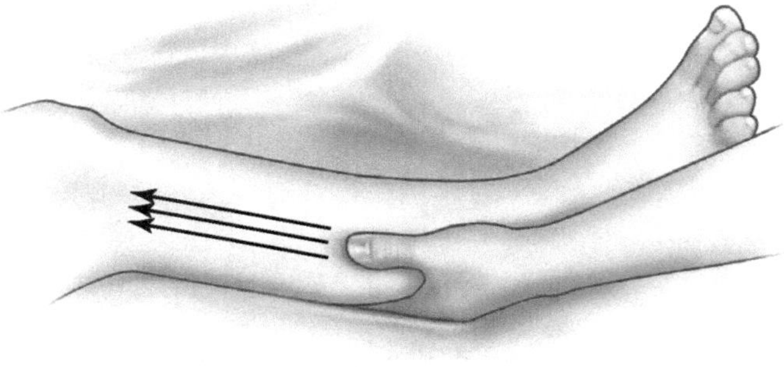

FIGURE 7–4. Stripping is performed with deep pressure along the length of a muscle to its attachment. Parallel strips are applied to cover the entire muscle width.

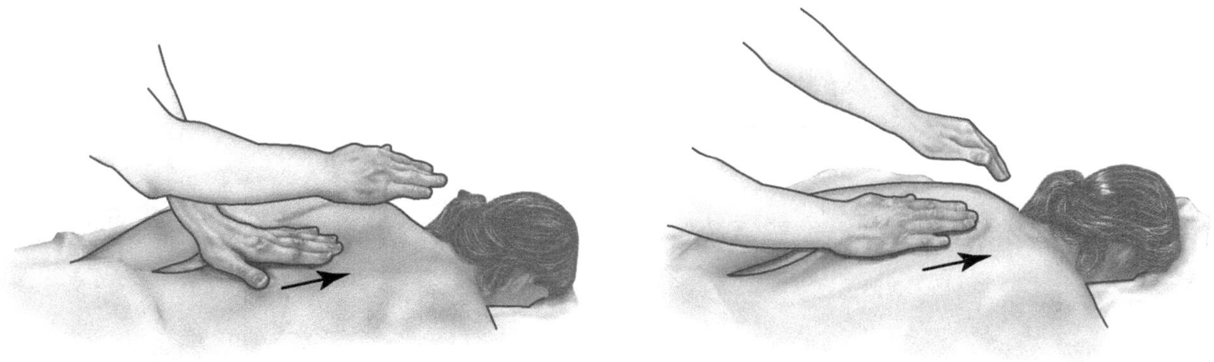

FIGURE 7–5. Shingles effleurage with hands parallel to the spine and to the direction of movement.

laterally to the insertion to complete the sequence. Figure 7–7 shows how the stroke is performed from the opposite side. The entire three-count sequence is repeated several times. This particular method of stroking the whole trapezius is rhythmic and relaxing when well done. It must be timed so that in spite of the lost contact as each hand is raised, the receiver feels unbroken contact.

Horizontal stroking is usually applied to broad, rounded areas like the thigh, abdomen, or lower back. The movement is across the width of the body part, rather than over the length. Horizontal stroking may be considered a hybrid form of effleurage and petrissage because in addition to sliding, there may be a lifting and pressing motion.

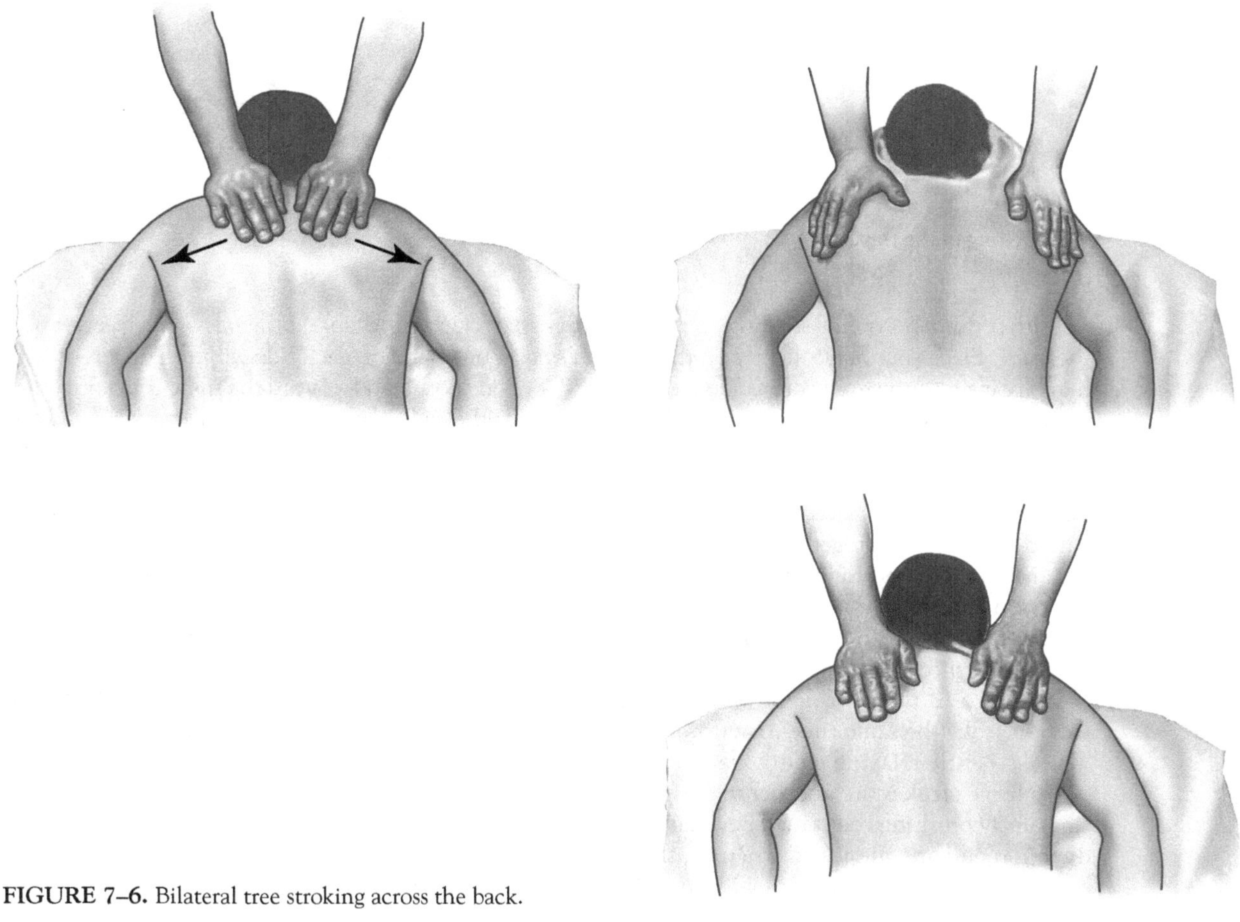

FIGURE 7–6. Bilateral tree stroking across the back.

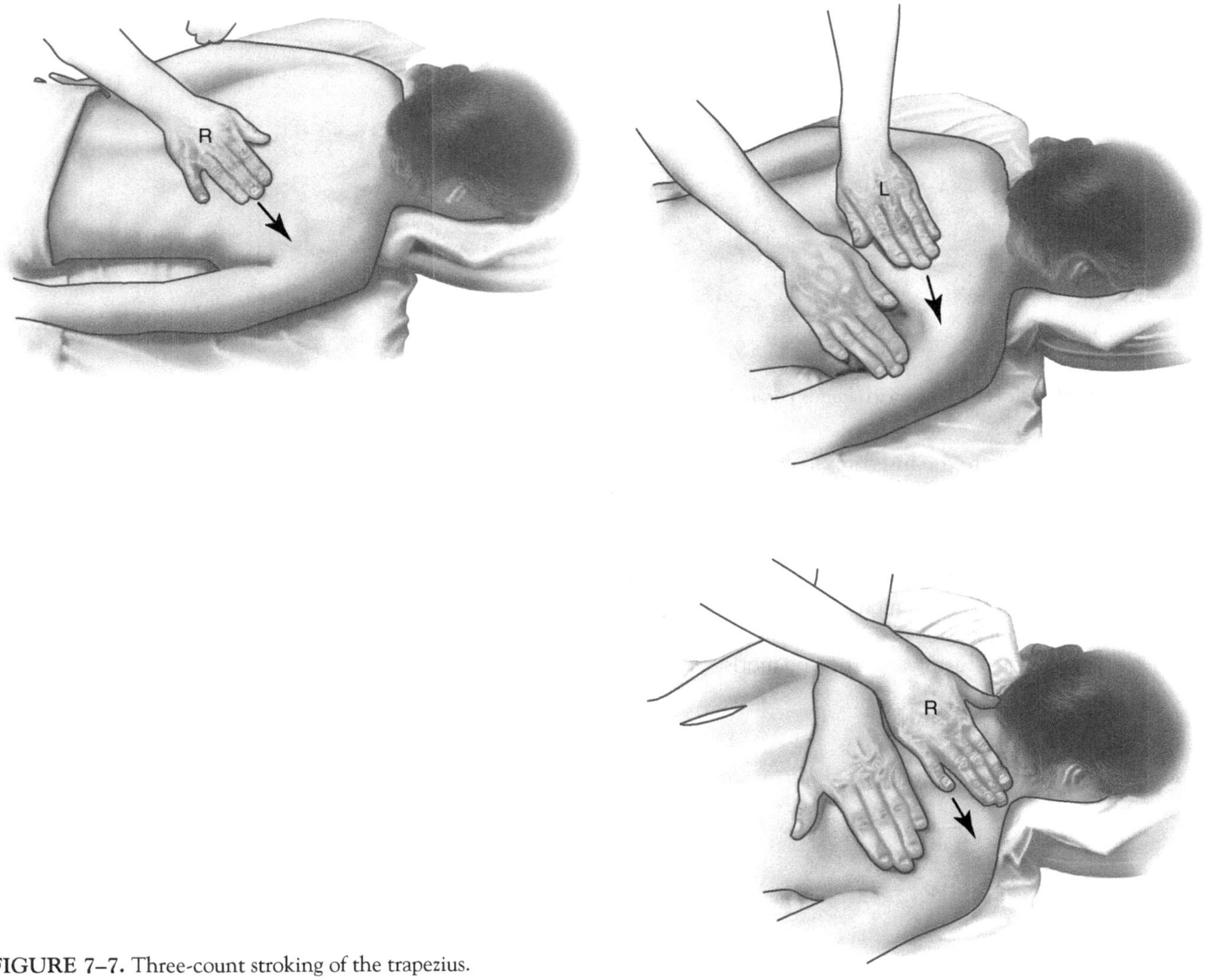

FIGURE 7–7. Three-count stroking of the trapezius.

To perform horizontal stroking on the lower back, stand facing the table at the side of the receiver near the waist. Place your hands lightly on the receiver's back, one hand on each side with the fingers of both hands pointing away from you, as shown in Figure 7–8. Slide both hands toward the spine using firm pressure, and then continue the movement all the way to the other side. One hand will move forward and one hand backward, crossing at the spine. The motion is then reversed without changing the position of the hands. As the hands slide from side to side, they execute a lifting and pushing together of the soft tissues. No pressure should be placed over the spinous processes as the hands pass over them. Greatest pressure comes with the lift and push together of the tissues as the hands move upward and inward to meet and cross over.

Mennell's superficial stroking is very light effleurage usually performed on a limb, moving in one direction either centripetally (distal to proximal) or centrifugally (proximal to distal), but never in both directions. To perform it on the arm with the recipient prone, slide your hand from the recipient's wrist to the shoulder while maintaining full contact and using the lightest pressure possible. See Figure 7–9. Return to the starting position through the air just over the skin surface in a controlled even rhythm. Take the same time to perform the return movement as the stroke that contacts the receiver. This is a gentle relaxing technique.

Nerve strokes are another very light effleurage movement. They are performed with the fingertips gently brushing the skin. They may also be done on top of the drape. Nerve strokes can go in any direction and are often used when finishing a section of the body or when ending the session. A few seconds of nerve strokes are usually enough to create a relaxing effect.

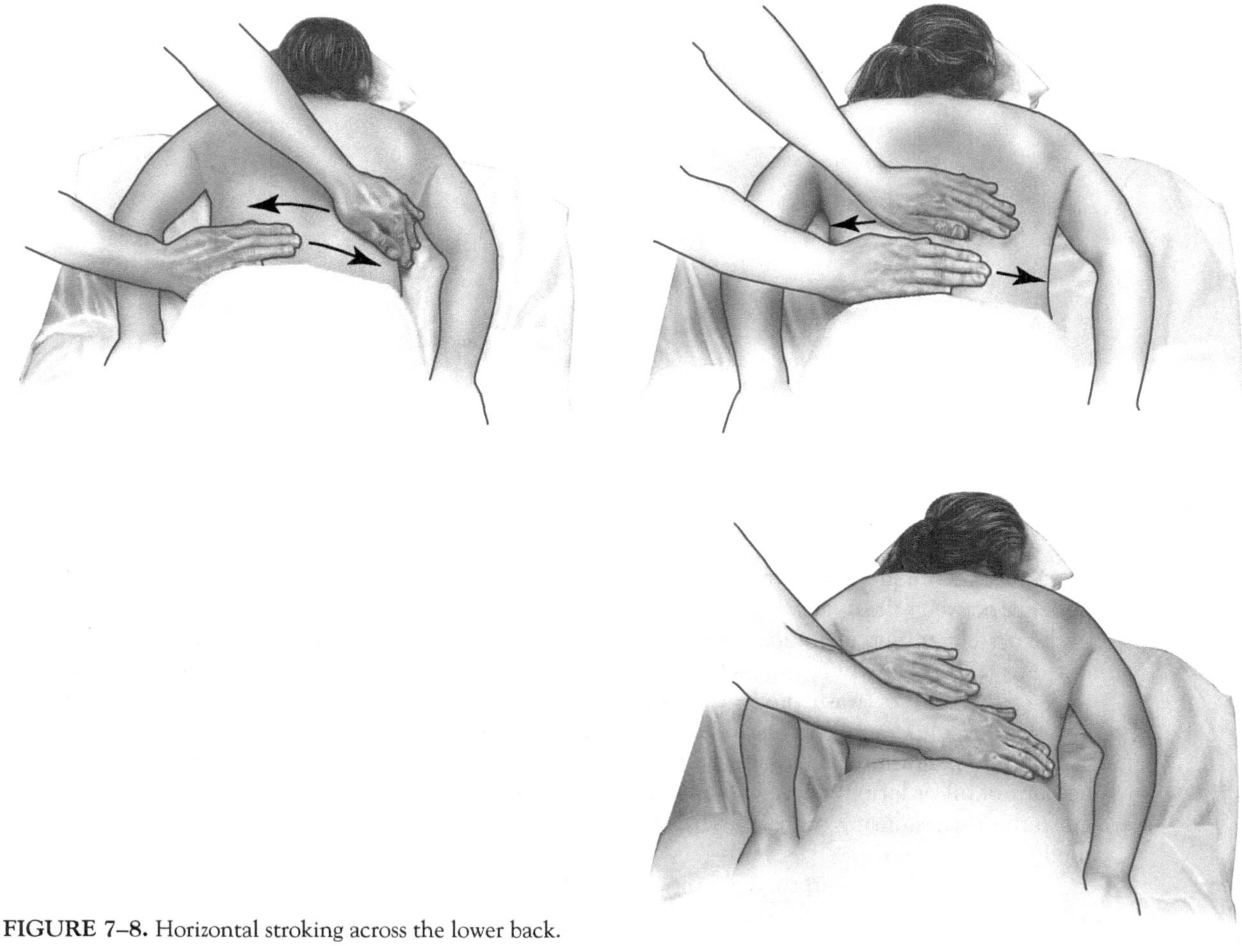

FIGURE 7–8. Horizontal stroking across the lower back.

Knuckling is an effleurage variation taught by Hoffa in which the pressure is first applied with the back of the fingers in a loose fist, gradually turning the fist over as it slides over the skin, and finishing with the palm of the hand. See Figure 7–10. Hoffa describes knuckling further.

> Gradually bring the hand from plantar (flexion) to dorsal (hypertension) flexion. Pressure is not continuous, but swells up and down, starting lightly and becoming stronger, then decreasing again in pressure. The hand must not adhere to the part but should glide over it lightly. Knuckling should only be used where there is enough room for the hand to be applied (Hoffa 1900).

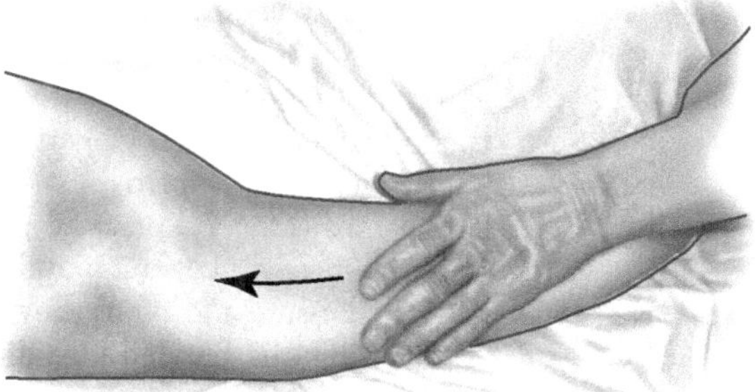

FIGURE 7–9. Mennell's superficial stroking over the arm with the recipient prone.

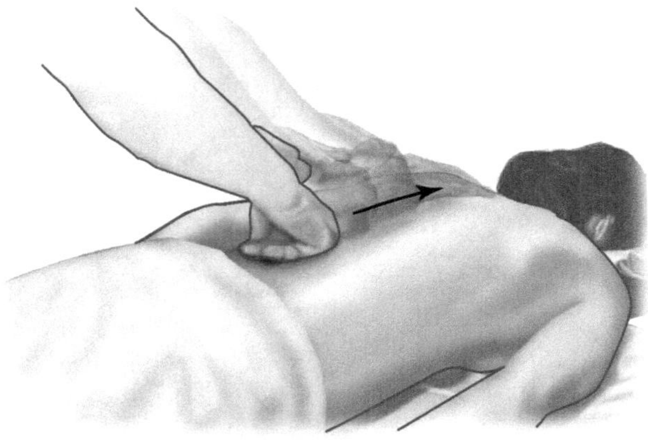

FIGURE 7–10. Knuckling effleurage (knuckle to palm) performed on the back.

PETRISSAGE

Petrissage techniques lift, wring, or squeeze soft tissues in a kneading motion or press or roll the tissues under or between the hands. Petrissage may be performed with one or two hands, depending on the size of the muscle or muscle group. There is minimal sliding over the skin except perhaps in moving from one area to another when using lubricant. The motions of petrissage serve to "milk" a muscle of accumulated metabolites (waste products), increase local circulation, and assist venous return. Petrissage may also help separate muscle fibers and evoke muscular relaxation.

Before performing petrissage, prepare and warm an area, usually with effleurage. Use only a small amount of oil or lotion when warming up the area, since too much lubricant will make it difficult to grasp the tissues during petrissage. If you are working without lubricant, light compressions may be used to warm an area.

Care should be taken to avoid pinching or bruising the tissues and to not work too long in one area. Adjust the amount of pressure used to match the condition of the recipient. Muscular and physically strong receivers will enjoy harder pressure, while less pressure should be used for smaller or frail individuals.

Variations of Petrissage

Basic two-handed kneading is performed by lifting, squeezing, and then releasing soft tissues with hands alternating in a rhythmical motion. Graham (1884) described the fingers and hands as slipping on the skin during kneading, while Kellogg (1929) discouraged letting the hands slide. In basic kneading, tissues are lifted with the whole hand in firm contact as shown in Figure 7–11, rather than with just the fingertips. The movement is a lifting away from the underlying bone. Two-handed kneading works well on the larger muscles of the arms, shoulders, and legs.

One-handed kneading may be used on smaller limbs, for example, arms and children's legs. Place your hand around the part, picking up the muscle mass using the whole hand. The kneading movement may be described as circular—grasping the tissues on the up motion, and relaxing the hand on the down motion without losing contact. As with two-handed kneading, the rhythm should be slow and regular. Progression to a new position should follow three or four repetitions in the same place. In general, the movements should be performed distal to proximal, and effleurage may be interspersed with petrissage or may follow it, to enhance venous return.

The biceps is a good place to practice one-hand kneading. Grasp the biceps with one hand as shown in Figure 7–12. Let the muscle belly fit firmly into the palm of the hand while the thumb and fingers apply pressure and lift as they begin the kneading motion.

Alternating one-handed kneading may be used to work flexors and extensors at the same time. For example, on the upper arm, grasp the biceps with one hand and the triceps with the other hand. Alternate lifting and squeezing first the biceps and then the triceps in an even rhythm. See Figure 7–13. Perform this technique rapidly when stimulation is desired.

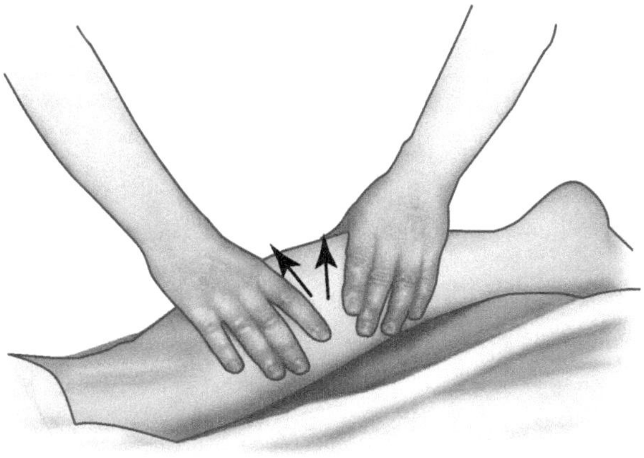

FIGURE 7–11. Basic two-handed kneading. Tissues are lifted with the whole hand in firm contact.

Circular two-handed petrissage is best performed on broad, flat areas like the back. This technique may be applied to one side of the spine after warming the area using deep effleurage. Stand facing the receiver from the side and near the hips and be ready to move along toward the head while performing the technique. Place both hands firmly on one side of the receiver's back, with the hand nearest the hips ready to start the movement over the upper portion of the gluteals. Each hand will describe a counterclockwise circle, timed so that when the hands pass each other, the soft tissues are picked up and pressed between the hands. The hands are almost *flat* as they shape themselves to the contours of the back. Pick up tissues between the hands (not with the hands) as they pass each other as shown in Figure 7–14. After about three repetitions of this technique in one place, slide the lower hand up to where the upper hand has just been working, while the upper hand slides to a new position closer to the head. Eventually, the technique progresses from lower back to upper back, ending over the shoulders. This technique may also be performed on the forehead using the thumbs.

Alternating fingers-to-thumb petrissage is very useful for following the direction of the fibers of the more superficial muscles such as the trapezius. In this technique, the soft tissues are pressed between the thumb of one hand and the first two fingers of the other hand. The hands alternate back and forth with an even rhythm.

To perform the technique, the fingers of one hand pick up the tissues and press them against the opposite thumb. At the same time, the thumb is moving toward, and pressing the tissues against, the fingers of the opposite hand. See Figure 7–15. This same motion is repeated alternating hands and working from the distal to the proximal (or lateral to medial) aspects of each muscle.

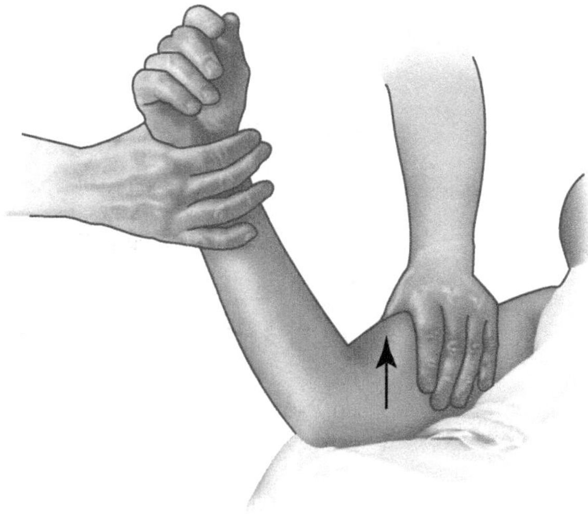

FIGURE 7–12. One-handed kneading. Tissues are lifted with the whole hand in firm contact.

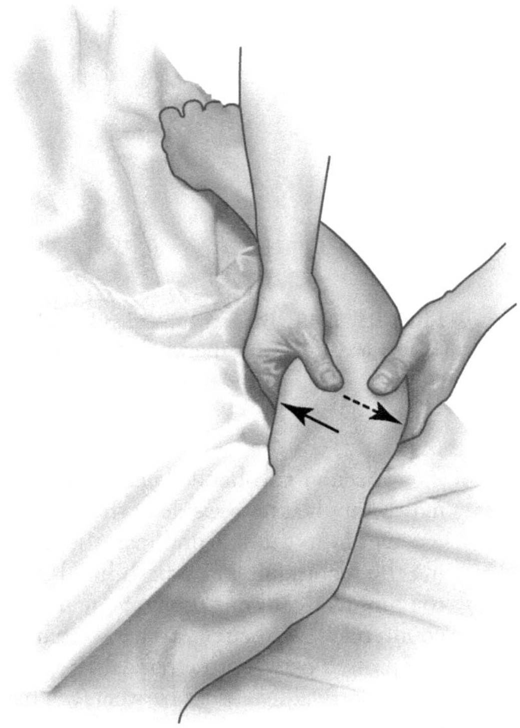

FIGURE 7–13. Alternating one-handed kneading. Alternate lifting and squeezing biceps and triceps in an even rhythm.

Skin rolling is a technique in which the skin and subcutaneous tissue are picked up between the thumb and the first two fingers and gently pulled away from the deeper tissues. Once the skin is pulled away, the thumbs may push forward, lifting the tissues in a smooth, continuous motion and causing a rolling effect. Skin rolling stretches the underlying fascia and increases superficial circulation. It is considered a basic myofascial massage technique. It is often performed on the back, but may be applied to almost any part of the body. Figure 7–16 shows skin rolling on the back.

In **compression** techniques, tissues are pressed or rolled against underlying tissues and bone in a rhythmic motion. The effects are similar to other petrissage techniques as the tissues are compressed under the hands. Figure 7–17 shows compression using the palm of one hand, while the other hand pro-

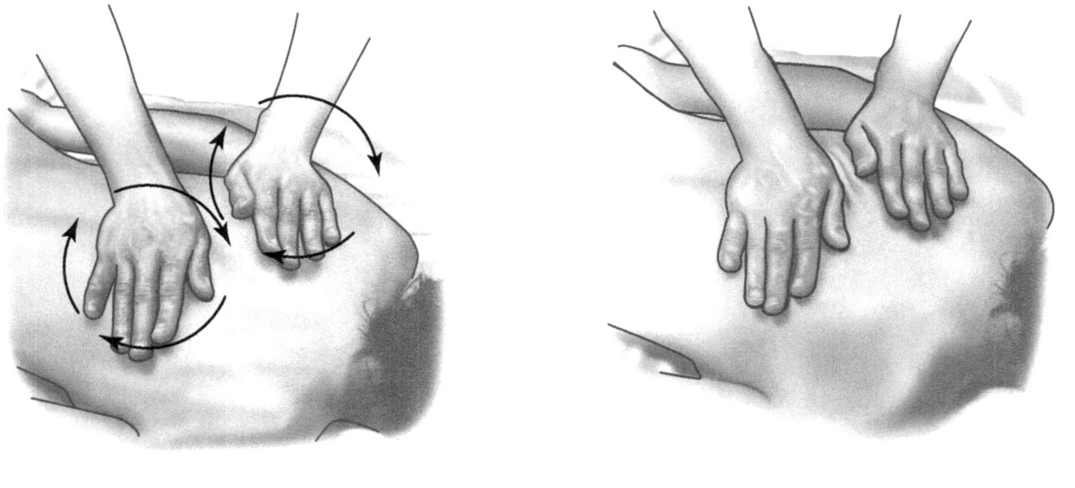

FIGURE 7–14. Circular two-handed petrissage. Tissues are picked up between the hands as they pass each other.

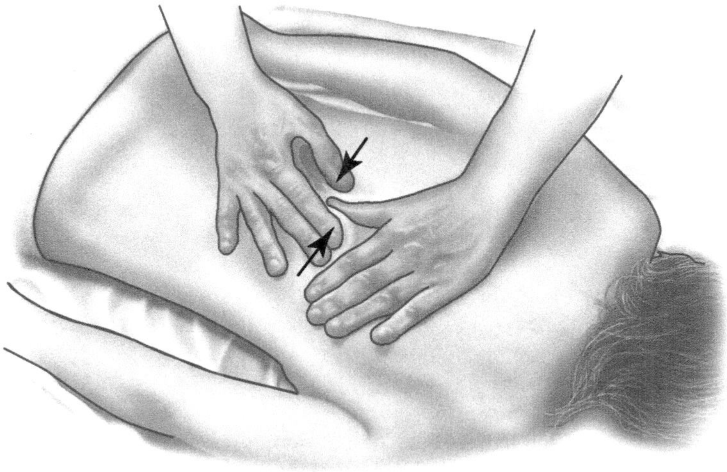

FIGURE 7–15. Alternating fingers-to-thumb petrissage. The soft tissues are pressed between the thumb of one hand and the fingers of the other hand.

vides additional force from above. Note that the heel of the top hand is placed so that it does not put pressure on the wrist of the bottom hand. The compressing force is applied through the palms, as you lean into the movement with your body weight. Avoid using just your arms and shoulders to perform compression techniques. Review the principles of good hand and body mechanics for compression in Chapter 6. A variation useful in working the buttocks is compression with a fist.

Rolling is a form of petrissage performed on the limbs. Grasp the limb lightly on opposite sides between the palms of the hands. The muscles of the limb are compressed against each other as the hands press in and perform an alternating back-and-forth motion. Rolling progresses from proximal to distal. In addition to compressing tissues, rolling causes movement in the shoulder or hip joint. The larger your hands are in proportion to the limb, the easier rolling is to perform.

FRICTION

Friction is performed by rubbing one surface over another repeatedly. For example, the hand is used to rub the skin for superficial warming, as in a traditional rubdown. The resistance to the motion provided by the surfaces creates heat and stimulates the skin.

Friction may also be created between the skin and deeper tissues. In *deep friction*, the practitioner's fingers do not move over the skin, but instead move the skin over the tissues underneath. Deep friction addresses one small area at a time and adds specificity to the massage by affecting specific structures, such as a particular section of a muscle or tendon. Cross-fiber, parallel, and circular friction are common forms of deep friction.

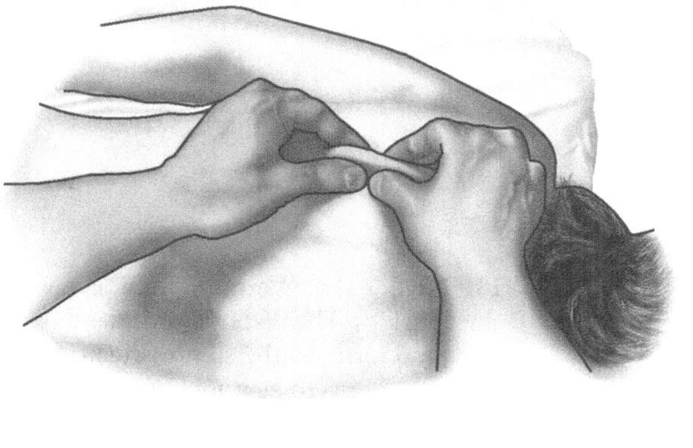

FIGURE 7–16. Skin rolling. Superficial tissues are picked up and gently pulled away from deeper tissues.

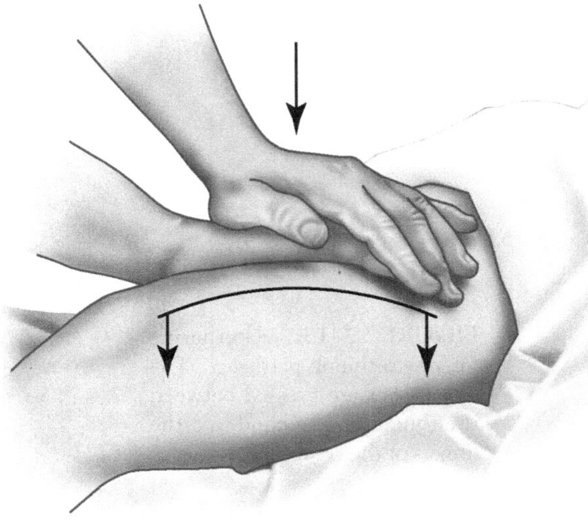

FIGURE 7–17. Compression using reinforced palm. The heel of the top hand is placed to avoid putting pressure on the wrist of the bottom hand.

Variations of Friction

In **superficial warming friction,** the palm or some other part of the practitioner's hand is rubbed briskly over the skin. This generates heat and stimulates superficial circulation. Variations of warming friction use different parts of the hands to create the friction. Greater pressure may be applied to affect deeper tissues such as when using the knuckles (Figure 7–18) and in **sawing,** also called ulnar friction (Figure 7–19). Warming friction is best done "dry" or with little lubricant, since oil or lotion reduces the amount of resistance between the two surfaces and thus reduces the amount of friction.

Deep friction is used to create movement between the deeper tissues and helps keep them from adhering to one another. For example, tissues of the musculoskeletal system are designed for smooth and efficient movement and should slide over each other without sticking. With lack of movement, stress, or trauma to an area, muscle fibers may stick together or tendons stick to tissues they come in contact with. Deep friction can help keep tissues separated and functioning smoothly.

Deep friction may also be used to create movement in tissues around joints such as the ankle and knee, reach into small spaces like the suboccipital region, or be used in areas that lack muscle bulk such as on the head. Areas that don't lend themselves well to petrissage (e.g., at tendonous attachments) may be massaged with deep friction. See Figure 7–20.

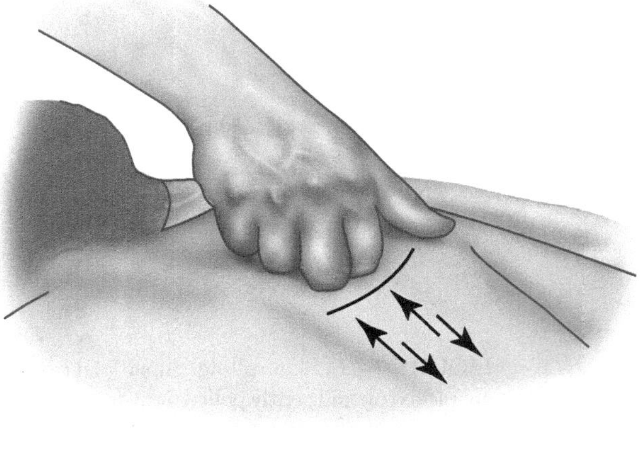

FIGURE 7–18. Warming friction using the knuckles. The first two knuckles move back and forth on the skin to create friction in the area to be warmed.

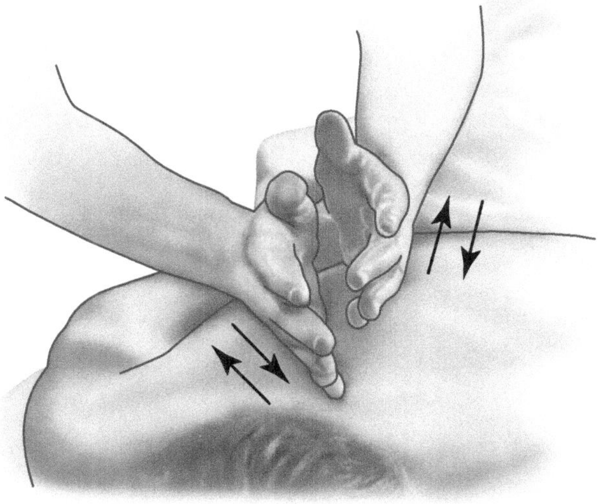

FIGURE 7–19. Warming friction created with a sawing motion, i.e., ulnar friction. The ulnar sides of the hands move back and forth on the skin to create friction in the area to be warmed.

Deep friction may be performed in a cross-fiber, parallel, or circular motion. Cross-fiber refers to deep friction applied across the direction of the fibers, while parallel friction is applied in the same direction as the fibers. Circular friction is performed using circular movements, which move the underlying tissues in many directions. Figure 7–21 shows cross-fiber friction being applied to the paraspinal muscles.

Deep friction is performed with the tips of the fingers, the thumb, or the heel of the hand, depending on the size of the surface to be covered. For example, small tendons in places such as the wrist or around the ankle may be frictioned with the fingertips. In Figure 7–22, circular friction is applied with the heel of the hand to free up the broad iliotibial band on the side of the leg.

Before deep friction is applied, the area must be warmed up thoroughly, usually with effleurage and petrissage. The lubricant used in the warming-up phase may have to be wiped off before performing friction, to allow the practitioner's hands to move the skin without sliding over it. Deep friction is a three-dimensional technique. Practitioners must be keenly aware of the depth at which they are

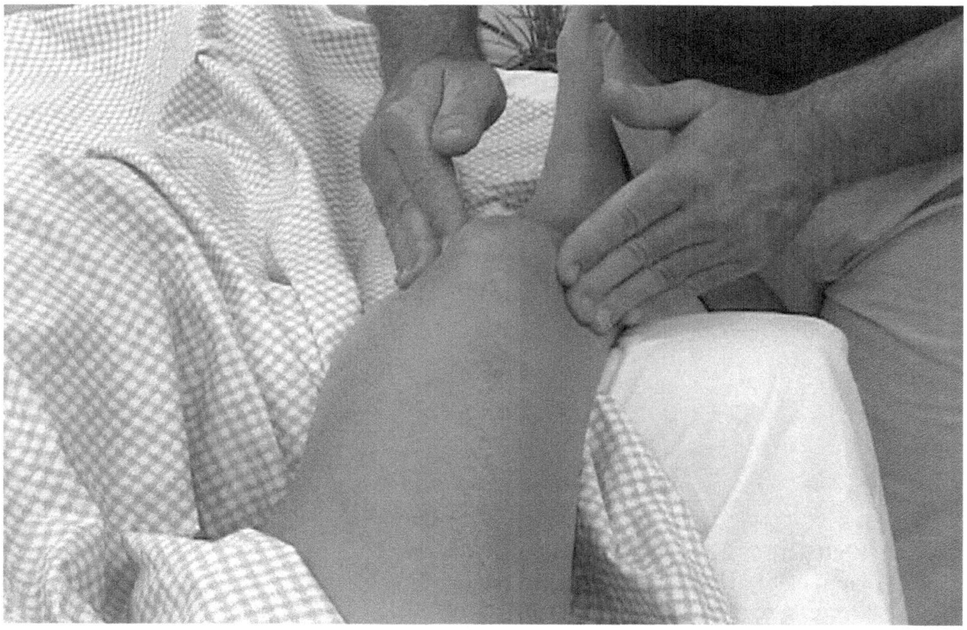

FIGURE 7–20. Circular friction around the knee with the fingertips.

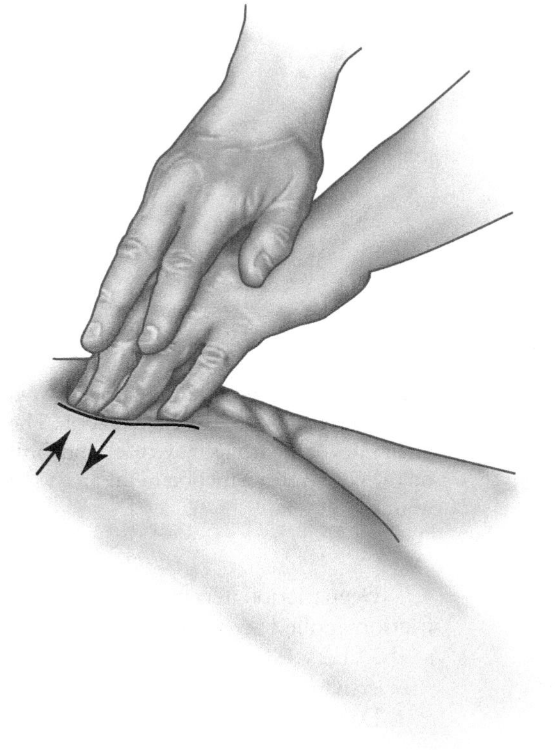

FIGURE 7–21. Cross-fiber friction to the paraspinal muscles. Friction is created by moving the skin and superficial tissues over the deeper tissues underneath.

working, and the depth of the tissues they wish to affect. If the tissues are just beneath the skin, then lighter pressure may be effective. If the tissues are deep or under other tissues, then you must "work through" the more superficial tissues. It is helpful to visualize the tissues in cross-section and to develop palpation skills that will allow you to feel the layers of tissue. Care must be taken in applying deep pressure. Do not try to "muscle through" more superficial tissues, but instead soften them layer by layer. This process takes patience and sensitivity.

Friction Used in Rehabilitation

Deep transverse friction or **Cyriax friction** is a specific type of cross-fiber friction that is applied directly to the site of a lesion. It is used to facilitate healthy scar formation at an injury site. The mechanical action across tissues causes broadening and separation of fibers. Deep transverse friction encourages a

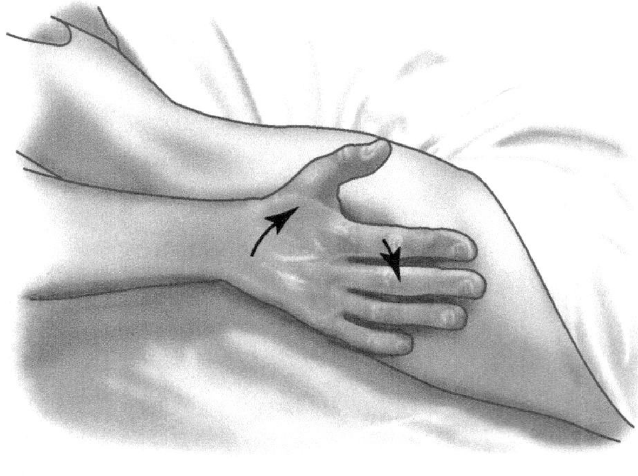

FIGURE 7–22. Circular friction to the broad iliotibial band. The heel of hand is used to create friction between the skin and the underlying tendon, and between the tendon and underlying muscles.

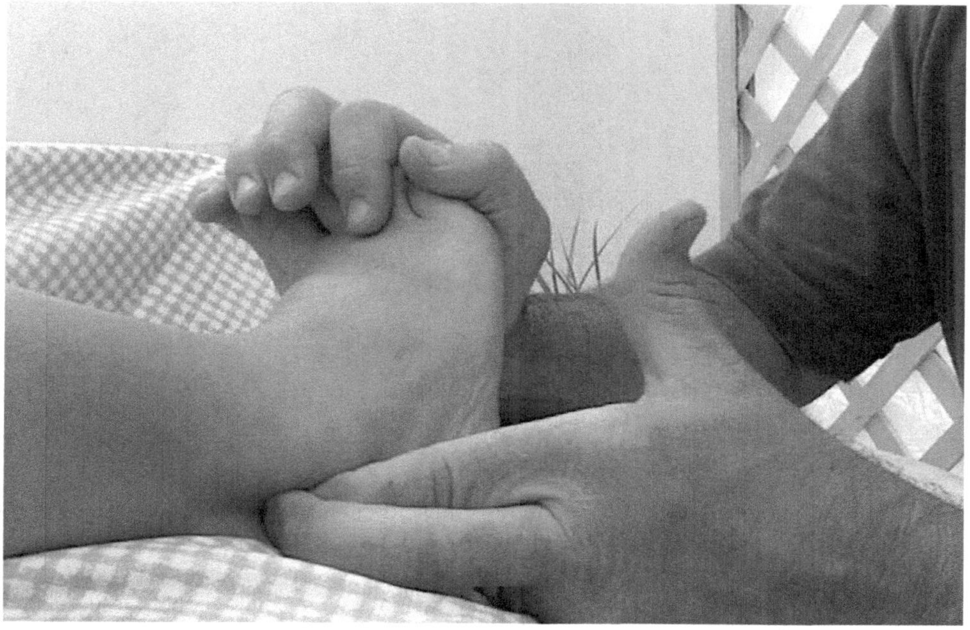

FIGURE 7–23. Deep transverse friction (i.e., Cyriax friction) on an ankle ligament.

more parallel fiber arrangement of scar tissue and fewer cross-connections that limit movement. See Figure 7–23.

James Cyriax popularized the use of deep transverse friction in injury rehabilitation. In the *Illustrated Manual of Orthopedic Medicine* (1993), the following principles were given for treating muscle and tendon lesions:

- The fingers and skin move together to affect deep tissues.
- The effect of friction is most important, not the amount of pressure used.
- The movement must be over the precise site of the lesion.
- The tissue must be in the appropriate tension.
- Do 6 to 12 sessions of 20 minutes each on alternate days for best results.

In addition to promoting healthy scar formation, circular and cross-fiber friction around an injury site can help keep normal tissues from adhering to the scarred area. Such adhering of tissues may cause chronic pain or inflammation. This is especially important where there is a large wound, such as in a cesarean section or other surgery.

TAPOTEMENT

Tapotement consists of a series of brisk percussive movements following each other in rapid, alternating fashion. Tapotement has a stimulating effect and is pleasant to receive if performed skillfully. The most common forms of tapotement are hacking, rapping, cupping, clapping, slapping, tapping, and pincement.

The movement of tapotement is light, rapid, and rhythmic. The hands should "bounce off" of the surface as they make contact, lightening the impact. The recipients should not feel like they are taking a beating, but should feel pleasantly stimulated. The percussive sound itself can be pleasing and can add to the therapeutic effect. Different hand positions create different sounds, and different parts of the body sound different when struck. Quacking and squishes described below are nontraditional forms of tapotement that make distinctive, interesting sounds.

Tapotement takes a certain rhythmic ability and much practice to master. The effort to learn it, though, is well worth while for the diversity it can bring to your work. Experiment with varying rhythms and hand positions for different effects.

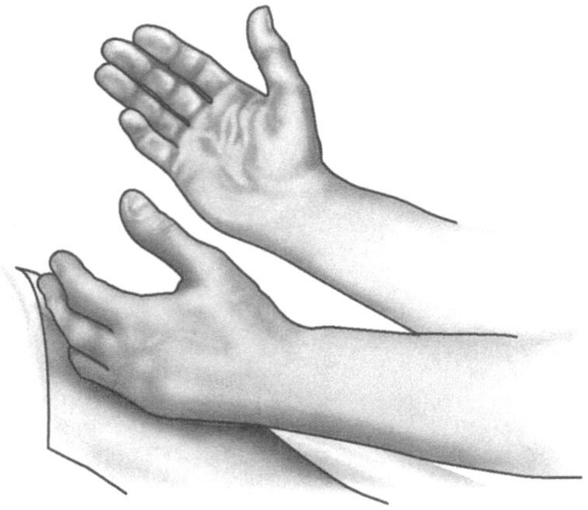

FIGURE 7–24. Hacking. Tapotement performed with the ulnar side of relaxed hands.

Tapotement is often used in finishing either a section of the body, a side of the body, or the session itself. Because it can be stimulating if received for a short period of time, tapotement is useful in situations in which the receiver must be alert when leaving the session. For example, it may be used if the receiver must drive directly after a session or go back to work. Athletes benefit from tapotement before a competition. Some people simply like the tingling and alive feeling that tapotement can leave with them.

While performing tapotement, the amount of force to use and the degree of stiffness of the hands depends on the area receiving the technique. Heavily muscular areas like the back and thighs can withstand more force, while more delicate areas like the head need a light touch. When performing tapotement over a broad area, as in ending a session with tapotement over a whole side of the body, the amount of force used will vary as you move from one section to another.

Variations of Tapotement

Hacking is performed with the hands facing each other, thumbs up. The striking surface is the ulnar surface of the hand and sometimes the sides of the third, fourth, and fifth fingertips. See Figure 7–24. The wrists, hands, and fingers should be held loosely during the rapid percussion movement. Alternate hitting with the left and right hands. Performed correctly, the effect of hacking is one of pleasant stinging and stimulation.

To practice hacking, shake your hands letting the wrists, hands, and fingers relax and "flip up and down." No attempt should be made to hold the fingers together or the hands and wrists in any particular position. If relaxation is complete, you will notice that the hands fall into a neutral plane of mo-

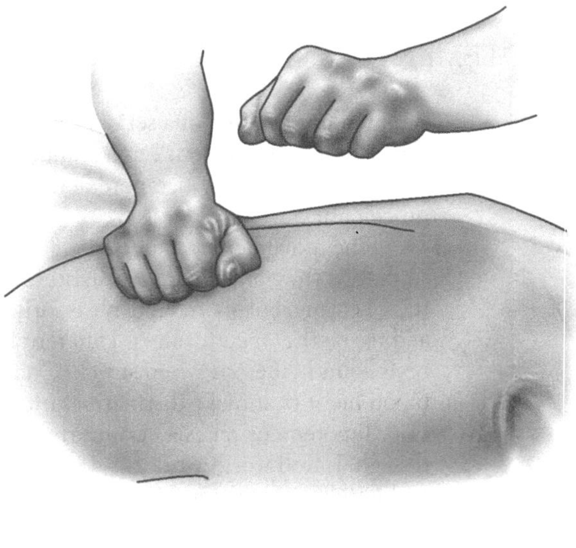

FIGURE 7–25. Rapping. Tapotement performed with the knuckles of a loosely closed fist, as if rapping lightly on a door.

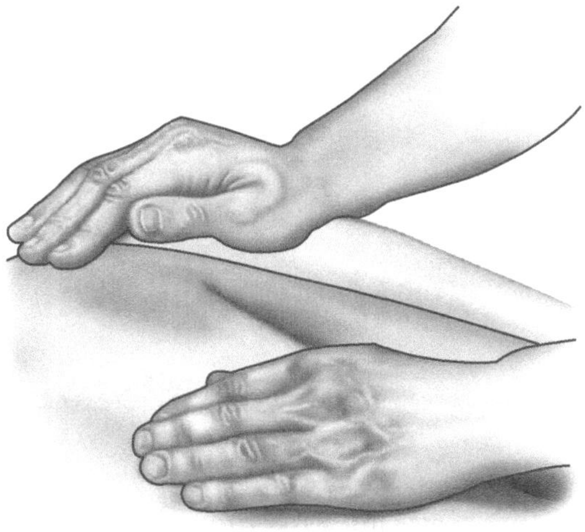

FIGURE 7–26. Cupping. Tapotement performed with the outside rim of a cupped hand.

tion that neither supinates nor pronates the forearms. Move the hands rapidly alternating one up and one down keeping the hands relaxed and shaking them. Practice on the back moving from the hips to the shoulder, and then back to the hips again. Never hit hard over the kidneys.

A similar movement, called **rapping,** may be performed using lightly closed and loosely held fists. The fists may be held palms down as in rapping on a door as shown in Figure 7–25. In side-rapping (sometimes called *beating*), the striking surface is the ulnar side of the fist. Keep the force of the blows light and "rebounding" in effect rather than jarring.

Cupping and **clapping** are applied with the same rhythmic, rapidly alternating force. For both techniques, cup the hand so that the thumb and fingers are slightly flexed, and the palmar surface contracted. The thumb is held tightly against the first finger. For *cupping,* strike the body surface with the outside rim of the cupped hand, keeping the palm contracted, as shown in Figure 7–26. There will be a hollow sound. A sight vacuum is created with each blow, which some believe may loosen broad flat areas of scar tissue or fascial adhesions. Cupping is also used for loosening congestion in the respiratory system.

Let the palm contact the body surface for **clapping.** This produces a less hollow sound and provides a broader contact surface. **Slapping** is performed with an open hand, the fingers held lightly together. Strike gently and briskly with the palmar surface of the fingers, rather than with the whole hand.

Tapping is done with the ends of the fingers. Sharp, light taps are done either with the edge of the fingernails or padding of the fingers. See Figure 7–27.

Pincement is a rapid, gentle movement in which superficial tissues are picked up between the thumb and first two fingers. It might be described as "plucking." A rhythm is established alternating left and right hands. See Figure 7–28.

Quacking is done with the palms together and fingers loosely apart. The striking surface is the lateral edges of the tips of the fourth and fifth (little) fingers as shown in Figure 7–29. As the fingers hit the bony surface, they come together, making a quacking sound.

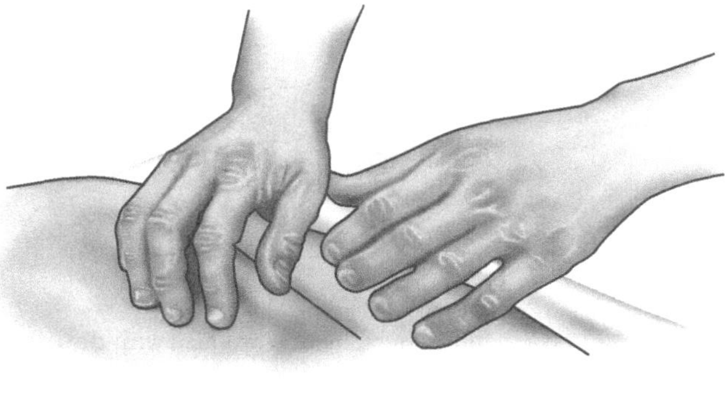

FIGURE 7–27. Tapping. Tapotement performed with the fingertips of a relaxed hand.

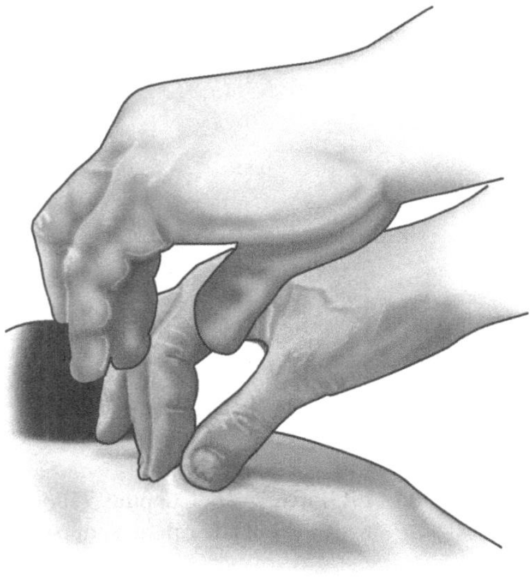

FIGURE 7–28. Pincement. Tapotement performed by gently picking up superficial tissues between the thumb and first two fingers with a light rapid movement.

Squishes are done with the hands loosely folded, making an air pocket with the palms. The striking surface is the back of one of the hands. As the back of the hand hits, the palms push out the air between them, creating a "squishing" sound.

VIBRATION

Vibration may be described as an oscillating, quivering, or trembling motion, or movement back and forth or up and down performed quickly and repeatedly. The vibration may be fine, and applied to a small area with the fingertips. Or it may be coarse, and involve shaking a muscle belly back and forth.

Vibration over the abdomen is sometimes used to stimulate the organs of digestion and elimination. Coarse vibration, in the form of jostling, may be used to help a recipient become aware of holding tension, to bring greater circulation to a muscle, and to help it relax. Fine vibration techniques impart an oscillating motion to the soft tissues and have a stimulating effect. They may also numb or relax specific muscles.

Electric vibrators may be used to impart fine vibration to tense muscles. The motion of vibration can be sustained for a longer period of time with a machine than if performed by hand. There are many types of hand-held electric vibrators. Some impart a coarser vibration, others a finer oscillation. One type of vibrator straps to the back of the hand and causes vibration in the fingers. This allows the

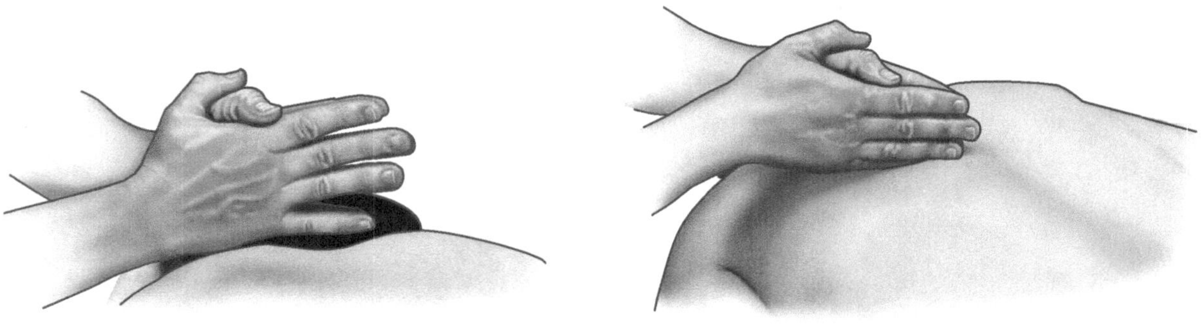

FIGURE 7–29. Quacking. Tapotement performed with the hands together and fingers loosely apart. Fingers come together as the little finger strikes, making a "quacking" sound.

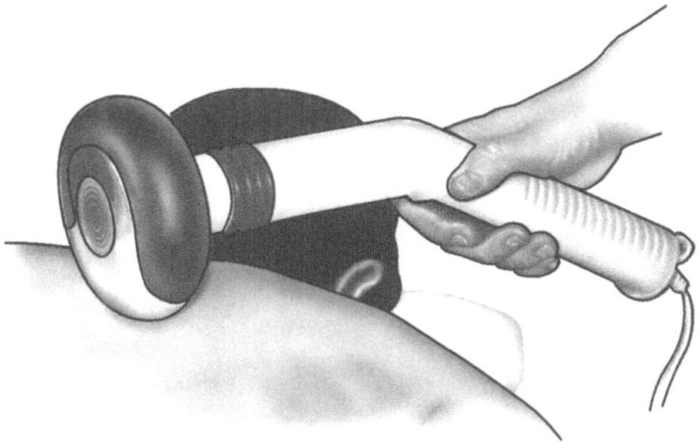

FIGURE 7–30. Fine vibration applied with a hand-held electric vibrator.

practitioner to stay in direct contact with the receiver and perform another technique such as light effleurage or friction. A standard hand-held vibrator is shown in Figure 7–30. A still finer vibration may be created by sound waves. There are devices that impart a lower frequency wave than ultrasound and are within the scope of practice of most practitioners.

Variations of Vibration

A **fine vibration** or trembling motion is imparted through the fingertips, but generated by the forearm. To practice fine vibration, place one hand on a muscle with the fingertips slightly apart. The trembling movement comes from the whole forearm, through the elbow, and the wrist and finger joints are kept in a fixed position. The elbow should be slightly flexed. This vibrating motion should be more in and out than side to side. The fingers remain in contact with the same spot during the vibration and are then lifted off of the skin and replaced to a new spot. Heavy pressure should be avoided. Fine vibration on the abdomen is shown in Figure 7–31.

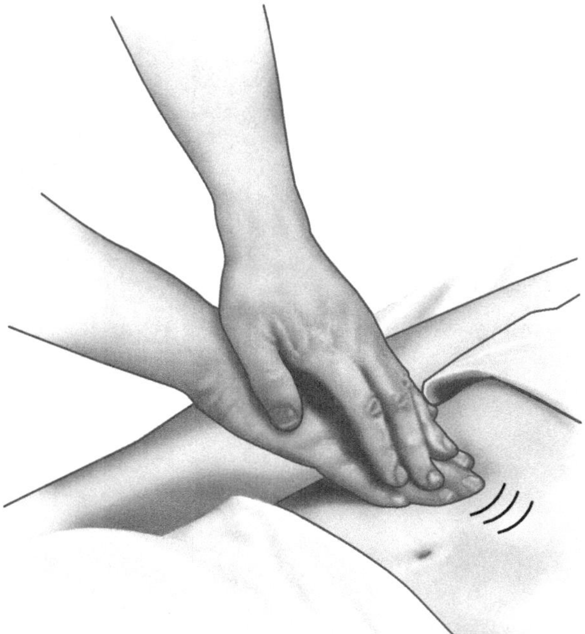

FIGURE 7–31. Vibration applied with fingertips to the abdomen.

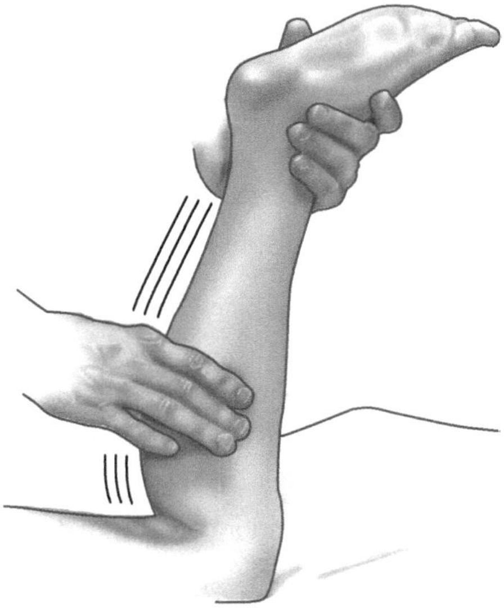

FIGURE 7–32. Shaking. A form of coarse vibration to a muscle or muscle group.

Light effleurage with vibration may be used for a soothing effect. While performing a light effleurage movement, add a sight vibration back and forth with the fingertips. Pressure can be so light that there is slight contact between the hand and the skin. It is a light brushing movement. In cases of hypersensitive nerves, this technique has been credited with having a soothing effect.

Shaking is a coarse form of vibration that can assist muscular relaxation. For example, a muscle such as the biceps or gastrocnemius may be grasped with one hand and shaken gently back and forth. Figure 7–32 shows shaking of the muscles of the leg.

In **jostling** the upper leg, two hands are used, one on each side of the leg. In this case, the muscle movement is back and forth from hand to hand as shown in Figure 7–33. It is helpful at times to jostle the entire limb gently to mobilize the surrounding joints and encourage relaxation and "letting go" of the whole area.

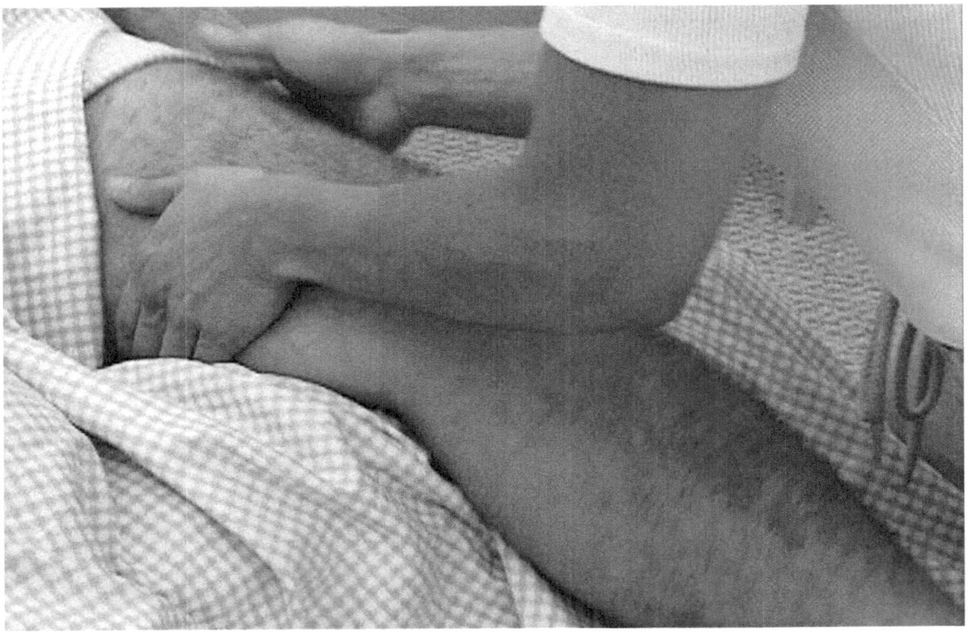

FIGURE 7–33. Jostling. A form of coarse vibration that includes mobilizing joints.

TOUCH WITHOUT MOVEMENT

Touch without movement is a unique massage technique category. It is defined by touch with the hands, but without any visible movement. Touch without movement is not casual or social touch, but is skilled touch with intention. Kellogg cautions that this is not ordinary touch, but "touch applied with intelligence, with control, with a purpose; and simple as it is, is capable of producing decided physiological effects" (p. 52).

Passive Touch

Passive touch is simply laying the fingers, one hand, or both hands lightly on the body. Passive touch may impart heat to an area, having a calming influence on the nervous system, or as some believe, help balance energy. Historically, the effects of passive touch have been attributed to "hypnotic" or "electrical" effects, "magnetism," and "subtle qualities of manner, a peculiar softness of the hand, or other personal quality not easy to describe" (Kellogg, 1929, p. 53). The use of passive touch to balance energy is more fully developed in systems of massage outside of classic Western systems.

Passive touch is often used to begin or end a session, or before turning over. It is used effectively for its calming effects when applied to the feet or to the head, as shown in Figure 7–34 and 7–35.

Direct Pressure

Direct pressure, also called direct static pressure, may be applied with a thumb, finger, knuckle, or elbow. Tissues are compressed using light to heavy pressure. Once tissues are compressed, the technique is held for 5–30 seconds, depending on the intent. There is no movement after the initial compression.

Although this text categorizes direct pressure as touch without movement, it might also be considered "static friction," or a form of compression. **Ischemic compression,** a form of direct pressure applied with enough force to cause blanching, causes vasodilation upon release of pressure, thus increasing local circulation.

Pressure should be applied slowly and carefully to avoid bruising or damaging tissues. Direct pressure is often preceded by warming the area with effleurage or rhythmic compressions, and followed with effleurage to "smooth out" the area or transition to another place. Figures 7–36 and 7–37 show two different uses for direct pressure.

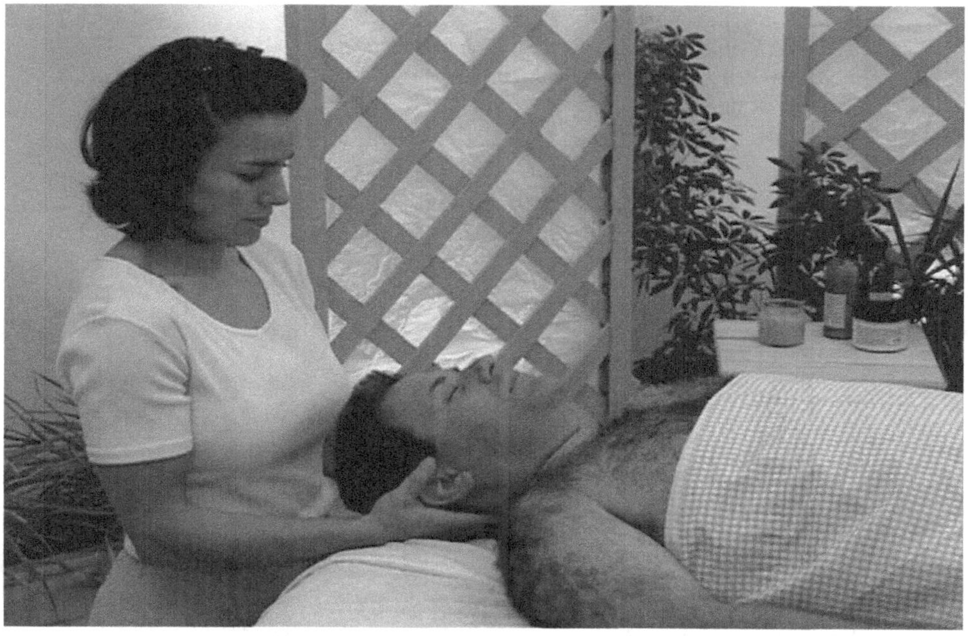

FIGURE 7–34. Passive touch by holding the head lightly.

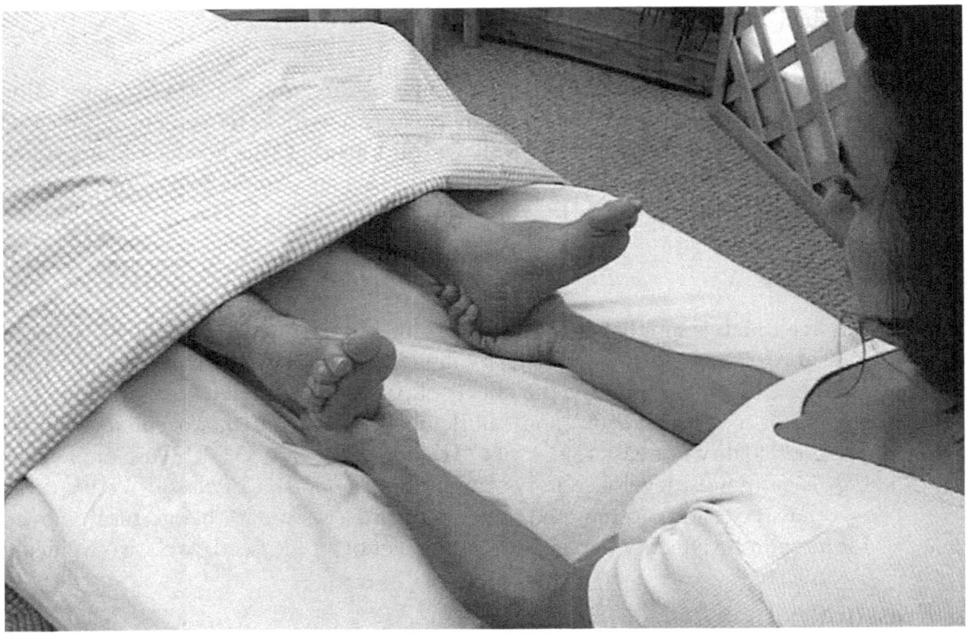

FIGURE 7–35. Passive touch by holding the feet lightly.

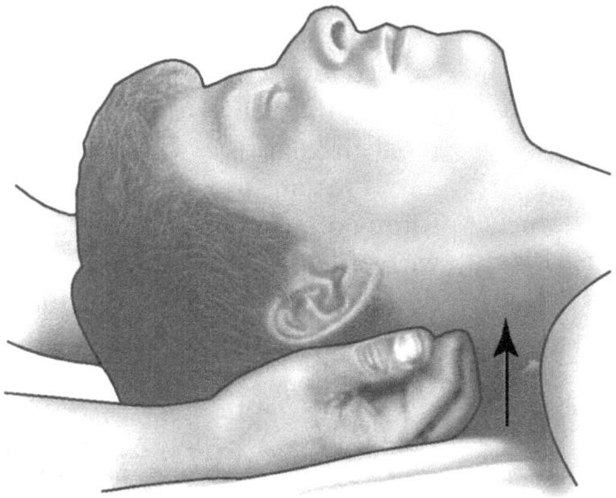

FIGURE 7–36. Direct pressure to suboccipital muscles. Fingers press up into the cervical muscle attachments along the occipital ridge.

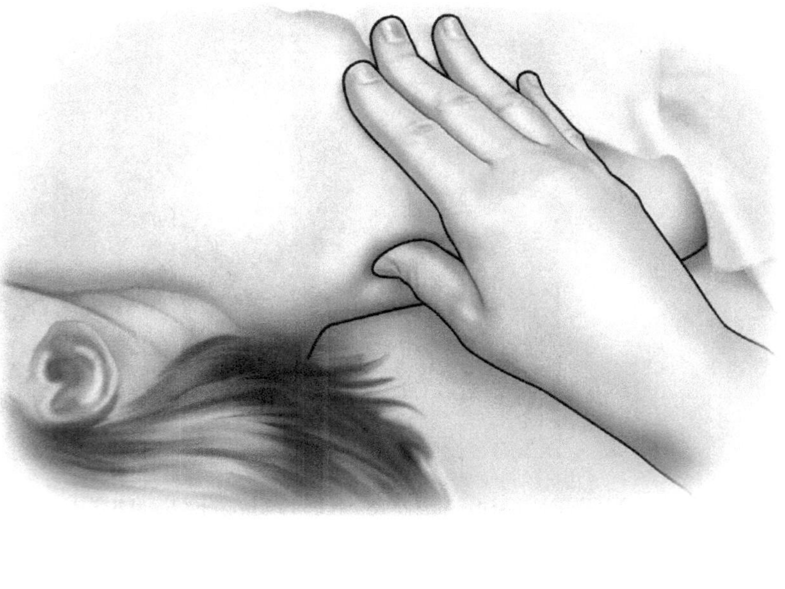

FIGURE 7–37. Ischemic compression (i.e., direct pressure) to a trigger point in the trapezius muscle.

Direct static pressure to various points is known to relieve pain, diminish congestion, and help muscles relax. Theories about how it works have evolved over the years and include the concepts of zone therapy, motor points, stress points, reflex points, trigger points, and acupressure points. The intentions of practitioners using direct static pressure may differ, and the amount of pressure used, location of areas pressed, and duration of pressure may also vary.

SUMMARY

Western massage is the most common form of massage found in spas, health clubs, and private practice, and is the foundation for therapeutic applications within the professions of massage therapy, physical therapy, and nursing. It is the legacy of historical figures such as Pehr Ling of Sweden, Johann Mezger of Amsterdam, J. Harvey Kellogg of the United States, and Mary McMillan of Britain and the United States. Swedish massage is a popular form of Western massage.

Western massage is understood in terms of Western science, and Western beliefs about health and disease. It is recognized as valuable for improving circulation, relaxing muscles, improving joint mobility, inducing general relaxation, and promoting healthy skin.

Western massage techniques fall into seven broad categories: effleurage, petrissage, friction, tapotement, vibration, touch without movement and joint movements. There are an endless number of variations of massage techniques, and the ones presented in this text are merely representative of many possibilities. Soft tissue techniques will be described in this chapter, while joint movements will be described in Chapter 8.

Effleurage techniques slide or glide over the skin with a smooth continuous motion. Effleurage is used to begin a session, apply lubricant, accustom the receiver to touch, connect or transition from one body region to another, assess the condition of tissues, and conclude work on an area. The application of effleurage, e.g., pressure, rhythm, pace, is varied for different effects. Variations of effleurage include basic sliding effleurage, stripping, shingles effleurage, bilateral tree stroking, three-count stroking of the trapezius, horizontal stroking, Mennell's superficial stroking, nerve strokes, and knuckling.

Petrissage techniques lift, wring, or squeeze soft tissues in a kneading motion, or press or roll the tissues under or between the hands. Petrissage is used to increase local circulation, "milk" tissues of accumulated waste products, assist venous return, separate muscle fibers, and evoke muscular relaxation. When applying petrissage, avoid pinching or bruising tissues, and working too long in one area. Variations of petrissage include basic two-handed kneading, one-handed kneading, alternating one-handed kneading, circular two-handed petrissage, alternating fingers-to-thumb petrissage, skin rolling, compression, and rolling.

Friction is performed by rubbing one surface over another repeatedly. Superficial friction is used for warming tissues, and is performed by rubbing the palms briskly over the skin. Deep friction is used to separate tissues, break adhesions, form healthy scar tissue, or to create movement in less-muscled areas such as around joints and over the head. Deep friction is performed in cross-fiber, parallel, or circular motion. Cyriax friction is a form of deep cross-fiber friction used in injury rehabilitation.

Tapotement consists of a series of brisk percussive movements following each other in rapid, alternating fashion. Tapotement is used for stimulation, and as a finishing technique. Variations of tapotement include hacking, rapping, cupping, clapping, slapping, tapping, pincement, quacking, and squishes.

Vibration is an oscillating, quivering, or trembling motion, or movement back and forth or up and down performed quickly and repeatedly. Fine vibration is applied with the fingertips, or with an electric vibrator. Coarse vibration is applied with the whole hand over a larger area and includes light effleurage with vibration, shaking, and jostling.

Touch without movement is defined by touch with the hands, but without any visible movement. Touch without movement is used to impart heat, have a calming effect, or balance energy. Variations of touch without movement include passive touch and holding. Direct pressure, e.g., ischemic compression, is applied to points for a number of effects including to relieve pain, diminish congestion, relax muscles, and stimulate points according to zone therapy, motor points, stress points, reflex points, trigger points, or acu-point theories.

A look ahead . . .

While soft tissue manipulation techniques are the most recognizable aspect of massage, joint movements are equally important for their therapeutic effects and have always been an important part of Western massage. Chapter 8 describes mobilizing and stretching techniques within the scope of massage therapy for each region of the body.

REFERENCES

Cyriax, J. H., & Cyriax, P. J. (1993). *Illustrated manual of orthopedic medicine*, 2nd ed. Boston: Butterworth & Heinemann.

Graham, D. (1884). *Practical treatise on massage*. New York: Wm. Wood and Co.

Hoffa, A. J. (1900). *Technik der massage*, 3rd ed. Verlagsbuchhandlung, Stuttgart: Ferdinand Enke. As translated by F. M. Tappan and Ruth Friedlander.

Kellogg, J. H. (1929). *The art of massage: A practical manual for the nurse, the student and the practitioner.* Battle Creek, MI: Modern Medicine Publishing Co.

CHAPTER EIGHT

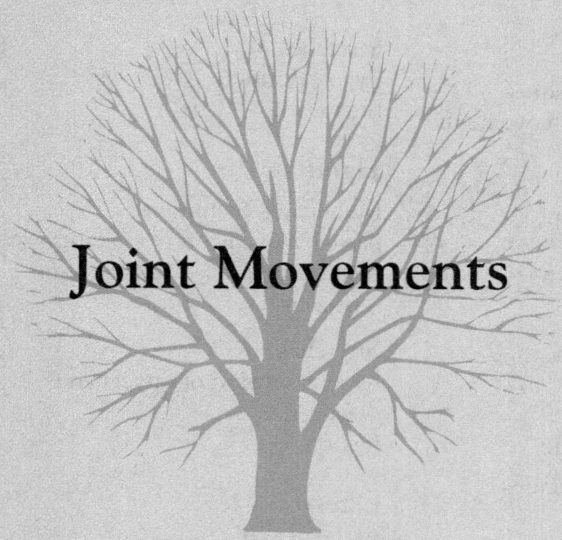

Joint Movements

LEARNING OUTCOMES

After studying this chapter, the student will have information to:

1. Describe the different categories of joint movements.
2. Compare mobilizing techniques and stretching.
3. Perform three methods of stretching: static, contract-relax-stretch, using reciprocal inhibition.
4. Explain the therapeutic benefits of joint movements.
5. Apply the general principles for joint movements.
6. Perform joint movement techniques for different areas of the body.

KEY TERMS/CONCEPTS

Assisted movements
Contract-relax-stretch (CRS)
Free active movements
Joint manipulations/adjustments
Normal range of motion
Mobilizing techniques
Passive movements
Reciprocal inhibition
Resisted movements
Static stretch
Stretching
Swedish movements

LINK LIBRARY TERMS

Medical Massage • *Massage Business* • *Massage Regulations*

MEDIALINK

A companion CD-ROM, included free with each new copy of this book, supplements the techniques presented in this chapter. Insert the CD-ROM to watch video clips of massage techniques being demonstrated. This multimedia feature is designed to help you add a new dimension to your learning.

JOINT MOVEMENT TECHNIQUES

Neck

Mobilizing Techniques
simple mobilizing movements
finger push-ups
melt-down
wavelike movement

Stretches
lateral flexion
rotation
forward flexion
cross-arm stretch

Shoulder Girdle

Mobilizing Techniques
wagging
shaking
passive shoulder roll
scapula mobilizing (prone)

Stretches
horizontal flexion
overhead stretch

Elbow

Mobilizing Techniques
pronation and supination
circling the forearm

Stretching
overhead stretch

Wrist

Mobilizing Techniques
passive movement through full range of motion
waving

Stretches
hyperextension
flexion

Hand

Mobilizing Techniques
passive movements of all joints
figure-eights
scissoring

Stretches
hyperextension of fingers and wrist
flexion

Chest

Mobilizing Techniques
rocking rib cage

Stretches
overhead stretch

Hip

Mobilizing Techniques
rhythmic rocking of straight leg
passive movement through full range of motion

Stretches
knee to chest flexion
straight leg flexion
diagonal adduction with flexed knee
straight leg hyperextension in side-lying

Knee

Mobilizing Techniques
wag
leg toss
circling the lower leg

Stretches
heel to buttocks

Ankle

Mobilizing Techniques
dorsiflexing foot with thumb pressure to bottom
passive movement through full range of motion
side to side mobilizing

Stretches
dorsiflexion
plantar flexion

Foot

Mobilizing Techniques
figure eights of toes
scissoring metatarsals
straightening toes with effleurage

Stretches
hyperextension of toes
foot widening at metatarsals
interlocking finger and toes

OVERVIEW OF JOINT MOVEMENTS

Western massage traditionally includes joint movements, as well as soft tissue manipulation. Pehr Ling's original system of medical gymnastics included passive movements of both the soft tissues and joints (Roth 1851). The term **"Swedish movements"** was commonly used in the United States to refer to joint movements up through the 1950s.

Categories of Joint Movements

Joint movements are categorized as active (i.e., free, assisted, and resisted) and passive (McMillan, 1925). **Free active movements** are performed entirely by a person without assistance from a practitioner. In **assisted movements,** recipients initiate the movement, while practitioners help them perform the movement. In **resisted movements,** practitioners offer resistance to the movement, thereby challenging the muscles used. **Passive movements** refer to movements initiated and controlled by the practitioner, while the recipient remains totally relaxed and passive.

Mobilizing techniques or joint mobilizations, within the context of massage therapy, are passive movements performed within the normal range of joint movement. Mobilizing techniques are nonspecific movements of the joints and surrounding soft tissues that free up motion at the joints involved. They can be easily integrated into a massage routine.

Stretching is a type of passive joint movement that is performed to the limit of the range of motion, with a slight stretch beyond. It is used to increase flexibility at the joint, as it elongates the muscles and connective tissues that cross the joint. Stretching may also be used for muscle relaxation.

Joint manipulations or adjustments (sometimes called *chiropractic adjustments*) are not within the scope of massage therapy. By joint manipulations and adjustments, we mean techniques that take a joint beyond its normal range of motion and that are specific attempts to realign a misaligned joint, or free a frozen joint, usually using a thrusting movement. They should be performed only by those trained to do so within their legal scope of practice. "Cracking" necks and backs and "popping" toes are potentially dangerous and should not be performed as part of standard Western massage.

In this chapter, we will describe simple passive joint movements that fall under the categories of nonspecific joint mobilizing techniques and stretching. These movements may be incorporated into a general massage session or might be used for specific therapeutic goals.

Uses of Joint Movements

Practitioners use joint movements for a variety of reasons including to stretch surrounding soft tissues, increase range of motion, stimulate production of synovial fluid, increase kinesthetic awareness, stimulate muscle relaxation, and build muscle strength. Both active and passive joint movements are applied to increase flexibility, and improve posture and body alignment. Athletes find joint movements particularly beneficial for improving performance, preventing injuries, and for rehabilitation.

Some contemporary systems of bodywork, such as Trager Psychophysical Integration®, use joint movements to affect the nervous system, re-educate muscles, and integrate function. Receivers can also learn to let go of tension they are unconsciously holding onto during passive joint movement. Joint movement adds a kinetic dimension to a massage session and provides diversity of technique.

GENERAL PRINCIPLES OF JOINT MOVEMENTS

Massage practitioners should be familiar with the bony structure and muscles that move each joint. Together these determine the movements possible at the joint. **Normal range of motion** refers to the degree of movement commonly found at a joint, and is useful knowledge to generally assess the degree of flexibility at a joint. Knowing the normal limitations to movement at each joint will decrease the likelihood of inadvertently damaging a joint or the surrounding tissues, and increase safety for the recipient.

Caution is advised in cases of abnormality of the bony structure, hypermobility, recent injury, and diseases of the joints such as bursitis and arthritis. A past trauma may have caused some unusual conditions around a joint, including shortening or loss of muscle tissue, scarring in connective tissues, and abnormal joint structure. Sometimes "hardware," such as metal pins and plates, is present from past injuries. Joint replacements are becoming more common, and movement around artificial joints may be restricted. Hip and knee replacements are important to know about, especially in the elderly. Take the time to learn about the condition from up-to-date medical references, the recipient, from available medical records, or from the recipient's physician to ensure a safe application of joint movements. Remember that massage and joint movements are contraindicated when acute inflammation is present.

Palpation skills are very important for learning how joints move. Practitioners can learn much about the condition of the joint and surrounding tissues from the kinesthetic feel of the movement. Sensations like "drag" and "end feel" offer clues to restrictions to normal range of motion, areas of tightness, patterns of holding, and the limits of stretches. Drag refers to resistance felt as the soft tissues around a joint are stretched, and end feel refers to resistance as the limit of the stretch is approached.

The stretches described in this chapter are passive movements applied as **static stretches.** Avoid sudden, forceful, or bouncing movements while performing the stretches. Move the part being stretched into position and hold at the limit of movement, which is determined by feeling for the point of resistance. Use feedback from the recipient for safety. The recipient should feel the stretch, but not feel pain. Hold for 10–15 seconds, and then try to increase the stretch. The muscles will often relax after a short time, allowing further stretch (30–45 seconds overall).

Stretches can be facilitated with techniques called **contract-relax-stretch (CRS),** and contract-relax-stretch using **reciprocal inhibition.** In CRS, the practitioner gets into position to perform the stretch, but first asks the client to contract the muscle to be stretched against a resistance (resisted movement). Immediately following the muscle's relaxation, the stretch is applied.

When reciprocal inhibition is used, the practitioner gets into position to perform the stretch, but first asks the client to contract the target muscle's antagonist against a resistance. The target or agonist muscle relaxes as its antagonist contracts. Immediately following the antagonist's relaxation, the stretch is applied.

Breathing may be used to help the recipient relax during a stretch. The body is more relaxed during exhalation than during inhalation, and holding the breath causes tension in the musculature and restricts movement. So it is better to stretch a muscle on the exhalation. Once you and the recipient are in position to apply a stretch, ask her to "take a deep breath and then let it out slowly." During the exhalation, apply the stretch.

The following is a summary of the general guidelines for performing passive joint movements:

- Stay within the normal range of motion of the joint.
- Qualities of mobilizing techniques are smooth, free, and loose.
- Warm surrounding soft tissues before stretching.
- Use breathing to enhance a stretch.
- Stay within the comfort range of the recipient.
- Be aware of abnormality of joint structure and adapt movements accordingly.

JOINT MOVEMENT TECHNIQUES

Neck

Structure and Movement. The "neck" is a general term for the region between the head and the trunk. It includes the seven cervical vertebrae and the surrounding soft tissues. The cervicals are the smallest, most delicate vertebrae and are designed to allow for a lot of movement but not bear a lot of weight. They are arranged vertically with an anterior convex curve.

The musculature in the neck region is complex with deeper, smaller muscles entirely within the neck, and larger and more superficial muscles attaching superior and inferior. The bony and muscular structures allow a variety of movements including flexion, extension, hyperextension, lateral flexion, and rotation.

Mobilizing Techniques. Mobilizing techniques for the neck are performed when the recipient is lying supine. The mobilizing movement occurs between the cervical vertebrae and in the suboccipital region. All of the following examples may be performed with the practitioner seated at the head of the recipient. It is useful to have an adjustable stool or chair on wheels so that you can get in good position, for both leverage and self-care.

Simple mobilizing movements of the neck may be performed by lifting the head slightly off the table, and moving the neck into lateral flexion, rotation, forward flexion, or hyperextension. Be sure to have a firm grip on the head. You may have to remind the recipient to relax, since it takes great trust to let someone hold and move your head. You may also assure them that you will not "crack" their neck, and that such manipulations are not part of this type of mobilization. Keep the movements small at first and gradually increase the range of motion as the recipient allows.

Finger push-ups may be used to produce gentle movement between the cervical vertebrae. First warm up the neck muscles with effleurage and circular friction along each side. Straighten the neck, so that the recipient is directly face up. Simply place the fingers at the base of the neck on either side, palms up, and push up with the fingers, applying direct pressure. Move your hands about an inch at a time along the neck, pressing up at each spot as you move along. You will feel movement between the vertebrae and notice movement at the head. Variations of finger push-ups include alternating pressing from side to side. The rhythm would be to press right, press left, move along; press right, press left, move along; repeating the sequence along the neck, moving toward the head.

The **melt-down** is a variation of the finger push-up applied in the suboccipital region. Place your hands, palms up, under the recipient's head, with fingers along the suboccipitals. Lift the head with the hands, and then lower the wrists to the table, while leaving the head balanced on the fingertips. Usually within 5–10 seconds, the neck muscles relax, the suboccipital tissues "melt," and the head hyperextends. You will notice the recipient's head falling back, and your fingers will be deep into the suboccipital space. This pressure usually feels good to the recipient. Finish by gently pulling on the occiput to straighten any hyperextension remaining from the movement.

A **wavelike movement** may be created in the neck by simply applying deep effleurage on both sides at the same time, moving from the base to the suboccipital region. You exaggerate the natural curve of the neck by pressing up as you slide along. The neck will return to its normal curve as you finish the movement. (See Figure 9–21.) At the end of the movement, give a gentle pull on the occiput to straighten any hyperextension remaining from the movement. The *wave* is a good technique to use to detect tension in the neck. The wavelike motion will not occur if the recipient is unconsciously holding tension in the neck or if the neck muscles are shortened and tight.

Stretches. Massage and simple mobilizing techniques are used to warm up the neck thoroughly before applying stretches. The following stretches may be performed when the recipient is lying supine on a table.

A stretch in **lateral flexion** helps lengthen the muscles on the sides of the neck. Place the head in position to one side at a point where you feel the tissues just starting to stretch. The head placement, either face up or turned to the side, will determine which muscles are stretched most. Place one hand on the shoulder and the other on the side of the head. You can create a gentle stretch of tissues by pushing the head and shoulders in opposite directions as shown in Figure 8–1. Guide the recipient to exhale as you apply the stretch. The head will move to a position of greater lateral flexion as the upper trapezius relaxes and lengthens. Repeat on the other side.

Range of **rotation** may be enhanced with a simple stretch. Position the head face up so that the neck is straight. Then rotate the head to one side, keeping the neck vertically aligned. Gently push the head into greater rotation, stretching the neck muscles. Repeat on the other side.

Position the head face up to stretch the neck in **forward flexion.** Lift the head with one hand, and with the other hand, reach under the head and across to the tip of the shoulder. The head rests on the

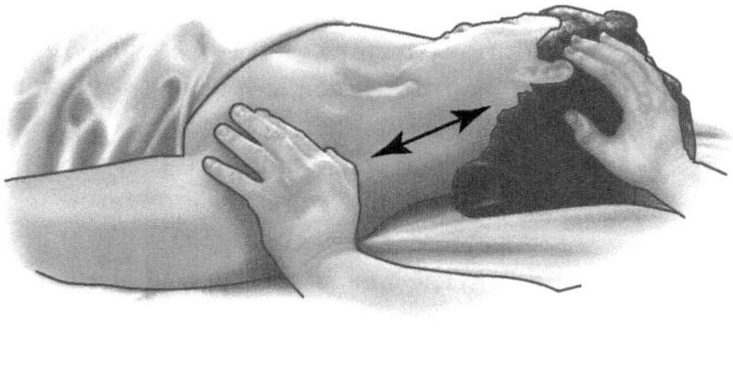

FIGURE 8–1. Stretch of trapezius and cervical muscles with neck in lateral flexion.

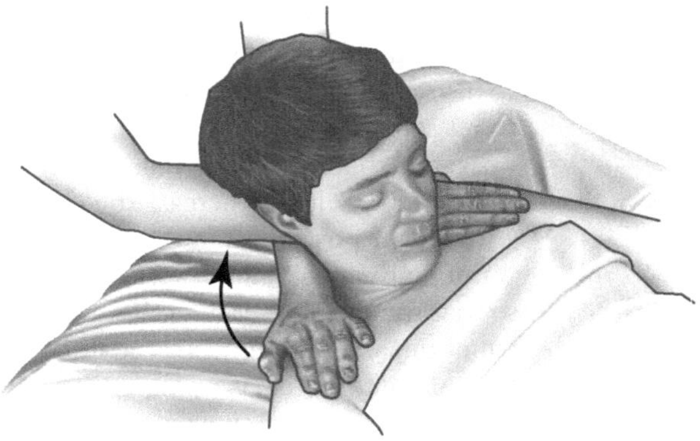

FIGURE 8–2. Cross-arm stretch of cervical muscles with neck in forward flexion.

forearm. Reach under that arm with the free hand and place it on the other shoulder. The head should be cradled safely at the place where the forearms cross, as shown in Figure 8–2. Slowly stretch the neck into forward flexion. Stand during this movement for best leverage.

The **cross-armed stretch** may also be performed with the head rotated. This will stretch neck muscles at a different angle. After forward flexion, return to the starting position and turn the head to one side. Repeat the forward flexion to each side with the head in rotation. For safety, be sure that the stretch is pain free.

Shoulder Girdle

Structure and Movement. The shoulder girdle is a complex region that can be defined in different ways. For our purposes, the shoulder girdle will be defined as including the glenohumeral, acromioclavicular, and scapulocostal joints. The glenohumeral joint is classified as a ball-and-socket joint, and the acromioclavicular joint as diarthrodial nonaxial. The scapulocostal juncture may be described as a gliding joint of the scapula with the rib cage separated by muscles and a bursa (Cailliet, 1981, p. 2).

The shoulder girdle is the most mobile area of the body. Movements possible in the shoulder girdle include the upper arm movements of flexion, extension, hyperextension, abduction, adduction, rotation, and horizontal flexion. Movements of the scapulae themselves include elevation, depression, upward and downward rotation and tilt, and retraction and protraction. The entire shoulder girdle is structured to accomplish circumduction.

Mobilizing Techniques. Mobilizing movements of the shoulder girdle may be performed with the recipient in supine, prone, side-lying, or seated position. Mobilizing the joints of the shoulder may be accomplished indirectly by movement of the arm or by movement of the scapula.

To mobilize the shoulder girdle with the recipient in the supine position, take hold of the hand and lift and wag the arm as shown in Figure 8–3. While **wagging** the arm, there will also be movement at the wrist and elbow. **Shaking** is performed by creating a slight traction of the arm toward the feet, holding onto the hand and leaning back as shown in Figure 8–4. Loosely shake the arm up and down. Movement will be felt at the wrist, elbow, and shoulder.

The **passive shoulder roll** may be used for mobilizing the shoulder. Hold onto the upper arm with one hand close to the glenohumeral joint, and the other hand at the tip of the shoulder. Simply move the shoulder through the full range of motion possible in the supine position. The quality of movement should be smooth, free, and loose. This same technique is effective in the prone, side-lying, and seated positions. Figure 8–5 shows the passive shoulder roll with the recipient supine.

With the recipient prone, **scapula mobilizing** may be accomplished using pressure applied at the top of the shoulder. Position the recipient's arm on the table with elbow bent and hand near the waist. Then place your hand on top of the shoulder near the tip and pressing lightly toward the feet. The scapula will move and lift if the attached muscles are relaxed as shown in Figure 8–6. Don't force the movement, but encourage relaxation by gentle motions and reminding the recipient to let go of tension in the area. Once the medial border lifts, you may apply effleurage to massage the muscles that attach there.

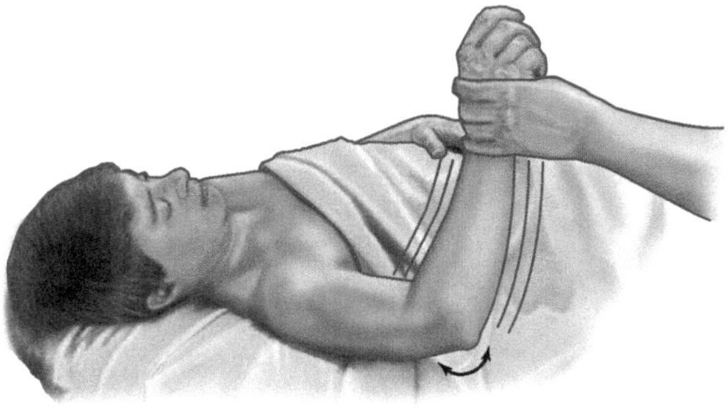

FIGURE 8–3. Wagging: an arm and shoulder mobilizing technique.

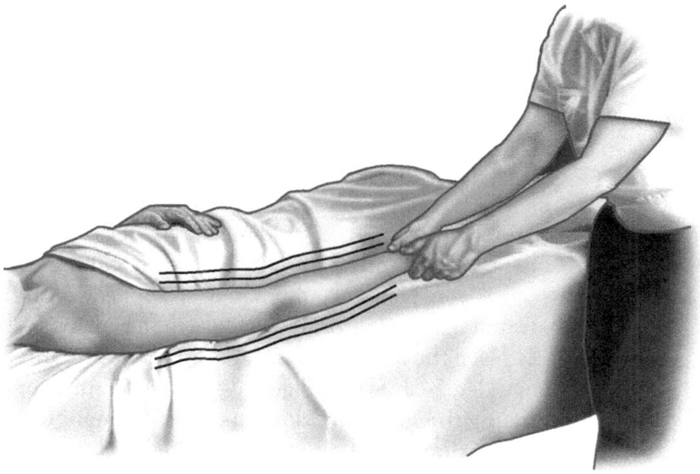

FIGURE 8–4. Shaking: an arm and shoulder mobilizing technique.

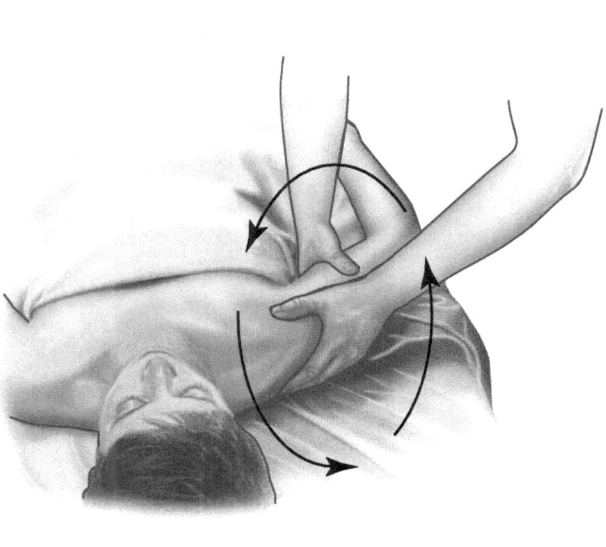

FIGURE 8–5. Passive shoulder roll. Mobilizing technique for the shoulder with recipient in supine position.

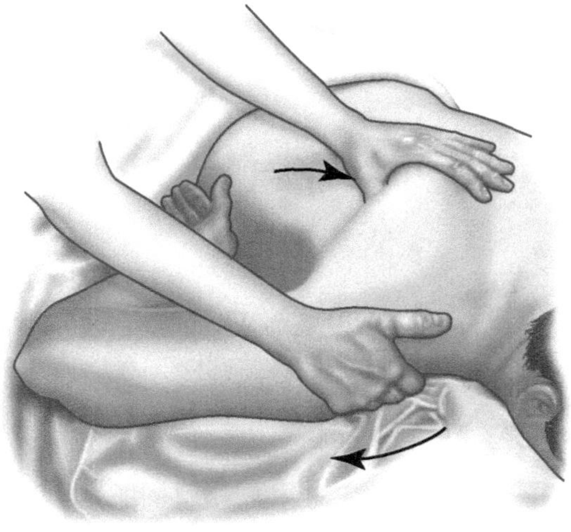

FIGURE 8–6. Scapula mobilizing technique. Move and lift the scapula by pulling back at the shoulder.

Stretches. Use massage and mobilizing technique to warm up the shoulder girdle before stretching. Shoulder girdle stretches are effective in the supine, prone, and side-lying positions. The muscles of the shoulder girdle are stretched primarily with movements of the upper arm.

In the supine position, a stretch in **horizontal flexion** may be performed by moving the arm over the chest. This elongates the muscles that attach to the medial border of the scapula, including the rhomboids, as well as the posterior shoulder muscles. Hold onto the recipient's lower arm near the wrist with one hand, while the other hand reaches under to the medial border of the scapula. Stretch the arm over the chest and enhance the stretch by gently pulling back on the scapula at the same time. See Figure 8–7.

A very pleasant stretch may be applied with the recipient's arms extended overhead. This **overhead stretch** may be performed one arm at a time or both arms at the same time. For a two-arm stretch, simply place the arms overhead, grasping the forearm near the wrist. Lean back to create the stretch at the shoulder, as shown in Figure 8–8. This technique stretches all of the muscles of the shoulder girdle, including the latissimus dorsi and pectoral muscles.

A similar stretch may be applied with the recipient seated in a massage chair. Grasp the forearm with both hands and move the arm overhead to a position in line with the angle of the body. You should be facing in the same direction as the recipient. Lift the arm upward and give it a gentle shake as shown in Figure 8–9.

Elbow

Structure and Movement. The elbow is formed by the junction of the distal end of the humerus and the proximal ends of the radius and the ulna. Movements of the humeroulnar joint are limited to flexion and extension. The bony structure of the joint further limits the range of motion in extension.

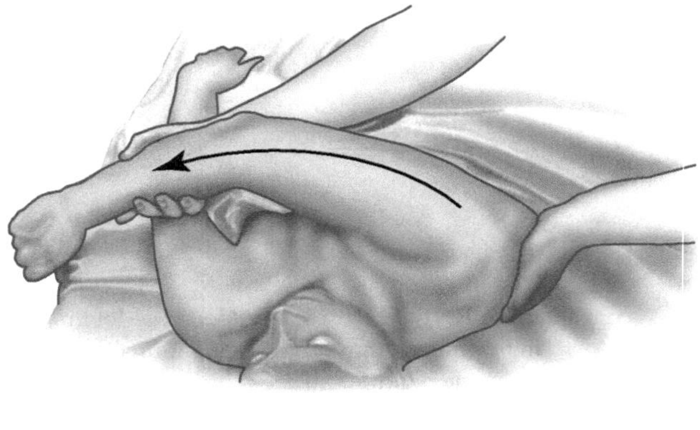

FIGURE 8–7. Stretching the shoulder muscles with arm in horizontal flexion.

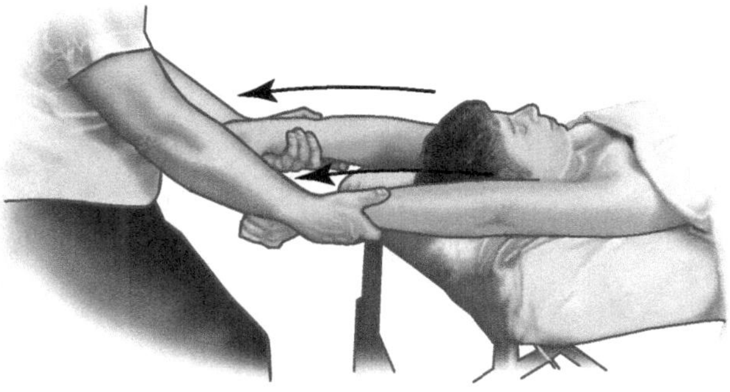

FIGURE 8–8. Overhead stretch for the shoulder muscles. Lean back to create the stretch using your body weight.

What we think of as the point of the elbow is the olecranon process of the ulna. The movements of pronation and supination of the forearm (palm-down and palm-up) occur as the head of the radius rotates over the surfaces of the capitulum of the humerus and the radial notch of the ulna. At the same time, the distal ends of the radius and ulna glide over one another.

Mobilizing Techniques. Movements at the elbow are limited by the structure of the joint. **Wagging** of the arm as described above offers some mobilization at the elbow. You may also **pronate and supinate the forearm** by holding the hand and turning it alternately palm up and palm down.

To perform a simple mobilizing technique at the elbow, bend the arm at the elbow so that it is perpendicular to the table. Hold the arm just below the wrist. Trace a circle with the hand (i.e., **circling the forearm**) creating movement at the elbow as shown in Figure 8–10.

Stretches. Stretches of muscles that cross the elbow are accomplished largely by stretching the whole arm as in the **overhead stretch** of the shoulder described above. If the biceps muscles are shortened, the stretch is created by simply straightening out the arm at the elbow.

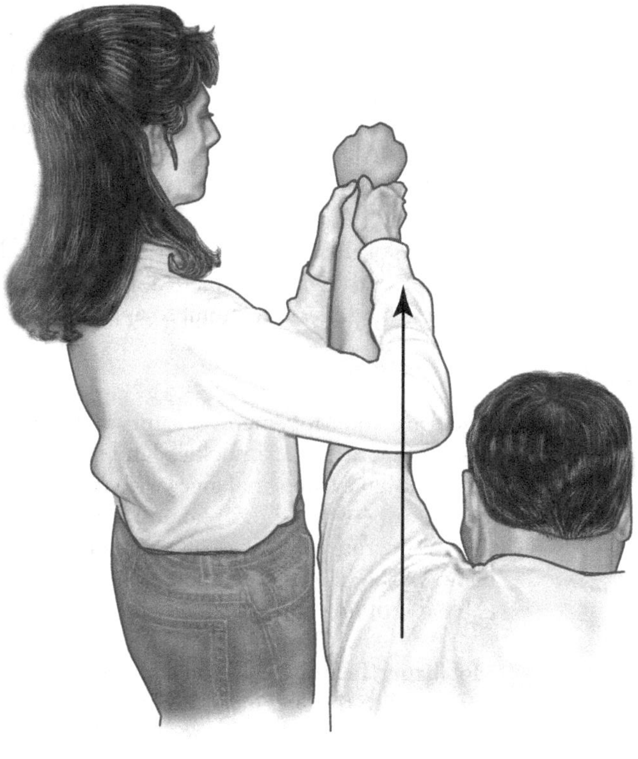

FIGURE 8–9. Overhead stretch of the shoulder muscles. Recipient in a massage chair.

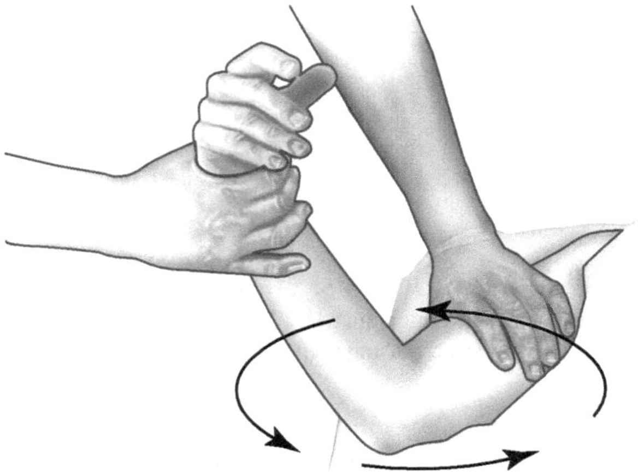

FIGURE 8–10. Circling the forearm to create movement at the elbow.

Wrist

Structure and Movement. The wrist joint is formed by the union of the slightly concave surface of the proximal row of carpal bones with the distal end of the radius and the midcarpal joint. What people commonly call the "wrist bone" is actually the distal end of the ulna. Movements possible at this juncture include flexion, extension, hyperextension, radial and ulnar deviation (side-to-side movement), and circumduction.

Mobilizing Techniques. Mobilizing of the wrist are best performed with the recipient supine. The soft tissues in the wrist area may be warmed up with small effleurage movements with the thumbs prior to mobilizing and stretching. A useful starting position for basic mobilizing techniques and stretching is achieved by clasping the recipient's hands, palms facing and fingers interwoven. The recipient's elbow is bent and may be resting on the table. In the hand-clasp position, you may move the hand through its entire range of motion at the wrist including flexion, extension, hyperextension, side-to-side in radial and ulnar deviation, and circumduction. Keep the passive movement well within the possible range of motion.

A light, quick mobilizing technique may be performed at the wrist with a **waving** movement. Face the head of the table and hold the forearm just proximal to the recipient's wrist (palm down) with both of your hands, the thumbs on top and index fingers below. Use the remaining fingers to cause the hand to *wave*, by pressing up against the heel of the hand quickly and repeatedly, letting gravity help it fall between times. Movement at the wrist also occurs during less specific mobilizations, including wagging the arm as shown in Figure 8–3, and supination and pronation of the forearm.

Stretches. Flexion and hyperextension are the major stretches performed at the wrist. Figure 8–11 shows stretching the flexors of the forearm by **hyperextending at the wrist.** Press down gently on the palm side of the fingers to create the stretch. Now **flex the hand at the wrist** and press down on the back side of the hand to create a stretch of the extensors of the forearm as shown in Figure 8–12. During these stretches, be careful to approach the limit of motion slowly.

Hand

Structure and Movement. Joints within the hand and distal to the wrist include the metacarpophalangeal juncture (i.e., knuckles) and the small joints between phalanges. The second through fifth fingers each have three phalanges with two joints, while the thumb has just two phalanges with one joint. The joint between the carpal and metacarpal of the thumb is designed to allow freer movement than similar junctures of the carpals and metacarpals. Movement may also occur between metacarpals. Movements of the fingers include flexion, extension, abduction, and adduction. The hand as a whole is capable of holding and grasping objects.

Mobilizing Techniques. Perform mobilizing techniques of the hand joints very carefully, matching the force used to the size and strength of the hand you are working with. Warm the muscles in the recipient's hands with effleurage and light frictions before performing mobilizing techniques and stretches.

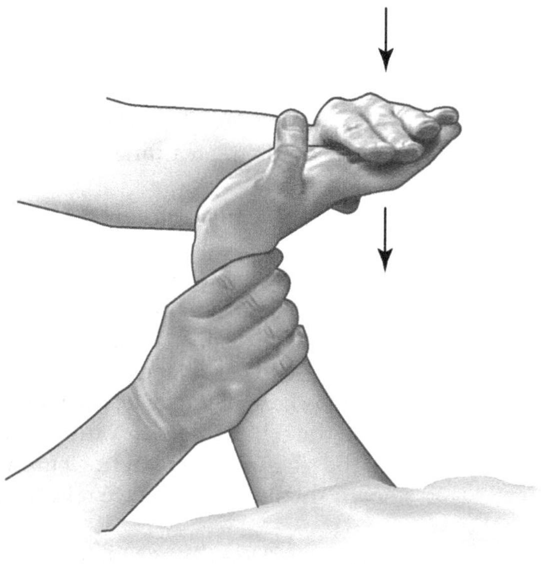

FIGURE 8–11. Stretching the flexor muscles of the forearm by hyperextending the wrist.

Mobilizing the knuckles, one at a time may be achieved making **figure eights.** Hold the recipient's hand with one of your hands, his fingers pointing toward you, palm down. With your other hand, grasp the fifth (little) finger firmly near the knuckle and move in a small figure eight pattern two or three times, mobilizing the joint. See Figure 8–13. Repeat for each knuckle joint. A similar, but lighter, mobilizing of the knuckles may be achieved by grasping the fingers more distally. Perform the figure eights as described above.

You can mobilize the tissues between the metacarpals with a **scissoring** motion. With the recipient's palm down, take hold of knuckles of the fifth and fourth fingers as shown in Figure 8–14. Simply move one knuckle up and the other down at the same time, alternating in a scissoring motion. Repeat along all of the knuckles.

Stretches. There are a few simple stretches for the joints of the hand. Perform them slowly and with care. The fingers can be **hyperextended** at the knuckles. Interlace your fingers with the recipient's, palm to palm, placing the tips of your fingers just below the recipient's knuckles. Gently press between the metacarpals, bending the fingers into hyperextension. This movement may also cause the metacarpals to spread out, stretching the tissues between them.

Taking the whole hand into **hyperextension** can stretch all of the flexor muscles within the hand and the wrist flexors in the forearm. Hold the forearm with one hand and, with the other hand, press back on the phalanges, causing hyperextension at the knuckles and at the wrist. Gently stretch the tissues of the hand and the forearm. See Figure 8–11.

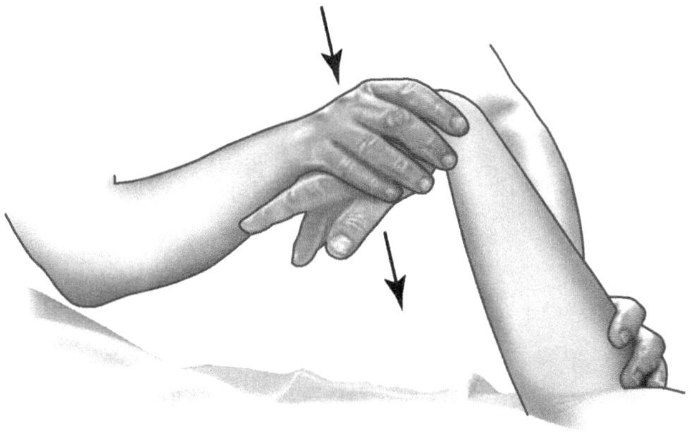

FIGURE 8–12. Stretching the extensor muscles of the forearm by flexing the wrist.

Chest

Structure and Movement. The "chest" is a common term for the area on the front and sides of the upper body generally defined by the ribs, sternum, and clavicle. It is the part of the thorax accessible when lying supine. The entire thorax, including the chest, expands and contracts with the inhalation and exhalation of breathing. The pectoral muscles are located on the chest.

Mobilizing Techniques. The rib cage may be mobilized by **gentle rocking** from the side. Stand facing the side of the table in line with the rib cage. Put one hand on top of the other and place them on the rib cage as shown in Figure 8–15. Gently rock the rib cage by repeatedly pushing and then letting up the pressure in a rhythmic manner. Move around on the rib cage to mobilize different areas. You will feel the elastic quality of the rib cage as it springs back after you push.

If you can reach far enough with your arms, you can cause movement in the chest from both sides. Facing the head of the table, reach over with one hand to the far side of the chest, fingers pointing down toward the table. Place the other hand on the near side, fingers pointing up. See Figure 8–16. Gently rock the rib cage by alternating pulling with the far hand and pushing with the near hand. Establish a smooth rhythm to encourage relaxation of the surrounding musculature.

Stretches. There are no highly movable joints on the chest itself. However, the pectoral muscles of the shoulder girdle attach there. Use the overhead stretch of the arms as shown in Figure 8–8 to lengthen the pectorals.

Hip

Structure and Movement. The hip joint is a typical ball-and-socket joint formed by the articulation of the head of the femur with the deep cup-shaped acetabulum of the pelvis. The large muscles that move the hip joint are located primarily on the thigh and the buttocks. The iliopsoas is a strong hip flexor that attaches to the lumbar vertebrae and inner surface of the ilium and the lesser trochanter of the femur. Movements possible at the hip joint include flexion, extension, hyperextension, abduction, adduction, diagonal abduction and adduction, outward and inward rotation, and circumduction.

Mobilizing Techniques. Most hip movements are performed with the recipient in the supine position. Mobilizing techinques are an excellent way to affect the deeper muscles that move the hip.

With the recipient supine, remove the bolster from under the knees. The legs should be straight and slightly apart. Stand facing the thigh at the side of the table. **Gently rock the leg** into rotation by placing the hands palms down on the top of the thigh and pressing down and away. See Figure 8–17.

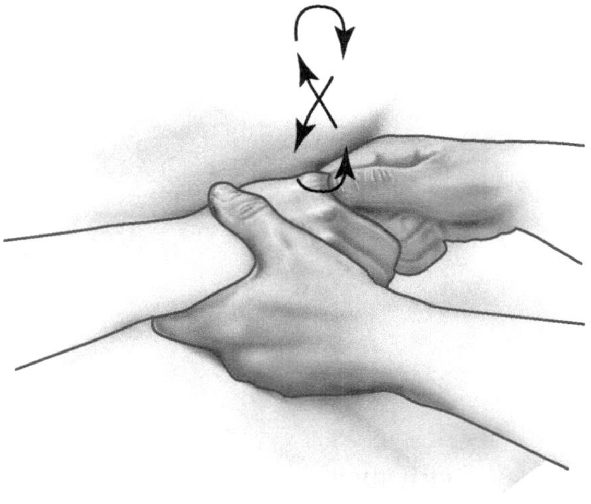

FIGURE 8–13. Figure 8s at the knuckles of the hand.

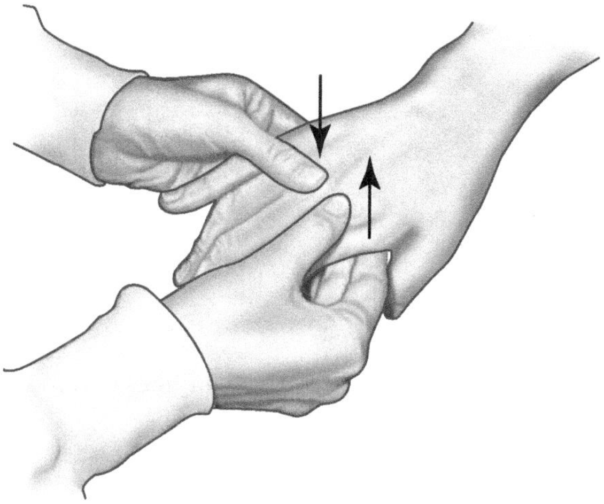

FIGURE 8–14. Scissoring motion to create movement between the metacarpals of the hand.

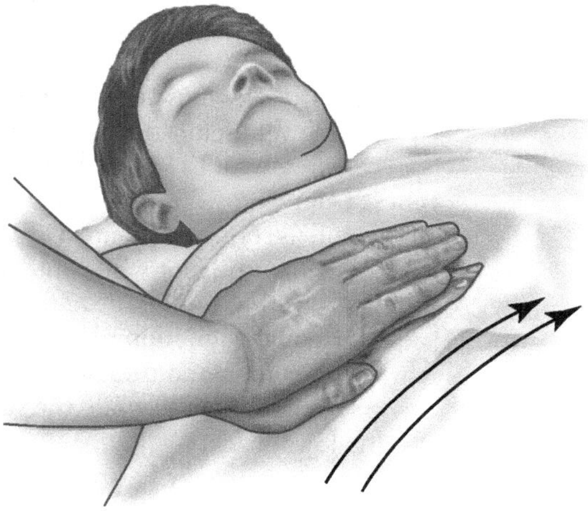

FIGURE 8–15. Placement of hands for mobilizing the rib cage from one side.

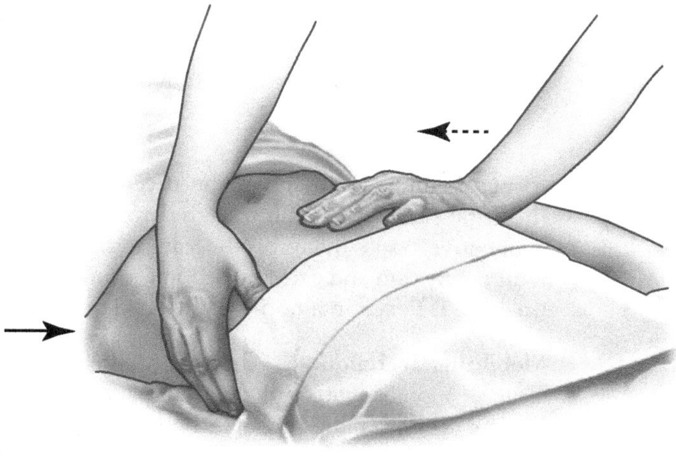

FIGURE 8–16. Placement of hands for mobilizing the rib cage from both sides.

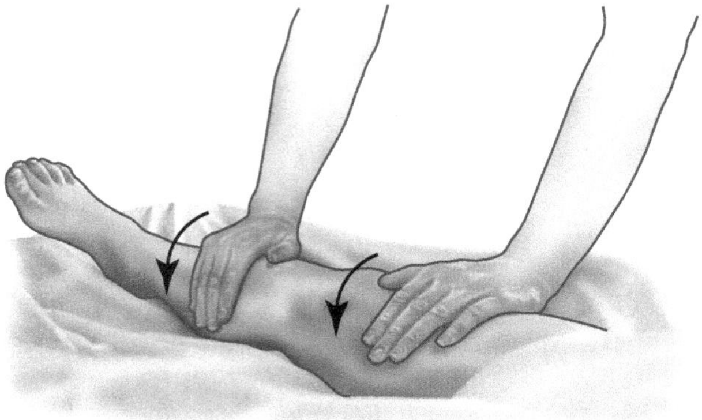

FIGURE 8–17. Rocking the leg to create rotation in the hip joint.

The leg will usually rotate back, especially if the gluteals are tight. The foot will wag from side to side if performed properly. Repeat with a rhythmic rocking motion.

To **move the hip through its full range of motion,** bend the leg, placing the foot in one hand, and using the other hand for support at the knee. See Figure 8–18. Let the knee trace a circle as the hip flexes, adducts diagonally, extends, abducts diagonally, and goes round again in circumduction. The movement should be smooth and loose.

Stretches. The muscles that move the hip can be stretched in many directions. The following are a few simple yet useful stretches for the hip joint.

A stretch for the gluteals may be applied with the hip in flexion by pressing the **knee toward the chest** (supine position). See Figure 8–19. The hamstrings may be stretched with the leg straight and in flexion as shown in Figure 8–20. To enhance the stretch and involve all of the gluteal and leg muscles, dorsiflex the foot while you bring the leg perpendicular to the table, and then as far toward the chest as possible.

Diagonal adduction of the thigh while lying supine will also stretch the gluteals. Bring the knee toward the chest, and then let it cross the body diagonally as shown in Figure 8–21. The shoulders remain flat on the table, while the supine twists and the hip muscles stretch. This is also a good stretch for the lower back.

The flexors may be stretched from the prone or side-lying position. With the recipient prone, stand at the side of the table facing the head. Bend the leg at the knee and grasp the thigh from underneath; the lower leg can rest against your shoulder. Lift the knee off the ground, putting the hip into hyperextension. You may anchor the hip with the other hand. This stretch takes some strength and is most easily performed if the recipient is smaller than you are.

The **stretch into hyperextension** can be more easily performed with the recipient in side-lying position. Stand behind the recipient facing the table at the hip. Cradle the upper leg with one arm while you stabilize the trunk with the other. Pull the upper leg back into hyperextension as shown in Figure 8–22. Because you are pulling the leg back, instead of lifting it up, this technique is more efficient and takes less strength. It primarily stretches the quadriceps and iliopsoas muscles.

Knee

Structure and Movement. The knee is classified as a hinge joint and is formed by the articulation of the distal end of the femur with the proximal end of the tibia. A large sesamoid bone embedded in the connective tissues that cross the joint forms the knee cap or patella. The major movements of the knee joint are flexion and extension. Some minor inward and outward rotation of the tibia is possible when the knee is flexed in a non–weight-bearing situation.

Mobilizing Techniques. The knee joint is best mobilized with the recipient in the prone position. For a simple mobilizing technique, stand facing the side of the table at the knee. Pick up the leg near the ankle with both hands, so that the lower leg is perpendicular to the table. Lift the leg slightly off the table and **wag** it back and forth. This also mobilizes the hip joint.

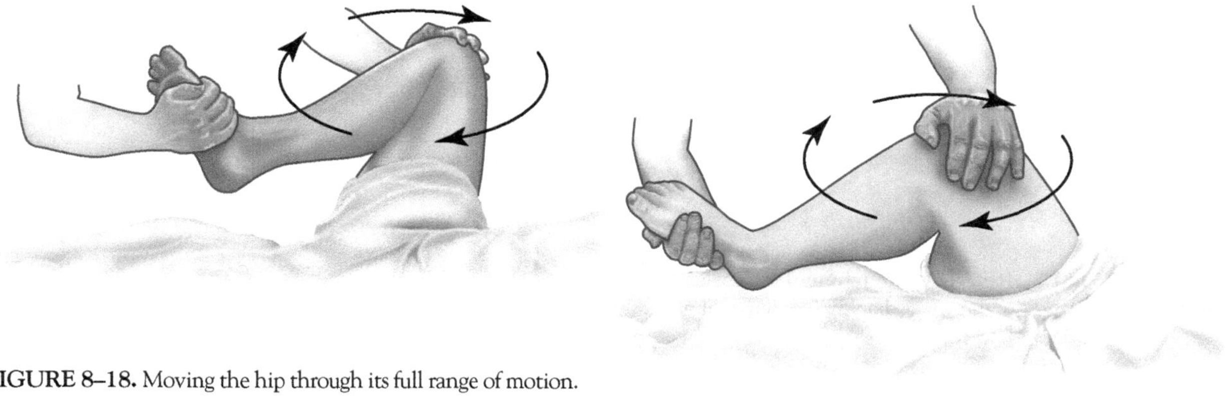

FIGURE 8–18. Moving the hip through its full range of motion.

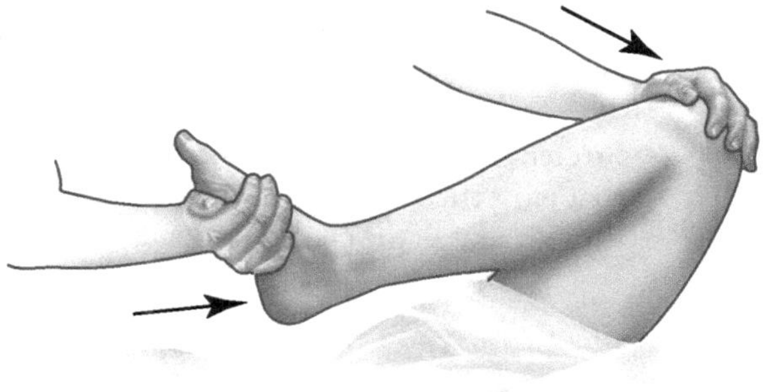

FIGURE 8–19. Stretching the gluteals by bringing knee to chest.

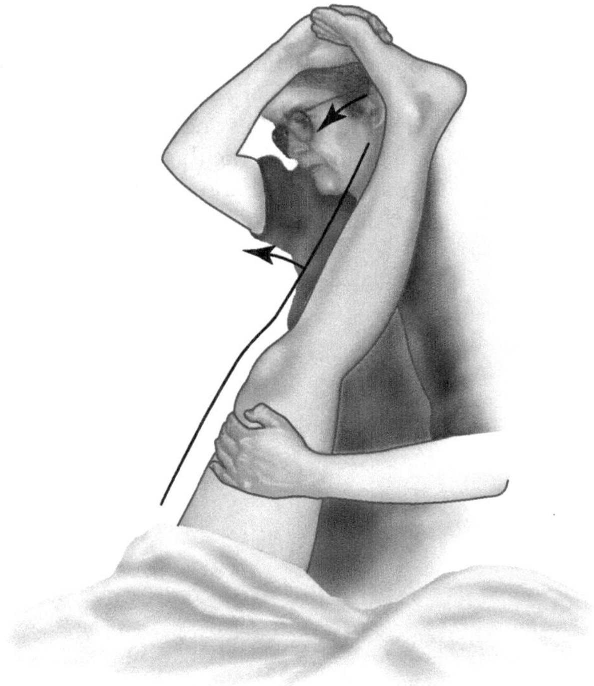

FIGURE 8–20. Stretching the hamstrings with straight leg flexion.

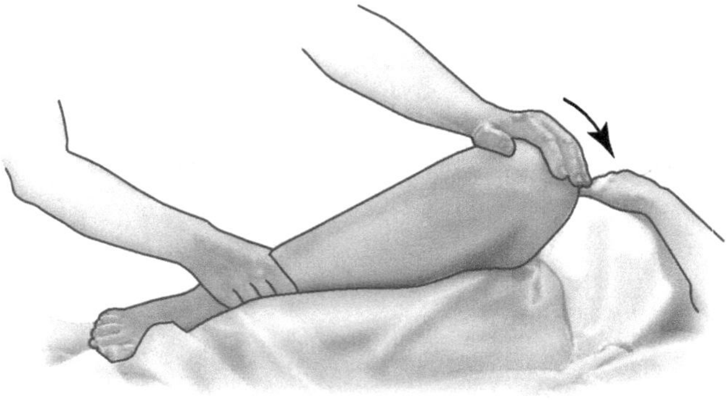

FIGURE 8–21. Stretching the muscles of the hip and lower back with diagonal adduction of the bent leg.

Another simple mobilization at the knee involves tossing the lower leg back and forth from hand to hand. This **leg toss** technique helps the recipient learn to relax and let go of tension in the legs. After the leg toss, you may perform a different knee mobilization by **circling the lower leg.** Place one hand on the thigh to steady it and grasp the lower leg near the ankle with the other hand. Make small circles with the lower leg. Stay well within the small range of this circular motion.

Stretches. A few of the stretches for the hip joint, performed with a straight leg, also stretch muscles that cross the knee. See Figure 8–20. An additional stretch for the knee extensors can be created with the recipient in the prone position by bringing the **heel of the foot toward the buttocks.** See Figure 8–23.

Ankle

Structure and Movement. The ankle is a hinge joint formed by the junction of the talus with the malleoli of the tibia and fibula. The structure is bound together with many ligaments for stability. The tendons of muscles of the lower leg that attach to the foot all pass over the ankle. They are bound neatly at the ankle by a band of connective tissue called the retinaculum. Movements possible at the ankle include dorsiflexion (flexion), plantar flexion (extension), pronation (eversion and abduction), and supination (inversion and adduction).

Mobilizing Techniques. When the recipient is prone, the ankle may be accessed by lifting the lower leg so that the foot comes off the table. For **mobilizing with dorsiflexion,** stand at the feet facing the end of the table. Lift one leg and place both hands on the foot, thumbs on the bottom of the foot. Lean into the foot with the thumbs in the arch, moving the foot into dorsiflexion as shown in Figure 8–24. Repeat the mobilization several times in a rhythmic manner, changing the location of the thumbs to affect different spots on the feet.

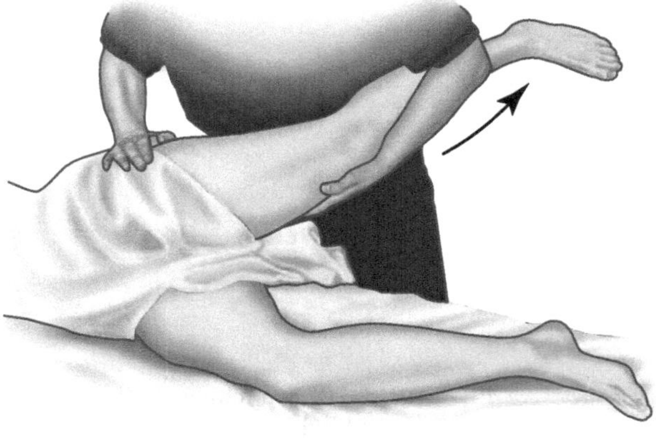

FIGURE 8–22. Stretching the hip flexors with the recipient side-lying.

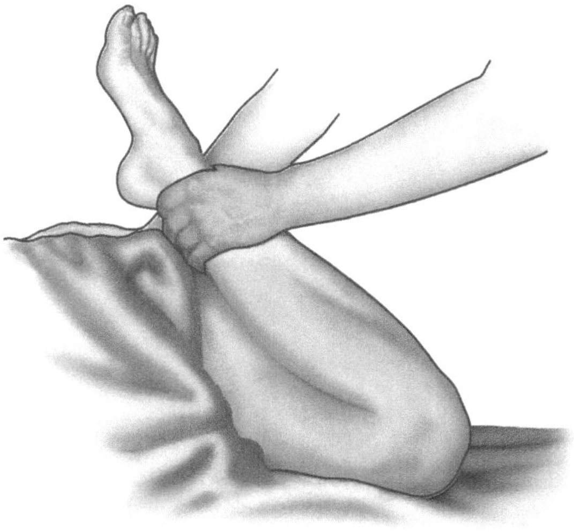

FIGURE 8–23. Stretching the quadriceps by bringing the heel of the foot toward the buttocks.

With the lower leg lifted so that it is perpendicular to the table, the ankle can be put through a full range of motion. Grasp the bottom of the foot from above and move the ankle through dorsiflexion, pronation, plantar flexion, and supination in a circular movement. This is also an excellent position from which to apply **simple dorsiflexion** and **plantar flexion.**

With the recipient supine, the ankle can be mobilized by placing the heels of the hands on the foot just under the malleoli of the tibia and fibula (ankle bones) and pressing in alternation one side and then the other. The movement is rapid, and causes the heel of the foot to move from side to side at the articulation of the talus and malleoli of the tibia and fibula. (See Figure 9–12.)

Stretches. Stretches at the ankle are primarily performed in dorsiflexion and plantar flexion and may easily be done with the recipient prone or supine. Stretches may be applied from any of the positions mentioned for mobilizations. Simply move the foot into dorsiflexion or plantar flexion and take it to the limit of range of motion. Figure 8–25 shows the ankle and foot stretching in **plantar flexion.** This movement helps elongate the foot flexors located on the front of the lower leg and may be felt across the top of the foot.

Foot

Structure and Movement. The foot may be described as an elastic arched structure made up of 26 bones and designed for support and propulsion. A foot has 7 tarsal bones (i.e., calcaneus, talus, navicular, cuboid, and 3 cuneiforms), 5 metatarsals, and 14 phalanges. There is a longitudinal arch, which extends from the heel to the heads of the 5 metatarsals, and a transverse arch, which extends side to side formed by the anterior tarsal bones and the metatarsals. The intertarsal joints are irregular joints and

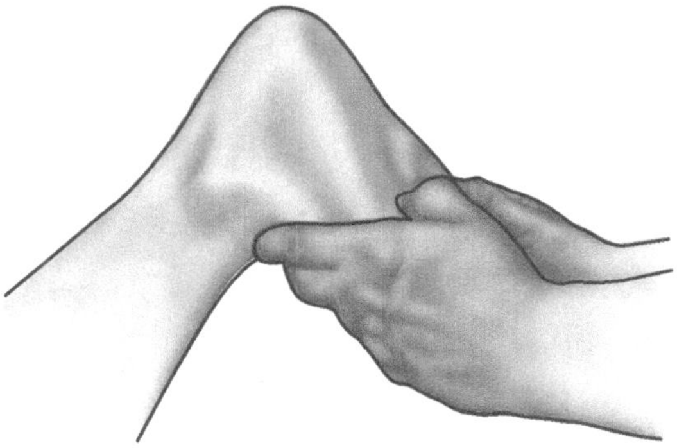

FIGURE 8–24. Dorsiflexion of the foot with direct pressure to bottom of foot with the thumbs.

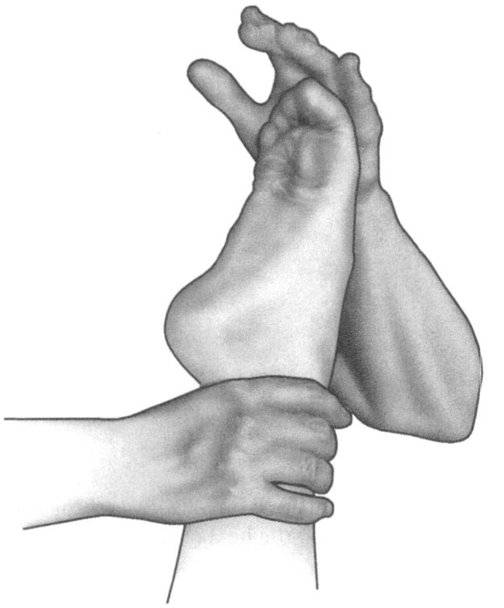

FIGURE 8–25. Stretching the flexors of the foot in plantarflexion. Lower leg perpendicular to the table.

allow slight gliding movements, and the interphalangeal joints of the toes are hinge joints that allow for flexion and extension.

Mobilizing Techniques. Mobilizing techniques for the feet are similar to those for the hands. They are best performed with the recipient supine. The soft tissues in the feet may be warmed up with small sliding effleurage movements with the thumbs or fingers, and compressions with the fist on the bottom of the foot.

Hold the foot steady with one hand and with your other hand, grasp the fifth (little) toe firmly near the knuckle and move in a small **figure eight** pattern two or three times, mobilizing the joint. Repeat for each knuckle joint. You can mobilize the tissues between the metatarsals with a **scissoring** motion. Take hold of knuckles of the fifth and fourth toes. Simply move one knuckle up and the other down at the same time, alternating in a scissoring motion. Repeat for all of the metatarsals.

Sometimes the toes curl under due to shortening of the toe flexors that are located on the bottom of the feet. The toes can be **mobilized into extension using effleurage** along the underside of the toes. This is usually performed with the thumbs. Do not "pop" or pull on the toes forcefully straightening them out, which is uncomfortable to most recipients and dangerous.

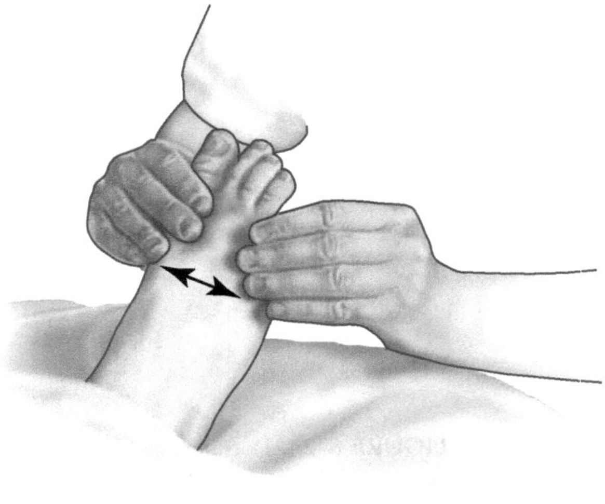

FIGURE 8–26. Creating space between metatarsals by pulling sides of foot away from each other.

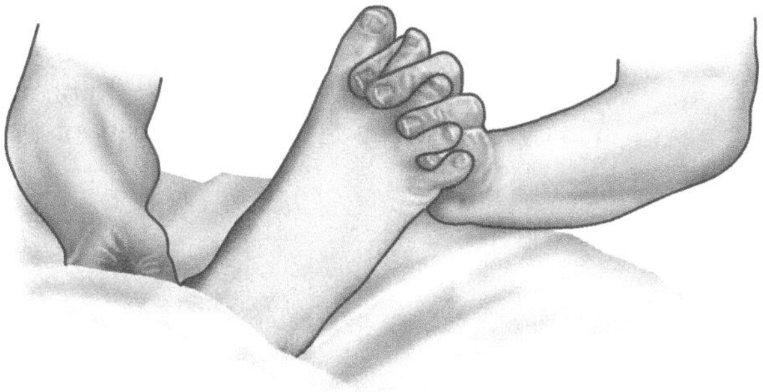

FIGURE 8–27. Creating space between metatarsals by interlocking fingers with recipient's toes.

Stretches. There are a few stretches for the intrinsic tissues of the foot itself. As described above, you can plantar flex the foot from either the prone or supine positions, stretching the tissues on the top of the foot, including the extensor muscles. The toes alone may easily be stretched back at the ball of the foot or pressed forward for a stretch. The foot may be spread stretching the spaces between the metatarsals, and the muscles that run across them. Simply grasp both sides of the foot and pull in opposite directions, **widening the foot and stretching** related tissues as shown in Figure 8–26.

You may also **interlock your fingers between the toes** of the foot. This in itself is usually enough to spread the toes and metatarsals into a stretch. See Figure 8–27. It will be ineffective if your hands are too small in relation to the recipient's foot, and may be painful if your hands are relatively big.

Since the foot is a small part of the body with many joints, it can be massaged thoroughly rather quickly combining soft tissue techniques with mobilizations and stretches. Joint movements help recipients regain a sense of their feet as having moving parts and help sharpen their kinesthetic sense. This is important especially for those who live in cultures where shoes are worn all day.

SUMMARY

Western massage traditionally includes joint movements as well as soft tissue techniques. Joint movements may be categorized as active (free, assisted, resisted) and passive. During passive joint movements the practitioner initiates and controls the movement, while the recipient remains totally relaxed and passive.

Mobilizing techniques are passive movements performed within the normal range of joint movement. Stretching is a type of passive joint movement that is performed to the limit of the range of motion, and then slightly beyond, to increase flexibility at the joint. Stretching approaches include static stretch, contract-relax-stretch, and using reciprocal inhibition. Mobilizing techniques and stretches can be easily integrated into a massage routine.

Joint manipulations or adjustments that involve thrusting movements are not within the scope of massage therapy. They should be performed only by those trained to do so within their legal scope of practice. Joint movements within the scope of massage therapy include simple passive and active joint movements, which fall into the categories of non-specific mobilizing and stretching techniques.

General guidelines for performing joint movements safely are as follows: Stay within the normal range of motion of the joint; qualities of movement for mobilizing techniques are smooth, free, and loose; warm the surrounding soft tissues before stretching; use breathing to enhance the stretch; stay within the comfort range of the recipient; be aware of any abnormality of joint structure and adapt movements accordingly.

The areas of the body for which passive joint movements are effective include the neck, shoulder girdle, wrists, hands, chest, hips, knees, ankles, and feet. Practitioners should have practical knowledge of the structure and the movement possible at each joint to ensure the safety of the recipient during joint movements.

Joint movements are used for a variety of reasons including to stretch surrounding soft tissues; increase joint range of motion; stimulate production of synovial fluid; increase kinesthetic awareness; induce muscle relaxation; and build muscle strength. Some contemporary systems of bodywork use joint movements to affect the nervous system, reeducate muscles, and integrate function. Receivers can learn to let go of tension during passive joint movements. Joint movements add a kinetic dimension to a massage session and provide diversity of technique.

A look ahead . . .

Massage techniques and joint movements are combined and applied to achieve the therapeutic goals of a massage session. In many settings (e.g., health club, spa, private practice) massage is offered in one-hour full-body sessions that focus on general health and wellbeing. Chapter 9 describes a typical full-body massage.

REFERENCES

Cailliet, R. (1981). *Shoulder pain*, 2nd ed. Philadelphia: F. A. Davis.
McMillan, M. (1925). *Massage and therapeutic exercise*. Philadelphia: W. B. Saunders.
Roth, M. (1851). *The prevention and cure of many chronic diseases by movements*. London: John Churchill.

CHAPTER NINE

Full-Body Western Massage

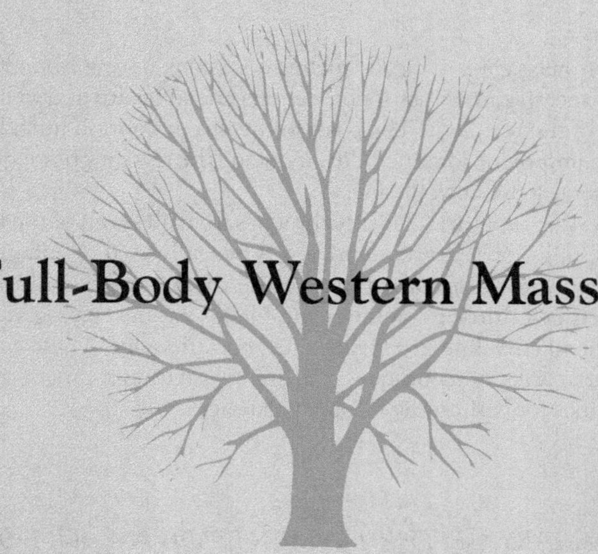

LEARNING OUTCOMES

After studying this chapter, the student will have information to:

1. Discuss the form and intent of a full-body Western massage.
2. Plan the sequence of the massage session from region to region.
3. Apply techniques in appropriate order within each body region.
4. Choose opening, warm-up, transition and finishing techniques appropriately.
5. Apply the principles of continuity, rhythm, pacing, and specificity.
6. Perform a one-hour full-body Western massage for health promotion.

KEY TERMS/CONCEPTS

Continuity
Draping
Eclectic
Finishing technique
Flow
Full-body Western massage
Opening technique
Order of techniques
Pacing
Rhythm
Routine
Sequence of body regions
Specificity
Technique combination
Transition technique
Warming technique

LINK LIBRARY TERMS

Swedish Massage • *Massage Business* • *Traditional Chinese Medicine/Traditional Asian Medicine* • *Massage Regulations*

MEDIALINK

A companion CD-ROM, included free with each new copy of this book, supplements the techniques presented in this chapter. Insert the CD-ROM to watch video clips of massage techniques being demonstrated. This multimedia feature is designed to help you add a new dimension to your learning.

OVERVIEW

Full-body Western massage is typically given in sessions lasting from 30 to 90 minutes. Performed from a wellness perspective, these sessions focus on general health and wellbeing as well as meeting the therapeutic needs of the recipient. The goals for health promotion include improving circulation, relaxing the muscles, improving joint mobility, inducing the relaxation response, promoting healthy skin, and creating a general sense of wellbeing.

A full-body session usually includes techniques from all seven of the basic Western massage technique categories. Oil, lotion, or other lubricant is typically used to enhance sliding over the skin and to prevent chaffing. Types of topical substances and their properties are described in Chapter 6.

Although each practitioner combines and blends various massage techniques in different ways, there are some general guidelines for giving a full-body massage. These guidelines address draping, sequence of body parts, order of techniques, continuity, rhythm, pacing, and specificity. Table 9–1 summarizes the guidelines for performing full-body massage.

Table 9–1 *SUMMARY OF THE ELEMENTS OF A FULL-BODY WESTERN MASSAGE ROUTINE*

Goals	General health promotion Improved circulation, relaxed muscles, improved joint mobility, relaxation response, healthy skin, sense of wellbeing Therapeutic needs (e.g., reduce muscle stiffness and soreness, relieve trigger points, injury recovery)
Length of Time	30–90 minutes (typically 60 minutes)
Draping	Full sheet or large towel Body regions uncovered for massage and then recovered Genitals and women's breasts covered at all times

Sequence of Body Regions	Starting point
	Direction (e.g., clockwise)
	Ending point
	
	Starting prone (example)
	  Start on back
	  Buttocks, legs
	  Turn to supine
	  Legs/feet, arms/shoulders, neck, chest, abdomen
	  End with head and face
	
	Starting supine (example)
	  Start on head and face
	  Neck, arms/shoulders, chest, abdomen, legs/feet
	  Turn to prone
	  Legs, buttocks
	  End with back

Order of Techniques on a Specific Body Region	Opening technique (e.g., effleurage to apply oil or compressions)
	Warming techniques (e.g., effleurage or compressions)
	Combination of techniques
	  For general health (e.g., effleurage, petrissage, superficial warming friction, joint movements
	  Specific therapeutic goals (e.g., deep friction, vibration, direct pressure)
	Transition techniques (e.g., effleurage, tapotement)
	Finishing techniques (e.g., effleurage, tapotement)

(continued)

Table 9–1 (Cont.)

Continuity	Sense of continuous touch throughout the session Avoid abrupt removal of touch
Flow	Orderly sequence and smooth transitions Skillful draping
Rhythm	Smooth and even rhythm
Pacing	Moderate speed
Specificity	For attention to specific muscle or small area Shorter length session = less specificity in full-body massage

GUIDELINES FOR FULL-BODY MASSAGE

Draping

Draping is done with a sheet or large towel, and body parts skillfully uncovered and recovered as needed. Genitals are covered at all times. Women's breasts are always covered, except when breast massage is performed by a practitioner with special training and then only with informed consent of the recipient. Breast massage will not be included in the general full-body routine described in this chapter.

Sequence of Body Regions

In a full-body session, the practitioner massages each region of the body (e.g., back, arm, and leg) in a particular **sequence.** The sequence usually includes supine and prone positions, and has a starting point, direction (e.g., clockwise), and an ending point. This establishes a routine way of working as discussed further below.

Recipients generally lie prone or supine for the first part of the massage, and then turn over for the second part. Whether they start prone or supine is a matter of preference for the practitioner and the recipient. Sometimes the side-lying position is used, for example, with pregnant women.

There are no hard and fast rules for sequence, but it should facilitate a smooth flow from one region of the body to the next. Some advocate moving clockwise around the table. The following are two suggestions for sequences in a full-body routine.

- If a session starts with the recipient in the prone position, a commonly used sequence of body sections would be the back, buttocks, and legs. The neck and feet are sometimes addressed prone, but are more easily accessed supine. Then turn over to the supine position with a sequence moving from legs and feet, to arms and hands, and then to shoulders, neck, chest and abdomen, and ending with the head and face.
- If the session starts with the recipient in the supine position, a commonly used sequence of body sections would be head and face, neck and shoulders, arms and hands, chest and abdomen, legs and feet. Then turn over to the prone position with a sequence moving from legs to buttocks and ending on the back.

The advantages of starting in the prone position include that it may feel safer to a recipient new to massage, back massage triggers the relaxation response sooner, and it allows those who need to be more alert at the end of the session to finish face-up. An advantage of starting in the supine position is that the practitioner can massage the head, face, and neck right away, which is good for recipients who do a lot of desk or computer work.

Order of Techniques

The general **order of techniques** for each region of the body is similar. Once a part is undraped, opening and warming techniques are applied. These are followed by a combination of techniques for general health promotion, as well as techniques for specific therapeutic effects. Finishing and transition techniques complete work on the region.

The most common **opening** and **warming technique** for each area to be massaged is effleurage. It is used to apply oil or other lubricant, to warm the area, and to facilitate circulation. It is applied first using lighter and then deeper pressure. Effleurage on the limbs should always be performed moving distal to proximal, unless the pressure used is very light. Compressions may also serve as an opening or warming technique.

The opening is followed by a combination of techniques to improve circulation, relax muscles, improve joint mobility, and other health promotion goals. **Technique combinations** at this stage usually include effleurage, petrissage, warming friction, and joint movements. Deep friction, vibration, and direct pressure are applied as appropriate for more specific work. Finish work on the area with effleurage and/or tapotement.

Transition techniques serve to provide continuity and flow from one section to another (see discussion below). For example, when moving from massage of the upper leg to the lower leg, a few effleurage strokes to the entire leg help tie the regions together kinesthetically for the recipient.

When ending work on a specific part of the body, the prone or supine side, or the entire session, some thought should be given to **finishing techniques.** Finishing techniques may be used to reconnect parts of the body that have been worked on more specifically or to further sedate or stimulate the recipient. Effleurage and tapotement are the usual finishing techniques that can be used to create a sense of wholeness. Light effleurage, sometimes called nerve strokes, is more soothing, while tapotement is more stimulating. Passive touch in the form of simple holding at the head or feet is calming and is sometimes used to end a session.

Continuity and Flow

A full-body session should have a sense of **continuity** and flow. Take care when establishing touch at the beginning of a session, and then create a sense of continuous touch throughout the session. Establishment or removal of touch should never be abrupt. This does not mean that you may never take your hands off a recipient during a session, but that doing so should be kept to a minimum and be done as imperceptibly as possible. A sense of **flow** is achieved through an orderly sequence and smooth transitions from one part of the body to the next. Skill in draping, including uncovering and recovering can add to the sense of smooth transitions.

Rhythm, Pacing, and Specificity

The **rhythm** of a classic full-body massage session may be described as smooth and even, and the **pacing** as moderate in speed. Trying to perform a full-body session in half an hour will necessitate a faster pace with less attention to detail. A session focusing on general relaxation will be slower paced and usually minimize or eliminate stimulating techniques such as tapotement. **Specificity** is required for attention to a specific muscle or small area. If the recipient requests more attention to certain parts of the body such as the back and neck, then those areas would receive more time and specific techniques, while the rest of the body would receive less specific massage.

FULL-BODY WESTERN MASSAGE ROUTINE

There is no one best way to perform a full-body Western massage. Practitioners usually develop their own styles and routine ways of performing a massage session. **Routines** generally involve a regular starting point and opening techniques, a specific sequence of body regions, a certain order of techniques in each body region, and a regular way of ending the session. These routines typically change with further training and experience, and are modified to meet the needs of the recipient on the table. Today's **eclectic** practitioners may use a full-body Western routine as a starting point and then integrate contemporary techniques as appropriate to accomplish the therapeutic goals of the session.

The following is an example of a one-hour full-body routine that may be used to practice the basic Western massage techniques on different parts of the body. By having a routine as a framework, the learner is free to focus on specific skills, including good body mechanics, draping, specific techniques, smooth transitions, continuity, rhythm, and pacing.

It is impossible to describe every single movement of a routine in writing. Use the routine described below as a framework but feel free to add variations of techniques as you become more attuned to the work. Experiment with what feels right to you. Most of the techniques described are illustrated in Chapters 7–10. To lengthen the routine you may repeat techniques or insert additional techniques as appropriate.

Prone Position (25 minutes)

Before leaving recipients alone to undress in private, request that when you return they be covered with the drape and lying face down on the table. Show them how the face cradle works, and position a bolster approximately where their ankles will be. Before you start the session, adjust the position of the face cradle and the bolster for safety and comfort.

Back (15 minutes). Uncover the back down to the waist. Standing at the head, begin applying oil or lotion on the back. Bilateral tree stroking is a good technique to use to apply oil (Figure 7–6). The movement should be smooth, and cover the entire back and sides. Use light to moderate pressure. Repeat the technique three or four times.

Without losing contact, move to the recipient's right side. Stand at the hip and face the head. Work this side of the back entirely before moving to the other side. Perform the "shingles" effleurage technique along the near side of the spine (Figure 7–5). Fingers point toward the head. Use moderate to deep pressure. Fully warm the erector muscles of the spine. Perform deep friction with the fingertips along the erector muscles moving from the sacrum to the neck (Figure 7–21). To apply deeper pressure, use both hands, placing one hand on top of the other, as shown in Figure 9–1.

Perform deep effleurage with the thumbs on the lower back between the iliac crest and the last three ribs to massage the quadratus lumborum. Be sure that the thumbs are in proper alignment. (Warming friction using the knuckles may be substituted as easier on the hands; Figure 7–18.) Repeat this technique in two or three strips moving out laterally from the spine. Use moderate to deep pressure.

Reconnect the lower back with the shoulder with a few light "shingles" effleurage strokes. Then perform a deeper effleurage over the upper back and shoulder. Place one hand over the other to apply greater pressure, and use a circular movement around the shoulder, as shown in Figure 9–2.

Perform circular two-handed petrissage over the entire upper back (Figure 7–14). Follow with basic kneading to relax the upper trapezius. Kneading with one hand works better with smaller recipients, as shown in Figure 9–3. Begin finishing this side of the back with three-count stroking of the trapezius (Figure 7–7). Follow with horizontal stroking of the back moving from lower back to shoulders.

Transition to the other side by performing light effleurage from waist to shoulders as you walk around the head of the table. Repeat the entire sequence on the other side, beginning with shingles effleurage.

When both sides of the back have been massaged, redrape the back. Finish the entire back with rapping or some other form of tapotement using moderate force (Figure 7–25).

Lower Limbs and Buttocks (10 minutes). Undrape the right leg up to the waist, being careful not to expose the natal cleft. Tuck the drape securely under the leg and at the waist (Figure 6–10).

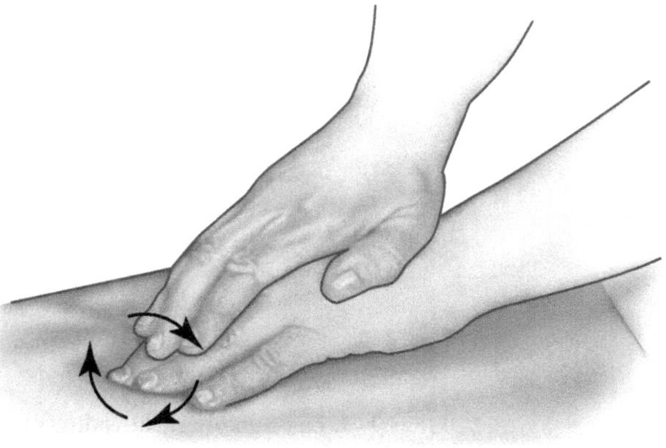

FIGURE 9–1. Circular friction with fingertips on erector muscles along side of the spine.

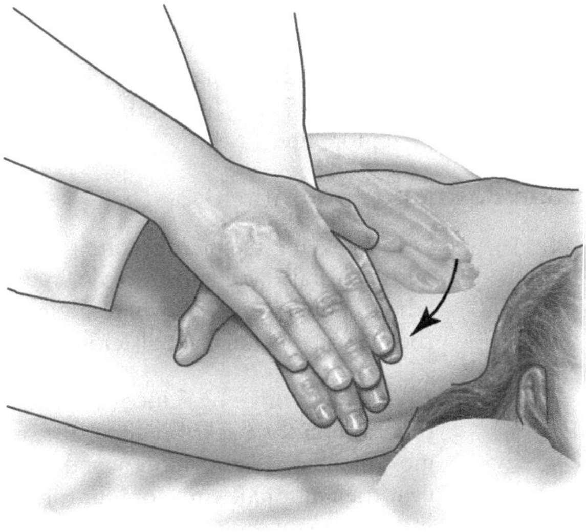

FIGURE 9–2. Deep effleurage over the upper back and shoulder.

Stand at the side of the table facing the head. Apply oil or lotion to the entire leg and hip with basic sliding effleurage using light to moderate pressure. Follow the curves of the leg in a continuous motion from foot to hip. Be sure to touch both sides of the leg, and not just the back of the leg. The inside hand will slide onto the back of the leg below the muscle attachments and follow the outside hand around the hip. Coordinate the movements of your hands so that as the outside hand starts to return down the leg, it is followed by the inside hand (see Figure 9–4). Both hands return to the ankle with a light sliding motion.

Note: Your hands should never touch or come unreasonably close to the genital area. Care should be taken when working on the inside of the leg to maintain ethical and comfortable boundaries. Skillful draping in this area will help to create a feeling of safety for both the recipient and the practitioner.

The lower limb and hip are massaged in this order: buttocks, upper leg, lower leg. Warm up the buttocks muscles using deep circular effleurage, one hand on top reinforcing the other as shown in Figure 9–5. Follow with compressions using the fist to reach deep gluteal muscles. Moderate to deep pressure may be used on these large muscles. Be sure to work the attachments along the iliac crest. Finish with circular effleurage as you started, using either the hand-over-hand position or the fist.

Two or three basic sliding effleurage strokes to the entire leg and hip help create a smooth transition to the upper leg. Perform deep effleurage with alternating fists on the hamstrings, from above the popliteal fossa to the attachments on the ilium, as shown in Figure 9–6. Continuing with one fist, perform effleurage along the iliotibial band and the tensor fascia lata muscle moving from the hip to the knee. This broad band of fascia and muscle can accept moderate to deep pressure.

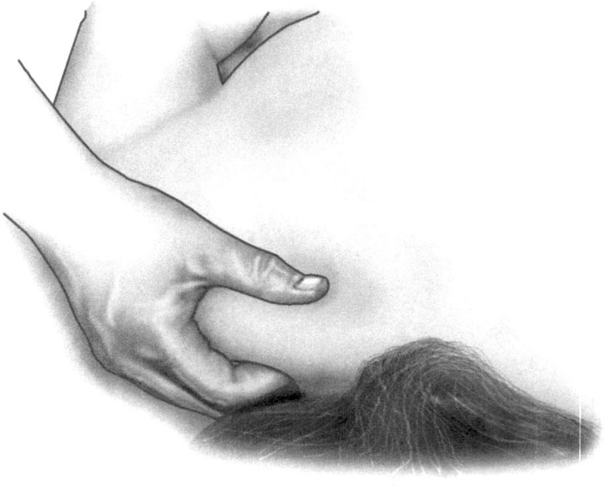

FIGURE 9–3. Basic one-hand kneading of the upper trapezius.

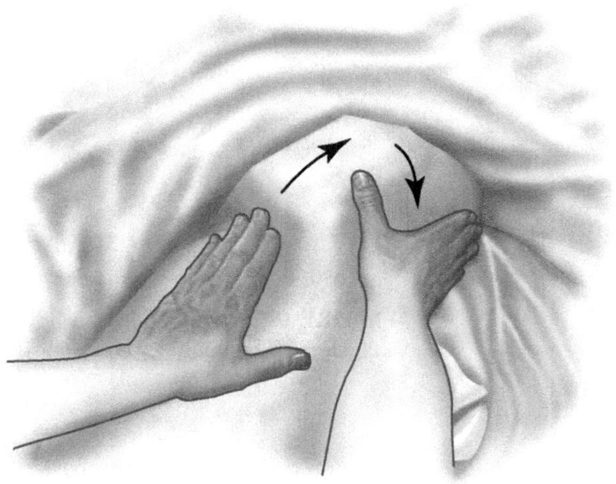

FIGURE 9–4. Applying oil to the entire leg, recipient in prone position.

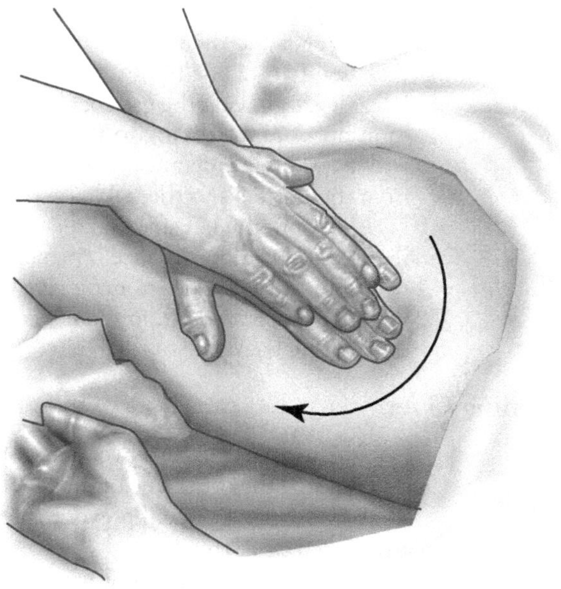

FIGURE 9–5. Deep effleurage to the gluteal muscles using reinforced fingertips.

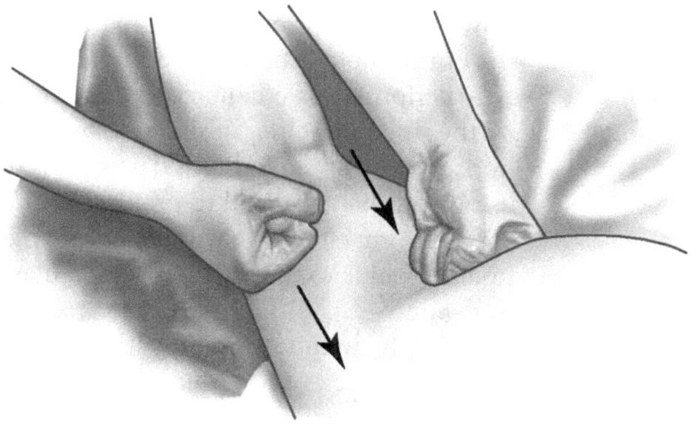

FIGURE 9–6. Deep effleurage to hamstring muscles using fists.

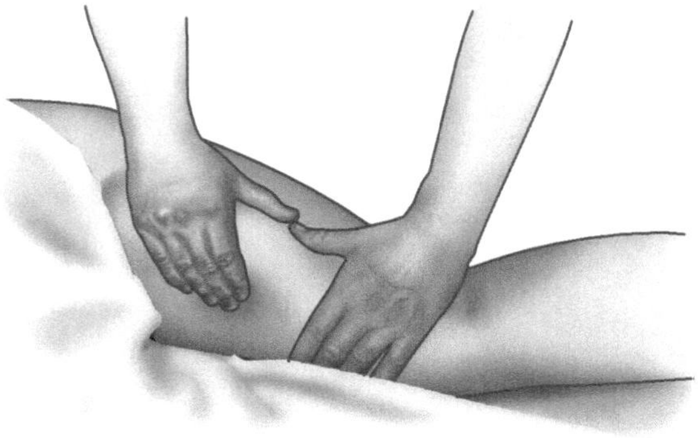

FIGURE 9–7. Two-handed kneading to adductors of the thigh.

Warm up the adductors with basic sliding effleurage using the palms. Reach to the medial side of the thigh, and then pull up and around to the back of the thigh in a smooth sliding motion. Alternating hands, move from the knee to just below the attachments of the adductors. Be mindful of boundaries as mentioned above when working the inside of the leg.

Perform basic two-handed kneading on the upper leg, including the back and both sides. Figure 9–7 shows kneading the adductors of the upper leg. Finish with basic sliding effleurage distal to proximal, first to the upper and then to the entire leg.

Use two-handed kneading to massage the lower leg. Finish with basic sliding effleurage to the lower leg, following the gastrocnemius to the attachments on either side of the knee (Figure 7–1). Perform horizontal stroking to the upper and lower legs, starting on the upper leg (Figure 7–8). Finish with a few basic effleurage strokes from ankle to hip. Redrape the leg. Finish this leg with nerve strokes from the buttocks to the ankle.

Move to the left side and repeat the entire leg sequence. Finish the back side of the body with the recipient fully draped. Place one hand on the back and the other hand on a lower leg, and gently rock the body. Switch hands from one leg to the other leg. This should take only 5–10 seconds. Perform 2–3 light effleurage stokes from shoulders to feet as a connecting maneuver, and to signal the end of the massage on the back side of the body.

Turning Over

Ask the recipient to turn over. Assist by anchoring the drape with your leg against the side of the table and holding the other side of the drape up. This is called tenting (Figure 6–12). Have the recipient roll away from you. This will prevent the drape from getting wrapped up around the recipient during the turnover. Lower the drape.

Note that the recipient was out of your sight as he or she turned over under the tent. If there is more than one session going on in the room, be sure that you do not expose the recipient to others.

Supine Position (35 minutes)

Lower Limbs (10 minutes). Uncover left leg and tuck the drape securely (Figure 6–9). Apply oil to the entire limb using basic sliding effleurage.

Perform deep effleurage to the thigh using both hands. Follow this with two-handed kneading. Jostle the thigh muscles, causing passive movement in the hip and knee joints as shown in Figure 9–8. Use horizontal stroking to lift and compress the thigh muscles. Finish massage of the thigh with effleurage using both hands, distal to proximal.

Perform effleurage with moderate pressure to the entire limb as a transition, followed by effleurage from the ankle to the knee. Apply circular friction around the knee using the heels of the hands as shown in Figure 9–9.

Apply thumb stripping to the tibialis anterior as shown in Figure 9–10. Perform this technique on the lateral side of the lower leg from just above the ankle to the attachment on the lateral condyle of the tibia. You will complete two to four strips, depending on the size of the muscle. Follow the thumb

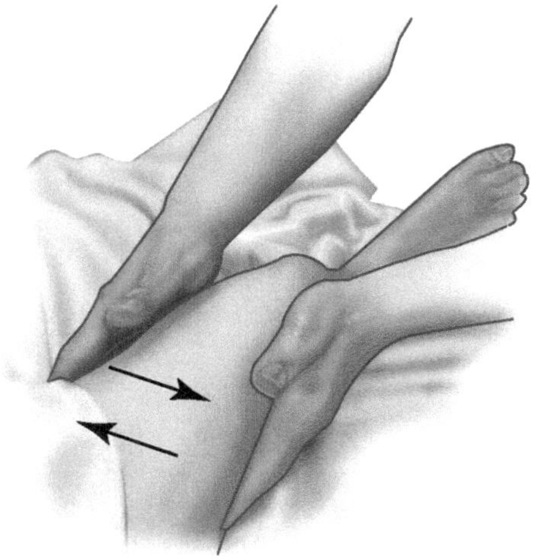

FIGURE 9–8. Jostling the thigh muscles, recipient in supine position.

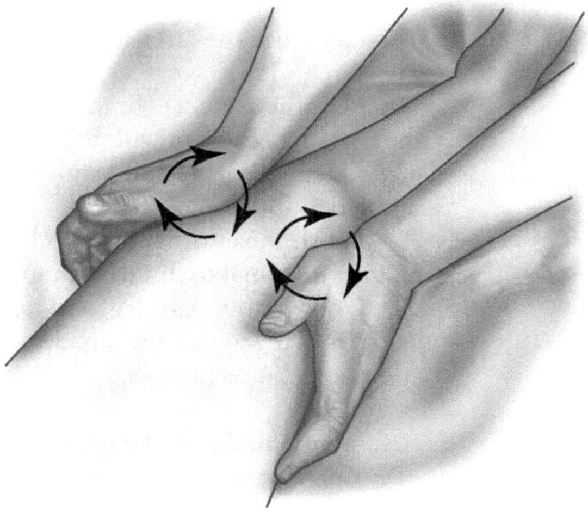

FIGURE 9–9. Circular friction around knee using the heels of the hands.

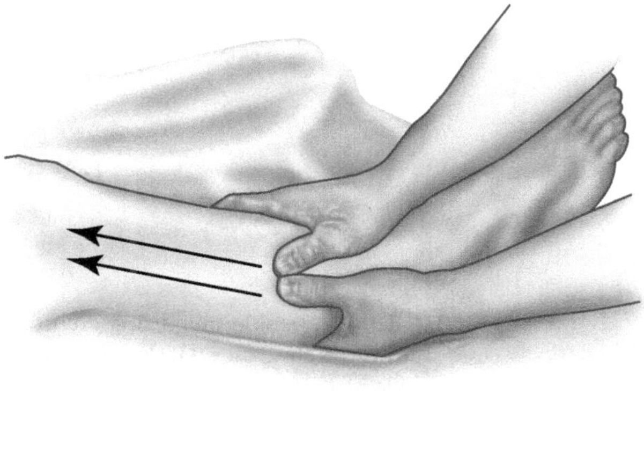

FIGURE 9–10. Thumb stripping along tibialis anterior.

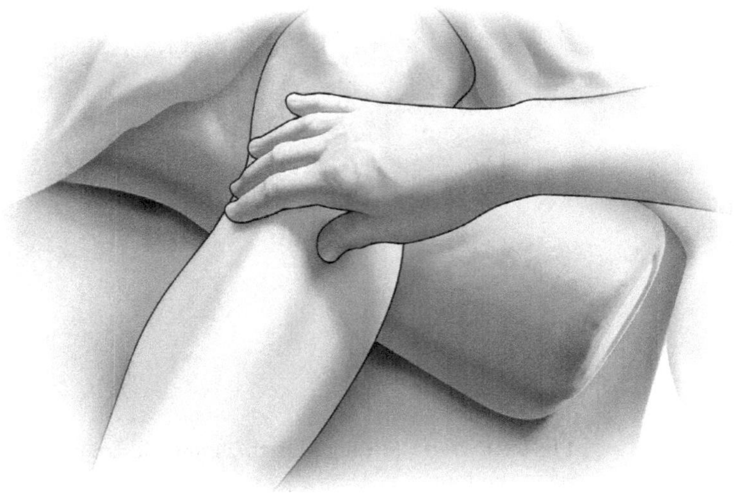

FIGURE 9–11. Direct pressure along tibialis anterior.

stripping with direct pressure along the tibialis anterior, moving about one inch at a time proximal to distal. Keep thumb and wrist in alignment as shown in Figure 9–11.

Slide down the lower leg and perform circular friction around the ankle with the fingertips. Then mobilize the ankle using the heels of the hands. The foot will wiggle back and forth as shown in Figure 9–12.

Perform effleurage between the metatarsals using the thumb or fingers (Figure 7–2). Slide along the bottom of the foot with the fist from the ball of the foot to the heel, as shown in Figure 9–13, using moderate to deep pressure. Finish with slapping tapotement on the bottom of the foot using the back of the hand.

Finish the entire limb with light effleurage moving distal to proximal, followed by nerve strokes moving proximal to distal. Redrape the leg.

Uncover the right leg, and repeat the entire sequence. After both legs have been massaged, and before moving to the upper body, some nerve strokes over the redraped legs may be used as a finishing and transition technique.

Arms and Shoulders (10 minutes). Uncover the right arm and shoulder (Figure 6–8). Apply lubricant to entire upper limb using basic sliding effleurage, moving distal to proximal. The movement should flow from the hand to the shoulder, including around the deltoid muscle.

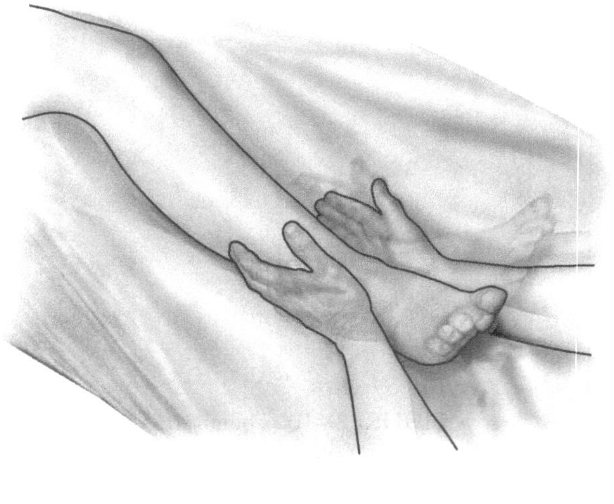

FIGURE 9–12. Ankle mobilizing technique using the heels of the hands. The foot moves from side to side.

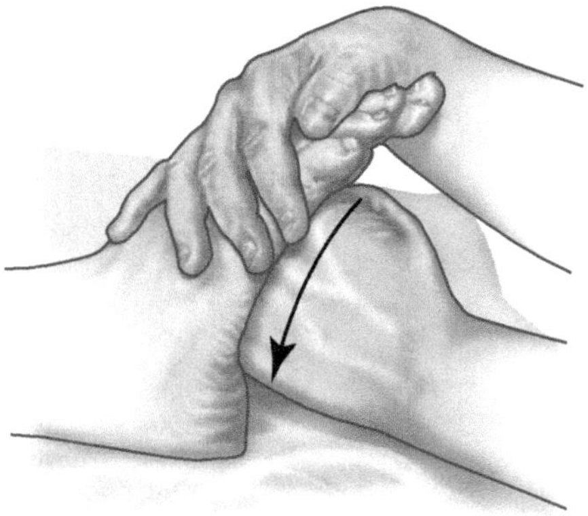

FIGURE 9–13. Effleurage to bottom of the foot using the fist.

Perform alternating one-hand petrissage to the upper arm. Squeeze the biceps side, then the triceps side, alternating in a rhythmical motion (Figure 7–13). Be sure to petrissage the entire upper arm from the shoulder to the elbow.

Mobilize the shoulder by grasping the upper arm with both hands just below the shoulder and moving the joint in a circle. This is a passive shoulder roll, in which the shoulders are brought forward, elevated, rolled back, and then depressed. Move both clockwise and counterclockwise (Figure 8–5).

After a few light effleurage strokes to the entire limb as a transition, perform one-hand effleurage to the lower arm as an additional warm-up using moderate to deep pressure. Knead the muscles of the lower arm, particularly near the elbow. Follow with thumb stripping to the flexor and extensor muscles on the lower arm, from the wrist to their attachments near the elbow. See Figure 9–14.

Interlock your fingers with the recipient's and press gently with your fingers to the back of his or her hand to mobilize the joints at the knuckle. Keeping the fingers interlocked, mobilize the wrist taking it through its normal range of motion. Apply effleurage to the back of the hand between metacarpals using your thumbs. Then lightly squeeze along each finger, moving proximal to distal. Turn the hand over so that it is palm up. Apply effleurage to the palm of the hand moving distal to proximal as shown in Figure 9–15. Grip the hand on the little finger and thumb sides, palm down, and gently squeeze the hand while broadening the palm and separating the metacarpals.

Use basic sliding effleurage from hand to shoulder to kinesthetically reconnect the arm. Lift the arm, holding just below the wrist, and perform effleurage on the pectoral muscles with a loose fist moving lateral to medial, and stopping at the breast tissue. See Figure 9–16.

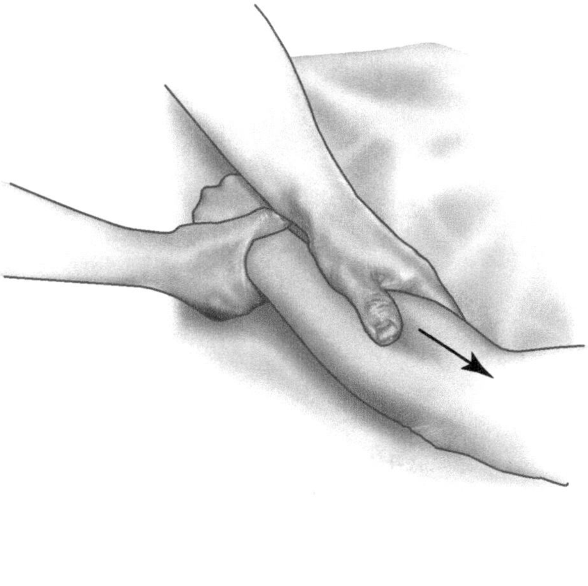

FIGURE 9–14. Thumb stripping along extensor muscles of the forearm.

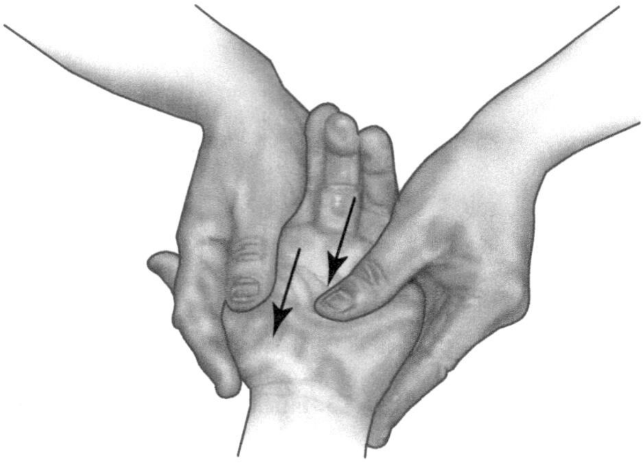

FIGURE 9–15. Effleurage to palm of the hand using thumbs.

A basic sliding effleurage stroke may be performed over the sternum as shown in Figure 9–17. Use good judgment in applying this stroke with women. It may be advisable to omit the technique if the woman has large breasts or if she might feel it as an invasion of her boundaries. Err on the side of omission, and ask permission if in doubt.

Finish with basic sliding effleurage to the entire upper limb using moderate pressure. Redrape the arm and shoulder. Repeat the entire sequence on the other arm.

Abdomen (5 minutes). The abdomen is a vulnerable area for many people. If the recipient is new to massage, or new to you, ask permission to work in this area. Explain to women that the breasts will be draped. You might also want to explain the purpose of massaging the abdomen. Find out if they have eaten within the past hour, and skip the area if that is the case. People experiencing constipation or gas in the bowels may be sensitive to pressure; however, massage of the abdomen may help relieve those conditions.

Cover a woman's breasts with an additional drape before you pull back the larger drape to the iliac crest exposing the abdomen (Figure 6–11). Do not expose the pubic area.

Begin by gently laying a hand on the abdomen to establish contact. Perform effleurage moving clockwise in a circular pattern. Use the fingertips of one hand, while the other hand rests on top. See Figure 9–18. Move in a large circle along the bottom of the ribs and around the outline of the pelvis, followed by smaller, then even smaller concentric circles. Check with the recipient to make sure the pressure is comfortable.

Perform vibration to the area with the fingertips moving from place to place in a clockwise pattern (Figure 7–31). Take care in areas that recipients report as feeling sore. Petrissage the abdomen

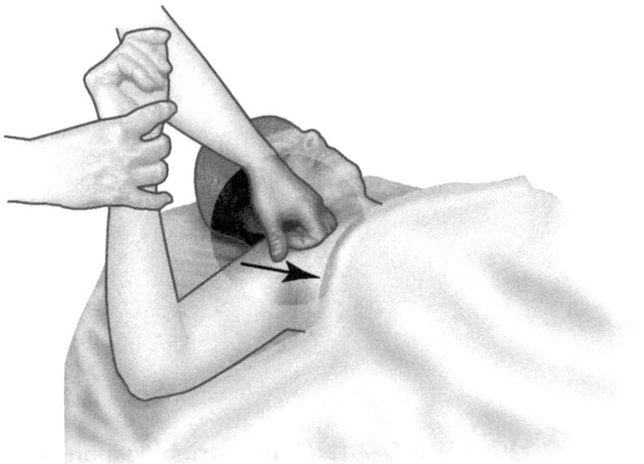

FIGURE 9–16. Effleurage to pectoral muscles using a loose fist.

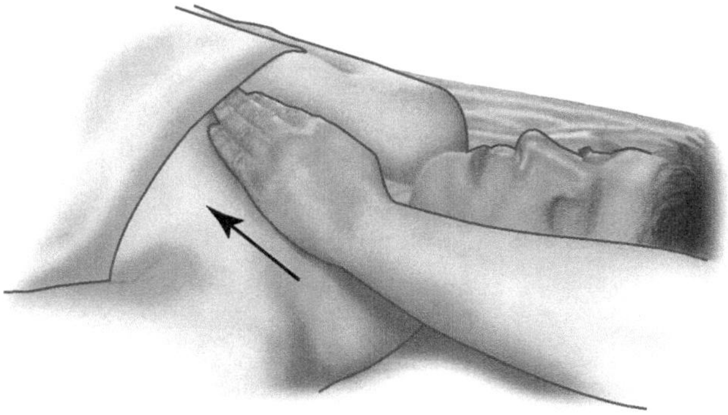

FIGURE 9–17. Basic sliding effleurage over sternum using palm of the hand.

with a flat hand, palm down, using an undulating or wavelike motion. Push in first with the heel of the hand, and then roll onto the fingertips. The soft tissues of the viscera are stimulated with the rhythmic compression. Move from place to place on the abdomen.

Repeat circular effleurage moving clockwise as a transition. Follow with horizontal stroking of the abdomen. Finish the area with passive touch in the center of the abdomen. Remove your hand and recover the recipient to the shoulders with the larger drape. The breast drape may remain in place for warmth or may be removed at this time.

Neck and Shoulders (5 minutes). You may sit at the head of the recipient to work on the head and shoulders. Maintain good body mechanics for sitting, as in Figure 6–21. Establish contact by mobilizing the shoulders with a "cat paw" movement, alternating pushing one side and then the other as shown in Figure 9–19.

Apply lubricant to both sides of the neck (one hand on each side), performing effleurage along the trapezius from the shoulder tips to the occipital ridge. Turn the head slightly to the right side, exposing the left side of the neck. Perform effleurage with the fist on the upper trapezius from the occipital ridge to the shoulder as shown in Figure 9–20. The upper trapezius will stretch mildly.

Continuing on the left side, use circular friction along the occipital ridge and the neck to warm the deeper muscles of the region. Start with the suboccipitals (medial to lateral) and then down the cervicals to the base of the neck. Follow this with stripping using fingertips or a knuckle, to the posterior cervicals from the occiput to the base of the neck. Finish the left side with effleurage with the palm of the hand, moving back and forth from the tip of the shoulder to the occiput. Turn the head slightly to the left, and repeat the sequence to the right side.

Create a wavelike neck mobilization. Place the hands palms up at the base of the neck, one on either side of the spine, with fingertips pressing up on the cervical muscles. Draw the fingers toward the occiput, maintaining pressure upward. The cervical vertebrae will rise and fall as the

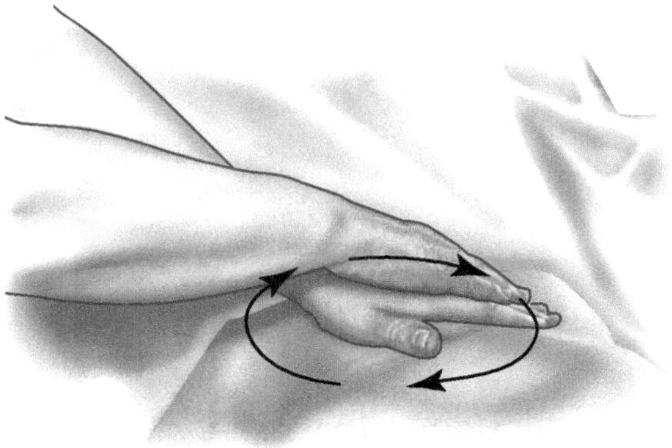

FIGURE 9–18. Effleurage in circular pattern applied to the abdomen.

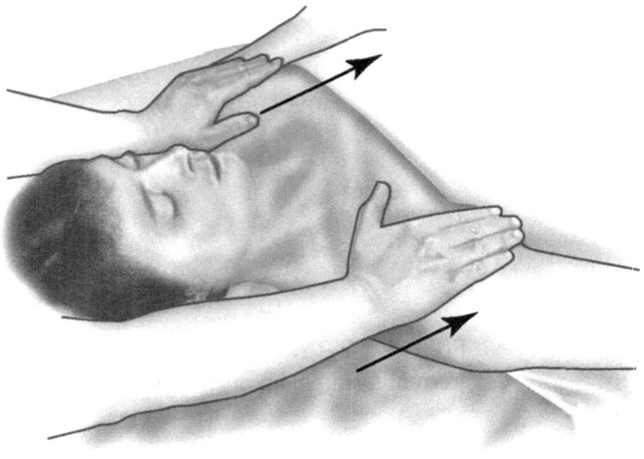

FIGURE 9–19. "Cat paw" motion to gently mobilize shoulders. Alternate hands pushing on shoulders.

fingers pass underneath. If the muscles are relaxed, this will create a wavelike motion in the neck. See Figure 9–21.

Finish with effleurage to both sides of the shoulders and neck. Start the movement at the tips of the shoulders and draw the hands toward the base of the neck and up to the occiput. Mobilize one shoulder at a time, holding the head with one hand and pushing on the tip of the shoulder with the other hand. Cradle the head briefly in both hands to end this section.

Face and Head (5 minutes). Use very little or no lubricant on the face. Ask the recipient what he or she prefers. Lotion may offer an acceptable solution; however, the entire face and head sequence can usually be performed quite well without using lubricant.

Place the hands gently on the face with fingertips at the jaw. Draw the hands toward the temples in an effleurage stroke using the full palm-side of the hands as shown in Figure 9–22. Repeat two or three times. Perform circular friction with the fingertips over the masseter and then the temporalis muscles. Stroke the muscles of the forehead using effleurage with the thumbs moving medial to lateral.

Petrissage the forehead using a circular motion of the thumbs. The movement is timed so that the tissues are lifted and pressed as the thumbs move by one another. This is similar to the two-handed circular petrissage described in Figure 7–14.

Stroke alongside of the nose and continue the effleurage movement along the cheekbones. Press up under the cheekbones with the fingertips using light to moderate pressure. Loosen the scalp with circular friction over the entire hair area. A relaxed scalp will have a greater degree of movement than a "tight" scalp. Loosening the area will improve blood supply to the skin and hair follicles.

Finish the entire session by holding the head without movement as shown in Figure 9–23. Hold for a few seconds until you can feel the recipient completely relax.

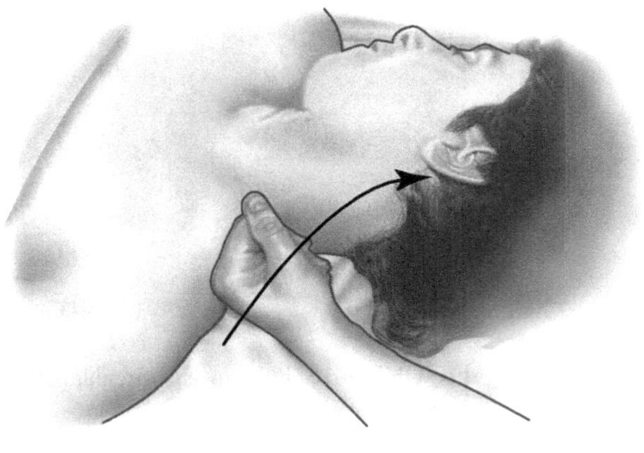

FIGURE 9–20. Effleurage to upper trapezius using fist.

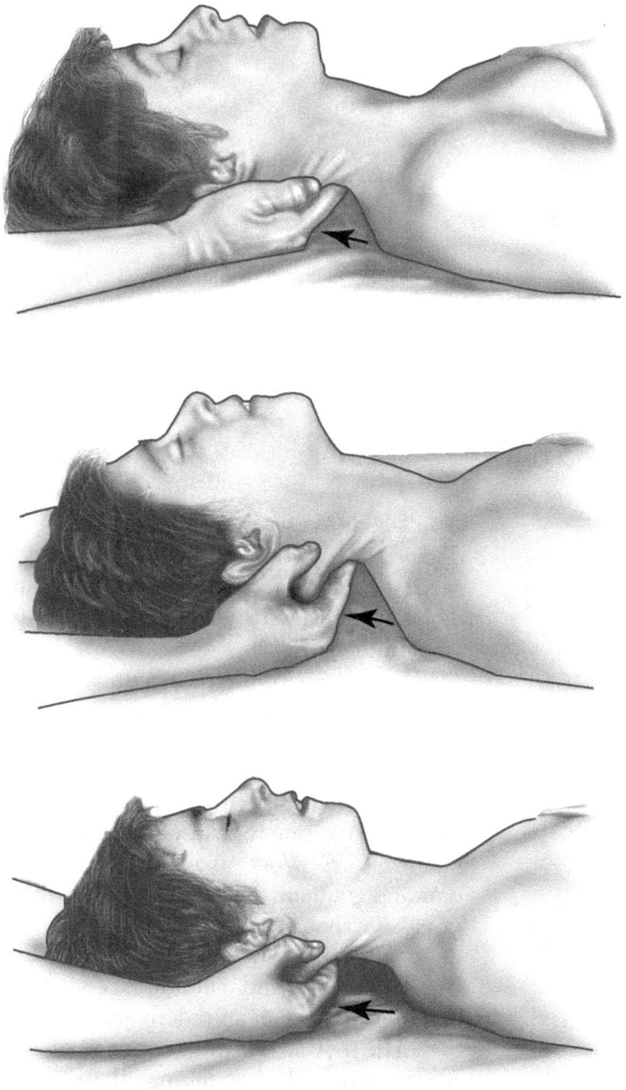

FIGURE 9–21. Wavelike neck mobilizing technique. Draw the fingers toward the occiput while maintaining pressure upwards.

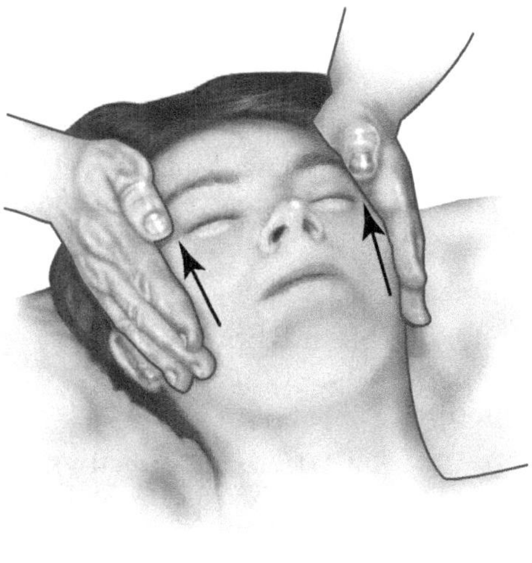

FIGURE 9–22. Effleurage to the face using palms.

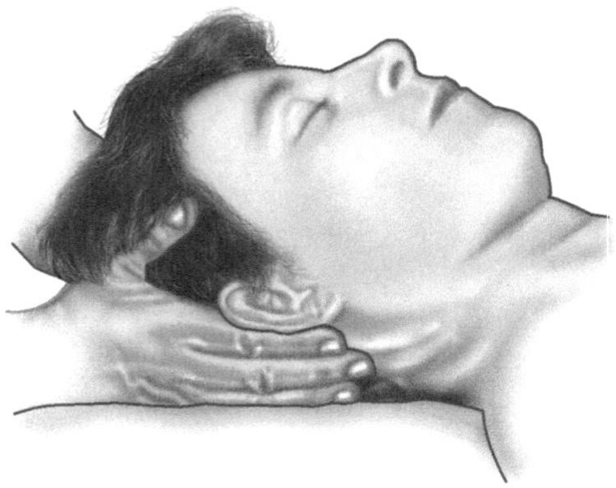

FIGURE 9–23. Cradling the head to finish the session.

SUMMARY

A full-body Western massage lasts from 30 to 90 minutes, and includes massage of the back, legs, abdomen, chest, arms, neck, and head. Performed from a wellness perspective, these sessions focus on general health and wellbeing as well as meeting the therapeutic needs of the recipient. Practitioners develop their own styles and routine ways of performing a massage session; however, some general guidelines apply.

The recipient is typically unclothed and draped with a sheet for modesty. The practitioner blends the seven basic Western massage techniques into a sequence to create a routine. The sequence usually includes both supine and prone positions, and has a starting point, a direction (e.g., clockwise), and an ending point. Oil or lotion is used to enhance movement over the skin and to prevent chafing.

The order of techniques for each part of the body includes opening and warming techniques like effleurage or compressions, followed by technique combinations for general health and specific therapeutic effects. Work on a particular area is concluded with finishing techniques to reconnect, smooth out, and gradually lighten touch. Finishing techniques typically include light effleurage, tapotement, or passive touch such as holding.

A full-body massage should have a sense of continuity and flow. Touch is established at the beginning of a session and maintained continuously throughout, with minimal interruption. A sense of flow is achieved through an orderly sequence and smooth transitions from one part of the body to the next.

The rhythm of a full-body massage is smooth and even, and the pacing is moderate in speed. Specificity is required when giving attention to small areas, or applying techniques for specific therapeutic purposes. Eclectic practitioners may use full-body Western massage as a starting point, and then integrate other massage forms as appropriate to meet the client's needs.

A look ahead . . .

A client will oftentimes need more specific attention to certain areas of the body, for example, the neck and shoulders, or legs and feet. Chapter 10 describes technique combinations for more specific therapeutic results in different areas of the body.

ADDITIONAL RESOURCES

Video

"Body massage for the day spa." (1997) Erica Miller Professional Education Series. Mile Ranch, British Columbia: Spa Expertise Canada LTD.

"Therapeutic Massage." Santa Barbara, CA: Real Bodywork. (*www.deeptissue.com*)

C H A P T E R   T E N

Regional Applications

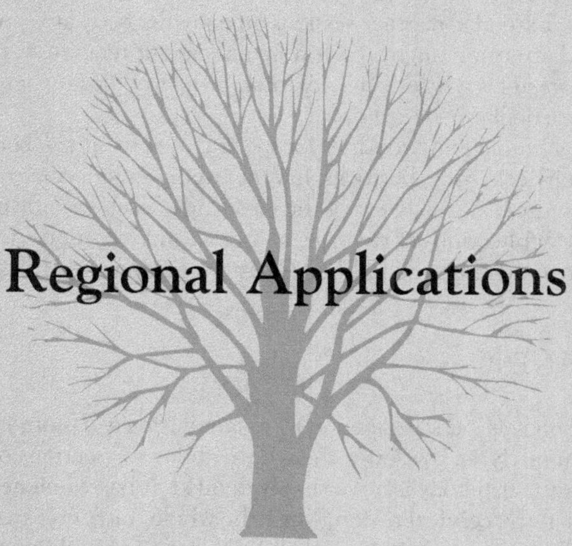

LEARNING OUTCOMES

After studying this chapter, the student will have information to:

1. Discuss the "wholeness" of the human body.
2. Describe the human meaning of different regions of the body.
3. Describe the general anatomy of different regions of the body.
4. Explain the applications of massage for different regions of the body.
5. Perform massage technique variations for different regions of the body.

KEY TERMS/CONCEPTS

Human meaning

Regions of the body

Wholeness

LINK LIBRARY TERMS

Swedish Massage • *Massage Business* • *Traditional Chinese Medicine/Traditional Asian Medicine* • *Massage Regulations*

MEDIALINK

A companion CD-ROM, included free with each new copy of this book, supplements the techniques presented in this chapter. Insert the CD-ROM to watch video clips of massage techniques being demonstrated. This multimedia feature is designed to help you add a new dimension to your learning.

Practitioners may focus more time and attention on a particular region of the body, for example, on the back, neck or feet. Extended massage sessions on a smaller body area provide an opportunity for greater specificity. Added attention might result from a recipient request, or practitioner observation and assessment. Information on a health history form, or referral from a health care provider, could prompt more focus on a particular body region.

Advanced techniques and routines for specific **regions of the body** are described in this chapter. The face and head, neck, back, buttocks, lower extremities, upper extremities, chest, and abdomen are the regions represented. A discussion of the meaning of each specific part of the body in human terms is followed by the applications of massage, anatomy, and technique descriptions. The techniques presented can be integrated into the full-body Western massage described in Chapter 9.

WHOLENESS AND MEANING

Even though the body is massaged region by region during a session, its interconnectedness should always be kept in mind. Note that even though the following sections of this chapter focus on different regions of the body, a real body is not so easily divided. It has **wholeness** or integrity. For example, the upper trapezius is in the cervical region, while the whole trapezius extends down the spine through the thoracic region. For someone with rounded shoulders, you would want to address all anterior muscle shortening, as well as in the pectorals. More than just the most obvious muscles may be involved. You cannot isolate a region entirely and be effective. Work in a specific area will necessarily flow into the surrounding regions, and sometimes to the entire body.

Another consideration is that different regions of the body have special significance in human terms. Their **human meaning** is determined by what they allow us to do and to be in this world, their social and emotional associations, and their specific use in a particular person's life (e.g., a musician's hands or a runner's legs). Practitioners should keep in mind that they are not just working on body parts such as shoulders or legs, but that they are in relationship with human beings, who give meaning to their bodies and body regions. As you interact with a client, be aware that you are not just touching a body, you are touching a person.

HEAD AND FACE

Much of human consciousness is focused in the head and face. The head is the center for thinking and processing information. Our senses of sight, hearing, taste, and smell are housed here. The structures for bringing food into our bodies are here. We communicate with others through the structures of speech, and our faces convey our feelings and emotional states through facial expression. The muscles of the face are part of the process of thinking, as seen in furrowed brows and frowns of concentration. Relaxing the muscles of the head and face helps bring clarity of mind and release of mental and emotional stress.

Applications of Massage

Massage can help release tensions in the face and head acquired in daily living. This may be an area of tension for people whose jobs involve a lot of thinking or require extensive use of the eyes. Reading, writing, looking at a computer monitor, and doing activities that require fine hand–eye coordination such as needlework or drawing put strain on the muscles of the face, especially around the eyes. People who wear eyeglasses may feel strain from the weight of the glasses on the nose and ears.

Emotional distress may also lead to tension in the face and head. Worry and anxiety may create tension in the forehead and temporal area. Habitual clenching of the jaw can cause tension in the masseter and temporalis muscles and lead to TMJ pain syndrome. While crying can lead to a healthy release of emotions, it can also create strain around the eyes. Holding back emotions, and holding back tears, is accomplished by tension in the face, throat, and diaphragm.

The muscles of the face and head may also be affected by certain pathologies, such as stroke and Bell's palsy. Face and head massage can help relieve muscle tension from these conditions.

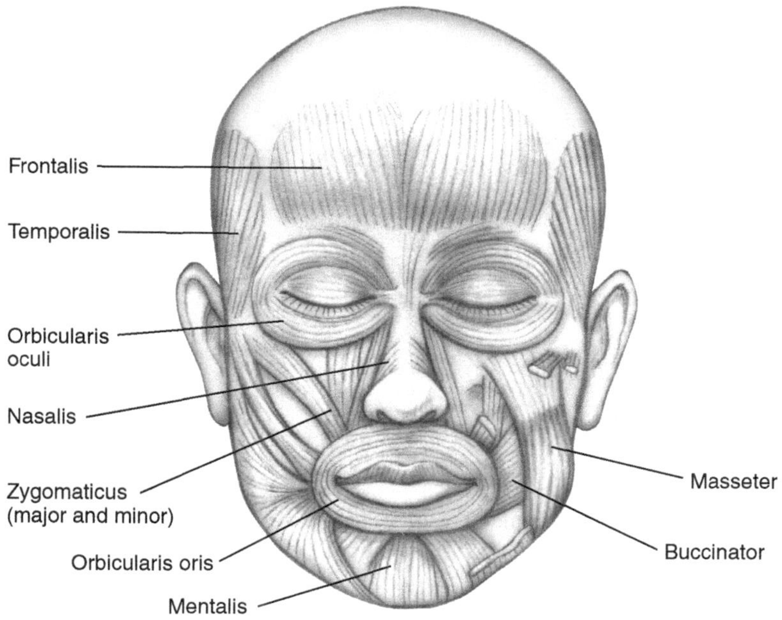

FIGURE 10–1. Major muscles of facial expression.

Anatomy

The musculature of the face and head is complex and includes muscles of expression, mastication, and movement. Some muscles are skeletal muscles that create movement, such as the masseter. The muscles of expression in the face are embedded in the cutaneous tissue and move the skin itself, such as in wrinkling the forehead, frowning, and smiling. These muscles are relatively thin and more delicate than skeletal muscles. Some of the major muscles of facial expression are pictured in Figure 10–1.

Techniques

The following techniques may be integrated into a basic face and head massage. They provide more specific attention to the facial muscles, skin, and scalp.

Always ask the recipient if they are wearing contact lenses, since some of these techniques may dislodge them. A general rule is to avoid movements around the orbit, or over the eyes, if a person is wearing contact lenses.

Squeeze to Eyebrows. The tissues in the eyebrow area become tense in people who squint, are sensitive to light, or use their eyes a lot in their work (e.g., computer work, reading, or activities that require fine hand–eye coordination). Congestion in this area often accompanies tension headache. The corrugator supercilii muscle, which draws the eyebrow downward and medially, is located there.

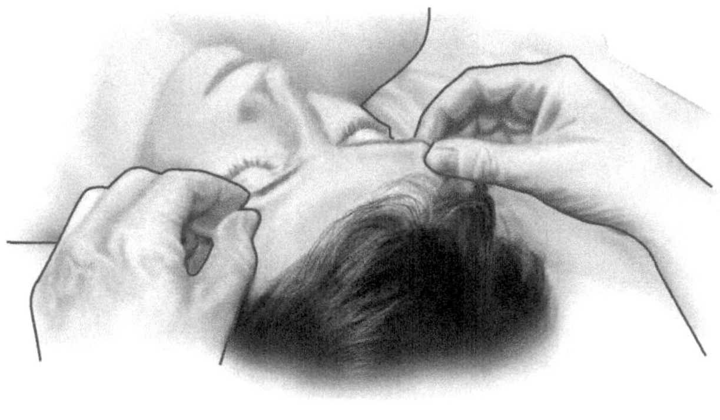

FIGURE 10–2. Gentle squeezing of tissues along the eyebrow line.

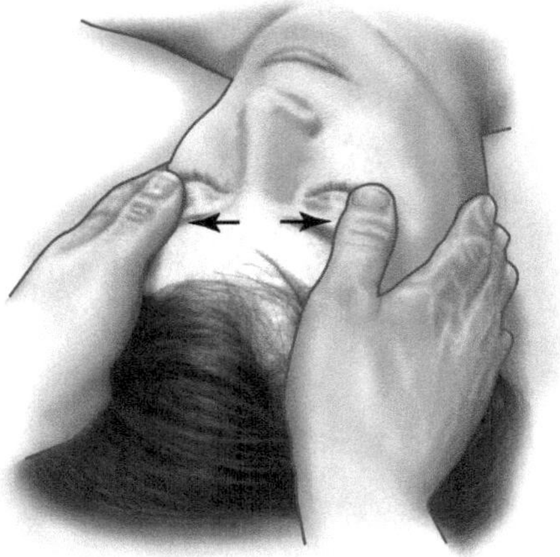

FIGURE 10–3. Very light effleurage over eyelids with the thumbs.

Gently squeeze the tissues between the thumb and the forefinger, beginning at the nose and moving laterally to the outside edge of the eye orbit. See Figure 10–2. Pressure should be light to moderate.

Effleurage over the Eyelids. This technique is similar to the common gesture of rubbing the eyes when tired. It massages orbicularis oculi, the sphincter muscle of the eyelids. Gently, using very light pressure, stroke the closed eyelids with your thumbs as shown in Figure 10–3. The movement is medial to lateral. Stroke once near the top, once in the middle, and once near the bottom of the eyelid.

Thumb Slides along the Nose. People who wear glasses often rub or squeeze the tissues between the eyebrows at the bridge of the nose to relieve pressure where the glasses sit. Procerus, a small muscle located there, draws the medial angles of the eyebrows downward and produces transverse wrinkles over the bridge of the nose. Those with sinus congestion may also feel tenderness in the external tissues of the upper nose area.

Using light to moderate pressure, slide a thumb over the procerus muscle, and then use both thumbs to slide along the outline of the nose from the eyes to the little depression at the base. See Figure 10–4.

Direct Pressure along the Zygomatic Arch. Pressure to the zygomatic or cheekbone area will sometimes help relieve congestion there. Perform effleurage with the fingertips along the underside of the zygomatic arch starting at the base of the nose and moving laterally. Apply direct pressure to the little depression at the base of the nose, and then moving laterally as before, press up and under the zygomatic arch with the index and third fingers. See Figure 10–5. Use light to moderate pressure. The area will be tender if the sinuses are congested.

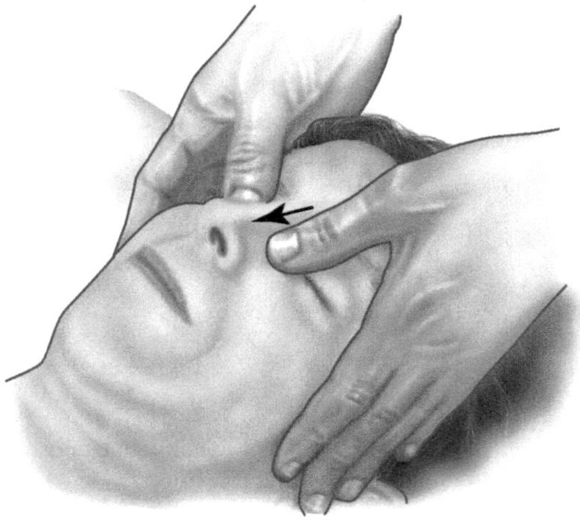

FIGURE 10–4. Thumb slides along the side of the nose.

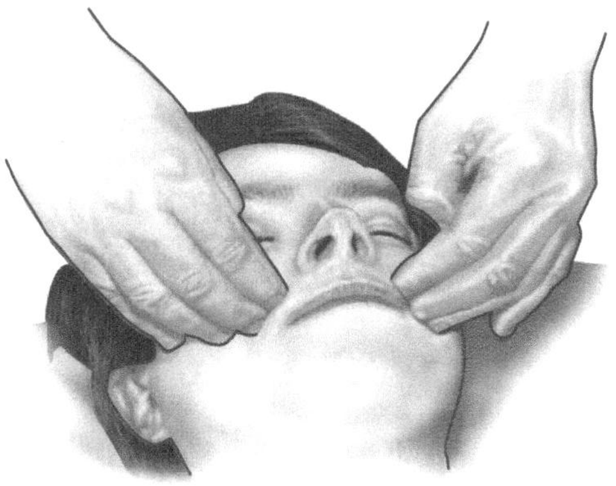

FIGURE 10–5. Direct pressure under zygomatic arch with the fingertips.

Massage Around the Mouth and Jaw. There are a number of muscles around the mouth and jaw, which create movement for eating, speaking, and expression. For example, chewing, sipping, whispering, singing, smiling, frowning, and sneering all involve muscles around the mouth and jaw. Muscles that aid in mastication include the masseter, pterygoid muscles, and the temporalis.

Begin specific work around the mouth and jaw with effleurage using the thumbs to outline the upper lip (i.e., moustache area) and then the lower lip as shown in Figure 10–6. Knead the tissues on the chin and along the jawline with the thumb and first two fingers. Deep circular friction is effective on the strong jaw muscles such as the masseter.

Massaging the Ears. The ears are made of soft cartilage and have many curves and folds. People who wear glasses, clip-on earrings, or any heavy earrings usually enjoy massage to the ears. Take care around hearing aids.

The ears may be massaged between the thumb and index finger. Follow the curves to rub the entire ear, including the ear lobes. As you approach the outer edges of the ear while rubbing, give a gentle pull to stimulate the area as shown in Figure 10–7. Perform circular friction all around the base of the ears to massage the small auricular muscles attached there. See Figure 10–8.

Mobilizing the Scalp. The skin that covers the top of the head (i.e., the scalp) moves freely on most people. Stress can lead to tension in the muscles of the head, causing the scalp to be less mobile. Mobilizing the scalp has similar effects to skin rolling, which frees the underlying fascia and increases superficial circulation. Since circulation to hair follicles is increased, this helps promote healthy hair.

The scalp can be mobilized using a friction-like technique in which fingers placed on the scalp move the skin over the underlying muscle and bone. As the skin moves, the fingers stay in place on the skin surface. See Figure 10–9. Mobilize the entire scalp, including the back of the head. The pressure used is much lighter than deep friction, since the object is simply to move the scalp.

The hair may also be used to move the scalp. Grasp the hair close to the skin and use it as a handle to move the scalp back and forth. This works best with thick hair. It will not work if the recipient has hair that is too thin or too short to grasp.

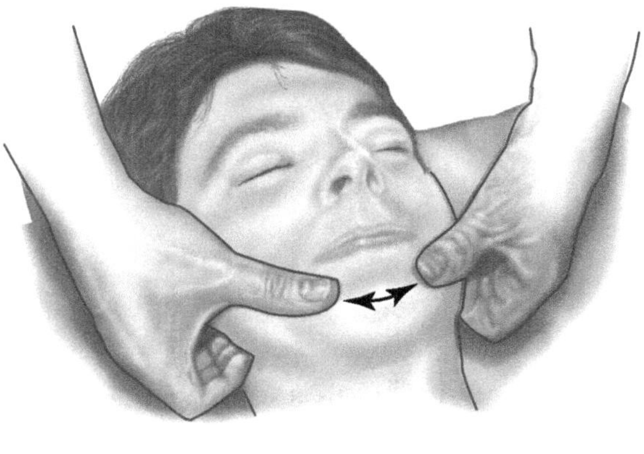

FIGURE 10–6. Thumbs outline the lower lip with effleurage.

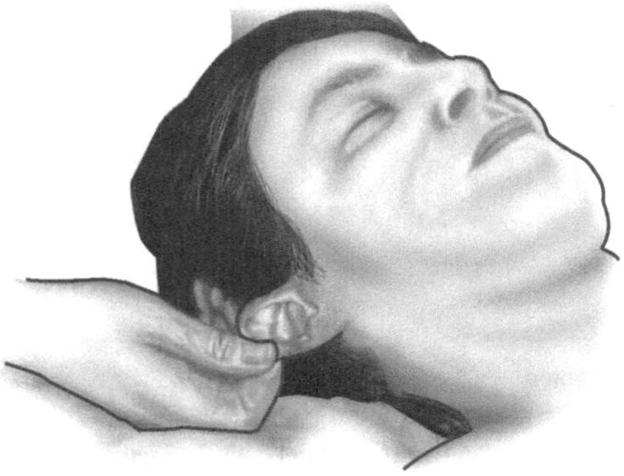

FIGURE 10–7. Gentle pull on the ear.

Muscles on the Head. There are several broad thin muscles on the head. Some of these move the scalp, for example, the occipitofrontalis and temporoparietalis. The large temporalis muscle, found above the ears, elevates the mandible and aids in mastication. These muscles are massaged somewhat in the process of mobilizing the scalp as described above. Moderate pressure may be applied using circular friction with the fingers.

Passive Touch over the Eyes. Placing the hands gently on the face with palms over the eyes can be soothing. It is similar to the self-comforting gesture of holding your face in your hands. See Figure 10–10. Pressure should be very light.

Pressing or Holding the Sides of the Head. Pressing the sides of the head near the top as shown in Figure 10–11 can help relieve tension. Use the full hand, and press in with moderate to heavy pressure depending on the recipient. Slowly release the pressure. It is the sensation of compression, and then letting go, that is relaxing.

Simply holding the head as in Figure 9–23 can be relaxing and is a good finishing technique. Pressure should be light, since the idea is to give the impression of holding, not pressing.

NECK

The cervical or neck region is "pivotal" in many senses of the word. It links the head with the torso and houses the delicate spinal cord. Nerves and blood vessels going to the brain pass through the neck. It contains the muscles that hold the head in position during upright posture and movement in different planes. It is the pivot point for the head and provides the structure and musculature that allows us to access sensation as we turn our heads to look, listen, smell, and taste.

For some, the neck and throat are areas to be protected from touch by others. People who have experienced choking, near suffocation or drowning, neck trauma, or who fear such occurrences may respond negatively to touching the neck, especially the anterior neck, in any way. Protective responses

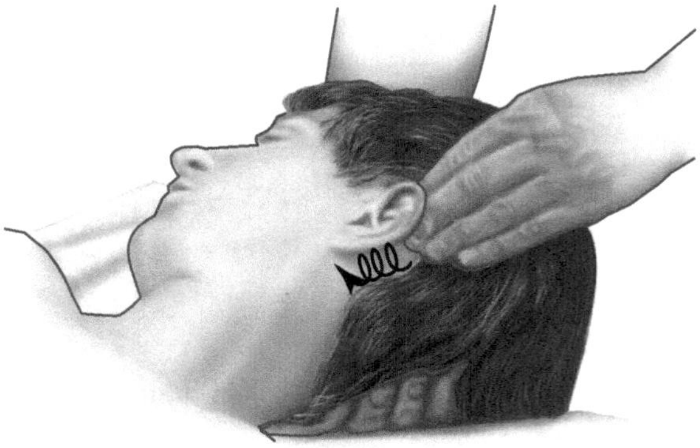

FIGURE 10–8. Circular friction around the base of the ear.

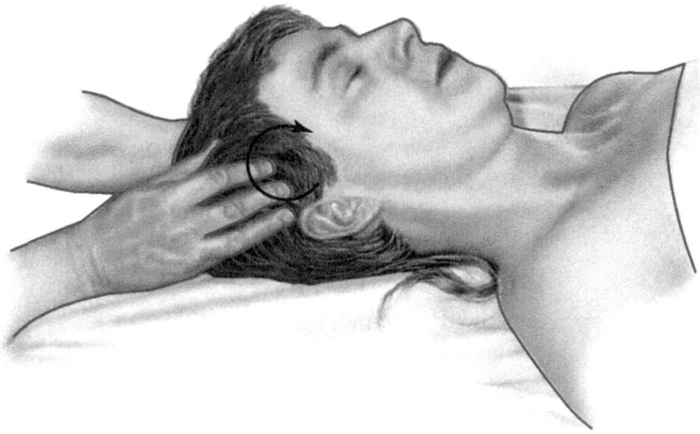

FIGURE 10–9. Mobilizing the scalp with the fingertips. The skin moves over underlying muscle and bone.

may include tightening the shoulder and neck muscles, raising the shoulders, lowering the chin, covering the throat with the hands, or even pulling the practitioner's hands from the neck.

Applications of Massage

Poor posture and body mechanics can lead to excessive tension in the neck. The *head forward* posture and poor sitting posture at workstations are two common sources of chronic neck tension. A cold draft on the back of the neck or sleeping in a cramped position can sometimes cause neck stiffness. Long airplane or automobile rides can also leave neck muscles painful and stiff.

Stressful life situations may aggravate cervical tension and may literally be a "pain in the neck." A major cause of tension headache is hypertonicity of the cervical muscles, which refer pain into the head. Trigger point work on the cervical and upper back muscles may be integrated into a Western massage routine for effective relief of a tension headache. The contraction of muscles and pain in the neck region from whiplash or wryneck (torticollis) may be relieved with massage.

Anatomy

The major muscles in the neck include the upper trapezius, splenius capitis and cervicis, semispinalis capitis and cervicis, longissimus capitis, levator scapulae, sternocleidomastoid (SCM); and the deeper smaller muscles of the suboccipitals (rectus capitis posterior major and minor, oblique capitis superior and inferior), multifidi and rotatores. Generally speaking, the more superficial muscles are larger and thicker, and the deeper ones are smaller and thinner. Some of the deeper muscles of the posterior neck are shown in Figure 10–12.

Cautions. Endangerment sites in the cervical region include the anterior neck and throat, and the arteries and veins that supply the brain. The carotid artery and jugular vein are located on the sides of

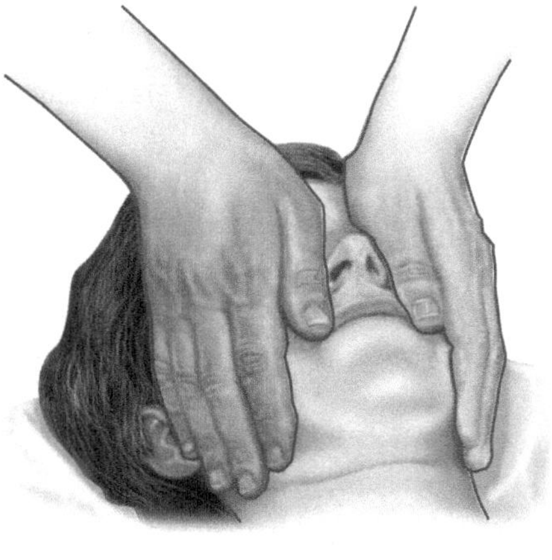

FIGURE 10–10. Passive touch over the eyes with the palms of the hands.

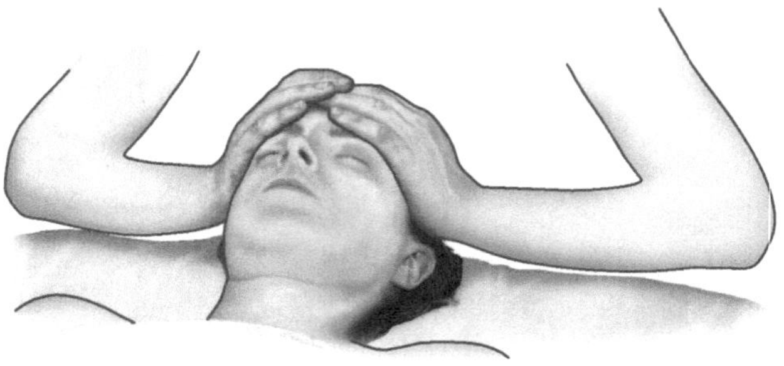

FIGURE 10–11. Pressing the sides of the head with the palms of the hands.

the neck. These areas should be avoided, especially in the elderly or anyone with a history of atherosclerosis, i.e., hardening of the arteries.

Techniques

The following techniques may be integrated into a basic massage of the neck. When working in the cervical area, attention should be given first to relaxing the superficial muscles, allowing better access to the deeper muscles. The area should be thoroughly warmed up before deeper techniques are performed.

Direct Pressure to the Cervical Muscles. With the recipient in the supine position, direct pressure may easily be applied to the cervical muscles on either side of the spine. Use the index finger to apply moderate pressure upward as shown in Figure 10–13. Apply pressure to both sides at the same time, or alternating back and forth from one side to the other. Start at the base of the neck and apply the direct pressure to one spot then the next, moving toward the suboccipital area. A slight movement of the neck will occur.

Deep Pressure to the Suboccipitals. With the recipient in the supine position, apply direct pressure to the suboccipital muscles using all of the fingers. Place the fingers along the suboccipitals and simply apply pressure upward. The chin will elevate, and the head will fall back slightly into a mild hyperextension.

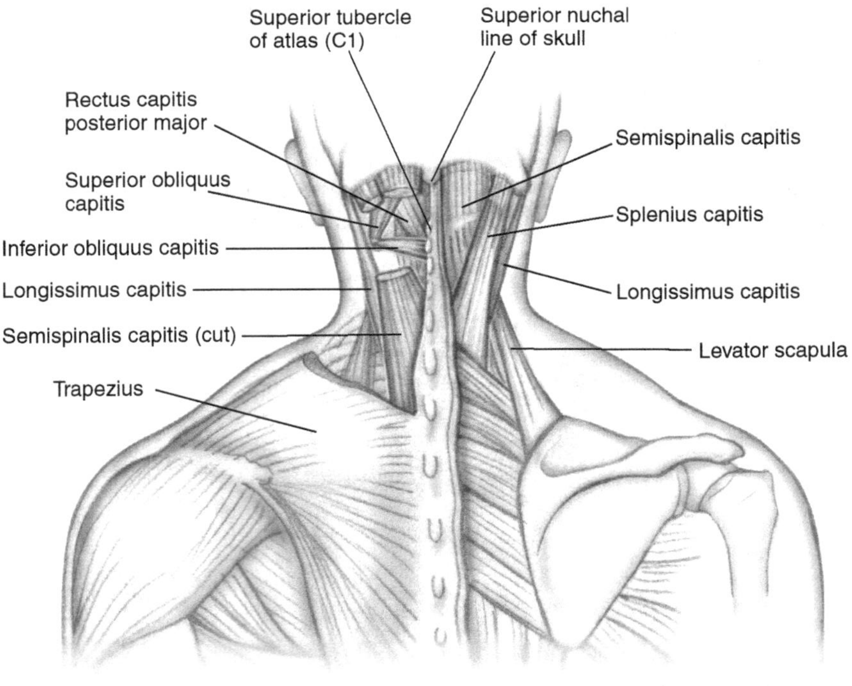

FIGURE 10–12. Deep muscles of the posterior neck.

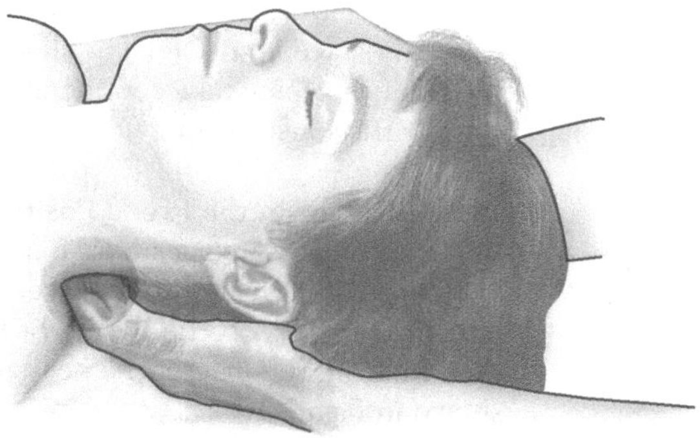

FIGURE 10–13. Direct pressure to posterior cervical muscles using fingertips with recipient supine.

Deeper pressure may be applied to the suboccipital muscles with the thumb. This is a useful technique when working with stiff or tense neck muscles. Cradle the head in one hand and rotate it away from the side you are working on. With the thumb of the other hand, slowly apply pressure into the suboccipital space. You can deepen the pressure by carefully accentuating the natural extension of the head. Instruct the recipient to take slow deep breaths to enhance relaxation. Hold the pressure for 1–2 breath cycles and then slowly release. Do not hold too long or press so deep that more pain is elicited. See Figure 10–14.

Direct pressure may be alternated with cross-fiber friction for a thorough and deep massage of the suboccipitals. This should be followed by gentle stretching for more lasting effects.

Direct Pressure to Thoracic Attachments—Supine. Some of the muscles of the neck attach to the thoracic spine or ribs. Direct pressure to these attachments can help improve flexibility of the neck. When performing passive forward flexion of the neck, you can sometimes feel a resistance at the lower attachments of the cervical muscles. These attachments are affected during upper back massage, but may also receive attention with the recipient in the supine position.

Reach under the trunk, palms up, to about the fourth thoracic vertebra, and place the fingers on both sides of the spine. Press up at one spot, and then the next, moving upward toward the base of the neck. The weight of the trunk will offer resistance and allow deep pressure to be applied.

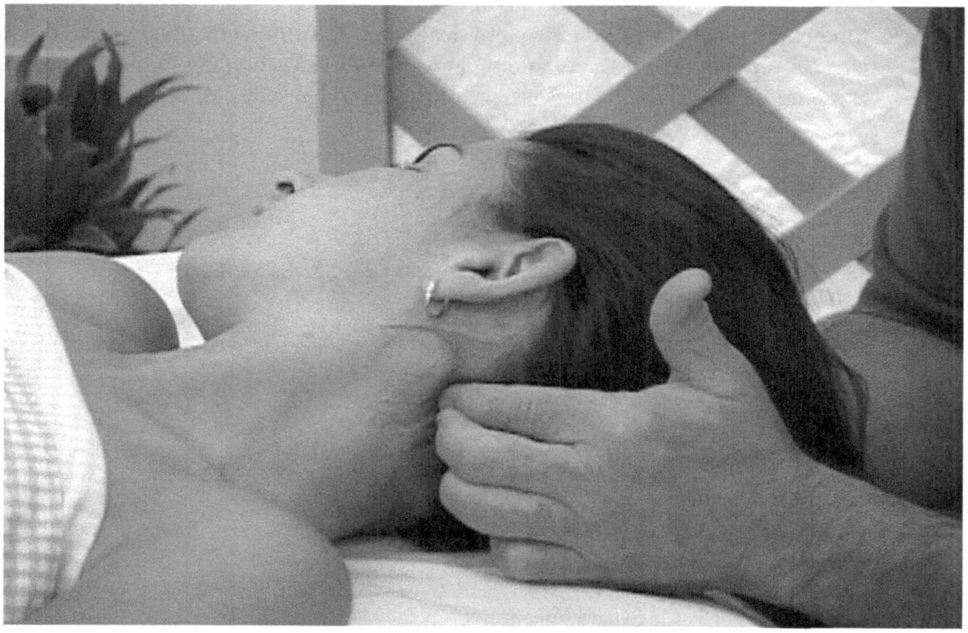

FIGURE 10–14. Direct pressure to suboccipital muscles with the thumb with recipient supine.

A variation of this technique is to use the same hand placement, but slide the fingers along the spine using deep pressure. The slide will help stretch tissues. Note that these techniques applied with the receiver supine take considerable strength on the part of the practitioner and should be performed only by those with strong flexors in the hands and wrists.

Neck Massage in the Prone Position. The cervical muscles may be massaged when the recipient is in the prone or seated position. If using an adjustable face cradle, tilt it down so that the neck is slightly stretched. This creates more space.

Effleurage with the thumb or fingertips can be used to warm the cervical muscles. Perform effleurage from the base of the neck to the suboccipitals. Follow this with kneading using one hand as shown in Figure 10–15.

Once the muscles are warmed up, the thumb or the fingers may be used to apply direct pressure at an angle into the suboccipital space and toward the top of the head. Care should be taken not to apply so much pressure that the recipient's face feels smashed into the face cradle. Direct pressure may be applied with the thumbs or elbow over the thoracic attachments of the cervical muscles.

BACK

"Spend more time on my back" is a frequent request from recipients of massage. The back is the core area for maintaining upright posture, and the place of attachment for muscles that move the arms and legs. It is a heavily muscled area that works hard and is prone to tension, aches, and stiffness. Poor body mechanics when sitting, lifting, playing sports, or during physical activities such as gardening can cause backache.

The back is a common place where worry and anxiety are held, which is sometimes experienced as Atlas carrying the weight of the world on his shoulders. A bent-over posture evokes the image of weakness, discouragement, and defeat; a straight back presents the image of strength, self-confidence, and vigor.

Applications of Massage

Soothing back massage is associated with the qualities of nurturing, sympathy, and deep relaxation. Perhaps because the nerves of the parasympathetic nervous system exit the posterior vertebrae, the relaxation response is easily triggered during massage of the back. Back massage is often used to help people go to sleep.

Deep massage of the back muscles can help release tension held there and relieves the stiffness and soreness that accompanies heavy physical labor. Joint movements improve the mobility of the scapulae (i.e., shoulder blades), enhancing movement in the shoulder girdle. Tension in the upper trapezius can refer pain into the head. Massage of the shoulders can help relieve tension headache.

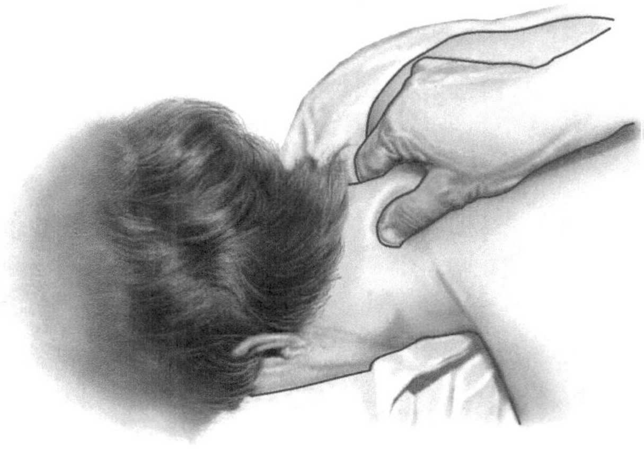

FIGURE 10–15. One hand kneading to posterior cervical muscles, recipient prone.

Anatomy

It is important for practitioners to develop a three-dimensional concept of the back. This includes the recognition that the "back" is the posterior portion of the torso, which also has sides. The back is thick with layers from large broad superficial muscles to the tiny deep muscles of the spine. The scapulae, or shoulder blades, located on the upper back are an integral part of the shoulder girdle. They glide over the posterior ribs and have numerous muscular attachments, which generate the free movement of the shoulder complex. Practitioners work at various depths of penetration during massage of the back.

The large superficial muscles of the back include the trapezius and latissimus dorsi. Spinal muscles include the erector spinae (iliocostalis, longissimus, spinalis), the deep posterior spinal muscles (multifidi, rotatores, interspinales, intertransversarii, and levatores costarum), and the semispinalis thoracis. Muscles surrounding the scapulae include subscapularis, upper trapezius, posterior deltoid, supraspinatus, infraspinatus, serratus anterior, teres major and minor, levator scapulae, and the rhomboids on the medial border. The quadratus lumborum is in the lower back, with attachments on the last rib, the transverse processes of the upper four lumbar vertebrae, and the iliac crest.

Techniques

The following techniques may be integrated into a basic back massage. They focus on muscles that move the spine and techniques for the back overall. Massage and movements for the shoulders are covered in more detail in the section on the upper extremities.

Skin Rolling. Skin rolling is an excellent technique to help relieve tension in the back. It helps restore elasticity to the subcutaneous connective tissues and improves superficial circulation.

First perform a general warm-up of the area with effleurage or compression. Skin rolling is performed by lifting the cutaneous tissues from the underlying muscles. It may be applied sequentially by lifting the tissues in one place and then the next, eventually covering the entire back. It may also be performed in strips using a continuous motion, by lifting the tissues and, without letting go, sliding the hands along in a line. The tissues are lifted as the hands slide along by the pressure between the thumbs and fingers. Skin rolling is also described in Chapter 7, Figure 7–16.

Warming Friction of the Back. Warming friction may be used to create heat in any relatively flat area. It is effective over the erector muscles on either side of the spine, over the rhomboids, and on the muscles covering the scapulae. Lubricant will reduce the effect of the friction and so should be used sparingly or wiped off before performing warming friction.

Sawing friction is performed with the ulnar side of the hands, palms facing each other. The hands are moved back and forth in a sawing motion, sliding over the skin and creating friction on the skin. Deeper pressure will create friction in deeper tissues. The skin will appear red as the superficial blood vessels dilate. Sawing friction is also described in Chapter 7, Figure 7–19.

Warming friction may also be performed with the knuckles. Figure 7–18 in Chapter 7 shows knuckling friction over the erector muscles of the thoracic region.

Effleurage Between the Ribs. Effleurage of the intercostal muscles with the fingertips helps relax these tiny muscles. This facilitates easier and deeper breathing by allowing the rib cage to expand more. Find the intercostal spaces using palpation skills, and slide the fingers in the spaces moving from the spine laterally and around the sides of the rib cage. See Figure 10–16.

Therapeutic Sequence for the Lower Back

The muscles of the lower back can get stiff and sore from sitting for long periods of time, especially in chairs or car seats with poor lumbar support. The following sequence of techniques helps relax the muscles of the lower back and relieve general fatigue of the area. A summary of the technique sequence for the lower back can be found in Table 10–1.

Warm up the entire back with effleurage and circular friction as described in the full-body Western massage. For the lower back portion of the routine, insert the following five-part combination of techniques. Position yourself at the client's hip, facing the head of the table for techniques applied inferior to superior, or at that lower back facing the side of the table for direct pressure, rocking, and horizontal stroking techniques.

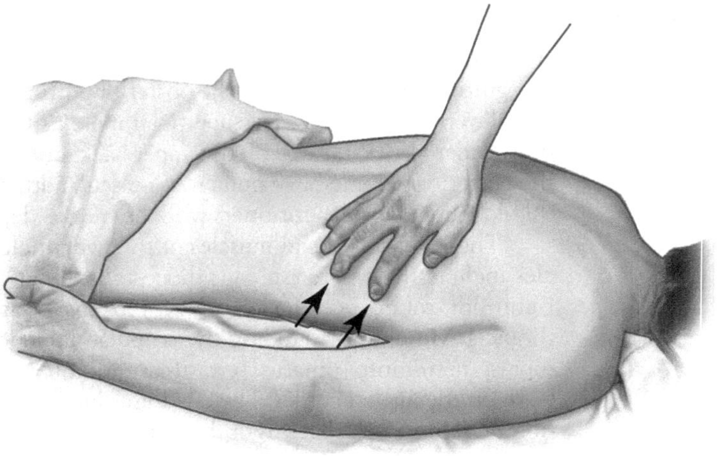

FIGURE 10–16. Effleurage of intercostal muscles using fingertips, recipient prone.

Once the lower back is warmed up, apply stripping in the space between the iliac crest and the twelfth rib (i.e., quadratus lumborum) using moderate to deep pressure. The first strip is applied just laterally to the spinous processes. Each strip is performed just laterally to the one before. See Figure 10–17. Stripping lengthens and broadens the muscle fibers.

Follow this with circular friction to the paraspinal muscles using the fingertips. Then apply direct pressure with the thumbs to the paraspinal muscles using moderate to heavy pressure. Begin at the 12th rib and press in at about one-inch intervals along the muscles, up to and along the iliac crest. See Figure 10–18.

Apply knuckle friction to the muscles in the region to further warm and bring blood to the lower back. Joint movement may be applied to the lower back by placing the thumb on one side of the spine and the fingers on the other, and gently rocking the spine from side to side. Apply rocking for a few seconds.

*Table 10–1 THERAPEUTIC SEQUENCE FOR THE LOWER BACK**

General Description:
Massage to relieve tension and fatigue in the muscles of the lower back. Goals include relaxation and lengthening muscles in the lumbar region.

Note: Figures cited below illustrate the technique, but it may be performed on a different part of the body in the picture.

Warming Techniques

1. Effleurage to entire back (Figure 7–6, 7–7)
2. Effleurage to right side of spine, hips to shoulders (Figure 7–5)
3. Circular friction to paraspinal muscles on right side of spine (Figure 9–1)

Therapeutic Combination—Lower Back

4. Stripping between the 12th rib and the iliac crest (quadratus lumborum) (Figure 10–17)
5. Cross-fiber friction over paraspinal muscles (Figure 7–21)
6. Direct pressure along paraspinal muscles and iliac crest at 1-inch intervals (Figure 10–18)
7. Knuckle friction over lumbar region (Figure 7–18)
8. Gentle rocking of lower back

Finishing and Transition Technique

9. Horizontal stroking across lumbar region (Figure 7–8)
10. Effleurage from hips to shoulders to reconnect the back kinesthetically (Figure 7–5)

*This is an example of a therapeutic sequence for the lower back. It can be altered to meet the needs of an individual recipient. There are many variations of this sequence, and many more techniques that can be incorporated to achieve the overall goal of relieving tension and fatigue in the lower back.

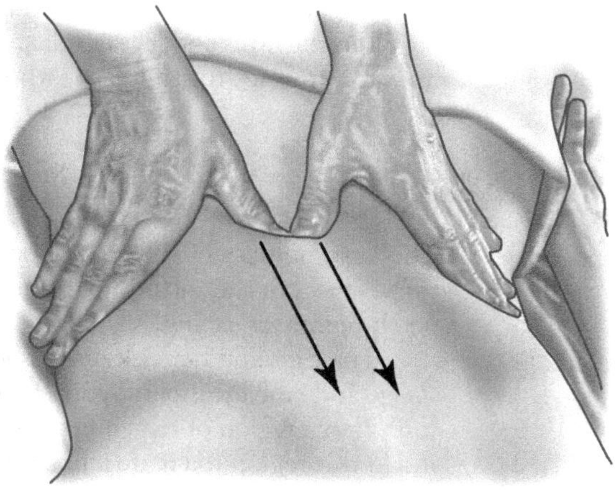

FIGURE 10–17. Thumb stripping along the lower back on quadratus lumborum.

To finish massage of the lower back and transition to the next phase of the session, apply horizontal stroking across the lower back. Follow with effleurage to the entire back to reconnect the lower back kinesthetically to the rest of the body.

Back Massage for Relaxation

If the purpose of back massage is general relaxation, either avoid specific painful work on the back altogether, or spend at least five to seven minutes after painful work on lighter, soothing techniques. Use long flowing effleurage strokes with oil, maintaining full contact with the palm of the hand throughout the stroking. Use moderate to slow continuous motion. The movement should feel "seamless."

Vary the pattern to avoid boredom. Mix up vertical, circular, and horizontal patterns of effleurage. Some petrissage of the shoulder may be integrated for variety. Avoid tapotement, and finish either with nerve strokes or passive touch over the scapulae.

Sedating Effleurage of the Back

Back massage is sometimes used in hospitals and nursing homes for those having trouble falling asleep. Sedating effleurage may be performed without oil or lotion. It is very effective for evoking the relaxation response, and promoting sleep. The movement consists of long gliding strokes directly over the spine that start at the base of the skull and go all the way to the coccyx. Hands alternate. As one hand is about to complete its motion near the coccyx, the other hand begins the next stroke starting at the base of the skull. Pressure must be light but firm and the rhythm monotonous. Pressure that is too light might stimulate rather than sedate. This gives the recipient the feeling of continuous contact, with one hand beginning the next stroke before the other hand finishes. Keep the

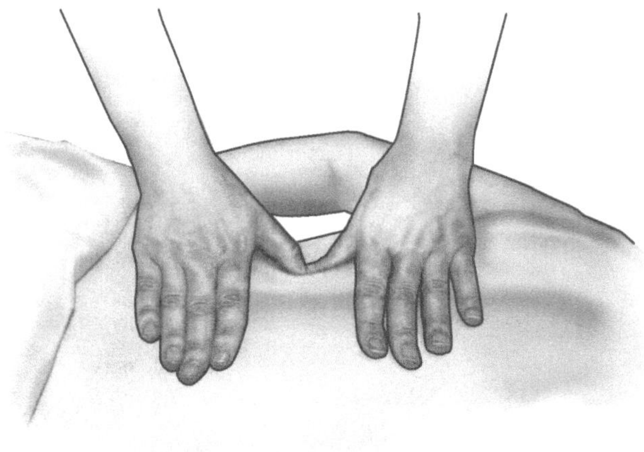

FIGURE 10–18. Direct pressure to muscles in the lower back using the thumbs.

motion going for a minute or two to help the recipient relax completely. A tingling sensation may be felt in the arms and legs as relaxation occurs. If this technique is applied for more than two or three minutes, it tends to stimulate rather than relax, so it should not be continued for too long.

BUTTOCKS

The large muscles of the hip region help support the entire body and provide the power for locomotion. They are the most important and the most stressed muscles in many sports. They are also the perch points for sitting.

The hips and buttocks are associated with sexual appeal. They may also be a source of poor self-image and embarrassment, particularly in women. For those physically or sexually abused as children, it is often a region of remembered pain and suffering. Practitioners should take great care when working in this region to create a feeling of safety and modesty.

Applications of Massage

Sports and fitness participants are often stiff and sore in the hip area from the strain of physical activity. On the other hand, those who are more sedentary may also experience stiffness from lack of movement. Tight buttock muscles can impinge on the sciatic nerve and cause leg pain. Soft-tissue manipulation and joint movements improve circulation to the area, relax muscles, and improve mobility at the hip joint. The elderly may especially benefit from improved hip mobility and, therefore, improved locomotion.

Anatomy

The more superficial muscles of the hip region are the large gluteals (maximus, medius, minimus), which run superior and inferior. The smaller, deeper hip rotators include the piriformis, gemelli, quadratus femoris, and obturator internus and externus. The deeper muscles run medial to lateral as shown in Figure 10–19.

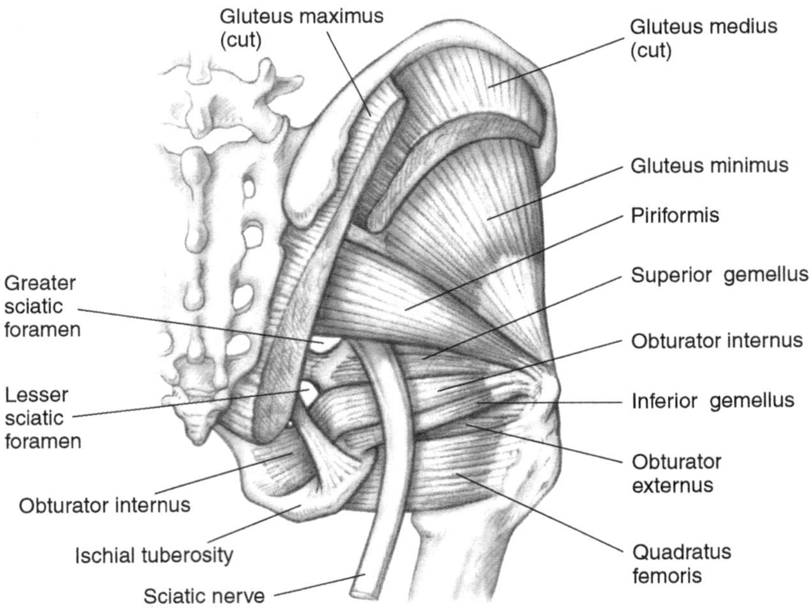

FIGURE 10–19. Deep muscles of the buttocks.

Techniques

The following techniques may be integrated into the basic massage of the lower limbs and buttocks. Some practitioners massage the buttocks as part of a back routine, while others include the buttocks in a lower limb sequence. Since most of the attachments are on the ilium and femur and create movement in the thigh, it may make more sense to treat the buttocks when massaging the lower limbs.

Use of the Elbow and Forearm. Because you must work through the large superficial muscles to reach the smaller deeper muscles, it is useful to use the elbow or forearm to apply some techniques to the buttocks. You can apply more pressure and avoid straining the hands. However, care should be taken not to use too much pressure, especially around the sciatic nerve outlet in the buttocks. Palpatory sensitivity should be developed so that you can feel the condition of the tissues as you would with your hands. The elbow or forearm is not used to "muscle through" the tissues, but to apply more pressure skillfully.

The elbow or forearm may be used for broad strokes, and the point of the elbow (olecranon process) for more specific techniques such as direct pressure to a spot. The elbow or forearm may be used to apply effleurage, direct pressure, and circular or transverse friction. Figure 10–20 shows direct pressure to the deep buttock muscles using the elbow.

Use of the Fist. The fist is useful for applying deep pressure during compressions or effleurage on the large muscles of the buttocks. Figure 10–21 shows compressions applied to the gluteal muscles using the fist. One advantage of this technique over using the palms is that the wrist can be kept straight, thus avoiding potential wrist damage when applying deep pressure.

Direct Pressure to Gluteal Attachments. Direct pressure to the gluteal attachments helps relax the muscles and facilitates a better stretch. Use the thumbs, knuckles, or elbow to press along the attachments along the iliac crest and sacroiliac junction. Follow with effleurage to the area using the fist.

Mobilizations and Stretching. A thorough treatment of the muscles of the buttocks should include both massage and joint movements. Mobilizing techniques and stretching help condition the deep rotators of the hip joint, which are difficult to reach directly with massage. While massage of the buttocks is necessarily performed with the recipient prone, most joint movements are done supine. If one of the major goals of the session addresses mobility in the hips, it may be useful to begin prone to warm up the muscles, and finish supine for the joint movements described in Chapter 8.

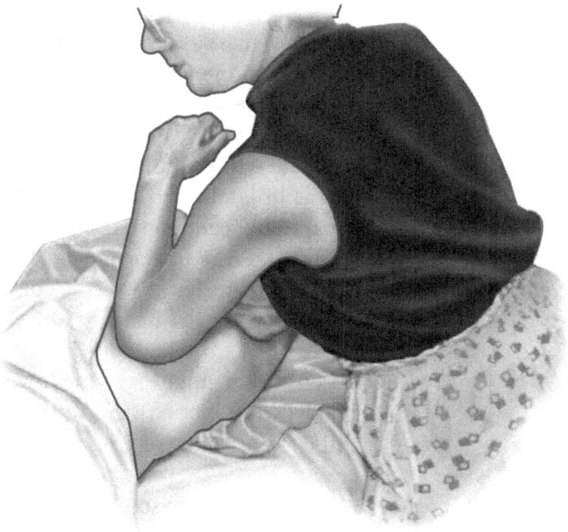

FIGURE 10–20. Use of the elbow to apply direct pressure to deep buttocks muscles.

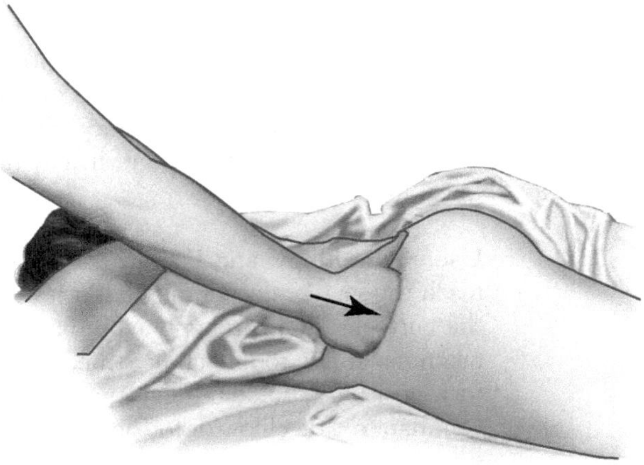

FIGURE 10–21. Compression to the gluteal muscles using the fist. Note the wrist alignment.

LOWER EXTREMITIES

The lower extremities are the principal means of locomotion for bipedal human beings. They afford us a great degree of independence as we can get from one place to another on "our own power." Loss or diminished use of the legs, through disease, accident, or old age, can result in greater dependence and loss of freedom. Having "a spring in your step" is a sign of vitality and positive outlook. Athletes depend on their legs to play their sports, and walking has become the premier fitness activity today.

In Western culture, shoes are worn for protection, and also confine the feet. It feels good to free the feet and kick off your shoes after wearing them all day. Going barefoot or wearing sandals is a sign of leisure and relaxation. If your feet hurt, you hurt all over. Foot massage is valued as a pleasurable treat.

Applications of Massage

People who stand long hours in their jobs often experience stress and pain in the legs and feet. Women especially tend to wear shoes with little support, and often wear high heels, which puts the feet and legs in a strained position. Those who sit a lot typically have problems with loss of leg strength, muscle shortening, and poor circulation. With age there is loss of strength, flexibility, and "spring," and muscles are more frequently stiff and sore. Massage and stretching can help the legs and feet feel and function better by improving circulation, joint mobility, and muscle relaxation.

Anatomy

For purposes of massage, the lower extremities may be thought of in three sections, that is, thigh, lower leg, and feet. In the prone position, the buttocks are often included with the lower extremities. There are three large joints in the lower extremities (i.e., hip, knee, and ankle), and several small joints within the feet.

Thigh. The major muscles of the anterior thigh include the quadriceps (rectus femoris, vastus intermedius, vastus lateralis, vastus medialis), and sartorius. Muscles found on the medial thigh include the adductors, that is, adductor brevis, adductor longus, adductor magnus, gracilis, pectineus. High on the lateral thigh is tensor fasciae latae. The posterior thigh includes the hamstrings (i.e., biceps femoris, semimembranosus, semitendinosus). The iliopsoas (i.e., psoas and iliacus muscles), act on the hip joint, but, for the purposes of massage, are palpated in the abdomen. See Figure 10–22.

Lower Leg. The muscles of the lower leg act largely on the ankle joint and include the anterior muscles (tibialis anterior, peroneus tertius, and the extensors), the lateral muscles (peroneus longus and brevis), and the posterior muscles (gastrocnemius, soleus, tibialis posterior, and the flexors).

Feet. There are many small muscles intrinsic to the feet, most of which are on the plantar side or bottom. The plantar muscles include a superficial layer (abductor hallucis, flexor hallucis longus, flexor dig-

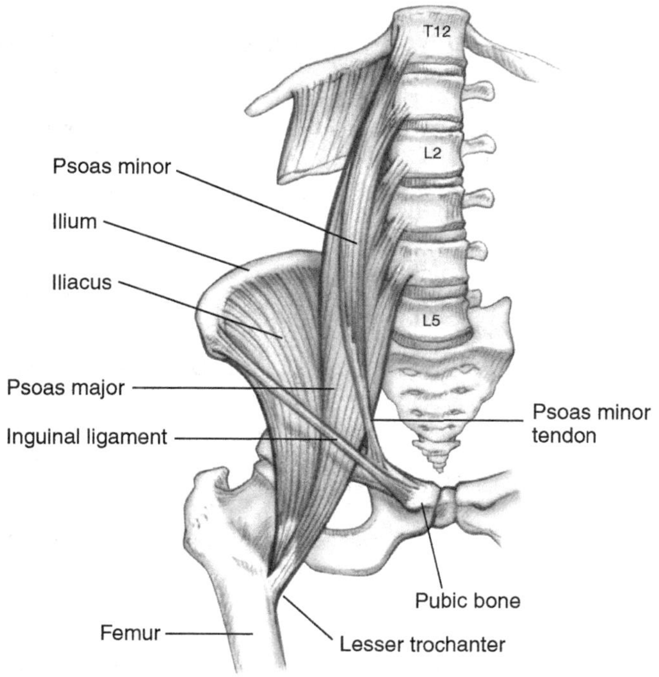

FIGURE 10–22. Components of the iliopsoas muscle.

itorum brevis, abductor digiti minimi brevis), a middle layer (lumbricales, flexor digiti minimi brevis, quadratus, flexor digitorum longus), and a deep layer (adductor hallucis, interossei plantares, flexor hallucis brevis, ligamentum plantarum longum). The plantar aponeurosis is a superficial strong fibrous band of fascia that runs from the heel to the ball of the foot and binds the longitudinal arch. It is the central part of a broad band of fascia that covers the muscles on the plantar side of the foot. The dorsal surface of the foot is fairly bony. The extensor digitorum brevis and the dorsal interossei are accessible to massage.

Cautions. One of the major endangerment sites in the lower extremities is the popliteal fossa located behind the knee. Care should be taken not to apply pressure in this area. However, attachments of muscles may be followed around the area.

Avoid deep pressure over varicose veins, which are common in older adults. Do not massage the legs if blood clotting or phlebitis is present.

Avoid irritating bunions found at the base of the great toe. Watch for athlete's foot and other fungal infections that may be spread through touch. Avoid massaging feet with active infections.

Techniques

The following techniques can be integrated into the basic massage of the lower extremities. Detailed attention is given to the feet, lower leg, and thigh.

Foot Massage. A thorough foot massage can make you feel good all over. It touches all of the small intrinsic muscles of the feet, as well as attachments of muscles of the lower leg, and mobilizes the many joints found there. It relaxes the muscles, improves circulation, and restores feeling to a part of the body encased in shoes most of the time.

The following foot massage routine uses techniques described in more detail in Chapters 8 and 9. The sequence includes soft-tissue manipulation and joint movements for the complex musculoskeletal structure of the foot. A summary of the therapeutic sequence for foot massage can be found in Table 10–2.

Begin by applying lubricant to the foot and ankle. Special lubricants are available for the feet that contain cooling substances such as peppermint and menthol. Be sure to cover the whole foot and each toe.

*Table 10–2 THERAPEUTIC FOOT MASSAGE SEQUENCE**

General Description:
Massage to relieve sore tired feet, and improve mobility to joints in the feet. Relaxes muscles, improves local circulation, and restores feeling to the feet.

Note: Figures cited below illustrate the technique, but it may be performed on a different part of the body in the picture.

Warming Techniques
1. Apply lubricant to the entire foot with effleurage

Therapeutic Combination
Joint Movements (Caution: Do not snap or pull toes)
2. Mobilize the ankle using the heels of the hands (Figure 9–12)
3. Basic sliding effleurage on dorsal surface of the foot between metatarsals (Figure 7–2)
4. Scissoring movement between metatarsals (Figure 8–14)
5. Figure 8s on metatarsal-phalangeal joints (Figure 8–13)
6. Squeeze along each toe gently (proximal to distal)—top/bottom, sides
7. Thumb strokes to underside of each toe to "unflex" the toe
8. Pull on sides of the foot or interlock fingers and recipient's toes to create space between metatarsals (Figure 8–26, 8–27)

Soft Tissues
9. Broad pressure to foot bottom with fist (Figure 9–13)
10. Basic sliding effleurage with fist (Figure 9–13)
11. Direct pressure to points on foot bottom (Figure 10–23)
12. Repeat basic sliding effleurage with fist (Figure 9–13)

Finishing and Transition Techniques
13. Slapping foot bottom with back of hand
14. Holding the foot for a few seconds

*This is an example of a therapeutic sequence for the feet. It can be altered to meet the needs of an individual recipient. There are many variations of this sequence, and many more techniques that can be incorporated to achieve the overall goal of relieving sore and tired feet.

Mobilize the ankle using the heels of the hands. Using your thumb, apply basic sliding effleurage between the metatarsals on the dorsal surface of the foot, and then mobilize the space between metatarsals with a scissoring action. Mobilize each metatarsal-phalangeal joint with figure eights, and then gently petrissage each toe with a gentle squeezing action along the length of the toe moving proximal to distal. Do one length squeezing top and bottom, and then another squeezing the sides. Do not snap or pull the toes.

The toes are sometimes curled under into flexion. You may spend a little time straightening the toes with effleurage using thumb strokes to the underside of the toe while bracing the dorsal surface. Or you may prefer thumb on dorsal surface and index finger on the underside.

Use the fist to apply broad pressure to the bottom of the foot. Hold the dorsal surface of the foot with one hand while the other applies the pressure. You may shape the foot around the fist, stretching the top of the foot and accentuating the longitudinal and transverse arches. Basic sliding effleurage may also be applied to the bottom of the foot with the fist (Figure 9–13).

More specific pressure may be applied to the bottom of the foot with fingertips, knuckle or thumb. Pressing points on the bottom of the foot is thought to improve energy flow to the rest of the body (acupressure theory), and stimulate and increase circulation to corresponding body parts (reflexology theory). It also helps relax the small muscles found there. Figure 10–23 shows some areas on the bottom of the feet to press to stimulate healthy function of different regions of the body. Also see Chapter 15.

Space can be created between metatarsals by holding on to the sides of the foot and pulling the hands away from each other or by interlocking your fingers with the recipient's toes (Figures 8–26, 8–27). These techniques help relieve the feeling of the feet being squeezed inside of shoes.

Finish by slapping the bottom of the foot with the back of your hand. This should create a pleasant stimulating sensation. To finish, hold the feet. Repeat the entire sequence on the other foot.

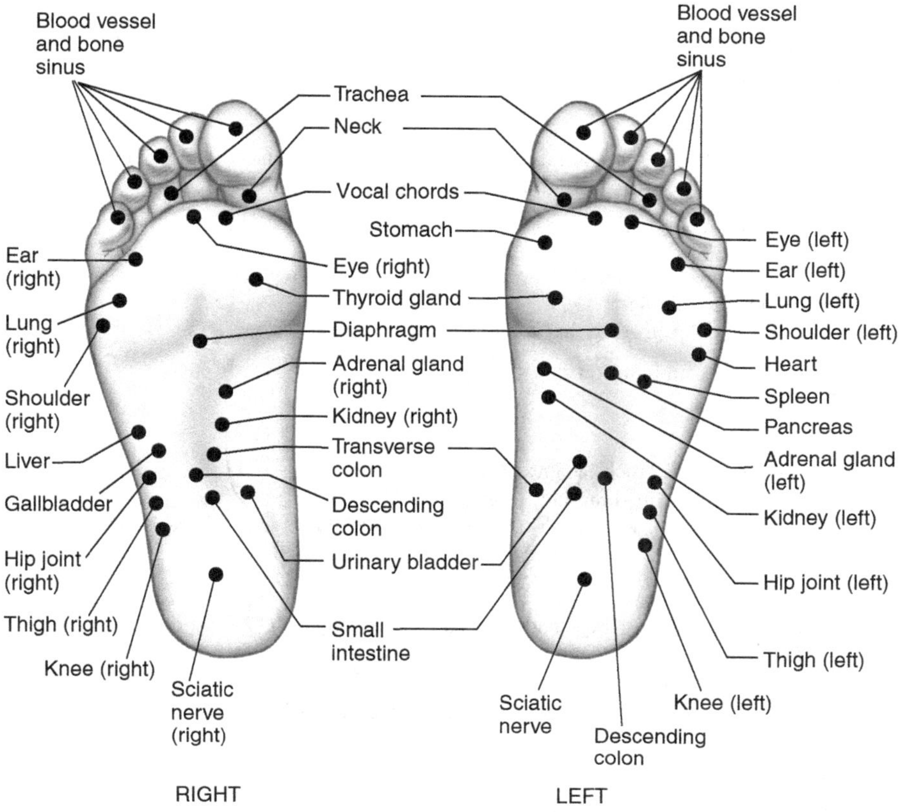

FIGURE 10–23. Areas to press on the bottoms of the feet to stimulate healthy function of different parts of the body.

Enhancing Mobility in the Lower Extremities. Mobility in the lower extremities may be restricted for a number of reasons. Overuse and shortening of muscles in athletes and physical workers, underuse and aging, recuperation from an extended illness or injury, or a sedentary lifestyle can all contribute to stiff joints and lack of fluid movement in the lower limbs.

For best results, all the muscles of the hips, thighs, lower legs, and feet should be thoroughly massaged with effleurage and petrissage and lengthened with stretching; major tendons should be loosened with friction to the point of attachment; and joints should be taken through their full range of motion. Direct pressure along muscles and tendons is used to help loosen them. The following techniques may be added to the basic full-body massage to further enhance mobility in the lower extremities. A technique sequence for enhancing mobility in the lower extremities can be found in Table 10–3.

Hips. After general massage of the buttocks, mobility at the hip joint may be further enhanced by pressing specific pressure points along the sacroiliac joint, the iliac crest, and around the trochanter at the hip joint. This may be done with the thumbs, an extended knuckle, or the elbow. Figure 10–24 shows some points to be pressed.

When the recipient is supine, take the upper leg through a full range of motion. The hip may be stretched by bringing the knee to the chest, out to the side in abduction, and across the body in adduction (Figures 8–18 to 8–21).

Thighs. After general massage of the thigh, perform deep effleurage along each major muscle, including the adductors, to the point of proximal attachment. Figure 10–25 shows the technique for reaching the proximal adductor attachments. You may perform cross-fiber friction near the point of attachment for further effect. Get the recipient's consent to work the attachments in the groin area, and provide secure draping of the genitals.

Table 10–3 THERAPEUTIC SEQUENCE FOR ENHANCING MOBILITY IN THE LOWER EXTREMITIES*

General Description:
Massage to relax muscles and restore mobility in the hips and legs. Relieves tension, increases circulation, and improves flexibility in the lower extremities.

Note: Figures cited below illustrate the technique, but it may be performed on a different part of the body in the picture.

Warming Techniques
1. Effleurage of the entire leg and hip

Therapeutic Combination
Prone

Hip
2. Effleurage of buttocks (Figure 9–5)
3. Petrissage of gluteal muscles (Figure 10–21)
4. Direct pressure to points along sacroiliac joint, iliac crest, and around the trochanter at the hip joint (Figure 10–24)

Thigh
5. Effleurage of hamstrings, adductors, abductors (Figure 7–3, Figure 9–6)
6. Petrissage to thigh (Figure 9–7)
7. Friction to muscle attachments
8. Stretch bringing heel of foot to buttocks (Figure 8–23)

Lower Leg
9. Effleurage to lower leg (Figure 7–1)
10. Petrissage to lower leg (Figure 7–11)
11. Dorsiflexion at ankle with direct pressure to foot bottom (Figure 8–24)

Supine
Thigh
12. Effleurage to quadriceps muscles, adductors, abductors (Figure 7–1)
13. Petrissage of thigh muscles (Figure 7–11)
14. Friction to muscle attachments at knee (Figure 7–20)
15. Friction to iliotibial band (Figure 7–22)

Lower Leg
16. Effleurage to lower leg (Figure 7–1)
17. Friction along tibialis anterior (Figure 7–18)
18. Direct pressure along tibialis anterior (Figure 9–11)

Foot
19. Foot massage sequence in Table 10–2

Joint Movements
20. Move hip through its full range of motion (Figure 8–18)
21. Knee to chest stretch (Figure 8–19)
22. Straight leg stretch in flexion (Figure 8–20)
23. Move ankle through full range of motion
24. Stretches at ankle in dorsiflexion and plantarflexion.

Finishing and Transition Techniques
25. Effleurage to reconnect the leg kinesthetically
26. Rocking the leg (Figure 8–17)

*This is an example of a therapeutic sequence for the lower extremities. It can be altered to meet the needs of an individual recipient. There are many variations of this sequence, and many more techniques that can be incorporated to achieve the overall goal of enhancing mobility in the lower extremities.

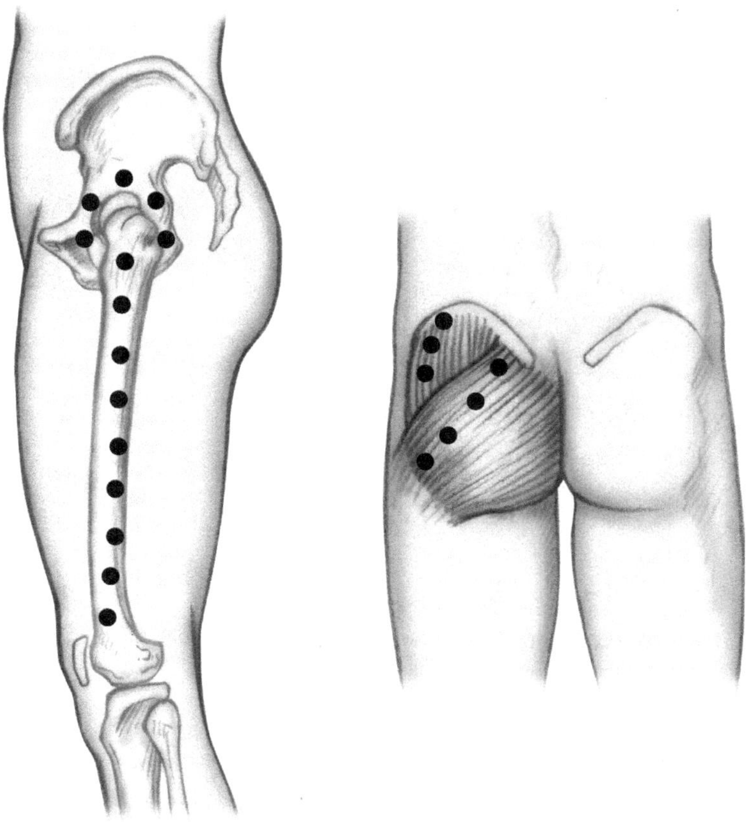

FIGURE 10–24. Points to press to improve mobility of the hip joint.

Perform circular friction over the muscle attachments at the knee, first with the heels of the hands, and then with the fingertips (Figure 9–9). These attachments are frequently sore to the touch. Cross-fiber friction may be performed over areas in which the tissues are adhering.

Lower Legs. Perform general massage of the lower leg in the prone position. Loosen the Achilles tendon using direct pressure along its length, especially at the point of juncture with the muscle. See Figure 10–26. The tendon may be further loosened by moving it back and forth with the fingers after creating slack in it by slightly plantar flexing the foot. Perform mobilizing techniques at the ankle and stretch the muscles of the lower leg.

Feet. The foot massage described previously will provide a nice finish to a thorough leg massage.

UPPER EXTREMITIES

Upright posture is thought to be an adaptation in the evolution of human beings to free us to use our hands for grasping and manipulating objects. Everyday activities such as cooking and eating, personal grooming, cleaning the house, and gardening are performed using the arms and hands. Hobbies and sports and most work activities also depend on the upper extremities.

The upper extremities are also important in communication. Some ethnic groups are known for using their hands to augment verbal expression. The hearing impaired use their hands for sign language. To be friendly or affectionate we shake hands, give pats on the back, and hug. Loss of the use of the arms or hands can be personally and socially devastating.

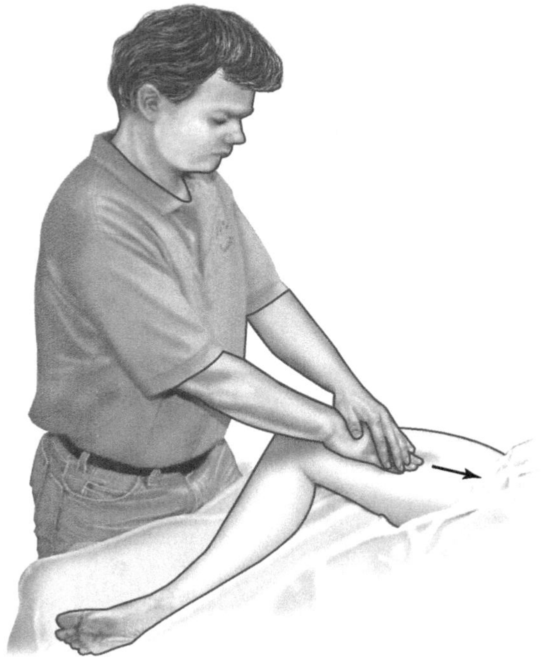

FIGURE 10–25. Position for reaching proximal adductor attachments. Be sure draping is secure.

Applications of Massage

People who work at computer terminals, or who perform other repetitive movements with the arms and hands often experience tightness and soreness in the upper extremities. Tennis elbow and golf elbow are repetitive strain injuries (RSI) common in those sports, and also in activities requiring similar movements of the arms. Massage and stretching can help keep muscles of the arms and hands relaxed and in good condition and help prevent overuse injuries. Massage is used with ice and rest to treat tennis and golf elbow.

Massage and joint movements can also help maintain shoulder flexibility. They can help restore mobility lost by poor posture, overuse, aging, or accident. The hands can be massaged and mobilized to help retain their function in old age.

Anatomy

For purposes of massage, the upper extremities may be thought of in four sections, that is, the shoulders, upper arms, forearms, and hands. The shoulders may be addressed as part of the upper back during massage, since the shoulder blades are located there. Functionally, however, the shoulder blades are part of the shoulder girdle and designed to facilitate use of the arms and hands. The joints of the upper extremities include the complex shoulder girdle, the elbows, wrists, and several small joints in the hands.

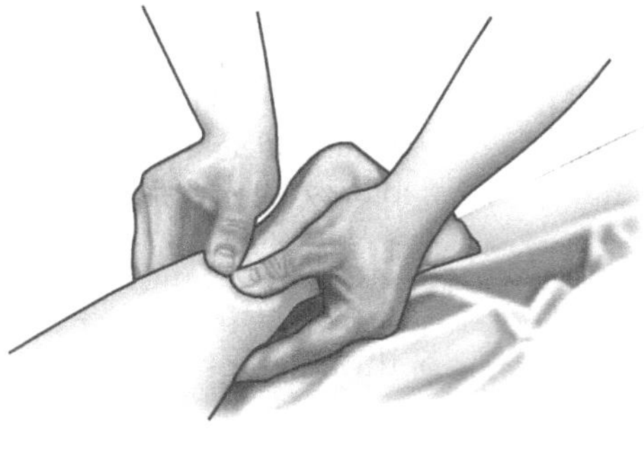

FIGURE 10–26. Direct pressure to Achilles tendon.

Shoulders. The muscles that move the shoulder include pectoralis major and minor, deltoid, subscapularis, supraspinatus, infraspinatis, teres major and minor, serratus anterior, levator scapulae, rhomboid major and minor, and trapezius. Latissimus dorsi is located on the back, but functions primarily to move the upper arm.

Arms and Hands. Muscles of the upper arm and forearms include the biceps brachii, triceps brachii, brachialis, the smaller muscles of pronation and supination (pronator teres, pronator quadratus, supinator), anconeus, coracobrachialis, and brachioradialis. The anterior forearm also contains the wrist flexors and palmaris longus, while the posterior forearm contains the wrist extensors. There are many small muscles intrinsic to the hand, which move the fingers and thumbs.

Techniques

The following techniques may be used to supplement a general massage of the upper extremities. The primary movers of the scapulae are located on the back and are best addressed as part of a back massage when the recipient is prone. The upper arms, forearms, and hands are most easily accessed and mobilized when the recipient is supine.

Enhancing Mobility of the Shoulder Girdle. Mobility of the shoulder girdle may be restricted for a number of reasons. Overuse and shortening of muscles in athletes and physical workers, underuse, aging, and recuperation from a shoulder injury can all contribute to loss of mobility in the shoulder.

A general approach to enhancing shoulder mobility would include warming of the superficial and deeper muscles of the upper back and upper arm with effleurage and petrissage, followed by deep

Table 10–4 THERAPEUTIC SEQUENCE FOR ENHANCING MOBILITY IN THE SHOULDER*

General Description:
Massage to relax muscles and restore mobility in the muscles of the upper back and shoulders. Relieves tension, increases circulation, and restores mobility in the shoulder.

Note: Figures cited below illustrate the technique, but it may be performed on a different part of the body in the picture.

Warming Techniques

1. Effleurage and petrissage of the entire shoulder (Figures 9–2, 9–3)
2. Circular friction along paraspinal muscles (Figure 9–1)

Therapeutic Combination

Prone

3. Knuckle or sawing friction between and over the shoulder blades (Figure 7–18)
4. Deep effleurage over upper trapezius and levator scapula
5. Direct pressure along upper trapezius and medial scapula border (Figure 10–27)
6. Swinging pendulum movement of arm
7. Scapula mobilizing technique (Figures 8–6, 10–28)

Supine

8. Direct pressure to subscapularis (Figure 10–29)
9. Deep effleurage and compressions to pectoral muscles and anterior deltoid (Figure 10–31)
10. Direct pressure to pectoral muscles (Figure 10–32)
11. Passive shoulder roll (Figure 8–5)
12. Arm stretches across the body and overhead (Figures 8–7, 8–8)

Finishing and Transition Technique

13. Effleurage over entire arm and shoulder

*This is an example of a therapeutic sequence for the shoulder. It can be altered to meet the needs of an individual recipient. There are many variations of this sequence, and many more techniques that can be incorporated to achieve the overall goal of enhancing mobility in the shoulder.

friction on muscles, on tendons, and at attachments. Direct pressure on muscles and tendons, particularly at tender or trigger points, helps muscles to relax and lengthen.

The shoulders and upper arms should be mobilized and taken through their full range of motion. Care should be taken not to force movement, potentially damaging tissues. Mobility that has been restricted for some time will take time to regain. The following techniques may be added to the basic full-body routine described in Chapter 9 to further enhance mobility of the shoulder girdle. A technique sequence for enhancing mobility in the shoulder is summarized in Table 10–4.

Prone. After general massage of the upper back, create a deeper warming by knuckling or sawing friction between and over the shoulder blades. How much pressure to use will be determined by the size and sensitivity of the recipient. The more heavily muscled the receiver, the more pressure you will use to affect deeper tissues.

Deep effleurage along upper trapezius and over the levator scapula will help loosen those muscles further. It may be useful then to apply vibration to the upper trapezius with an electric vibrator.

Direct pressure along the upper trapezius, and along the medial border of the scapula, will help relax these muscles. Apply pressure slowly, meeting the resistance offered by the tissue, then move along to another spot at about one-inch intervals. The reinforced thumb-over-thumb technique may be used for the large upper trapezius as shown in Figure 10–27.

With the receiver in the prone position, a gentle mobilization of the shoulder may be created by simply lifting the upper arm above the elbow, letting the forearm hang down toward the floor, and then swinging the forearm back and forth like a pendulum. This creates movement in the glenohumeral joint, as well as in the scapula. To create a larger and more controlled movement, place the recipient's arm alongside the body on the table. Grasp the upper arm just below the glenohumeral joint and move the shoulder superior and inferior, and then in a circle in a passive shoulder roll (Figure 8–5).

The scapula may be isolated for movement by placing the recipient's hand behind the back, which causes the scapula to lift away from the rib cage. Take care not to force this position, which may cause some discomfort. See Figure 10–28. You may modify this position by placing the hand next to the body with the elbow bent as shown in Figure 8–6. In either position, the scapula may be mobilized by placing a hand near the tip and on top of the shoulder and pressing lightly toward the feet. The other hand is placed at the inferior border of the scapula, assisting in the movement. The scapula will lift and move if the attached muscles are relaxed.

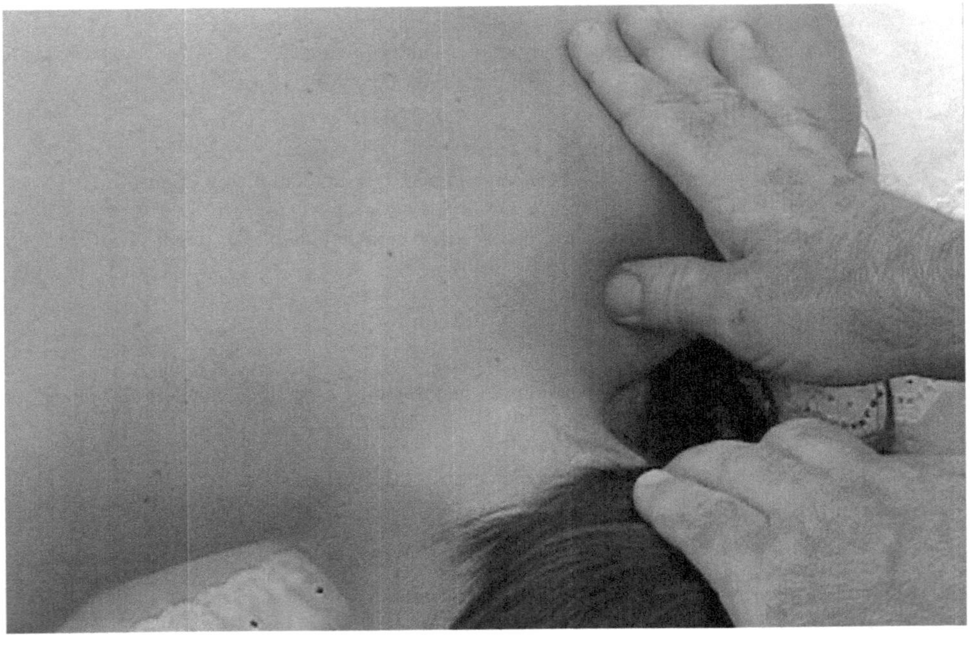

FIGURE 10–27. Direct pressure along upper trapezius with thumbs, recipient prone.

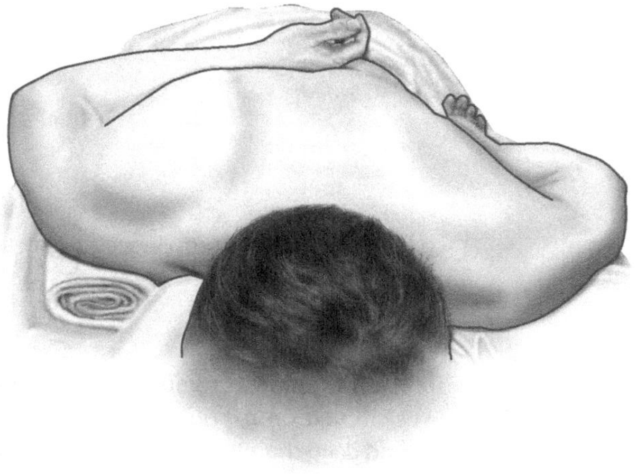

FIGURE 10–28. Mobilizing the scapula. Placing the recipient's hand behind the back causes the scapula to lift up.

Supine. The subscapularis muscle may be accessed with the recipient supine. Stand at the side near the shoulder and face the table. Bring the recipient's lower arm across the chest with the upper arm perpendicular to the table. This will expose the underside of the scapula somewhat. Locate the subscapularis in the axilla (i.e., armpit) and press into the subscapularis muscle with the fingertips as shown in Figure 10–29. This is usually very tender, so proceed gently.

Teres major and latissimus dorsi may be located by passively extending the recipient's arm overhead. Grasp the lateral edge of these muscles near the armpit. Gently knead the muscles, and then pull along their length for a gentle stretch.

Mobility in the shoulder girdle may be restricted anteriorly by the pectoral muscles and the anterior deltoid. After general warming, apply deep effleurage to these muscles. Direct pressure along the length of the pectorals at half-inch intervals may help to loosen them further. Care should be taken, since the pectorals will likely be sore if hypertonic. Follow the more specific massage with stretches of the upper arm across the body and overhead.

Preventing Forearm Strain. The muscles of the forearms create movement at the wrist and the hands. Certain occupations and activities tend to stress these muscles and produce chronic tension in them. Regular specific massage of the hands and forearms can help prevent overuse injuries in this area. A complete prevention program would also include regular resting time, stretching and self-massage, and biomechanically safe performance of the movements. Massage therapists themselves are prone to such overuse.

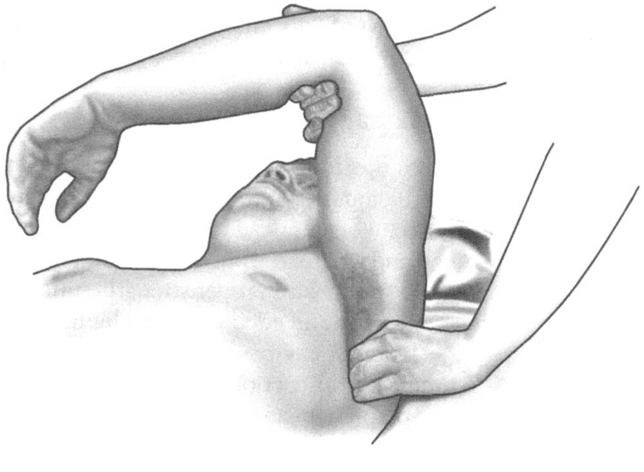

FIGURE 10–29. Accessing the subscapularis, recipient supine.

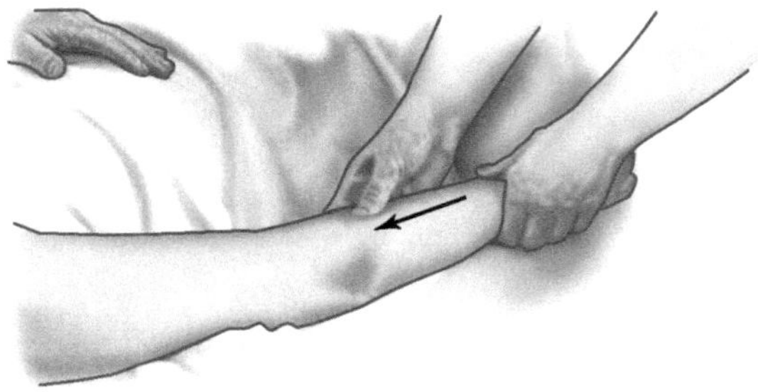

FIGURE 10–30. Deep stripping effleurage to the forearm muscles.

Warm the forearms and hands with general massage. Skin rolling over the wrist and forearm improves circulation to the area.

Add deep thumb stripping to the anterior and posterior forearms, following the long muscles from the wrist to their attachments at the elbow. See Figure 10–30. Apply deep circular friction to the attachments at the elbow. Direct pressure along the belly of the muscles of the forearms may help them relax. Mobilize the wrist joint and stretch the forearm muscles by passive flexion and hyperextension at the wrist.

To finish, perform the hand massage and joint movements described in Chapters 8 and 9. This will affect the forearm muscles that attach on the hand as well as muscles intrinsic to the hand itself.

CHEST AND ABDOMEN

The front of the body includes the chest and the abdomen. These areas are usually addressed separately during massage. However, they are connected for certain functions such as respiration and movements involving forward trunk flexion.

The expansion and contraction of the chest for breathing is evidence of life itself. Because it is the location of women's breasts, the chest is associated with both nurturing and sexual appeal. The chest is also associated with strength and power, as when the pectorals are more developed in men.

In the United States, women's breasts are kept covered in public and, therefore, should be draped to maintain modesty and proper professional boundaries. Practitioners can access the pectoral muscles and intercostals of women working around a small drape. When working on women with large breasts, it may be difficult to get to the muscles underneath.

Massage of the breast tissue itself is becoming more common as both a general health measure, and for certain clinical applications. Breast massage can be a valuable complementary therapy for women in treatment for breast cancer. It should be performed only after special training and with informed consent. (For further information, refer to *Breast Massage* by Debra Curties, 1999.)

The abdomen is a relatively vulnerable area extending from the diaphragm to the pubis. It contains the viscera, that is, the internal organs of digestion, elimination, and reproduction. It lacks the bony protection afforded the lungs and heart in the chest. The abdomen is contained and supported principally by the abdominal muscles. It is the soft belly exposed in humans because of our upright posture.

The word "visceral" has come to mean deeply felt, instinctive, or having to do with elemental emotions. This area is sensitive for many people and should be approached with care.

Applications of Massage

Poor posture, long periods of sitting at a desk, and carrying objects in the arms can all lead to shortening of the muscles of the chest and abdomen. A chronic slumped posture can inhibit the functions of the visceral organs, lead to back and neck tension and fatigue, and restrict breathing. Massage can help stretch and lengthen shortened anterior muscles that are the result of and contribute to chronic slumped posture. Along with proper strengthening exercises for the back and abdominal muscles, massage can help one maintain good postural alignment.

The chest cavity expands to accommodate expansion of the lungs during inhalation. Therefore, any muscular restriction in the area can adversely affect breathing. The major muscles of respiration are the diaphragm and intercostals. Forced inhalation and exhalation also involve the abdominal muscles, and muscles that move the rib cage such as pectoralis minor, serratus anterior, scalenes, and sternocleidomastoid. Massage can help maintain the muscles of respiration in optimal condition and relieve tension caused by poor posture or stress.

Breast massage is a specialized technique performed as a wellness measure for female breast health, and to address discomforts associated with the menstrual cycle, pregnancy and nursing. (Refer to *Breast Massage* by Debra Curties, 1999.)

Anatomy

The chest is defined by the rib cage, sternum, and muscles of the shoulder girdle that attach to them. The prominent muscles of the chest are pectoralis major and minor. Muscles located on the chest with the primary function of respiration include the diaphragm (separates the chest from the abdomen) and intercostals.

The breast structure sits over the muscles of the chest wall. It is "a specialized gland structure which evolves essentially as an appendage of the skin." The female breast is made up of fat tissue, and mammary glands and ducts with supporting connective tissue (i.e., fascia and ligaments). Breast tissue lies beyond the obvious contour of the breast, and extends inferior and laterally on the chest (Curties, 1999, p.19).

The abdomen lies between the thorax or chest and the pelvis. The abdominal cavity contains the stomach, liver, spleen, pancreas, small and large intestines, kidneys, bladder, reproductive organs in females, and other visceral organs. The abdominal muscles surrounding and supporting the viscera include the rectus abdominus and internal and external obliques.

Techniques

Rounded Shoulders. When the pectoral and anterior deltoid muscles shorten, the effect is rounded or forward shoulders. A program of stretching the muscles of the chest and shoulders, while strengthening the muscles of the upper back, is needed to truly correct rounded shoulders. During a massage session, rounded shoulders may be addressed by relaxing and stretching the pectorals and anterior deltoid.

Warm up the anterior deltoid with effleurage and petrissage. Apply compression over the anterior deltoid with a loose fist as shown in Figure 10–31. Warm up the pectorals using effleurage with the fist. Start superficially and gradually deepen the pressure. Once the muscles are warmed up, you may apply circular friction along the sternal and clavicular attachments of pectoralis major. Apply deep effleurage with the thumbs along the length of pectoralis minor, pausing to hold static pressure over the attachment on the third, fourth, and fifth ribs. See Figure 10–32.

Stretch the arm overhead to lengthen pectoral muscles. At the end of the session, have the recipient sit on the edge of the table with his hands behind his head. Get up onto the table behind the

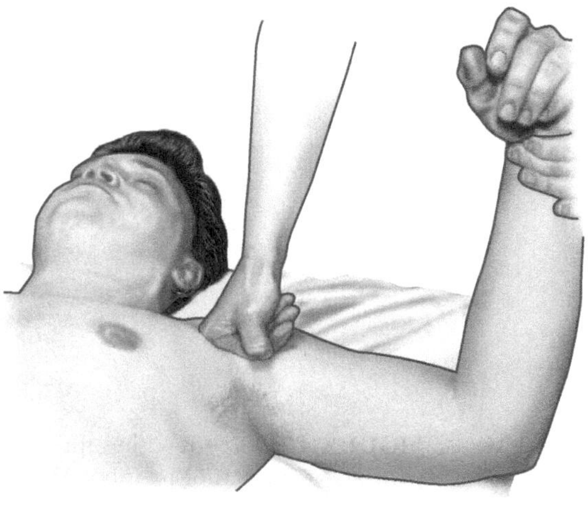

FIGURE 10–31. Compressions over anterior deltoid with loose fist.

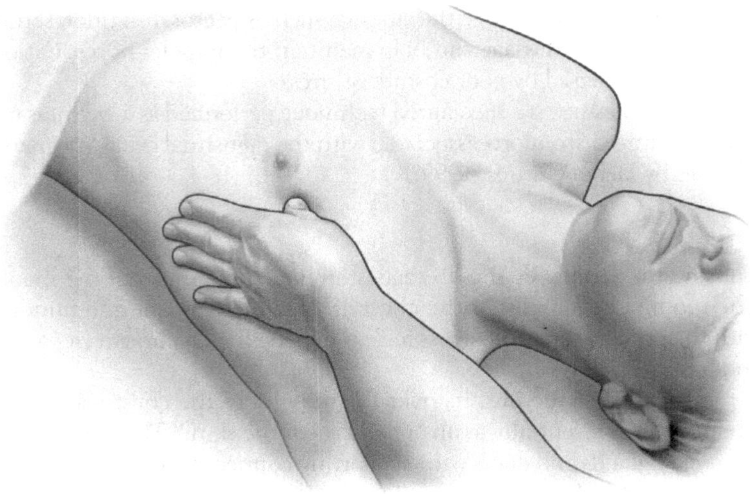

FIGURE 10–32. Direct pressure on attachments of pectoralis minor.

recipient and brace his back with your hip. Pull back on the elbows for a stretch of the pectorals as shown in Figure 10–33. Have the recipient inhale as you pull back and expand the chest.

Enhancing Respiration. Breathing is easier when muscles of respiration are relaxed. Muscular tension in the diaphragm, intercostals, abdominals, scalenes, and levator scapulae can inhibit proper expansion and lifting of the chest during inhalation. A therapeutic sequence for enhancing respiration is described in Table 10–5.

During massage of the cervicals, perform effleurage specifically over the scalenes with the thumb or fingertips to help relax them. When the recipient is prone, perform thumb stripping along the

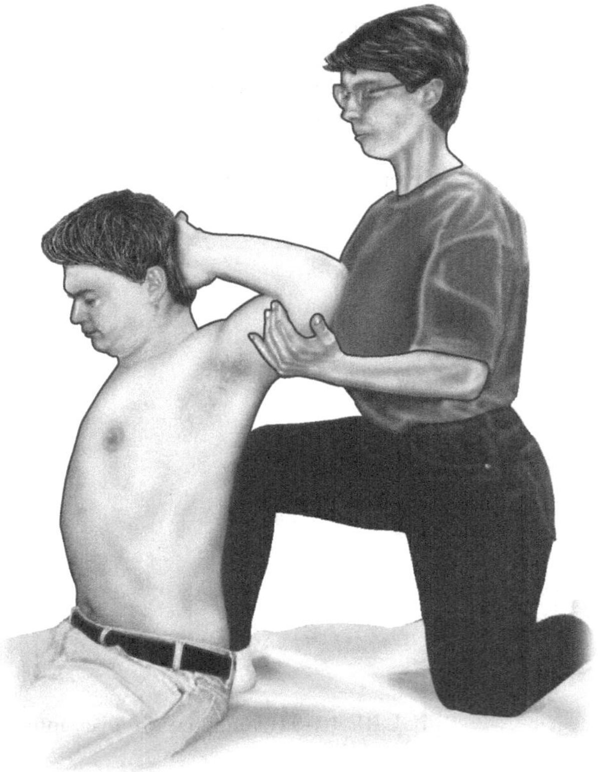

FIGURE 10–33. Stretching the pectorals with recipient in sitting position. Also used to enhance inhalation during deep breathing.

Table 10–5 THERAPEUTIC SEQUENCE FOR ENHANCING RESPIRATION*

General Description:
Massage to relieve muscular tension in the muscles of respiration to allow for greater expansion of the rib cage. General relaxation to encourage deep diaphragmatic breathing.

Note: Figures cited below illustrate the technique, but it may be performed on a different part of the body in the picture.

Warming Techniques

1. Effleurage and petrissage to the cervical muscles and upper trapezius (Figure 9–2, 9–3)

Therapeutic Technique Combination

Prone

2. Kneading of upper trapezius (Figure 9–3)
3. Direct pressure to points along upper trapezius (Figure 7–37)
4. Deep effleurage to levator scapula muscle moving superior to inferior
5. Friction of levator scapula muscle and attachments
6. "Cat paw" mobilizing technique to shoulders (prone version of Figure 9–19)
7. Effleurage of intercostal muscles (Figure 10–16)

Supine

8. Effleurage to upper trapezius using fist (Figure 9–20)
9. Effleurage with thumb or fingertips over scalene muscles, moving superior to inferior
10. Deep effleurage over pectoral muscles, moving superior to inferior (Figure 9–16)
11. Direct pressure on pectoral muscle attachments (Figure 10–32)
12. "Cat paw" mobilizing of shoulders (Figure 9–19)
13. Effleurage to intercostal muscles (supine version of Figure 10–16)
14. Rocking the rib cage (Figures 8–15, 8–16)
15. Slide along diaphragm attachment and lift side (Figures 10–34, 10–35)

Finishing and Transition Technique

16. Effleurage over shoulders and neck
17. Cradle head to encourage relaxation and deep diaphragmatic breathing (Figure 9–23)

*This is an example of a therapeutic sequence to enhance respiration. It can be altered to meet the needs of an individual recipient. There are many variations of this sequence, and many more techniques that can be incorporated to achieve the overall goal of improving breathing.

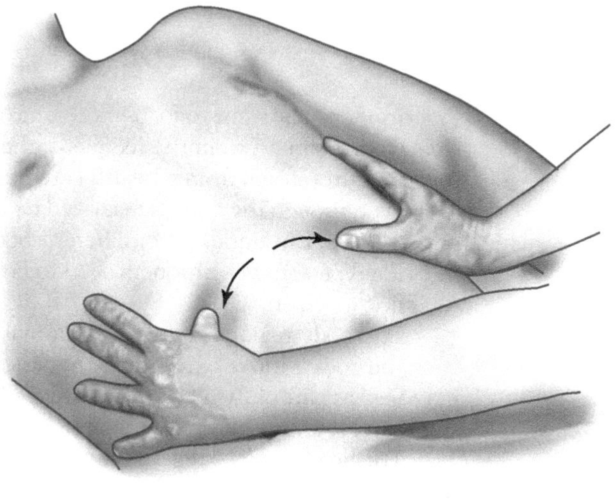

FIGURE 10–34. Sliding the thumbs along the attachment of the diaphragm.

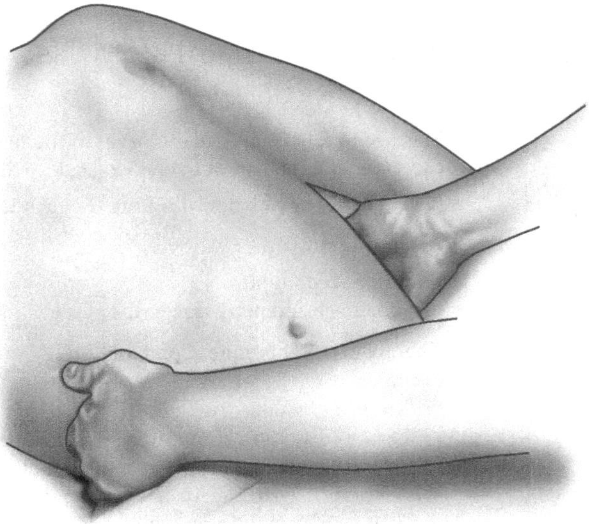

FIGURE 10–35. Lifting the abdominal muscles around the waist.

levator scapula to its point of attachment on the superior medial border of the scapula, lengthening the muscle. These are the muscles that elevate the shoulders and help expand the chest. They may be tense in people who are stressed and are breathing shallowly from the shoulders.

When the recipient is supine, lengthen the pectorals as described above to create space across the chest. Then perform effleurage over the rib cage from the opposite side of the table. Reach around as far as you can and pull up and over the rib cage with spread fingers. Try to find the spaces between the ribs to massage the intercostals. Rock the rib cage to further relax the area.

Stand at the waist of the recipient facing the head. Place your thumbs just beneath the sternum and have the recipient take a deep breath in. As he exhales, press in and slide your thumbs along the attachment of the diaphragm along the outline of the rib cage as shown in Figure 10–34. Be careful to avoid pressure on the xiphoid process. Finish by lifting up and around the sides of the abdominals. See Figure 10–35.

You may want to spend some time with the recipient practicing diaphragmatic breathing, or taking a full breath beginning with the diaphragm and expanding the chest. The stretching exercise shown in Figure 10–33 can also be used to help the recipient feel the expansion of the chest during inhalation.

Abdominal Massage. Abdominal massage is described in Chapter 9 as part of full-body massage. Techniques include effleurage in a circular pattern moving clockwise around the abdomen, fingertip vibration in the same pattern, and gentle undulating compression of the area, followed by effluerage, horizontal stroking, and finishing with passive touch. These techniques help stimulate movement of the contents of the lower digestive tract.

SUMMARY

Practitioners may want to focus more time and attention on a particular region of the body. This could stem from a request from the recipient, the practitioner's own judgment, information on a health history form, or referral from a health care provider.

Even though the body is massaged region by region during a session, its interconnectedness should always be kept in mind. Also, different body regions may have significance or human meaning to an individual person. Practitioners need to be aware that they are not just touching body regions, but are touching a person.

The body regions addressed in a massage session are usually divided into head and face, neck, back, buttocks, lower extremities, upper extremities, chest and abdomen. The scapula is commonly massaged as part of the back. Knowledge of each region in terms of its human meaning, anatomy, cautions, and relevant massage applications and techniques is essential for meeting the recipient's needs.

The head and face region is the center for thinking and communication. The senses of sight, hearing, taste, and smell are housed there. Massage can release tension caused by job-related activities, by emotional distress, and by pathologies that affect the facial muscles. Specific techniques that can be integrated into a head and face massage include: squeeze to eyebrows, effleurage over eyelids, thumb slide along nose, direct pressure to zygomatic arch, massage around mouth and jaw, massage to ears, mobilizing the scalp, massage of head, passive touch over eyes, and holding the sides of the head.

The neck region links the head and torso, and contains the muscles that hold head in upright posture. Muscle tension in the neck may result from poor posture, stress, or injury. Endangerment sites in the region include the anterior neck, and arteries and veins to the brain. Specific techniques that can be integrated into massage of the neck include direct pressure to cervical muscles, deep pressure to suboccipitals, direct pressure to thoracic attachments, and neck massage in prone position.

The back region is the core area for maintaining upright posture, and the place of attachment for arms and legs. Soothing back massage helps elicit the relaxation response. Tension in the back may result from heavy labor, sports, poor posture, or stress. Specific techniques that can be integrated into back massage include skin rolling, warming friction, effleurage between the ribs, lower back massage, and back massage for relaxation.

The buttocks, or large muscles of the hip region, support the entire body and provide the power for locomotion. They can be a source of sexual appeal, as well as of embarrassment. Specific techniques that can be integrated into massage of the buttocks include use of elbow, forearm and fist, direct pressure to gluteal attachments, and mobilizing techniques and stretching.

The lower extremities are the principal means of bipedal locomotion. Stress and pain in the legs and feet may be the result of accident, old age, sports, or job requirements. Foot massage involves massage of intrinsic muscles of the feet and attachments of leg muscles, and mobilizing of joints. Mobility in lower extremities can be enhanced with massage of the hips, thighs, lower leg, and feet.

The upper extremities allow us to use our hands and manipulate objects. They are important for everyday and work activities, and for communication. Problems in the upper extremities can result from repetitive motion, poor posture, old age, or accident. Mobility of the shoulder girdle can be enhanced with massage.

The front of the body includes the chest and abdomen. The chest is the location of pectoral muscles and breasts, and is associated with both nurturing and sexual appeal in women and with strength in men. The abdomen is a relatively vulnerable region containing the viscera or internal organs. Applications of massage in the chest region include addressing poor posture, rounded shoulders, and enhancing respiration. Massage techniques performed on the abdomen help stimulate movement of the contents of the lower digestive tract.

A look ahead . . .

The effects of massage can be enhanced by hot and cold applications such as hot packs, ice packs, and by thermal facilities such as steam rooms. Chapter 11 provides information and guidelines for the safe and effective use of these adjuncts to massage.

REFERENCES

Curties, D. (1999) *Breast massage*. Moncton, New Brunswick, Canada: Curties-Overzet Publications.

ADDITIONAL REFERENCES

Videos

"Classical and innovative European facial massage." (1988). Erica Miller Professional Education Series. Mile Ranch, British Columbia, Canada: Spa Expertise Canada LTD.

"Head, Neck & Shoulder Massage." (2003). Massage Master Class™ Series. Riverside, CT: At Peace Media. (*www.atpeacemedia.com*).

"Japanese hand massage." (2001). With Shogo Mochizuki. Boulder, CO: Kotobuki Publications.

"Zoku shin do™, Volume 1: The art of Japanese foot massage." (1999). With Shogo Mochizuki. Boulder, CO: Kotobuki Publications.

CHAPTER ELEVEN

Hydrotherapy/Thermal Therapies

LEARNING OUTCOMES

After studying this chapter, the student will have information to:

1. Discuss the history of hydrotherapy.
2. Describe the healing properties of water.
3. Describe hydrotherapy facilities found in spas and health clubs.
4. Use hot packs within the scope of massage therapy.
5. Use cold and ice packs, and ice massage within the scope of massage therapy.
6. Compare the temperature ranges for different thermo- and cryo-hydrotherapy methods.
7. Observe the contraindications for hydro- and thermal therapies.
8. Use hydrotherapy facilities effectively and safely.
9. Use hot and cold applications effectively and safely.

HISTORICAL PEOPLE AND DEVELOPMENTS

Ancient Greek gymnasium
Battle Creek Sanitarium
European spas
Finnish sauna
Hippocrates
Hot springs
Kellogg, J. Harvey
Kneipp, Sebastian
Maya sweatbaths
Mineral springs
Mineral water hospitals
Natural healers
Naturopaths
Physical therapists
Priessnitz, Vincent
Roman baths
Turkish baths
Winternitz of Vienna

LINK LIBRARY TERMS

Massage Business • *Traditional Chinese Medicine/Traditional Asian Medicine* • *Shiatsu* • *Massage Regulations*

KEY TERMS/CONCEPTS

Cold pack	Ice cup	Steam cabinet
Cold shower	Ice massage	Steam room
Cryo-therapy	Ice pack	Swiss shower
Facial steam	Moist hot pack	Thermal therapy
Hydrocollator	Neutro-therapy	Thermo-therapy
Hydrotherapy	Sauna	Vichy shower
Hot tub	Shower	Whirlpool bath

Hydrotherapy is the use of water in health and healing practices. The trio of water, massage, and exercise is a natural combination found all over the globe in bath houses, spas, and health clubs. Water and other modalities are also used for local applications of hot and cold, called **thermal therapy.**

This chapter will explore some of the more common hydrotherapy methods, and hot and cold applications within the scope of massage therapy. For more in-depth information on the use of physical agents within the context of physical therapy, a much more extensive topic, refer to specialty textbooks. (Refer to *Evidence-Based Guide to Therapeutic Physical Agents* by Alain-Yvan Belanger, 2002, or *Physical Agents: A Comprehensive Text for Physical Therapists* by Bernadette Hecox et al., 1994.)

HISTORY OF HYDROTHERAPY

The use of water for bathing, relaxation and recreation is found all over the world. Wherever **mineral and hot springs** come to the earth's surface, people from time immemorial have enjoyed their soothing and cleansing properties. Hot, sometimes bubbling, mineral waters are collected in pools for bathers. People come to these spas and hot springs for relaxation and healing. Native Americans are said to have frequented natural springs for their healing effects. Later, in places like Saratoga Springs, New York; Hot Springs, Arkansas; and Calistoga, California, resorts were built where the hot and cold mineral waters were taken internally as well as used for bathing. (Refer to *Taking the Waters* by Alev Lytle Croutier, 1992.)

Archeologists studying the ancient Maya and Aztec civilizations have found the ruins of sweat baths throughout Central America. The oldest of the sweat baths date from about 1350 BCE. These structures called *temezcalli* are described in the first history of Mexico, written by Friar Diego Duran in 1567. Most were small buildings that had low ceilings and a small entranceway, and held about 10 people. Steam was created by pouring water over hot rocks. Herbs were used with the steam for their healing effects. Sweating was thought to purify the body. It was used for a variety of illnesses, and by women after childbirth. **Maya sweat baths** are the antecedents of today's *temescal* or sweat houses still found in Central America, and are reminiscent of sweat lodges common among North American natives (Benjamin 2004).

The **Finnish sauna** was developed as a health practice centuries ago. After sitting in the superheated rooms, hardy Finns would jump into cold rivers and snow banks to cool off. It is a practice that many believe builds stamina, energy, and strength.

Today's spas and health club facilities like whirlpool baths, showers, steam rooms, and sauna can be traced in Western civilization to the **ancient Greek gymnasium** and **Roman baths. Turkish baths** followed, becoming popular in Europe and the United States in the latter 19th century. Baths were also popular in ancient Asia—India, China, Korea and Japan. Massage and bodywork was and still is an integral part of the bath house experience.

Water-Based Therapies

The healing effects of water applications were known in ancient Greece.The famous Greek physician **Hippocrates** used compresses, spongings, bathing, and drinking water in his treatments (c. 460 BCE).

Water therapies of various kinds were among the natural healing methods that blossomed in the 1800s. **Vincent Priessnitz,** a farmer in the Austro-Hungarian Empire, was famous for the methods of water therapy he developed from 1829 to 1849. Priessnitz developed an entire system of baths, compresses, and other hot and cold applications to treat various diseases.

Sebastian Kneipp, born in 1821 in Bavaria, is perhaps the most famous water cure practitioner of his era. Kneipp was a priest who built on Priessnitz water-based therapies, and his own knowledge of herbal remedies, to become the foremost authority on the subject. His little book, *My Water Cure* (1889), was translated into many languages over the years. People flocked to him from all over Europe to be cured from a variety of ailments.

European spas, which cater to people seeking healing as well as relaxation, adopted the methods of Priessnitz and Kneipp. An example of a Kneipp treatment given at the Biltz Sanitarium in Weisbaden, Germany 1898 is shown in Figure 11–1. The great spas at Baden-Baden and Weisbaden in Germany, Montecatini Terme in Italy, and Evian-les-Bains and Eugenie-les-Bains in France, as well as many smaller hydrotherapy establishments, carry on the tradition of the water cure.

The idea of the natural healing resort was imported to the United States in places like the **Battle Creek Sanitarium** in Michigan. **J. Harvey Kellogg** wrote *Home Handbook of Domestic Hygiene and Rational Medicine* (1880), which covered hydrotherapy, electrotherapy, and Swedish remedial gymnastics. His book *Rational Hydrotherapy* (1900) described 200 water treatments.

Hydrotherapy in Medicine

Sir John Floyer, a physician in Lichfield, England wrote a treatise in 1702 titled *The History of Cold Bathing to the Ancient and Modern*. Later that century Dr. Currie of Liverpool, England wrote *Medical Reports on the Effects of Water, both Warm and Cold, as a Remedy in Fevers and Other Diseases* (1797). The use of water as a therapeutic agent was being recognized within the developing field of biomedicine by the 18th century.

Almost a century later, **Winternitz of Vienna** experimented with various forms of external water applications to treat a variety of diseases. He used the shower, spray, alternating hot and cold baths, along with manipulations and massage. He varied the temperature of the water and the force with which it was applied for his results (Graham 1923).

Mineral water hospitals were opened in England starting with Bath in 1738, Harrogate in 1824, Droitwich in 1836, and Buxton in 1858. Physicians controlled the larger spas, but had competition from lay natural healers whom they considered quacks. The medical-versus-lay split widened, although each side adopted methods of the other.

By the 1890s hydropathy had two main branches. At places like Nauheim, Bath and Malvern where the medical influence was strong, it became "hydrotherapy," a rational system of baths, exercises, and electricity. At continental mountain resorts, on the other hand, hydropathy tended toward "barefoot back-to-nature cults" masterminded by lay philosophers . . ." (Barclay 1994, p. 3).

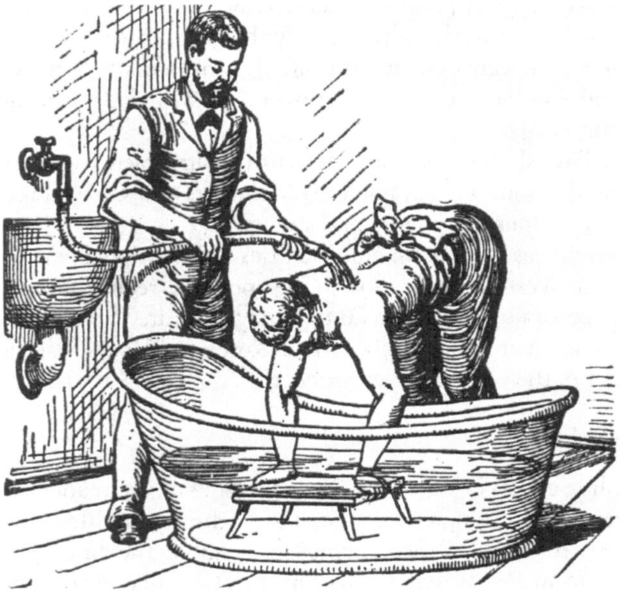

FIGURE 11–1. Kneipp treatment: Upper affusion with hose at the Biltz Sanitarium in Weisbaden, Germany, 1898.

Methods of natural healing and those of modern biomedicine were diverging into separate paths by the turn of the 19th century. Biomedicine opted largely for treatments with drugs and surgery. The old hydrotherapy became the province of **naturopaths** and other **natural healers.** Hydrotherapy retained its association with massage and movement therapies.

Physical Therapy

Members of the Chartered Society of Trained Masseuses (later Physiotherapy) in England treated injured servicemen during World War I (1914–1918) with hydrotherapy, massage, and related therapies (Barclay 1994). This idea was imported to the United States at about the same time, and the profession of physical therapy as we know it here was born. **Physical therapists** continue to research the therapeutic uses of water as a science.

HEALING PROPERTIES OF WATER

Water is relaxing to look at in rivers, lakes and ponds, and to listen to by the seashore, waterfall, or in a desk top water fountain. Flowing water feels pleasurable on the skin.

Taken internally and externally, water is the basis of many natural healing methods. The therapeutic use of water taken internally is outside of the scope of massage therapy, aside from encouraging clients to drink plenty of water, and perhaps filtering water to rid it of unhealthy contaminants. However, external applications of water in various forms, and immersion in water, have an association with massage that goes back to ancient times. Hydrotherapy and thermal therapy may be roughly divided into thermo-, neutro-, and cryo-. **Thermo-therapy** involves methods above normal body temperature. **Neutro-therapy** uses methods at about body temperature. **Cryo-therapy** involves methods below body temperature. Table 11–1 outlines the temperature sensations for these thermal ranges.

Methods within the scope of massage therapy include types of hydrotherapy used for health promotion such as those found in health clubs and spas. It also includes therapeutic uses of hot and cold applications in the forms of hot and cold packs, and ice. The general temperature ranges for these methods are listed in Table 11–2.

Healing properties of water are related to its use in cleansing the body, and its ability to raise and lower the core body temperature or the temperature of specific body tissues. Water can assume different forms—liquid, steam, and ice—each with its own contribution to healing. Water pressure from a shower, hose, or water jets is also used for a type of massage of the soft tissues.

Table 11–1 *TEMPERATURE SENSATIONS FOR THERMO-, NEUTRO-, AND CRYO-HYDROTHERAPY*

Descriptions are based on perception of temperature on the skin. These perceptions are subjective and vary from person to person.

Type	Description	Fahrenheit	Celsius*
Thermo	Very hot	111° to 120°	44° to 49°
	Hot	101° to 110°	38° to 43°
	Warm	94° to 100°	34° to 38°
Neutro	Neutral	90° to 93°	32° to 34°
Cryo	Tepid	80° to 92°	27° to 33°
	Cool	70° to 79°	21° to 26°
	Cold	55° to 69°	13° to 21°
	Very cold	31° to 54°	1° to 12°
	Freezing	32° and below	0° and below

*Temperature conversion Fahrenheit (°F) to Celsius (°C): °C = (°F − 32°)/1.8

Source: Adapted from *Day Spa Techniques* by Erica Miller (1996), Albany, NY: Milady Publishers; *Evidenced-Based Guide to Therapeutic Physical Agents* by Alain-Yvan Belanger (2002), Philadelphia: Lippincott Williams & Wilkins.

Table 11–2 *TEMPERATURE RANGES FOR HYDROTHERAPY AND THERMAL THERAPY METHODS FROM COLD TO HOT APPLICATIONS*

Method	Temperature range
Ice	23° to 32°F (−5° to 0°C)
Cold pack	33° to 50°F (1° to 10°C)
Cold water	50° to 80°F (10° to 27°C)
Bath—cool/cold	70° to 80°F (21° to 27°C)
Whirlpool bath—warm	95° to 104°F (35° to 40°C)
Whirlpool bath—hot	105° to 110° (41° to 43°C)
Steam room*	105° to 130° (41° to 54°C)
Sauna**	160° to 180° (71° to 82°C)
Hot pack—wet	165° – 170°F (74°–77°C)

* Wet heat with 100% humidity
** Dry heat with 6–8% humidity

Source: Adapted from *Day Spa Techniques* by Erica Miller (1996), Albany, NY: Milady Publishers; *Evidenced-Based Guide to Therapeutic Physical Agents* by Alain-Yvan Belanger (2002), Philadelphia: Lippincott Williams & Wilkins.

WHIRLPOOL BATHS, SHOWERS, STEAM ROOM, SAUNA

Typical spa and health club settings offer whirlpool baths, showers, steam rooms, and/or sauna in addition to massage services. Hot tubs and Esalen massage have been part of the California scene since the 1970s. Massage practitioners should know something about these facilities to be able to give their clients guidance, and to suggest their safe and effective use in relation to massage.

The benefits of warm to hot forms of hydrotherapy include raising the body temperature, producing sweating, cleansing skin pores, increasing superficial circulation, and general relaxation. These are best used before receiving massage.

The benefits of cool to cold forms of hydrotherapy include lowering body temperature, closing skin pores, decreasing superficial circulation, and general invigoration or stimulation. The cold shower is the most common form of cryo-hydrotherapy in the spa setting. Cold showers, or a contrasting hot to cold shower, are best taken after massage. See Table 11–3 for major effects of hot and cold hydrotherapy.

A **whirlpool bath** consists of a tub filled with water that has air or water jets causing movement or churning of the water. Private whirlpool bathtubs are deep enough that a person can lie down. In the spa, health club, or bath house, whirlpools are usually communal baths, where people sit on benches and are immersed with just their heads above water. Whirlpool baths within the context of physiotherapy may be smaller to accommodate an arm or a leg, and are made out of stainless steel.

The temperature of the water in a whirlpool bath is generally hot, but may vary considerably depending on the purpose of the bath, and the health of the patron. The recommended water temperature for relaxation ranges from about 95° to 105° (Miller, 1996).

The healing effects of the whirlpool bath stem from the water heat, and from the pressure of the water coming out of the jets and hitting the body. The churning of the water helps sustain the heat of the water on the skin, and stimulates the touch receptors of the skin.

A **hot tub** is a barrel-shaped tub made with wood slats, and a rubber or plastic liner. Hot tubs have water heaters, and may have whirlpool jets. They are especially popular on the West Coast. The guidelines for whirlpool baths apply also to hot tubs.

Showers are created by water streaming out of showerheads mounted on the wall. Showers may have no added pressure, i.e., falling like rain, or may have added pressure or pulsing pressure. Showers may be hot or cold. Hot showers have a similar effect as whirlpool baths, i.e., relaxation and increased superficial circulation.

Cold showers are stimulating and help reduce general body heat. They may be taken as a cool down after thermo-hydrotherapy or exercise.

Variations of the shower found in spas include the **Swiss shower** in which showerheads surround the bather at different levels from head to toe. The **Vichy shower** is given with the patron lying down

Table 11–3 *GENERAL EFFECTS OF HYDROTHERAPY COMPARING THERMO-HYDROTHERAPY AND CRYO-HYDROTHERAPY**

Hydrotherapy refers here to methods that are applied to the whole body, e.g., whirlpool, shower, steam room, and sauna.

Thermo-hydrotherapy
- Increase core body temperature
- Increase pulse rate
- Decrease blood pressure
- Increase respiratory rate
- Decrease muscle tone
- Induce sweating
- Relaxing/sedative effect

Cryo-hydrotherapy
- Decrease core body temperature
- Decrease pulse rate
- Increase blood pressure
- Decrease respiratory rate
- Increase muscle tone
- Induce shivering
- Invigorating/stimulating effect

*The actual effects of specific hydrotherapy methods depend on the health of the client, the actual temperature of the water or room, and the length of time a person is exposed to the heat or cold.

Source: Adapted from Table 14–4, Body Systemic Effects Generally Associated with Cryo-, Thermo-, and Neutro-hydrotherapy, in *Evidenced-Based Guide to Therapeutic Physical Agents* by Alain-Yvan Belanger (2002), Philadelphia: Lippincott Williams & Wilkins.

on a table with water showering down from about 4 feet above. The Vichy shower can be varied with pulsating water, with alternating hot and cold water, or with a salt or shampoo scrub. An attendant controls the water pressure and temperature from a panel (Miller 1996).

Steam rooms are generally tiled spaces from floor to ceiling with benches for sitting. Steam comes out from jets in the wall and fills the space with wet heat from 105° to 130°F (41° to 54°C) with 100% humidity. Patrons in the steam room inhale the steam, which helps clear sinuses and relieve respiratory congestion. Steam also raises the body temperature and causes sweating. It is a relaxing, cleansing experience.

A variation of the stream room is the **steam cabinet.** The patron sits on a stool in an enclosed box with the head sticking out. Steam is pumped into the box, raising core body temperature, and causing sweating. Since the head is out of the box, the steam is not inhaled. A cold shower following a steam room or cabinet experience can help wash off sweat and bring body temperature down to normal.

When raising the core body temperature is contraindicated or undesirable, **facial steam** may be beneficial. Facial steam devices focus steam to the face and are used in skin care as well as to improve respiration.

The **sauna** is a practice that originated in Finland, and involves sitting in a room with dry heat from 160° to 180°F (71° to 82°C) with 6 to 8% humidity. The sauna is typically a wood-lined room heated without steam, and the air is very dry. Patrons sit on wooden benches. Occasionally, water may be poured over hot rocks to produce steam, adding some moisture to the air. A cold shower or a plunge into a swimming pool or lake (or snow bank) after sitting in a sauna is stimulating, closes the skin pores, and helps reduce body temperature.

Contraindications for thermo-hydrotherapy are listed in Table 11-4. The most serious contraindications are related to heart, circulatory, and other systemic diseases. People with skin rashes should also avoid the increase in superficial circulation that results from immersing in hot water. Of course, people using public facilities should be careful not to spread contagious disease of any kind.

Although it is possible to overdo cryo-hydrotherapy causing adverse reactions, it is more common for people to stay too long in the hot hydrotherapy baths and rooms. First-time bathers should only stay

Table 11–4 CONTRAINDICATIONS FOR THERMO-HYDROTHERAPY

These contraindications apply to hydrotherapy methods that raise the core body temperature. In some cases, using water with lower temperature and/or limiting the time in the hot water or steam may make their use safer.

- High or low blood pressure
- Heart or circulatory problems
- Pregnancy
- Systemic diseases such as hepatitis
- Seizures
- Multiple sclerosis
- Infection or inflammatory condition
- Vascular problems associated with phlebitis, varicose veins, diabetes
- Skin rashes
- Allergies to water additives
- Contagious conditions
- Some cancers and cancer treatments

Certain medications may make hydrotherapy unsafe for a client. These include drugs that:

- Alter how blood vessels react to hot and cold
- Change skin sensitivity to hot and cold
- Alter the body's temperature control or cooling mechanisms

Source: Adapted from *Day Spa Techniques* by Erica Miller (1996), Albany, NY: Milady Publishers; *Massage Therapy and Medications* by Randall S. Persad (2001), Toronto: Curties-Overzet Publications; *Evidenced-Based Guide to Therapeutic Physical Agents* by Alain-Yvan Belanger (2002), Philadelphia: Lippincott Williams & Wilkins.

5–15 minutes in hot water, while healthy experienced bathers may stay up to 30 minutes. People who are weak or over 60 years old should limit their exposure to hot baths and steam to 5–15 minutes (Miller 1996).

If a client reports feeling lightheaded or dizzy, is nauseous, or develops a headache, they probably stayed immersed too long in hot water or steam. Take measures to reduce the body temperature gradually such as sitting or lying in a neutral temperature environment, and sipping tepid to cool water. If symptoms persist or get worse, consider medical evaluation. Guidelines for safe use of thermo-hydrotherapy facilities are listed in Table 11–5.

Table 11–5 GUIDELINES FOR SAFE USE OF THERMO-HYDROTHERAPY FACILITIES: WHIRLPOOL, SHOWER, STEAM ROOM, AND SAUNA

1. Check to make sure that no contraindications are present before using thermo-facilities. See Table 11–4.
2. Wait for at least one hour after eating before using thermo-facilities.
3. Avoid alcohol before or during use of thermo-facilities.
4. Wear sandals or shoes with non-slip bottoms to avoid slipping and falling.
5. Check temperature of the water or room (steam and sauna) for therapeutic range (Table 11–2), and for individual tolerance.
6. Limit use according to experience in thermo-facilities, and factors such as general health and age. In general less experienced, less healthy, weaker, or over age 60 limit use to 15 minutes, and otherwise 15–30 minutes.
7. Drink plenty of water or other fluids during and after thermo-hydrotherapy to replace loss through sweating.
8. Always have someone to call for help if needed.
9. Monitor how you feel, and if weak, dizzy, or nauseous get out of the water or room. Lie or sit down in a cooler place, and replace fluids by sipping a cool drink.
10. If reaction to heat is severe or lasts a long time, consider seeking medical evaluation.

Use before massage is beneficial for initiating general relaxation, muscle relaxation, and increased superficial circulation and connective tissue pliability.

Use after massage may continue benefits described above. Be sure to wash off oil and lubricant thoroughly before entering thermo-facilities. Lubricants can contaminate water, and leave slippery films on benches and floors.

The most commonly used methods of thermal therapy within the scope of massage therapy are hot packs, ice, cold packs, and ice massage. The focus of the following section is on local applications of thermal therapy.

HOT APPLICATIONS — THERMO-THERAPY

Healing Effects of Heat

Heat applied locally to muscles and related soft tissues not only feels good, but also helps muscles relax, increases local circulation, and makes connective tissues more pliable. Sore stiff muscles benefit from the increased circulation and heat.

Raising tissue temperature to between 104° and 113°F (40°–45°C) increases cell metabolism and blood flow for various therapeutic results. Lower temperatures have little therapeutic effect, and higher temperatures will damage cells (Belanger 2002).

Although heat is applied locally, use of hot packs can raise core body temperature. In that case, contraindications for thermo-hydrotherapy also apply. See Table 11–4. Local contraindications for the use of hot packs include burns, wounds, swelling, inflammation, and skin conditions (e.g., rashes) that could be made worse by heat. Check the area visually and/or by palpation for evidence of contraindications before deciding to use hot packs.

Hot Packs and Massage

The application of hot packs *prior* to massage can help begin muscle relaxation, enhance circulation locally, and prepare the area for deeper massage techniques. *After* massage of an area, hot packs can enhance muscle relaxation and prolong increased local circulation.

Heat sources may be from moist hot packs, or dry hot packs or pads. Moist hot packs are more penetrating. However, some newer types of dry hot packs heated in microwave ovens can be good heat sources, are generally easier to use, and can be used with warm, damp cloths to create moist heat.

Typical **moist hot packs** come in various sizes and shapes, and are heated in hot water. **Hydrocollator** units are metal containers with electrical heating elements used to keep the water within a constant range: 158°–168°F (51°–54°C). Hot packs are suspended in the hot water to a therapeutic temperature, and then applied to the client.

Table 11–6 SUMMARY OF GUIDELINES FOR SAFE USE OF MOIST HOT PACKS BEFORE AND DURING MASSAGE

1. Be clear about your goals for using hot packs in association with massage.
2. Check to make sure that no contraindications are present and that the client is not taking medications that reduce sensation or alter circulation.
3. Get informed consent from the client to apply hot packs.
4. Instruct the client on the need for feedback about how the hot pack feels to them, especially if it feels too hot.
5. Check hot pack to make sure it is correct temperature. Touch to own skin (e.g., wrist) to judge if it is hot enough or too hot, and how many layers of towels to use.
6. Apply layers of towels between the client's skin and the hot pack to help avoid burns. Use more layers for more sensitive skin and for clients over 60 years old.
7. Apply a towel over the hot pack to help keep heat from escaping.
8. Ask for feedback from client every 5 to 7 minutes or more if needed. Heat of tissues increases the longer the hot pack is applied.
9. Add additional towels beneath the hot pack if the client complains of too much heat.
10. Remove hot pack immediately if you judge potential for damage to skin or if client is having negative reaction to heat (e.g., dizziness, nausea).
11. Maximum time for hot pack use on a local area is about 20 minutes.

Always check how the hot pack feels on your own skin, e.g., at the wrist, prior to applying it to a client. Packs that have been sitting in the hydrocollator for a long time (i.e., over 60 minutes) will be hotter than packs that are used often, or that have been heating for only a few minutes.

Care must be taken not to burn the client's skin. This is accomplished by placing towels between the hot pack and the skin. Ask the client for feedback every 5 to 7 minutes about how the pack feels, i.e., if it feels too hot. A visual and tactile check is also a good idea. Clients taking medications that reduce skin sensation, or alter the reaction of blood vessels to heat, or reduce their body heat control mechanisms, are not good candidates for hot packs. See Table 11–6 for guidelines for the use of moist hot packs with massage.

COLD APPLICATIONS—CRYOTHERAPY

Healing Effects of Cold

Cold applied locally to muscles and related soft tissues causes vasoconstriction and decreased local circulation. There is also decrease in cell metabolism, nerve conduction velocity, pain, muscle spindle activity, and spasm in the cold area. After about 20 to 30 minutes of continuous application, cold-induced vasodilation is thought to occur. This may lead to increased circulation, but it is doubtful that circulation rises to a baseline of before the cold was applied. Cold applied locally can also act eventually to lower core body temperature (Belanger 2002; pp. 267–270).

Cold applications to tissues after trauma or injury can decrease secondary cell and tissue damage. This limits worsening of soft tissue injury, and prevents further swelling of tissues and edema.

First aid for a strain or sprain, or a blow to soft tissues, includes immediate application of cold, preferably as cold as ice. This limits hemorrhaging, swelling, and secondary cell hypoxia or damage. If a limb is involved, the R.I.C.E.S. first aid principle applies, i.e., rest, ice, compression, elevation, and stabilization.

Cryotherapy is used most often with massage in settings where clients are likely to have soft tissue injury or pain. These include sports medicine and rehabilitation settings, and chiropractic offices. However, any client may have had a recent injury or have muscle spasms, so knowledge of the use of cold applications can be useful. (Refer to *Cryotherapy in Sport Injury Management* by Kenneth L. Knight, 1995.)

Table 11–7 CONTRAINDICATIONS FOR CRYO-HYDROTHERAPY AND COLD APPLICATIONS

These contraindications apply to hydrotherapy methods that lower the core body temperature.

- Circulatory insufficiency or vasospastic disorders (e.g., Raynaud's disease, diabetes)
- Cardiac disorder
- Allergy to cold
- Cold hypersensitivity or chilling
- Multiple sclerosis
- Asthma
- Rheumatoid arthritis
- Osteoarthritis
- Some cancers and cancer treatments
- Infection
- Depression
- Pregnancy

Certain medications may make hydrotherapy unsafe for a client. These include drugs that:

- Alter how blood vessels react to hot and cold
- Change skin sensitivity to hot and cold
- Alter the body's temperature control or cooling mechanisms

Source: Adapted from *Cryotherapy in Sports Injury Management* by Kenneth L. Knight (1995), Champaign, IL: Human Kinetics; *Evidenced-Based Guide to Therapeutic Physical Agents* by Alain-Yvan Belanger (2002), Philadelphia: Lippincott Williams & Wilkins; *Massage Therapy and Medications* by Randall S. Persad (2001), Toronto: Curties-Overzet Publications.

Contraindications to local cold applications include circulatory insufficiency such as with Raynaud's disease and diabetes, allergic reaction to cold, cold sensitivity, or chilling. Clients with multiple sclerosis or asthma may not react well to cold. Take special care with clients taking medications that reduce skin sensation, alter the reaction of blood vessels to heat and cold, or reduce their body temperature control mechanisms. See Table 11–7 for a summary of contraindications for cryo-hydrotherapy and cold applications.

Cold Packs, Ice, Ice Massage

Cold packs of various kinds are commercially available. They are usually made of materials that hold cold over a period of time and stay pliable even when near freezing. They have coverings for comfortable contact with skin.

Ice packs are made with ice cubes or crushed ice inside plastic bags that can be sealed. A disadvantage of ice is that it melts over time, and plastic bags can leak water. Ice, water below 32°F (0°C), is also hard to the touch and may be less comfortable over injuries. However, ice is readily available, and generally stays cold longer than cold packs. Ice can be replaced in bags as needed to hold a freezing temperature.

Cold packs are used as adjuncts to massage to reduce muscle spasm or muscle pain, or if a client has swelling from a recent injury like a sprained ankle. Cold may be applied to reduce spasm and pain so that the area can be massaged. It can also be used instead of massage if massage would further aggravate the injury or spasm. Cold or ice may be applied to an area for up to 30 minutes at a time, during massage of other parts of the body.

Ice massage involves rubbing ice directly on the skin using an ice cube or ice cup. **Ice cups** are made by filling paper cups with water, and putting them in the freezer to harden. The paper is peeled back to expose the ice, and some paper left on for holding the cup.

Ice massage is usually performed in a circular motion over a small area for about 5–10 minutes, until the area becomes numb. Ice massage may be used to numb an area before performing deep transverse friction such as in a case of tendinitis. It allows the therapist to work deep enough without causing severe pain. Ice is also used after this treatment to continue to numb the area.

The person receiving the cold application will normally feel the following: (1) a sensation of cold, (2) tingling or itching, (3) pain, aching or burning, and (4) numbing or analgesia. It is good to inform the client about what they will feel, since some of the sensations can be uncomfortable.

Be careful not to apply very cold applications for too long (a one-hour maximum) to avoid tissue damage and frostbite. Guidelines for cold applications are found in Table 11-8.

Table 11–8 SUMMARY OF GUIDELINES FOR SAFE USE OF COLD AND ICE PACKS BEFORE AND DURING MASSAGE

1. Be clear about your goals for using cold applications in association with massage.
2. Check to make sure that no contraindications are present and that the client is not taking medications that reduce sensation or alter circulation.
3. Get informed consent from client to apply cold packs.
4. Instruct the client on the need for feedback about how the cold application feels to them.
5. Inform them of the stages of sensation to expect with cold applications, i.e., (1) cold sensation, (2) tingling or itching, (3) aching or burning, and (4) numbness or analgesia.
6. Apply the cold or ice pack directly to the desired area.
7. Do not apply cold-gel packs under a compression bandage, since it may cause frostbite.
8. Use the R.I.C.E.S. principle if injury on a limb, i.e., rest, ice, compression, elevation, stabilization.
9. Ask for feedback on the cold application every 5 to 7 minutes.
10. Remove cold pack immediately if it causes an adverse reaction, e.g., skin rash, chilling.
11. Maximum time for continuous cold application is one hour; 15 minutes is sufficient in the context of a massage session.

SUMMARY

Hydrotherapy is the use of water in health and healing practices. Water is also a medium for local applications of hot and cold called thermal therapies.

The history of the use of water in health and healing can be traced to ancient times in all parts of the globe. The European and Western traditions of water-based therapies include the names of Priessnitz, Kneipp, Winternitz, Kellogg, and the Chartered Society of Trained Masseuses in England.

Hydrotherapy and thermal therapy can be roughly divided into thermo-, neutro-, and cryo-therapy based on the temperature of the water or other medium. Water is used in form of liquid, steam, and ice. Water pressure from shower, hose, or water jets serves as a type of massage of the soft tissues.

Hot forms of hydrotherapy include whirlpool baths, showers, steam rooms, and sauna. Effects of hot hydrotherapy include raising the body temperature, producing sweating, cleansing skin pores, increasing superficial circulation, and general relaxation. These are best used before a massage session. Guidelines should be observed for safe use of these facilities.

Heat applied locally to muscles and related soft tissues feels good, helps muscles relax, increases local circulation, and makes tissues more pliable. Moist hot packs are typically used for thermo-therapy. Measures to avoid burning the client's skin include using towels as a safety barrier, and limiting the time the hot pack is applied.

Cold applications or cryotherapy causes vasoconstriction and decreased local circulation, cell metabolism, nerve conduction, and reduced pain and spasm. Cold applications are used in first aid for trauma and injury. Cryotherapy methods include cold and ice packs, and ice massage.

Contraindications and safety guidelines for all forms of hydrotherapy and thermal therapies should be observed to avoid harm to the client.

A look ahead . . .

A variety of contemporary massage and bodywork approaches have been developed to address specific body tissues and systems. Chapter 12 describes specialized techniques used to improve the health of the body's myofascial tissues.

REFERENCES

Barclay, J. (1994). *In good hands: The history of the chartered society of physiotherapy 1894–1994*. London: Butterworth-Heinemann.

Belanger, A.-Y. (2002). *Evidenced-based guide to therapeutic physical agents*. Philadelphia: Lippincott Williams & Wilkins.

Benjamin, P. J. (2004). "Massage and sweatbaths among the ancient Maya." *Massage Therapy Journal*, Spring, pp. 148–154.

Croutier, A. L. (1992). *Taking the waters: Spirit, art, sensuality*. New York: Abbeyville Press.

Graham, R. L. (1923). *Hydro-hygiene: The science of curing by water*. New York: The Thompson-Barlow Company.

Hecox, B., Mehreteab, T. A., & Weisberg, J. (1994). *Physical agents: A comprehensive text for physical therapists*. Norwalk, CT: Appleton & Lange.

Knight, K. L. (1995). *Cryotherapy in sport injury management*. Champaign, IL: Human Kinetics.

Miller, E. T. (1996). *Day spa techniques*. Albany, NY: Milady Publications.

Monastersky, R. (2002). "Plumbing ancient rituals: Sweatbaths in Maya cities provide a window into lives long ago." *The Chronicle of Higher Education*. 17 May 2002, pp. A22–23.

Persad, R. S. (2001). Massage therapy & medications: General treatment principles. Toronto: Curties-Overzet.

ADDITIONAL REFERENCES

Videos

"Day Spa 1: Hydrotherapy Treatments." (1997) Erica Miller Professional Education Series. Mile Ranch, British Columbia, Canada: Spa Expertise Canada LTD.

CHAPTER TWELVE

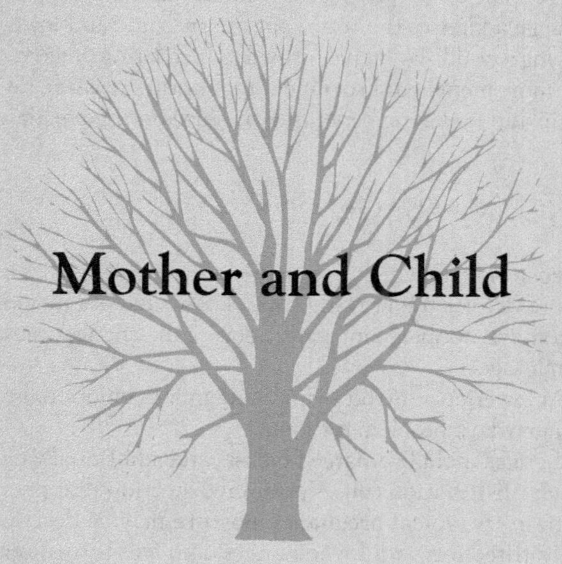

Mother and Child

LEARNING OUTCOMES

After studying this chapter, the student will have information to:

1. Plan a massage session to meet the special needs of pregnant women.
2. Take into consideration the physical and emotional changes women experience during pregnancy.
3. Identify contraindications and cautions for giving massage to pregnant women.
4. Provide an optimal environment for giving massage to pregnant women.
5. Position pregnant women comfortably on the massage table.
6. Include important elements and techniques in pregnancy massage.
7. Explain how massage can help ease labor, delivery, and recovery.
8. Discuss the benefits of massage for nursing mothers and women with small children.
9. Plan a massage session to meet the special needs of infants.
10. Perform massage for the optimal growth and development of infants.

KEY TERMS/CONCEPTS

Breast massage
Gall bladder channel
Infant massage
Kinesthetic stimulation
LI4 and Sp6
Pregnancy posture
Reclining position
Side-lying position
Tactile stimulation

LINK LIBRARY TERMS

Massage Business • *Traditional Chinese Medicine/Traditional Asian Medicine* • *Infant Massage* • *Pregnancy Massage* • *Massage Regulations*

MEDIALINK

A companion CD-ROM, included free with each new copy of this book, supplements the techniques presented in this chapter. Insert the CD-ROM to watch video clips of massage techniques being demonstrated. This multimedia feature is designed to help you add a new dimension to your learning.

Massage can relieve some of the physical and emotional stresses women experience during pregnancy. For example, massage addresses the strain put on the spine and lower extremities by the extra weight gained while carrying a child. Women confined to bed during pregnancy can benefit from the improved circulation, joint movements, and social contact during massage. Women are especially grateful for the anxiety reducing and relaxing benefits of massage during pregnancy.

BENEFITS OF PREGNANCY MASSAGE

Pregnancy is a special time in which a woman's body undergoes significant changes as it nurtures, carries, and prepares to deliver the growing baby. These changes include hormonal, structural, and postural deviations from the nonpregnant state. Some of the changes cause discomfort and distress that can be relieved with massage.

Many women experience mood swings and greater emotional reactions as hormone activity increases. Insomnia may be a problem for some.

Structural changes include enlarged breasts and additional weight anteriorly as the fetus grows. This shifting weight distribution causes postural distortion that puts pressure on the lower back, and results in neck strain. A typical **pregnancy posture** may be described as head forward, chest back, belly out, and hips tilted forward, locked knees, and feet turned out. Figure 12–1 shows the typical posture of a pregnant woman and major areas of stress. Pressure from the additional weight being carried and decreased physical activity as the pregnancy progresses may cause swelling of the hands, legs, and feet.

During pregnancy, there is a softening of the connective tissue of the body, including cartilage and ligaments. This facilitates normal delivery of the baby. It may also cause instability and pain in the joints.

The intent of pregnancy massage includes helping the mother relax and release emotional stress, and addressing the strain felt in the lower back, neck, legs, and feet. Massage may also help reduce edema in upper and lower extremities. Research shows massage to have potential for reducing obstetric and postnatal complications including lower prematurity rates (Field, T. et al 1999).

CONTRAINDICATIONS AND CAUTIONS

Because each woman is unique, and many complications are possible during pregnancy, it is best to get permission from the primary health care provider before giving massage. Massage may be contraindicated totally in a few cases, or there may be cautions or restrictions to take into consideration. It is important for practitioners working with pregnant women to understand what is happening in a woman's body during that time in order to give massage safely.

Abdominal massage is contraindicated during pregnancy. A few nerve strokes, passive touch, and some forms of energy work may be performed safely. It is best to use extreme caution in the area of the belly.

Elaine Stillerman, in her book *Mother-Massage* (1992), lists the following general contraindications for massage of pregnant women: morning sickness, nausea, or vomiting; any vaginal bleeding or discharge; fever; a decrease in fetal movement over a 24-hour period; diarrhea; pain in the abdomen or anywhere else in your body; excessive swelling in arms or legs; immediately after eating (wait two hours); over a bruise or skin irritation (local contraindication).

According to Chinese medicine, strong pressure should be avoided on the **gall bladder channel** at the top of the shoulders, and points **LI4** and **Sp6.** If there is worry about miscarriage in the early months of pregnancy, also avoid pressure on the Yin Channels on the inside of the lower legs (Lundberg 1992, p. 176).

SETTING THE ENVIRONMENT

There are some things about the general environment and your equipment to keep in mind when preparing to give massage to pregnant women. They are often warm, and so the room should generally be kept 5–10 degrees cooler than usual for massage. Good air flow and fresh air are desirable. The

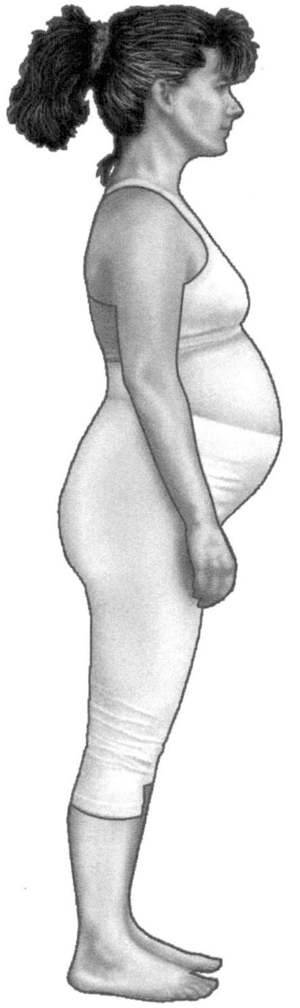

FIGURE 12–1. Typical posture of a pregnant woman—head forward, chest back, belly out and hips tilted forward, locked knees.

massage space should be near a bathroom if possible, because pregnant women feel the need to urinate frequently. The atmosphere should be relaxing, including any music played.

Your table height should be lower than usual, especially when the woman is further along in the pregnancy. As she gets larger, and especially in the side-lying position, you will be better able to use good body mechanics with a lower table. Have several bolsters or pillows to use as props for comfortable positioning of the pregnant recipient. A glass of water should be in reach for the recipient, and tissues handy.

A stepping stool may be useful for the woman to use to get up onto the table. You may also want to be present to assist the recipient and help her get into a comfortable position. This is especially true in the later stages of pregnancy.

POSITIONING OPTIONS

It is important for the recipient to be in a safe and comfortable position while receiving massage. The prone, supine, reclining, and side-lying positions each have their place in giving massage to pregnant women.

In the first few months, women may be comfortably prone or supine as usual for massage. Once the fetus has grown and the mother's belly starts to get larger, other positions may be more comfortable. Later in the pregnancy, the mother may not be able to lie supine without the fetus putting pressure on the descending aorta, impeding the flow of blood to the placenta and causing shortness of breath. Lying flat on the back may also put pressure on the inferior vena cava, resulting in feelings of lightheadedness, nausea, and backache. Lying prone may be difficult, although with proper bolstering, it may be quite comfortable.

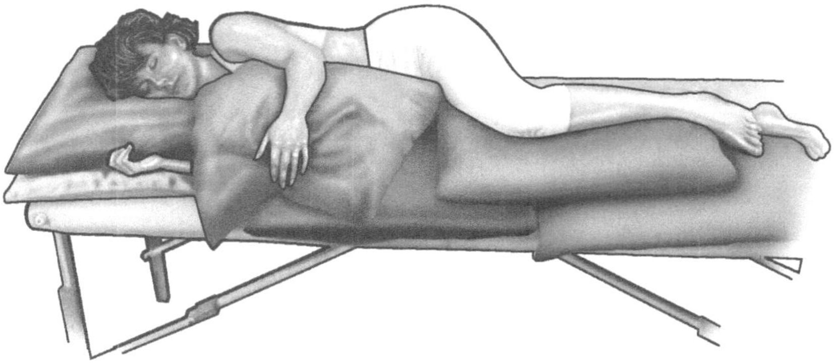

FIGURE 12–2. Props for side-lying position for pregnant woman; pillows under and around the belly, under the head, and under the top arm and leg.

Reclining, or half-sitting, may be a good alternative to lying supine. Bolsters may be used to prop the recipient into a half-sitting position. Some stationary massage tables have an adjustment to convert the flat tabletop into one with a back support.

Side-lying is perhaps the most common position for pregnant women receiving massage. Some doctors caution against pregnant women lying on the left side while sleeping. This may not be a problem for the short duration of massage, but it doesn't hurt to check with the woman's physician for his advice on positioning, especially if there is any complicating health factor.

A general rule of thumb for positioning and propping pregnant women is to fill in any spaces you find with bolsters, pillows, or rolled-up towels. In the supine and reclining positions, a bolster under the knees is useful to take pressure off of the lower back. In the prone position, props may be placed under the shoulders, under the ankles, and as needed around the belly. In the side-lying position, pillows are placed around the belly for support, under the top arm, and under the top leg or between the legs. A pillow may also be needed under the head. Figure 12–2 illustrates the props for the side-lying position, and Figure 12-3 shows draping in side-lying while massaging the legs.

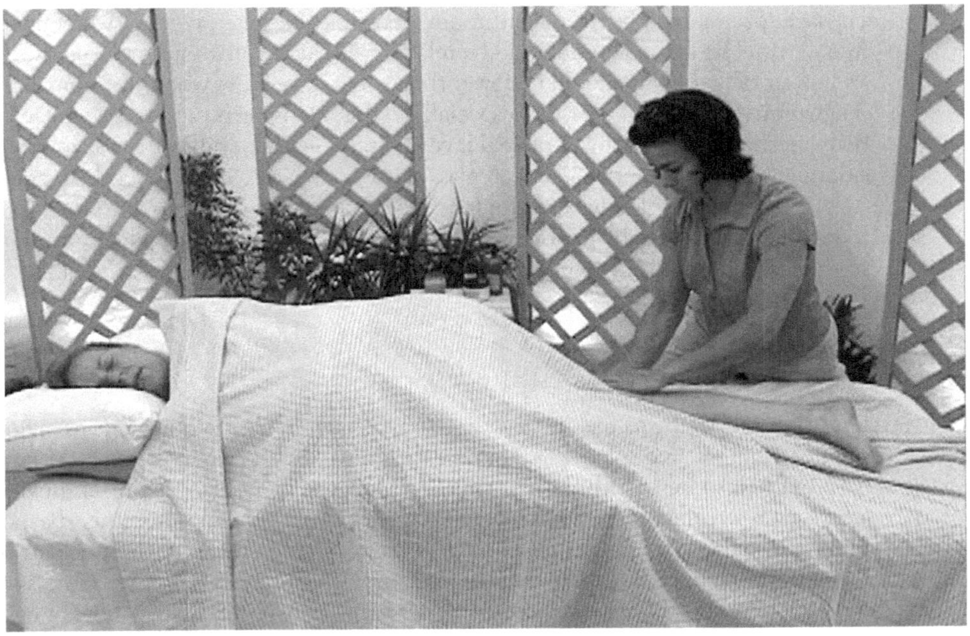

FIGURE 12–3. Draping in side-lying position for massage of legs.

PREGNANCY MASSAGE SESSION

The massage should generally be gentle and relaxing. Traditional Western massage and its variations, various forms of acupressure and other energy work, reflexology, and other forms of massage and bodywork may be used to address the wellness of pregnant women.

While there are no special techniques for massage during pregnancy, there are some places on the body that need special attention, for example, neck, chest, lower back, hips, legs, and feet. Suggestions for massaging specific areas are described below.

Because of the forward head posture, the neck and upper back may feel strained. This may also result in tension headache. The neck is most easily accessed in the supine or side-lying positions. Effleurage, deep friction, and compression are effective in reducing tension in the muscles of the neck and upper back. There may be trigger points to be relieved. Direct pressure to certain acupressure points can also reduce neck tension. Figures 12–4 and 12–5 show massage around the scapula and to the neck with pregnant client in side-lying position.

The chest may become sunken or depressed as the pregnancy progresses. The enlarged uterus also takes up a lot of room in the abdomen, making it hard for pregnant women to breathe. Therefore, massage that frees up the rib cage and diaphragm can be important. Massage of the skeletal muscles involved in respiration can relieve tension and promote easier breathing.

An exaggerated lordosis that puts pressure on the lower back often results from pregnancy. This can be addressed effectively in the side-lying position, which itself relieves pressure in the lower back. A simple technique to help relieve tension in muscles of the back is a firm effleurage with the palm of the hand from the upper back to the sacrum. When over the sacrum, apply a little more pressure to help reduce the lordotic curve. Repeat several times.

Childbearing puts strain on the entire lower body. The muscles of the hips and legs have to work harder to carry the added weight accumulated during pregnancy. The lower extremities are massaged as usual, ending with distal to proximal effleurage to help accumulated fluid move out of the area. Deep work on inner thighs should be avoided in advanced stages of pregnancy.

When massaging the feet, you may want to apply some reflexology. Areas to stimulate include along the medial border, which corresponds to the hips and spine, and on the inside of the foot below the ankle bone, which corresponds to the uterus. It is now considered a myth that reflexology can cause miscarriage. Kunz and Kunz believe that reflexology is safe for pregnant women and that it has never

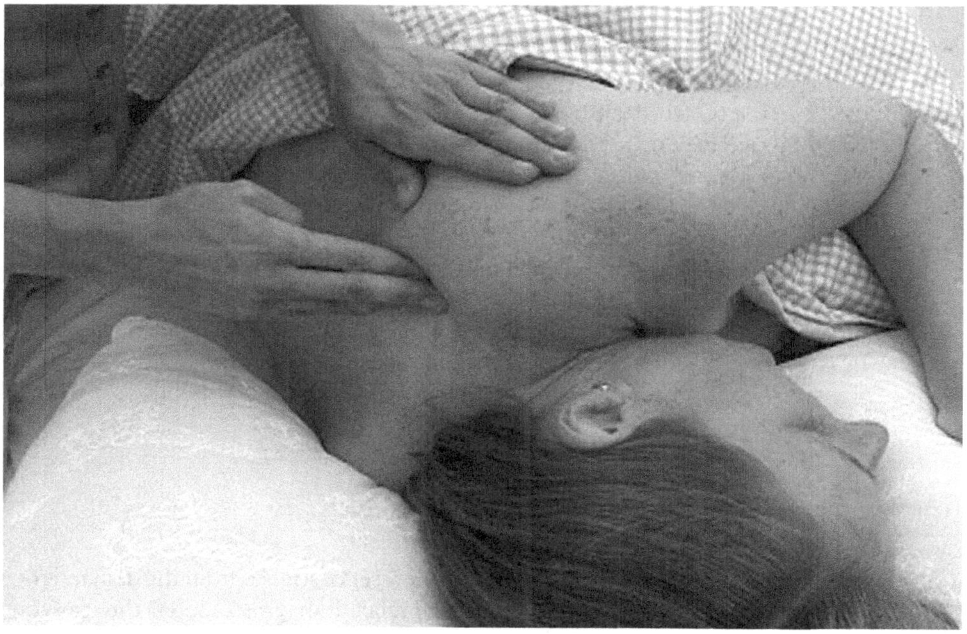

FIGURE 12–4. Friction around the scapula with pregnant client in side-lying position.

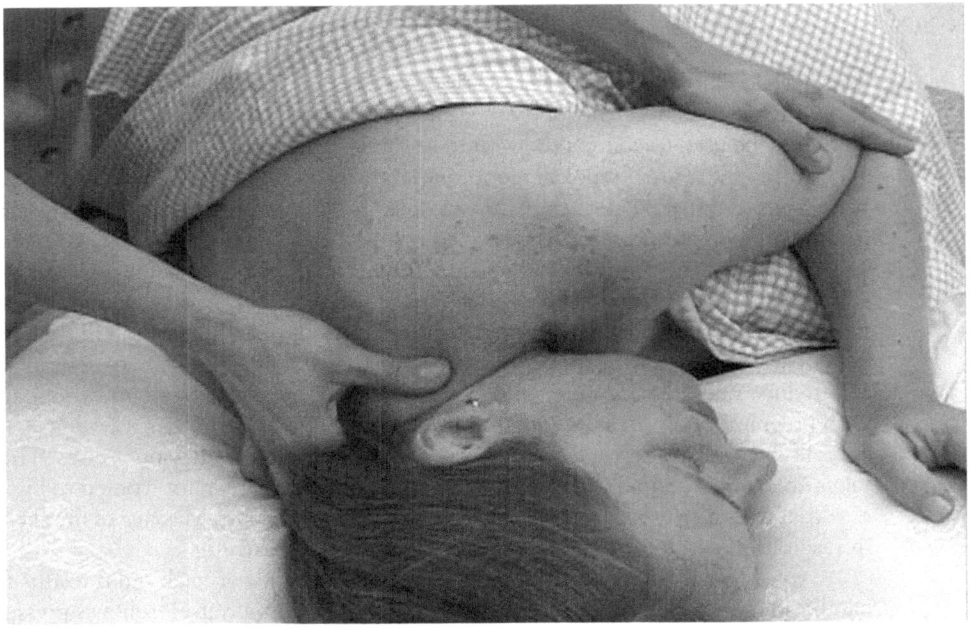

FIGURE 12–5. Kneading the neck with pregnant client in side-lying position.

been shown to have caused the body to do something it didn't want to do. It merely helps the body seek its own equilibrium (1980).

LABOR, DELIVERY, AND RECOVERY

Midwives, childbirth assistants, and others in the delivery room may use massage during labor and delivery, as desired by the mother. This may be as simple as gentle stroking to reduce anxiety. Massage has been shown to reduce anxiety and labor pain, and for some women to decrease the length of labor and need for medication (Field, T. et al. 1997).

There are also certain acupressure points that may be pressed to relieve labor pain. These include the Shoulder Well (GB21) on the trapezius; Sacral Points (GB 27–34); Hoku or Joining the Valley (LI4) in the web of the thumb; Bigger Stream (K3) near the Achilles tendon; and Reaching Inside (B67) on the little toe (Gach, 1990).

Massage may be used during recovery from labor and delivery. Traditional Western techniques help relax stressed and sore muscles and soothe nerves. Acupressure points to press for postpartum recovery include Sea of Energy (CV6) just below the navel; Inner Gate (P6) inside of the forearm just above the wrist; Sea of Vitality (B23 and B47) across the back at waist level; Womb and Vitals (B48) lateral to the sacrum; Three Mile Point (St36) just below the kneecap lateral to the shin bone; and Bigger Rushing (Lv3) on top of the foot between the big toe and the second toe (Gach, 1990).

After an appropriate amount of healing has taken place, women who have delivered their babies by C-section may benefit from abdominal massage and massage around and on the scar itself. Deep transverse friction can help prevent adhesions and promote mobile scar tissue as in any wound healing situation.

WOMEN WITH INFANTS AND TODDLERS

Women with infants and toddlers have a new set of stresses from the demands of motherhood. Massage affords an opportunity to take time out and relax. It may also address the stress on the upper back, neck, and arms from picking up, holding, and nursing the growing babies. Nursing mothers may find **breast massage** useful for relieving the discomforts of nursing. (Refer to *Breast Massage* by Debra Curties, 1999.)

INFANT MASSAGE

Benefits

Massage given by parents and other caregivers is an excellent way to provide the **tactile and kinesthetic stimulation** essential for the healthy growth and development of infants. A significant body of evidence confirms that massage not only contributes to the healthy development of normal infants, but is also effective in promoting recovery of preterm, cocaine-exposed, HIV-exposed, and other high-risk infants (Field 2000; Dieter, Emory 2002).

Massage has other benefits for infants, including releasing tension and learning to relax, bonding with parents, aiding digestion and elimination, improving sleep, easing growing pains, and helping calm colicky babies. In addition, touching and handling her baby promotes milk production in the mother by stimulating the secretion of prolactin. Massage can also provide fathers with an opportunity to touch and interact with their babies in a way that is satisfying and also builds confidence in handling the child (Schneider, 1982).

Infant Massage Techniques

Infant massage is a simple, gentle, yet firm application of stroking, pressing, squeezing, and movement of the limbs. Examples of infant massage techniques include soft circular motions with fingertips all over the baby's head; gentle but firm squeezing and twisting the soft tissues of the legs; strokes with the thumbs on the bottom of the feet; circular massage of the abdomen; broad strokes on the chest; milking the arms; and small circles all around the back with the fingertips.

It is important that the massage giver be relaxed and comfortable throughout the session. Givers may sit on the floor with legs extended and back straight, perhaps supported against a wall or piece of furniture. The infant is placed supine on or between the giver's legs, or prone across the legs. Figures 12–6 to 12–14 illustrate positioning and important infant massage techniques using a doll.

Figure 12–14 shows the squeeze and twist technique used on the legs and arms. Grasp the limb like holding a baseball bat, then gently squeeze and twist the hands in opposite directions. Continue the motion while traveling up the leg from buttocks to feet. This gentle twist primarily causes movement in the superficial tissues, and should not be confused with deep effleurage on adults that is always performed distal to proximal.

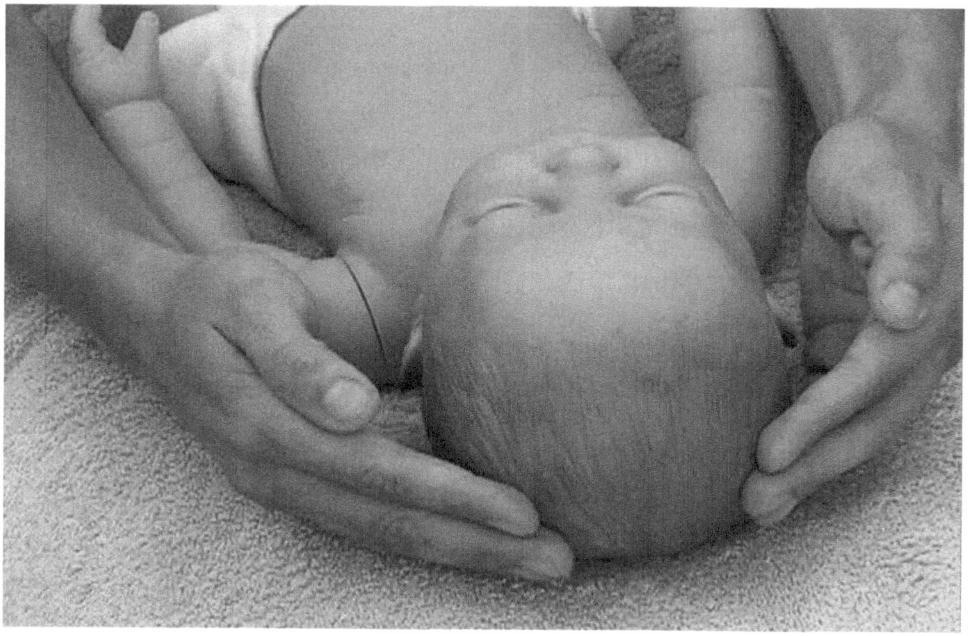

FIGURE 12–6. Gentle circles over the infant's head.

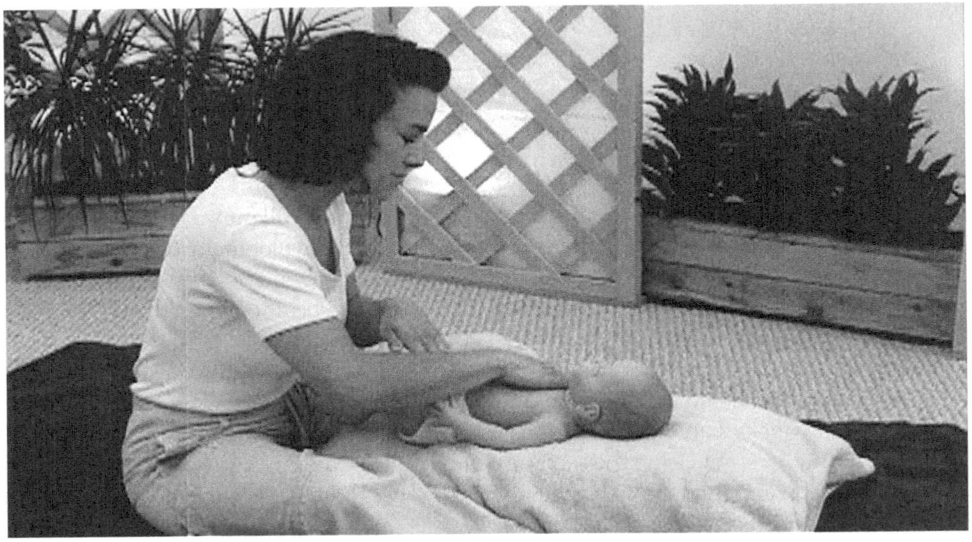

FIGURE 12–7. Applying oil to the chest with effleurage applied diagonally from rib cage to shoulder.

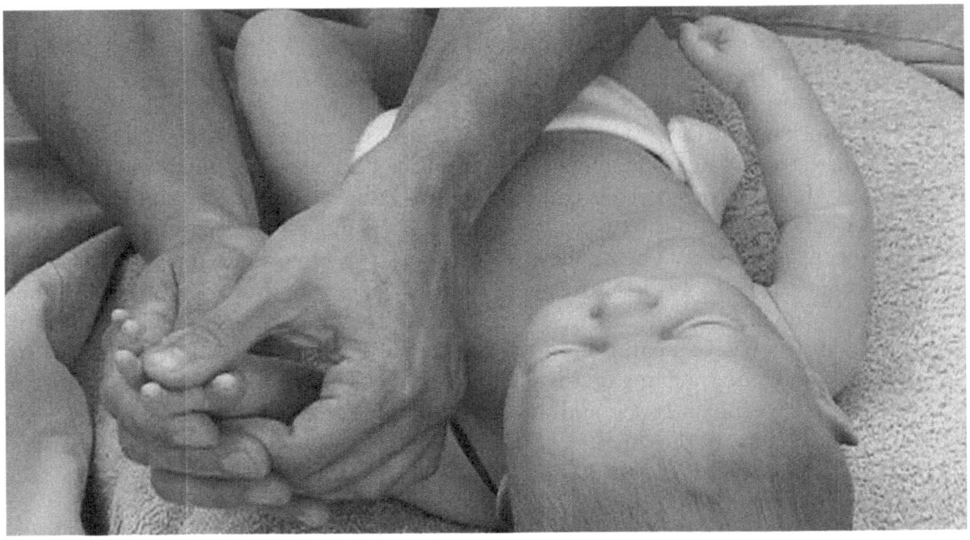

FIGURE 12–8. Thumb strokes to the infant's palms and fingers.

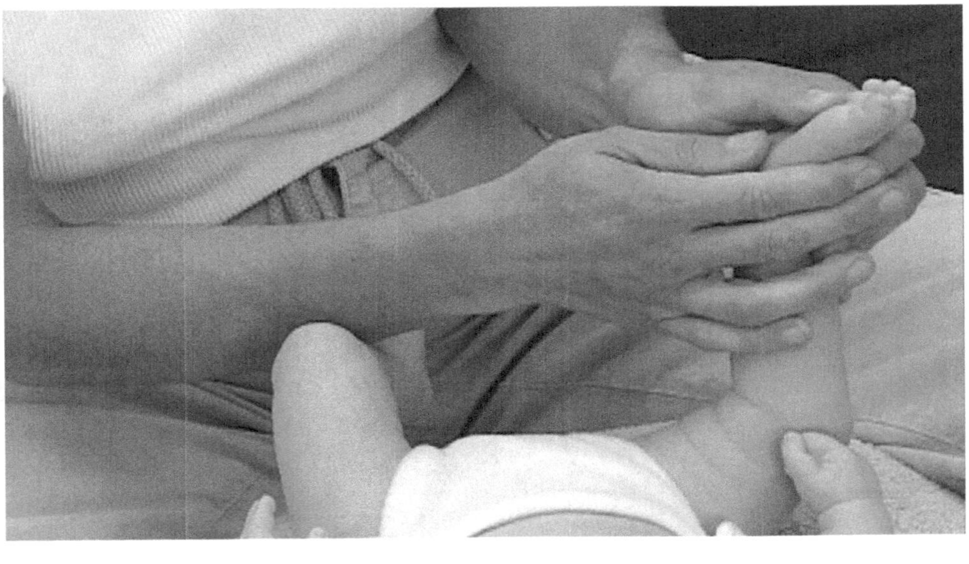

FIGURE 12–9. Thumb strokes to the bottoms of the feet.

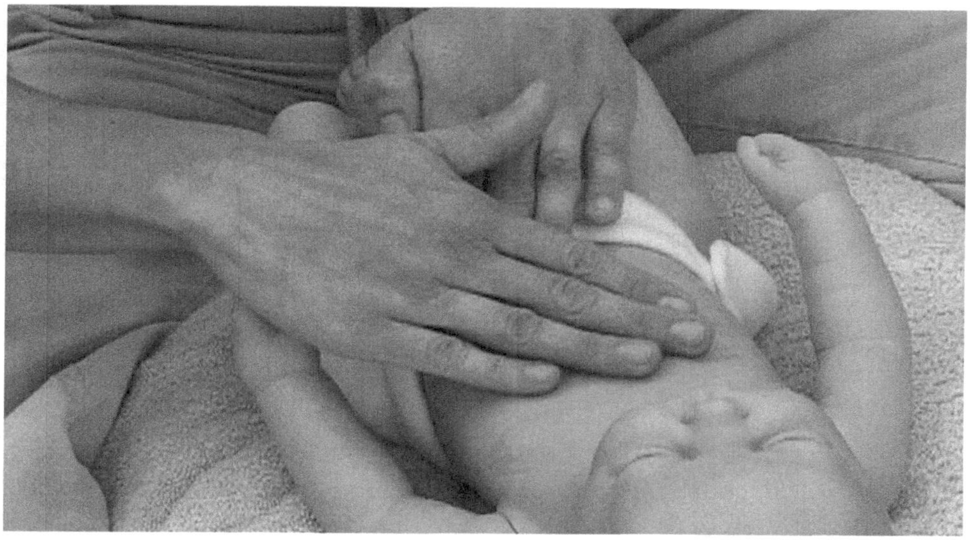

FIGURE 12–10. Circular effleurage clockwise over the abdomen.

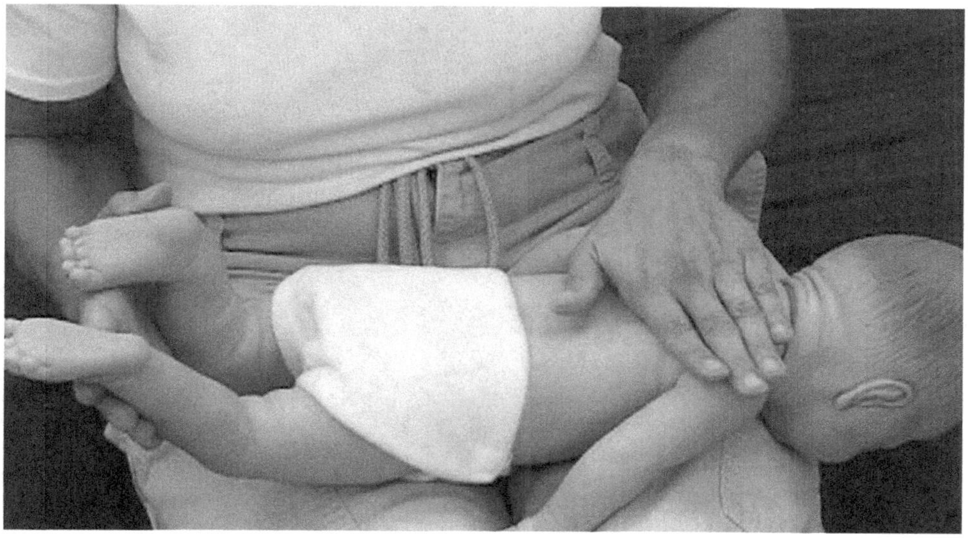

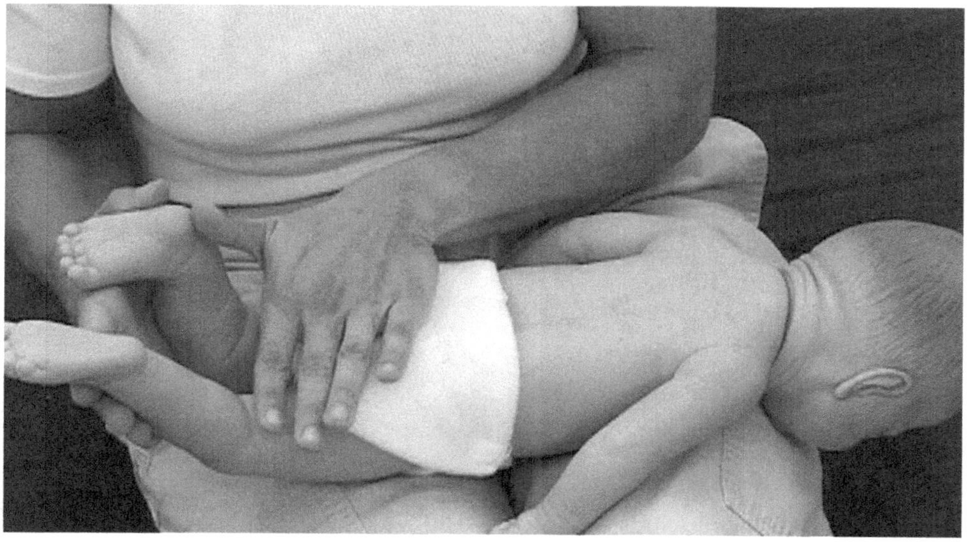

FIGURE 12–11 A–C. Long stroke over the back and legs with infant prone over the caregiver's thighs.

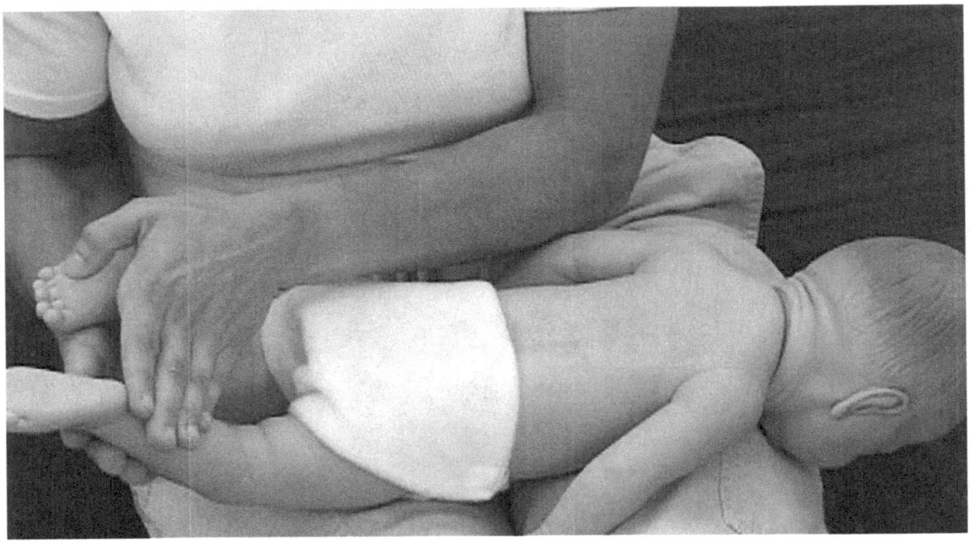

FIGURE 12–11. *(Continued)*

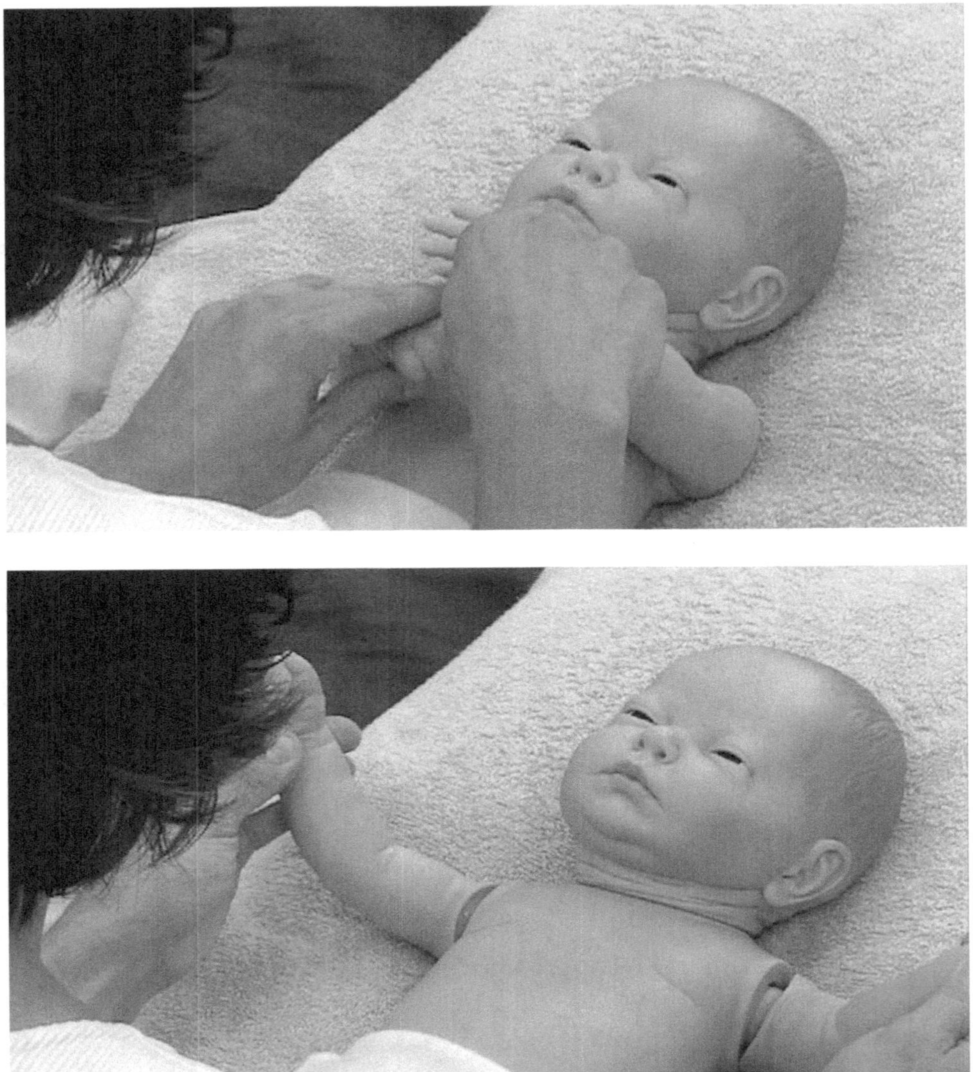

FIGURE 12–12 A, B. Arm movement across chest (hug) and then out to the side.

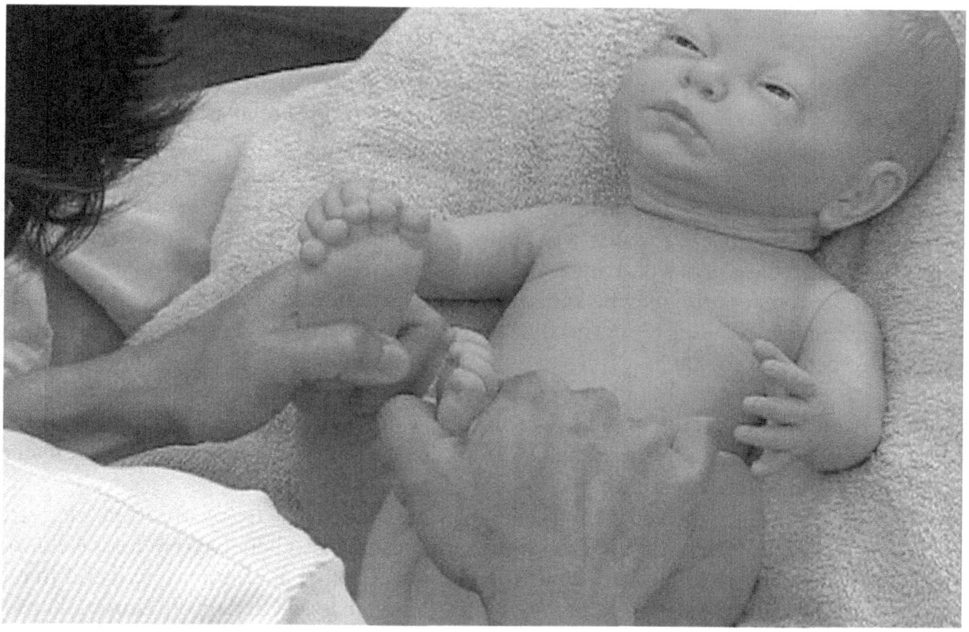

FIGURE 12–13. Leg movement with knees to abdomen and then straightening.

Caregivers should maintain eye contact and talk or sing to the child throughout the massage. It can be a time of connecting and playful interaction that helps in the infant's emotional and social development, as well as the physical.

Massage practitioners may include training in infant massage in their services to pregnant clients before or after delivery. Dolls may be used to introduce massage techniques before the baby is delivered.

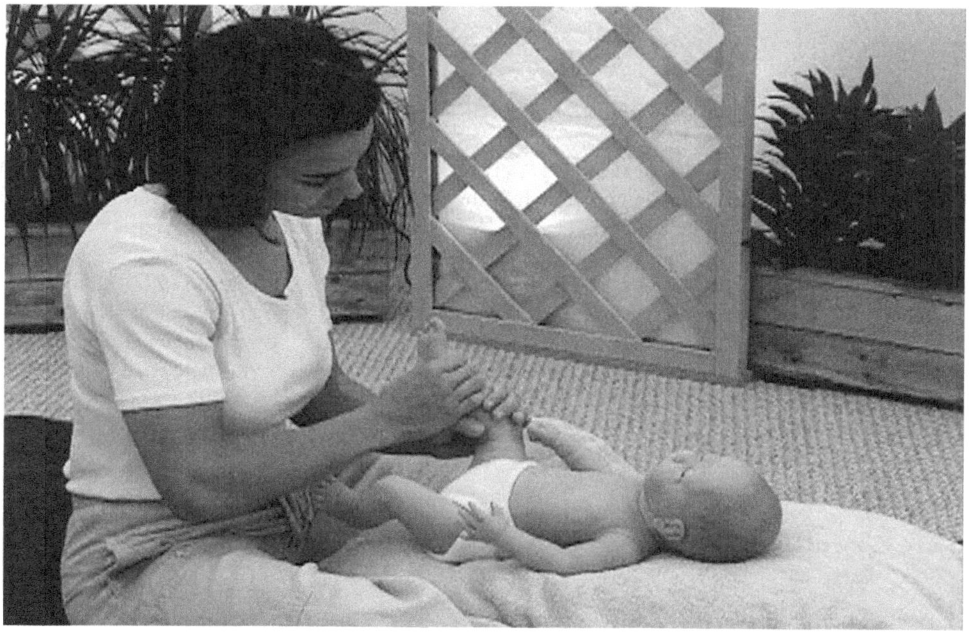

FIGURE 12–14. Gentle squeeze and twist of the muscles of the infant's leg.

SUMMARY

Massage helps relieve some of the stresses women experience during pregnancy, including strain on the spine and lower extremities. It can also be a time of relaxation and emotional relief. Massage is safe in most cases of pregnancy, but it is best to check with the mother's physician for any special cautions or directions. Abdominal massage is contraindicated, and massage should be avoided if the mother is experiencing nausea, vomiting, diarrhea, or any unusual pain, swelling, or bleeding.

In the first few weeks of pregnancy, women may lie supine or prone. As the belly gets larger, switch to the reclining or side-lying position. Use pillows and other props to support the body comfortably. The room temperature may be kept a little cooler than usual for massage. Air should be fresh and flowing, and music relaxing. A bathroom should be accessible. A stepping stool may be useful for the recipient to get onto the table.

Techniques should be gentle and relaxing. Western massage, acupressure, and reflexology have been found effective to address pregnant women's needs. Focus of the sessions is on neck, lower back, legs, and feet, and general relaxation. Massage may be performed during delivery to help reduce anxiety and ease labor pain.

Massage received during the weeks after delivery helps recondition areas stressed during the birth process. Women who have cesarean sections may also benefit from massage during recovery and from techniques that help form healthy scar tissue. Women with infants and children may benefit from taking time for themselves and receiving relaxing massage as part of their regular self-care.

Massage given to infants by parents and other caregivers is an excellent way to provide the tactile and kinesthetic stimulation essential for their healthy growth and development. Massage also helps infants to release tension and learn to relax, and bond with caregivers. It aids digestion and elimination, improves sleep, eases growing pains, and calms colicky babies. Massage techniques for infants include gentle stroking, pressing, squeezing, and movement of the limbs.

A look ahead . . .

Massage is also beneficial for those further along in the life cycle. Chapter 13 addresses the special needs of adults in midlife and beyond, and the applications of massage for maintaining lifelong health and vigor.

REFERENCES

Curties, D. (1999). *Breast massage*. Moncton, New Brunswick, Canada: Curties-Overzet Publications.

Dieter, J. N. I., & E. K. Emory (2002). "Supplemental tactile and kinesthetic stimulation for preterm infants." Chapter 7 in *Massage therapy: The evidence for practice*. Rich, G. J., Editor. New York: Mosby.

Field, T. (2000). "Enhancing growth." Chapter 1 in *Touch Therapy*. New York: Churchhill Livingston.

Field, T., Hernandez-Reif, M., Hart, S., & Teakston, H. (1999). "Pregnant women benefit from massage therapy." *Journal of Psychosomatic Obstetrics and Gynecology, 19*.

Field, T., Hernandez-Reif, M., Taylor, S., Quintino, O., & Burman, I. (1997). "Labor pain is reduced by massage therapy." *Journal of Psychosomatic Obstetrics and Gynecology, 18*, pp. 286–291.

Gach, M. R. (1990). *Acupressure's potent points: A guide to self-care for common ailments*. New York: Bantam Books.

Kunz, K., & Kunz, B. (1991). *The complete guide to foot reflexology*. Englewood Cliffs, NJ: Prentice-Hall.

Lundberg, P. (1992). *The book of shiatsu*. New York: Simon & Schuster.

Schneider, Vimala (1982). *Infant massage: A handbook for loving parents*. New York: Bantam Books.

Stillerman, E. (1992). *Mother-massage: A handbook for relieving the discomforts of pregnancy*. New York: Delta/Delcorte.

ADDITIONAL RESOURCES

Books

Osborne-Sheets, C. (1998) *Pre- and perinatal massage therapy: A comprehensive practitioner's guide to pregnancy, labor, postpartum*. San Diego, CA: Body Therapy Associates.

Videos

"Gentle touch infant massage." (2003) Goldhil Home Media.
"Infant massage: A gift of love." (1999) With Cheryl Brenman. Sedona, AZ: Brenman Productions.
"Infant massage: The power of touch." (1995). View Video.
"Living Arts massage practice for infants." Gaiam/Living Arts. (*www.gaiam.com*)
"Living Arts massage practice for pregnancy." (2000) With Michelle Kluck. Gaiam/Living Arts. (*www.gaiam.com*)

WEB SITES

www.bodytherapyassociates.com (Pre- and Perinatal Massage Therapy)
www.lovingtouch.com (International Loving Touch Foundation)
www.iaimi.com (International Association of Infant Massage Instructors)

CHAPTER THIRTEEN

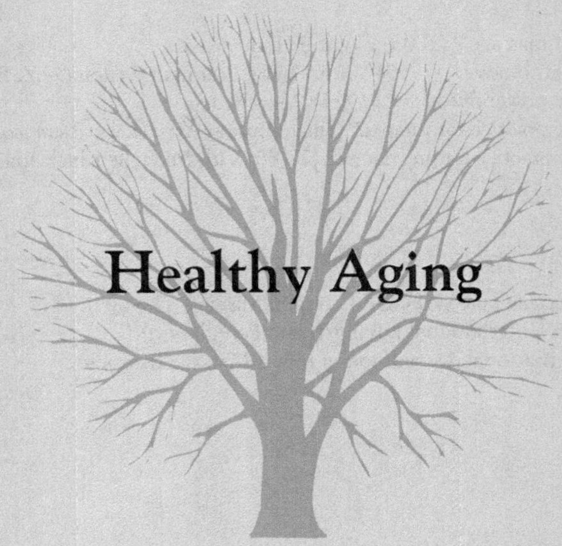

Healthy Aging

LEARNING OUTCOMES

After studying this chapter, the student will have information to:

1. Describe the effects of aging.
2. Explain the benefits of massage for healthy aging.
3. Identify the benefits of massage for elders.
4. Distinguish between physiological and chronological age.
5. Distinguish among robust, age-appropriate, and frail elders.
6. Plan a massage session to meet the special needs of elders.
7. Observe appropriate cautions in working with elders.

KEY TERMS/CONCEPTS

Age-appropriate
Chronological age
Elders
Frail elderly
Life-long wellness
Physical effects of aging
Physiological age
Robust elderly

LINK LIBRARY TERMS

Massage Business • *Traditional Chinese Medicine/Traditional Asian Medicine* • *Reflexology* • *Geriatric Massage* • *Massage Regulations*

MEDIALINK

A companion CD-ROM, included free with each new copy of this book, supplements the techniques presented in this chapter. Insert the CD-ROM to watch video clips of massage techniques being demonstrated. This multimedia feature is designed to help you add a new dimension to your learning.

Massage can be an important component of **life-long wellness.** It promotes general physical and emotional wellbeing, addresses conditions commonly associated with aging, and enhances the quality of life. Massage can help slow the aging process and maintain youthful characteristics longer.

Massage works best if received regularly and over a period of years. As we grow older, our state of wellbeing is a reflection of a lifetime of both good and poor health practices. Along with good eating and exercise habits, regular massage can help prevent or retard some of the decreases in condition and function associated with age. Massage can help improve an already deteriorated condition, but works best as a measure of prevention.

EFFECTS OF AGING AND BENEFITS OF MASSAGE

The **physical effects of aging** are perhaps the most visible, and begin noticeably for most around age 30. These include decrease in general mobility and muscular strength, slower nerve conduction, less efficient circulation, less tissue elasticity, thinner and drier skin, loss of bone mass, decreased function of the senses, and a less efficient immune system. This is experienced as general aches and pains, slower movement, and less stamina. Research has found that many of these "biomarkers" can be slowed considerably with a healthy lifestyle, including good nutrition and exercise (Evans & Rosenberg, 1991).

Massage addresses many of the effects of aging directly. For example, it promotes well nourished skin by increasing superficial circulation, and moisturizes skin through the use of oils and lotions. Massage improves general blood circulation, especially in the extremities. Immune system function is strengthened with improved lymph flow and general relaxation.

It has been found that chronic stress and inactivity accelerate the aging process (Evans & Rosenberg, 1991). Massage helps reduce the physical and mental effects of stress and anxiety. It is known to trigger the relaxation response, relieve muscular tension, reduce anxiety, improve sleep, and increase feelings of wellbeing. Older adults find massage useful for reducing the muscular tension, aches and stiffness that can accompany exercise programs. By keeping muscles more pliable and increasing flexibility, massage reduces the potential for injury during workouts. Chapters 3 and 4 review the research on the effects of massage discussed in this section.

BENEFITS FOR ELDERS

Massage has special benefits for **elders**, that is, people 65 years and older. Along with exercise, it helps elders keep the flexibility and strength needed to do simple things like get up out of a chair, dress and undress, climb stairs, and get in and out of a bathtub. Therefore, it contributes to maintaining independence.

Another physical benefit is improved digestion and elimination. Abdominal massage improves large intestine function, and helps alleviate constipation. See Figure 13–1.

Massage helps ease the pain of loss, frustration, and fear about the future. Elders are often confronted with loss of work, home, spouse, family, friends, independence, and financial security. The caring touch and relaxing benefits of massage help ease these emotional pains. Relaxing massage of the face is shown Figure 13–2.

Massage also provides an avenue for social interaction, especially for elders in nursing homes or homebound. The personal interaction with the practitioner helps reduce feelings of social isolation, and the inherent touch of massage provides a special connection to others.

In her book *Compassionate Touch,* Dawn Nelson lists some of the common conditions that the elderly experience and that massage can help alleviate. These include insomnia, loss of appetite, constipation, immobility, poor circulation, decreased immune system functioning, skin problems such as loss of elasticity and dryness, bedsores, physical discomfort and pain, chronic stress, chronic depression, feeling alone and useless (1994).

Some of the research about elders and massage in clinical settings is reviewed in Chapter 4 of this text. Studies have shown massage to be beneficial to those hospitalized for a number of conditions, including heart disease, cancer, and psychiatric problems. The benefits of back massage to institutionalized elderly included relaxation, improved communication, and reducing the common dehumanizing

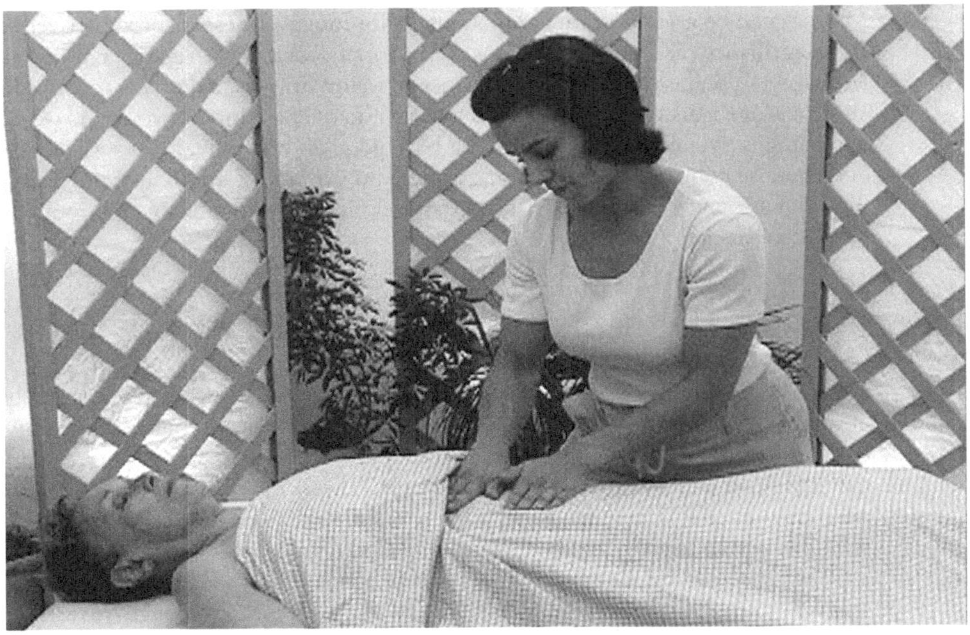

FIGURE 13–1. Abdominal massage aids elimination and relieves constipation.

effects of institutional care (Frazer & Kerr, 1993). These results were confirmed by another study of slow-stroke back rub for the elderly by nurses (Fakouri & Jones, 1987).

There is promising research on massage for the agitated elderly in institutions and for those with Alzheimer's disease and dementia. Several studies have found reduction in certain agitated behaviors with regular 10-minute massage. Massage performed in the studies can be characterized as using light pressure, even rhythm, and slow strokes (Remington 2002).

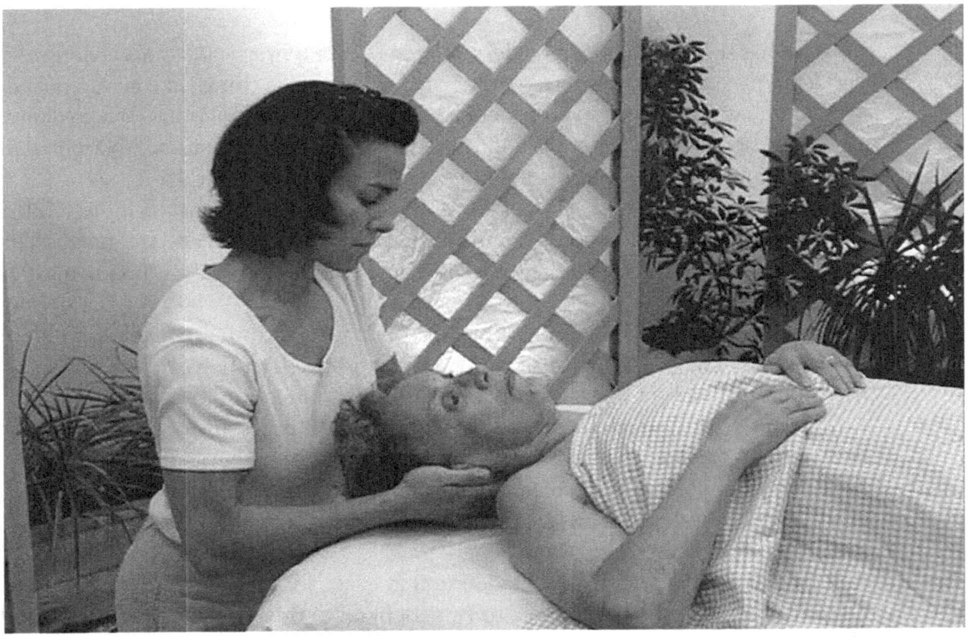

FIGURE 13–2. Massage of the face during general relaxation massage.

WORKING WITH THE ELDERLY

Elders are perhaps the most distinctive population to work with. Individuals in this age group are more different from each other than those in other age groups. By the time people have reached 65+ years of age, they exhibit the accumulated effects of a lifetime of good and poor health habits, diseases and injuries, and life experiences. They are more likely to have chronic health problems and to be on medications. Care should be taken in learning about each individual and in planning their massage sessions.

It is useful to think about older adults in terms of **physiological age,** rather than **chronological age.** People age at different rates depending on their genetic makeup, life-long health habits, and unusual life events such as car accidents, work accidents, and sports injuries. Diseases experienced earlier in life may have an effect later, such as the incidences of post-polio syndrome affecting people 40–50 years after the acute phase.

Elders may be thought of as falling into one of three categories: robust, age appropriate, and frail. **Robust elders** show few outward signs of impaired health, look younger than their chronologic age, are mentally sharp and physically active. People who show some of the typical signs of aging are considered **age appropriate. Frail elders** look and feel fragile to touch (Meisler, 1990).

Robust elders can generally be treated like the typical middle-aged recipient of massage. Information obtained on a health questionnaire can help you identify any areas of caution that are not obvious.

Age-appropriate elders will have some problems associated with aging. Information from a health questionnaire is useful to identify contraindications and areas of caution. Use pillows and bolsters to ensure maximum comfort and the least stress on joints. Limit the prone position to 15–20 minutes. After the session, help the recipient sit up, or at least stay until he or she is sitting up. Leave the room only when you are sure that the recipient is not lightheaded and can get off the table safely.

Frail elders need special care. Check with their physicians before massaging the very frail. Frail elders will probably need assistance getting onto and off of the table. You might find it necessary to massage them in a regular chair or on their beds. Limit the session to 15–20 minutes until you know that they can handle longer sessions. Watch them carefully in the prone position on the table to be sure that they can lie there comfortably. Be extra gentle in lifting frail elders, avoiding pulling on their arms to help them up. Cradle their bodies to help them change position (Meisler, 1990).

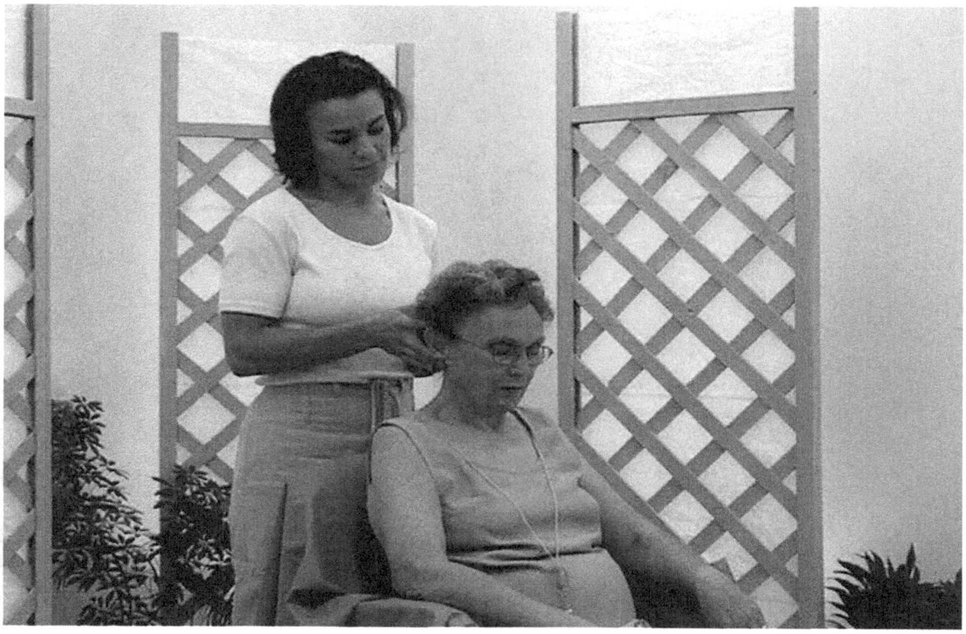

FIGURE 13–3. Massage of the head to a seated elder client.

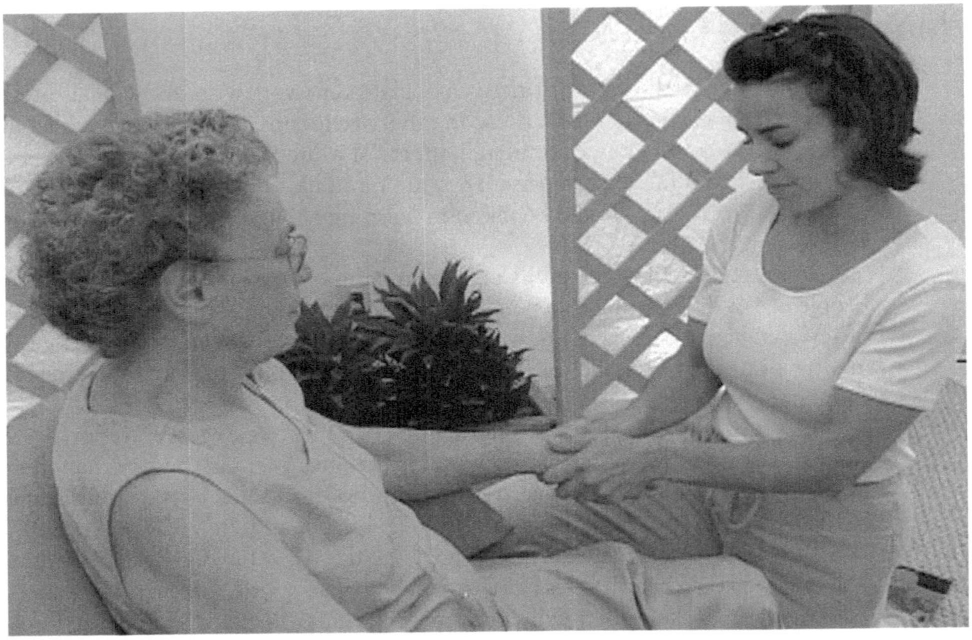

FIGURE 13–4. Massage of the hands of a seated elder client.

MASSAGE FOR ELDERS IN CHAIRS

Massage with the elderly client in a chair can be very pleasant and effective. Remember to use good body mechanics when giving massage to a seated client, keeping your neck and back in alignment. Massage of the head, hands and feet of a seated elder is shown in Figures 13–3, 13–4 and 13–5.

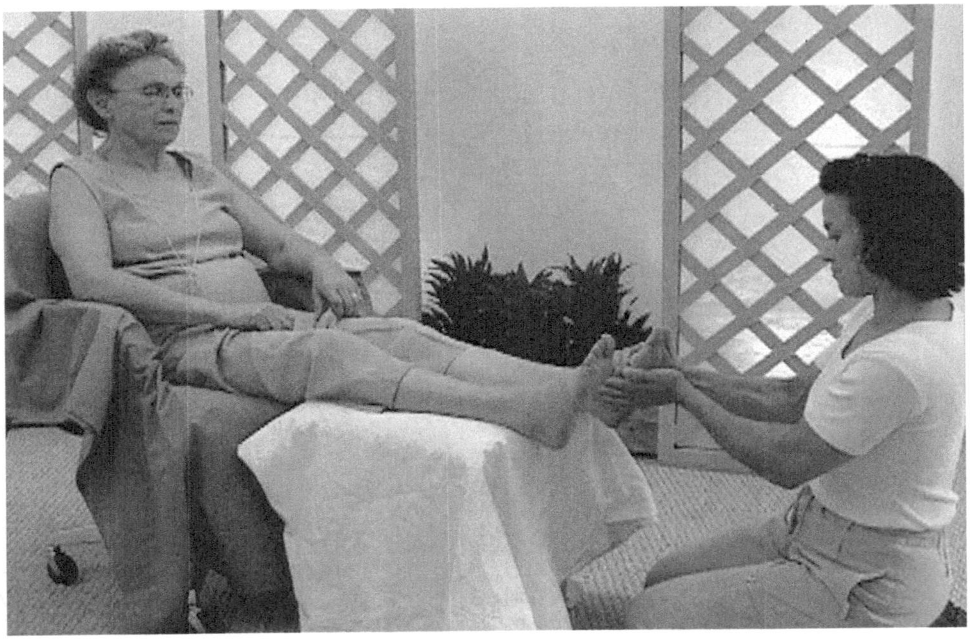

FIGURE 13–5. Massage of the feet of a seated elder client.

MASSAGE SESSION FOR HEALTHY AGING

There are no special massage "techniques" that slow the aging process. However, there are certain points to keep in mind in working with adults, and especially with the elderly.

Do include the following in a massage session for healthy aging:

- Techniques to improve circulation in the extremities. Effleurage moving distal to proximal enhances venous return, and relaxing the muscles with kneading and jostling improves local circulation.
- Kneading, compression, and other petrissage movements that help keep muscle and connective tissue pliable and elastic.
- Joint movements and stretches of the lower extremities for improved mobility and flexibility. Spend time on the feet to relieve soreness, improve circulation, and mobilize joints. Mobilizing the legs and feet can help increase kinesthetic awareness, and thereby improve movements such as walking and climbing stairs.
- Movements and stretches for the shoulders to help maintain some important daily living functions such as getting dressed and undressed and reaching for things overhead. The hands may benefit from special attention to help them to stay mobile and sensitive.
- Passive motion and stretches for the cervical muscles to help maintain normal range of motion in the head and neck. With declining peripheral vision, the ability to turn the head to see things in the environment is important. This is essential for the safety of elders who drive motor vehicles.
- Techniques that focus on lengthening the front of the body, especially abdominal and pectoral muscles, to help maintain an erect posture. Exercises are also needed to keep postural muscles strong and to avoid a bent-over or collapsed condition later in life.
- Abdominal massage for the viscera, which may be important for sedentary elders to improve digestion and elimination. Use gentle but firm pressure, always going clockwise during circular movements.

CAUTIONS

Some problem conditions are more common in older adults and warrant special awareness. Massage is rarely contraindicated totally, but certain cautions apply with the conditions mentioned below. It is important to take a thorough health history to identify the conditions that are contraindicated or for which cautions are important. Always consult the recipient's physician when in doubt about a condition or disease mentioned by a recipient of massage.

- Massage may be contraindicated with certain medications. If you work regularly with older adults and elders, it would be wise to have a reference book that explains the effects and possible side effects of common medications. (Refer to *Massage Therapy & Medications* by Randal S. Persad, 2001.) Check with the recipient's physician if in doubt about the advisability of his or her receiving massage while taking a certain medication.
- Elders usually have thin and delicate skin and bruise more easily than younger people. Pressure used in massage should be gentle to moderate depending on the recipient's general condition.
- Watch for varicose veins in the legs, and do not perform deep effleurage or strong kneading over them. Light effleurage and jostling movements are better for circulation in this case. Elevating the legs slightly when the recipient is supine will help venous return during the massage.
- Older adults and elders may have diagnosed or undiagnosed atherosclerosis, or hardening of the arteries. This is especially dangerous in the cerebral arteries, which pass through the neck. Avoid deep work in the lateral neck area. Avoid movements that put the neck in hyperextension or increase the cervical curve, since this position may further occlude blood vessels to the head and cause fainting.
- Use great care in performing joint movements and stretches involving the hip joint for those who have had hip replacements. Avoid movements involving abduction and circumduction.

Consult the recipient's health care provider for instructions. Extreme care should be taken in the case of any joint replacement because of the potential instability of the joint.

- In the case of cancer patients, always check with the physician before performing massage. Some types of cancer may spread with massage, while some will not be affected. It may be possible to perform massage away from the site of the cancer and do no harm. Observe appropriate cautions with those receiving chemotherapy or radiation cancer treatments.
- Older adults and elders tend to have problems in their joints, including osteo- and rheumatoid arthritis. Massage of the area should be avoided if the joint is inflamed. When there is no inflammation, massage of the surrounding muscles is indicated to help relieve stress on the joint. Holding and warming arthritic and sore joints can be soothing.
- Because massage is commonly done directly on the skin, practitioners may detect skin cancers of which recipients of massage are unaware. Basal and squamous cell carcinoma and malignant melanoma usually appear on sun-exposed areas of the body, including the face, arms, and chest. Malignant melanoma may develop at the site of a mole. Report any lesion or suspicious-looking skin condition to the recipient, or to the caregiver in the case of frail elders, and suggest that it be checked by a physician or dermatologist. Do not massage directly over the site.

SUMMARY

Regular massage can help retard some of the decreases in function and condition that are a part of the normal aging process. Massage promotes well nourished skin, improves general blood circulation and lymph flow, helps keep fascia and muscles more pliable, improves joint flexibility, and strengthens immune system function. It helps reduce physical and mental effects of stress that accelerate the aging process.

Massage is especially beneficial for elders of 65 years old or more. It helps them maintain mobility and independence longer, and eases the emotional pain of loss and frustration often experienced in later years. It alleviates some common problems such as insomnia, constipation, and depression. Massage offers regular caring touch, relaxation, and social interaction to homebound elders and those in institutions.

It is useful to think of older adults in terms of physiological, rather than chronological, age. Elders may be robust, age appropriate, or frail. Contraindications and conditions that warrant caution include certain medications, thinning skin, skin growths, circulatory problems, joint disease, and joint replacements.

There are no massage techniques that slow the aging process. However, massage sessions may be planned to meet the needs of aging adults: for example, to maintain healthy tissues, mobility, good posture, independence, and functions such as digestion and elimination. Massage can be an important part of a life-long personal wellness program, and an aid to caring for elders in institutions.

A look ahead . . .

Massage has special benefits for those at the end of their lives due to old age or illness. Chapter 14 will give information and guidelines for providing massage to this very unique population.

REFERENCES

Evans, W., & Rosenberg, E. H. (1991). *Biomarkers*. New York: Simon & Schuster.

Fakouri, C., & Jones, P. (1987). Relaxation ℞: Slow stroke back rub. *Journal of Gerontological Nursing, 13*(2), pp. 32–35.

Frazer, J., & Kerr, J. R. (1993). Psychophysiological effects of back massage on elderly institutionalized patients. *Journal of Advanced Nursing, 18*, pp. 238–245.

Miesler, D. W. (1990). *Geriatric massage techniques: Topics for bodyworkers no. 2*. Guerneville, CA: Day-Break Productions.

Nelson, D. (1994). *Compassionate touch: Hands-on caregiving for the elderly, the ill, and the dying*. Barrytown, NY: Station Hill Press.

Persad, R. (2001). *Massage therapy & medications: General treatment principles*. Toronto: Curties-Overzet Publications.

Remington, R. (2002). "Hand massage in the agitated elderly." Chapter 8 in *Massage therapy: The evidence for practice* by G.J. Rich, editor. New York: Mosby.

ADDITIONAL RESOURCES

Books

Nelson, Dawn (2001). *From the heart through the hands: The power of touch in caregiving*. Forres, Scotland: Findhorn Press.

Videos

"ABC's of Geriatric Massage." Day-Break Massage Institute (*www.daybreak-massage.com*).

WEB SITES

Aging Research Centre (ARC) *(www.arclab.org)*
American Society on Aging *(www.asaging.org)*
Day-Break Geriatric Massage Institute *(www.daybreak-massage.com)*
National Council on Aging (NCOA) *(www.ncoa.org)*
National Institute on Aging at the National Institutes of Health *(www.nia.nih.gov)*
U.S. Administration on Aging (AoA) *(www.aoa.gov)*

CHAPTER FOURTEEN

Terminally Ill and Dying

LEARNING OUTCOMES

After studying this chapter, the student will have information to:

1. Explain the value of massage for the terminally ill from a wellness perspective.
2. Describe different approaches to massage for the dying.
3. Seek knowledge and skills needed to work with seriously ill and dying people.
4. Plan a massage session for someone seriously ill or dying.
5. Practice self-care while working with the terminally ill and dying.

KEY TERMS/CONCEPTS

Comforting touch
Conscious self-care
Emotional distress
Hospice
Nonverbal communication
Nurturing touch
Palliative care
Touch deprivation

LINK LIBRARY TERMS

Massage Business • *Geriatric Massage* • *Massage Regulations*

MEDIALINK

A companion CD-ROM, included free with each new copy of this book, supplements the techniques presented in this chapter. Insert the CD-ROM to watch video clips of massage techniques being demonstrated. This multimedia feature is designed to help you add a new dimension to your learning.

Massage is used to bring caring and **comforting touch** to the terminally ill and dying. It is a valuable complementary therapy in hospitals, hospice, and home care. Simple massage techniques may be used by health practitioners, and taught to nonprofessional caregivers, to aid those seriously ill or approaching the end of their lives.

CARING TOUCH OF MASSAGE

From the wellness perspective, even those with terminal illnesses or nearing death continue to strive for optimal wellbeing in their unique life circumstances. Although massage will not cure or save someone from imminent death, it can help improve physical function and ease some of the pain and anxiety felt. As Dawn Nelson points out in her book *Compassionate Touch*, "attentive **nurturing touch** can be a significant therapeutic factor in treating despondency in the aging and/or the ill because of its multiple psycho-social, mental, emotional, and physical benefits" (1994, p. 12). Nurturing touch provides food for the soul as well as for the body and mind.

General relaxation, improved circulation of blood and lymph, reduced muscular tension, and skin stimulation are effects of massage with benefits for everyone. These effects are relevant to the special needs of those who have been physically inactive or bedridden for a long period of time. Massage helps alleviate problems with insomnia, digestion, constipation, difficulty in breathing, and skin degeneration. It can help prevent bedsores.

The terminally ill and dying experience **emotional distress** for a number of reasons. They may feel isolation, grief from the loss of freedom and friends, fear of abandonment, fear of the disease or aging, or fear of dying. Depression is common among the seriously ill and elderly, and may be caused or deepened by **touch deprivation**. Touch is essential nourishment for optimal wellbeing at all stages of life.

Gentle relaxation massage is known to reduce anxiety, provide a sense of connection, and generate feelings of general wellbeing. Massage may also facilitate a release of pent-up feelings, frustrations, sadness, and emotional energy. Pain that is aggravated by stress may be lessened with relaxing massage.

HOSPICE AND PALLIATIVE CARE

Hospice and **palliative care** programs are provided in freestanding facilities, hospitals, nursing homes, and other long-term care facilities. They provide compassionate care at the end of life, and typically involve a team-oriented approach to medical care, pain management, and emotional and spiritual support tailored to the needs of the dying. Hospice services include nursing care, personal care, social services, physician visits, counseling, and domestic services. The goal is to provide high quality palliative care. (Refer to National Hospice Foundation at www.hospiceinfo.org; and Center to Advance Palliative Care at www.capc.org.)

Massage therapy is one of the services increasingly available in hospice settings. The value of massage as a palliative care method has been studied and validated in integrative medical settings (Ellis et al., 1995; Howdyshell, 1998; Ruebottom, 1989).

MASSAGE FOR THE DYING

Near the end of life, massage can provide comforting touch, and communicate caring and love in a **nonverbal** way. The quality of touch for the dying should be gentle, and the techniques simple, such as stroking and holding.

In his book *Touching is Healing* (1982), Jules Older describes a program in New Zealand for the seriously ill and dying called the TLP Programme. TLP stands for Tender Loving Physiotherapy. The function of TLP is short-term rehabilitation and clearing the chest, and if appropriate, easing the transition from life to death. When death is near, smooth, soothing touch is used as a form of comfort and a means of communication. Some technical skills are needed to avoid causing pain or damaging delicate tissues.

Cathleen Farnslow, RN, describes how she uses Therapeutic Touch with the dying in *The Many Facets of Touch* (1984):

> When treating people near the end of the life continuum, I am drawn to place my hands on or near the heart, since this is the area of relationship and fear and requires life energy so that the dying can make

> amends and say good-bye, I'm sorry, or I love you before death occurs. As I hold my hands on or near the heart I am consciously sending thoughts of peace, love, and wholeness, which makes energy available for patients to finish their business with those who remain here and decreases pre-death anxiety. The elders feel deep warmth penetrating the heart area and report a sense of peace and deep calm (p. 187).

In hospice and home-care situations, family members and other caregivers can be taught simple ways of giving massage to the dying person. This has benefits for both parties, since it offers caregivers something active to do with their loved one and provides a means of connection even for those who may not be able to speak.

KNOWLEDGE AND SKILLS

A medical profile of the recipient is essential in working with the seriously ill and dying to protect both them and you. As with any other massage, identify contraindications and areas of caution before proceeding with a session. It may also be useful to understand the symptoms expected as a specific disease or condition progresses.

Specific techniques are less important than other essential skills when working with the terminally ill and dying. Dawn Nelson points out that:

> If you develop the ability to "see" an individual rather than just looking at a body, and if you reach out to that individual with a caring and open heart, your touch is likely to be far more effective than that of a highly trained professional who may be simply going through the mechanics of manipulating a physical body. Out of your real and pure contact with the individual, you will intuitively know what to do and how to proceed (1994, p. 43).

Intuition and sensitivity to others are important qualities for giving massage to the terminally ill and dying. Other characteristics and abilities recommended by Nelson (1994) include being touch oriented, able to adapt, open-hearted, able to focus energy, willing to face death, and able to focus on the individual. The skills she identifies as important include sensitive massage, active holding, listening and feedback, visualization and guided fantasy, guided meditation, shared breathing, and communicating with the dying. While some of these skills seem outside of the normal scope of a massage practitioner, they are useful in working with this special population.

In planning massage sessions for the terminally ill or dying, there are no specific procedures to follow or ironclad rules to memorize. Each individual will be different in how he or she experiences dying and in how massage might be of benefit. However, there are some general guidelines to keep in mind.

In general, massage sessions with the dying should be softer, gentler, and shorter. A person may only be able to benefit from 10–20 minutes of contact. Techniques may vary from simple hand holding to full-body massage. Massage may be given with the receiver lying on a standard massage table, sitting in a chair or wheel chair, or lying in bed. Patients may be in hospital beds with tubes or IVs in their bodies. Massage practitioners in these situations need to be versatile and able to adapt to the circumstances. Listening and feedback skills are important since communication may be a great need for someone facing death. The key is to be caring, supportive, and accepting.

Hand and arm massage is a useful approach for getting to know a new patient or client and for nursing home and hospice volunteers to give. The hands are easily accessible, relatively safe to massage, benefit from the application of lotion, and are a familiar place of contact with other people. Having the hands touched is comforting in itself and affords the opportunity for eye contact while talking.

SELF-CARE

Working with the terminally ill and dying can be physically and emotionally challenging. It is important to practice **conscious self-care** to help maintain your own wellbeing.

The actual massage techniques used with the seriously ill or elderly tend to be simple and light and easy on the practitioner's hands. However, maintaining good body mechanics may be difficult when working with people in chairs or in bed. The general principles of good mechanics apply here also, and you need to find ways to keep your back straight and spine and neck in good alignment.

If the recipient has a communicable disease, proper precautions and hygiene should be observed. Although potentially awkward, either latex or another type of glove should be worn if necessary for protection.

Maintaining emotional wellbeing involves a variety of factors. It helps to have confronted your own issues and fears around illness and death to a point of acceptance. Conscious awareness of how you feel when you are with someone seriously ill or nearing death can help you work through those feelings later with a friend, co-worker, or supervisor.

Eventual loss is expected in working with the dying. It is natural to develop caring relationships with your patients or clients. When one of them dies, be sensitive to your own process of grieving and letting go. Ongoing professional supervision or peer counseling may be of benefit when working with this special population.

SUMMARY

Massage brings comfort and caring touch to the terminally ill and dying. Simple massage techniques can be used by health practitioners, and taught to nonprofessional caregivers, to help improve the wellbeing of those approaching the end of life. Gentle, soothing stroking and holding are the main techniques used to relieve anxiety and produce a sense of calm. Massage has benefits related to improved circulation, healthy skin, and general relaxation. Touching itself communicates caring nonverbally, and helps those suffering from depression and touch deprivation.

Hospice and palliative care programs provide compassionate care at the end of life, and typically involve a team-oriented approach. The value of massage as a palliative care method has been studied and validated in integrative medical settings.

Massage sessions with the dying are softer, gentler, and shorter than with most other populations. Practitioners use intuition and sensitivity in determining how to approach each person. Knowledge of the recipient's medical profile helps practitioners plan effective massage sessions, and provide a safe environment for both giver and receiver. Physical and emotional self-care practices help practitioners maintain their own wellbeing while working under unique circumstances, and in facing loss encountered when working with the terminally ill and dying.

A look ahead . . .

The invention of the modern massage chair has brought massage into public places like trade shows, conferences, airports, shopping malls, and street fairs. Chapter 15 takes a look at the popularity of seated massage in an environment where millions of people spend a good portion of their waking hours—at their jobs.

REFERENCES

Ellis, V., Hill, & Campbell, H. (1995) Strengthening the family unity through the healing power of massage. *Journal of Hospice & Palliative Care*, V.12, pp. 19–20.

Fanslow, C. (1984). Touch and the elderly. In *The many facets of touch*, edited by C. C. Brown. Skillman, NJ: Johnson & Johnson Baby Products Company.

Howdyshell, C. (1998). Complementary therapy: Aromatherapy with massage for geriatric and hospice care for a holistic approach. *Hospice Journal*, V.13, pp. 69–75.

Nelson, D. (1994). *Compassionate touch: Hands-on caregiving for the elderly, the ill and the dying*. New York: Station Hill Press.

Older, J. (1982). *Touching is healing*. New York: Stein & Day.

Ruebottom, A., Lee, C., & Dryden, P. J. (1989). Massage for terminally ill AIDS patients. *International Conference on AIDS*, June.

ADDITIONAL RESOURCES

Books

Nelson, Dawn (2001). *From the heart through the hands: The power of touch in caregiving*. Forres, Scotland: Findhorn Press.

Videos

"Cancer massage video." Canada Institute of Palliative Massage. Nelson, British Columbia, Canada: Sutherland Massage Productions. (*www.sutherlandmassageproductions.com*)

"AIDS massage video." Canada Institute of Palliative Massage. Nelson, British Columbia, Canada: Sutherland Massage Productions. (*www.sutherlandmassageproductions.com*)

WEB SITES

Center to Advance Palliative Care (*www.capc.org*)
National Hospice and Palliative Care Organization (*www.nhpco.org*)
National Hospice Foundation (*www.hospiceinfo.org*)

CHAPTER FIFTEEN

Seated Massage in the Workplace

LEARNING OUTCOMES

After studying this chapter, the student will have the information to:

1. Trace the history of workplace massage.
2. Explain the benefits of massage in workplace wellness programs.
3. Choose and adapt techniques for seated massage.
4. Explain the popularity of workplace massage.

KEY TERMS/CONCEPTS

Ergonomics
Massage chair
On-site massage
Repetitive strain injuries (RSI)
Seated massage
Worker productivity
Workplace wellness programs

LINK LIBRARY TERMS

Massage Business • *Massage Regulations*

MEDIALINK

A companion CD-ROM, included free with each new copy of this book, supplements the techniques presented in this chapter. Insert the CD-ROM to watch video clips of massage techniques being demonstrated. This multimedia feature is designed to help you add a new dimension to your learning.

Massage is increasingly popular in **workplace wellness programs.** These employer-sponsored programs make services and activities available to employees to improve their overall health and wellbeing. Many businesses recognize the benefits of massage for their employees and are making massage available at the work site itself. Seated massage, in particular, is popular with businesses exploring ways to reduce stress on the job and to minimize job-related injuries.

HISTORY OF WORKPLACE MASSAGE

In the late 19th and early 20th centuries, massage was available at businesses such as large factories and retail stores as part of employee benefits. Industrial recreation programs provided fitness and sport activities that likely included massage. Large businesses often had on-site medical departments, including physiotherapy. Some large companies provided massage for their executives. These in-house programs largely disappeared by the mid-20th century.

In the 1980s, businesses began to rediscover the importance of employee health, and to implement programs to encourage healthy life habits. These include programs such as exercise, weight loss, smoking cessation, and stress reduction. Healthy employees are more productive and lose less work time due to illness or injury. Workplace wellness programs have been found to reduce workers' compensation claims and absenteeism.

The invention of a specially designed chair that allows people to receive massage in a seated position has had a dramatic impact on the availability of massage in offices and other work settings. The first modern **massage chair** was designed in the 1980s by David Palmer of San Francisco, CA, and promoted as the foundation for on-site massage. **On-site massage** means that the massage practitioner goes to where the potential clients are (e.g., at work, in stores, at airports, on the street), making massage more accessible. One of the first large corporations to provide on-site massage for their employees in 1985 was Apple Computer Corporation (Palmer, 1995).

The idea of the massage chair was to make receiving massage more readily available to the general public. It can be transported easily, takes up less room than a massage table, and allows recipients to receive massage sitting up and with their clothes on. Massage techniques that do not need oil, such as compression, direct pressure and kneading, are generally used for seated massage.

BENEFITS OF MASSAGE IN THE WORKPLACE

Many of the tasks performed by workers in the past are now done by sophisticated machines run by computers. However, many workers still sit at workstations for long periods of time performing repetitive tasks such as using computer keyboards, and sorting or assembly. Tradesmen, craftsmen, artists and musicians repeat certain movements over and over, stressing their bodies. Repetitive tasks can cause aching, tenderness, swelling, tingling and numbness, weakness, loss of flexibility, or spasms in the muscles affected.

Repetitive strain injuries (RSI) are common in a number of occupations. RSIs include tendinitis (inflammation of tendons), bursitis (inflammation of fluid sacs around a joint), ganglion cysts (a mass formed over a tendon), and nerve impingement.

Attention to **ergonomics** (i.e., good posture and body mechanics) in the work environment has alleviated some potentially damaging conditions. For example, computer keyboards and monitors are placed in the proper spacial relationship to the user to reduce strain, adjustable chairs that support good sitting posture are used, and phone headsets help prevent neck strain. While these practices can lessen the negative impact on employees, they do not eliminate problems altogether.

The stress level of employees is also a major wellness factor. The dizzying pace of modern times, at work and in everyday life adds to the stress of employees. A high level of chronic stress is known to have a negative effect on health. Tension headaches are common at work.

Massage can help address many of the potentially harmful conditions mentioned above, and it has also been found to increase mental clarity and alertness (Field 1993; *Massage* 1996). This can only enhance **worker productivity.** Practitioners can adapt massage sessions to address the needs of workers, and the use of massage chairs makes offering this service in the workplace convenient.

A recent study on work-site acupressure massage (WSAM) found that the group receiving the specific massage protocol enjoyed significant health benefits. The massage was a 20-minute session received twice weekly for a period of eight weeks. The recipients were fully clothed. Techniques included Western massage, acupressure and reflexology. Results showed that people receiving massage had a significant decrease in anxiety, increase in emotional control, decrease in perceived sleep disturbances, decreased blood pressure, improved cognition, and a decrease in perception of muscle tightness (Hodge et al. 2002).

A summary of the benefits of workplace massage, especially seated massage, are listed below. The list was adapted from the information brochure, *On-Site Therapeutic Massage: Investment for a Healthy Business* (Benjamin, 1994):

- Reduces the physical and mental effects of stress; thus helps prevent burnout and stress-related diseases
- Reduces the adverse effects of sitting for long periods of time in the same position, such as at a desk or other workstation
- Relieves physical problems associated with repetitive tasks such as computer keyboard use, sorting, filing, and assembly-line tasks
- Improves alertness and ability to focus, an antidote for work slumps
- Helps relieve common problem conditions such as tension headaches and stiff and sore muscles
- Improves immune system functioning for better general health and resistance to colds and other illnesses
- Employees feel revitalized and ready to return to work.

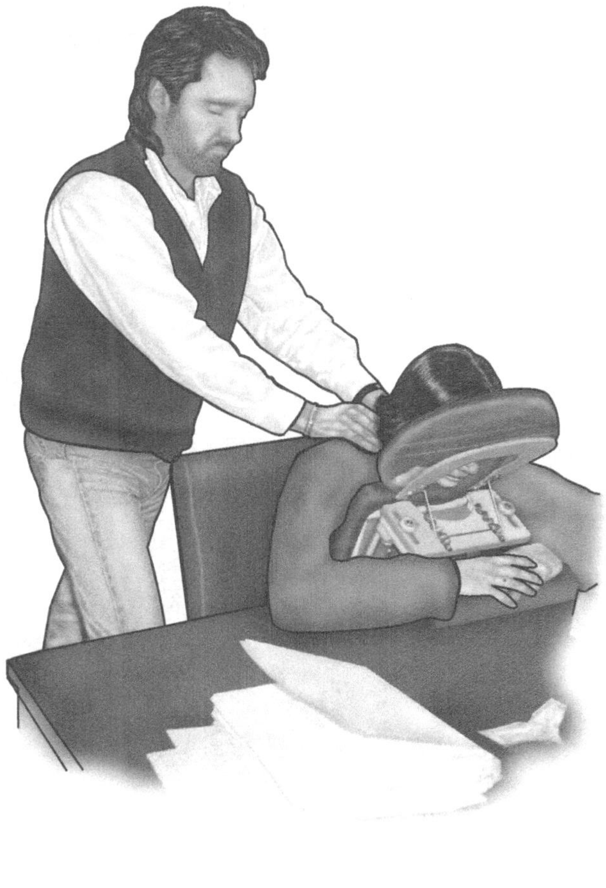

FIGURE 15–1. Portable table-top equipment that provides support for recipients receiving massage at their workstations.

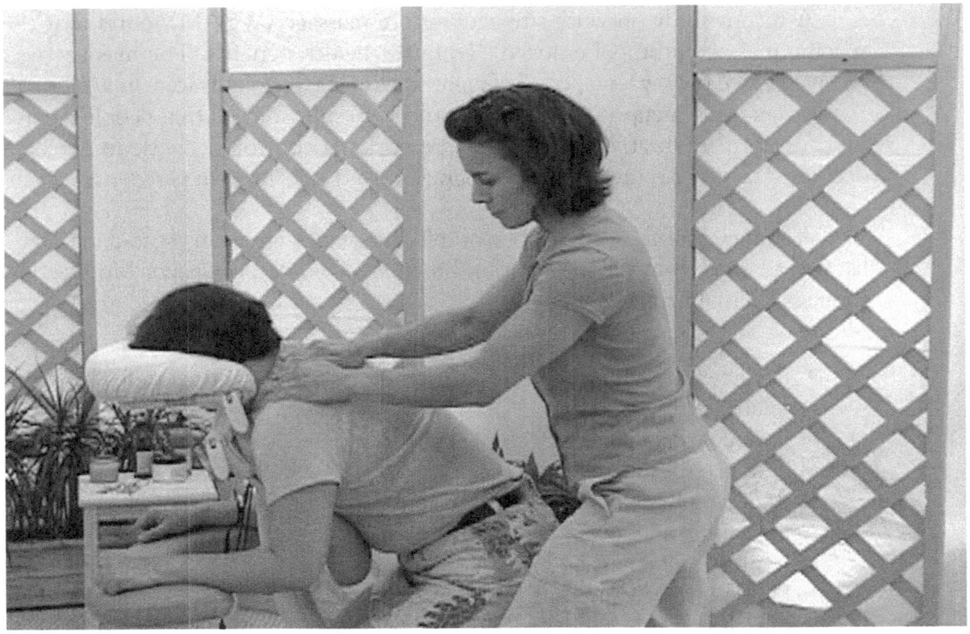

FIGURE 15–2. Kneading the shoulders during seated massage.

SEATED MASSAGE FOR OFFICE WORKERS

Seated massage is massage given to a recipient in a seated position. It may be given at a workstation, in an empty office or cubicle, or in any small space such as the corner of a conference or workroom. Seated massage sessions for office workers typically last from 15 to 20 minutes. Recipients may be seated at their workstations or may be in portable massage chairs. Figure 15–1 shows a tabletop unit that offers recipients support when receiving massage at desks.

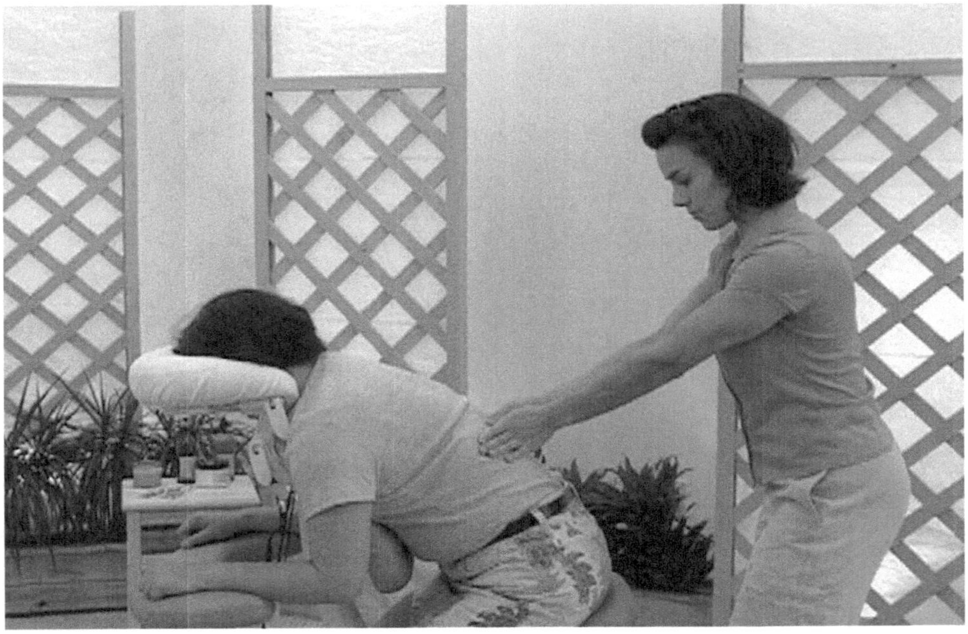

FIGURE 15–3. Direct pressure to muscles along the spine during seated massage.

The recipient is clothed, but removes his or her jacket, tie, large jewelry, or other things that might interfere with the massage. Practitioners should ask permission to work on the face if the recipient is wearing makeup, or on the scalp if massage would disturb the hair.

Seated massage sessions focus on the upper body. Areas of concern are the neck and shoulders, head and scalp, upper back, and forearms, wrists, and hands. Techniques that are effective without the use of oil are used; for example, forms of petrissage (i.e., kneading and compression), friction, tapotement, light stroking, and joint movements. Forms of energy balancing such as polarity therapy may be incorporated into a session. Shiatsu and other forms of Asian bodywork are particularly adaptable for seated massage, since they are given without lubricant and include techniques such as direct pressure, compressions, and percussion.

Seated massage includes kneading the shoulders (Figure 15–2), and direct pressure to points on either side of the spine (Figure 15–3). The upper extremities can be accessed with the arms hanging down or relaxing on the arm rest. Hand and wrist massage using the arm rest is shown in Figure 15–4.

Neck massage can be performed with the client positioned in the face cradle (Figure 15–5). Friction to the small muscles of the head and scalp is shown in Figure 15–6. A combination of kneading the neck and shoulders, pressure points along the trapezius and cervical muscles, and friction to the head and scalp can help relieve tension headache.

Light tapotement to the head as shown in Figure 15–7 is stimulating and increases alertness before getting back to work. (Refer to TouchPro Institute—www.touchpro.org —for information on chair massage training.)

POPULARITY OF WORKPLACE MASSAGE

Massage is popular with employers and employees for a number of reasons. It has immediate positive effects, since recipients usually feel better right away. It may alleviate some of the physical aches and pains developed from sitting long hours doing deskwork. In contrast to other wellness practices,

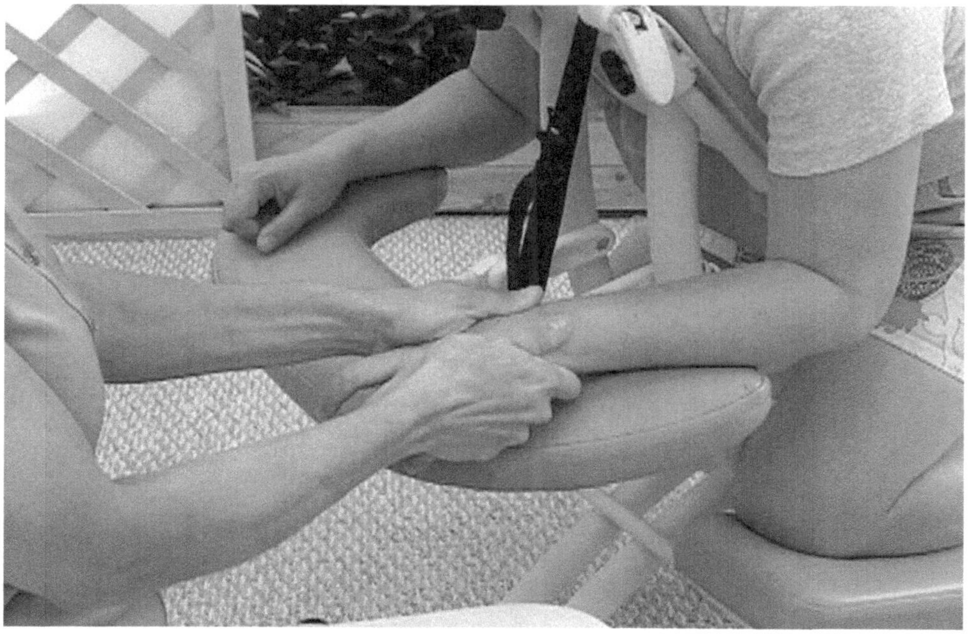

FIGURE 15–4. Hand and wrist massage with arms relaxing on the arm rest during seated massage.

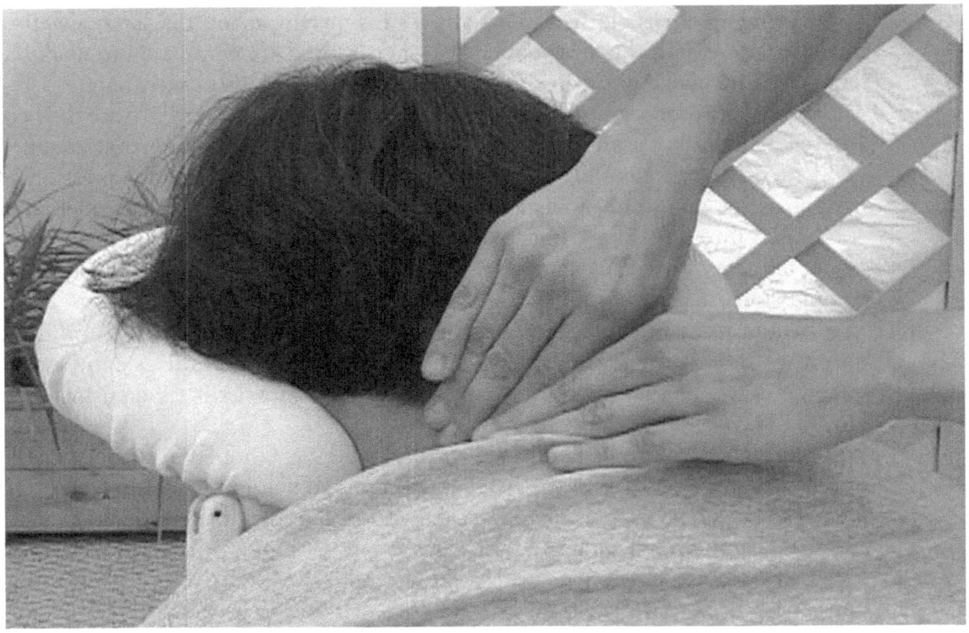

FIGURE 15–5. Neck massage with client positioned in the face cradle during seated massage.

massage requires no practice or effort on the part of the recipient. It complements other health practices such as exercise and stress-reduction programs.

Massage programs help increase good feelings about the workplace and loyalty to businesses that show caring for their employees' wellbeing. They boost productivity, and may be taken advantage of by most workers (Benjamin, 1994).

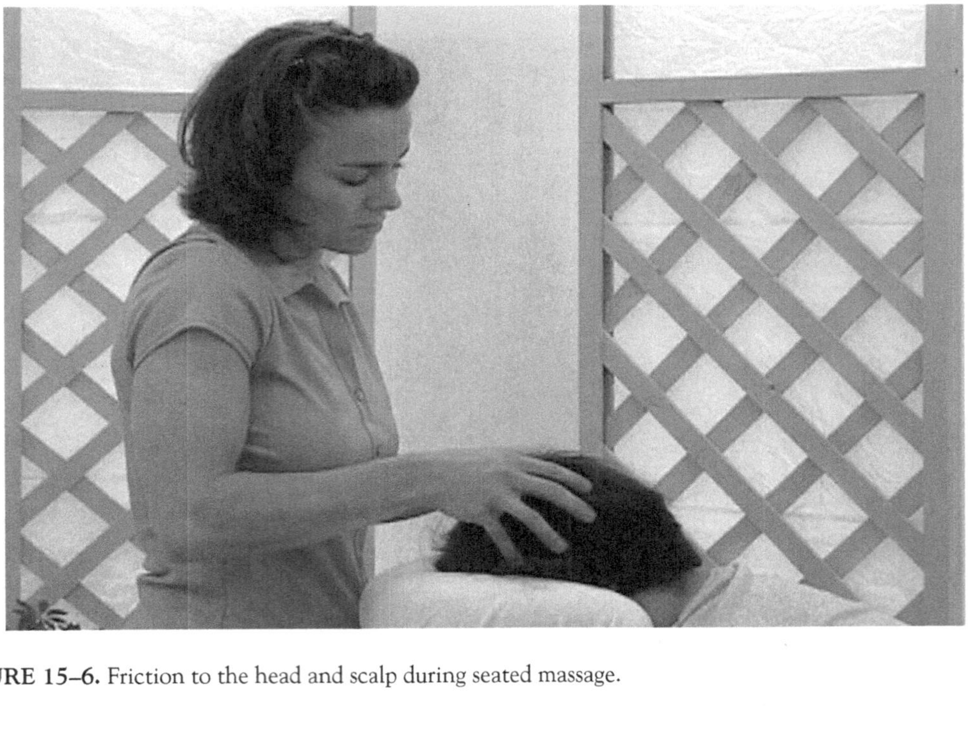

FIGURE 15–6. Friction to the head and scalp during seated massage.

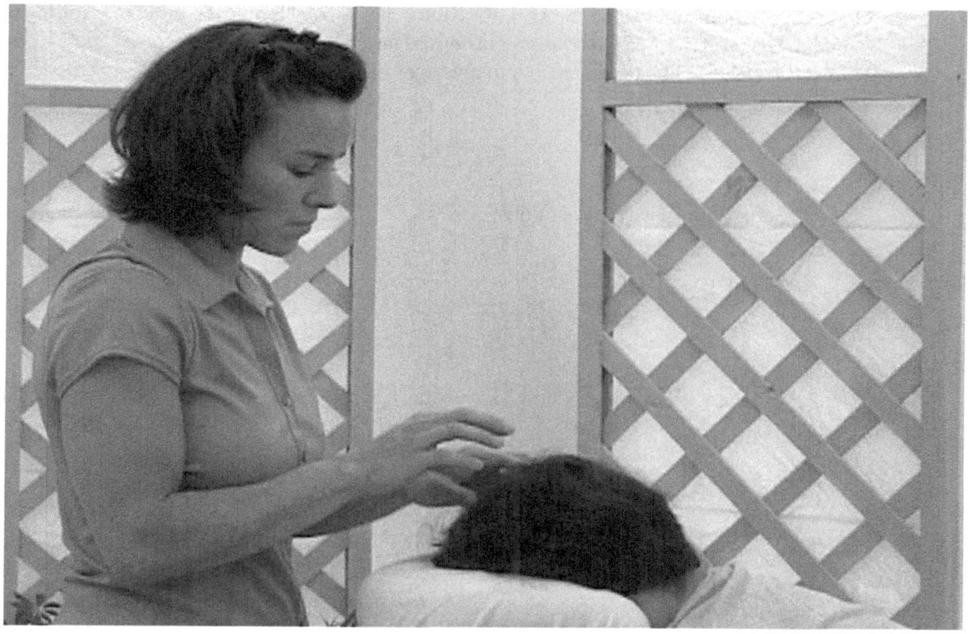

FIGURE 15–7. Light tapotement to the head to conclude seated massage session.

SUMMARY

Massage is an increasingly popular part of workplace wellness programs. Employers recognize the benefits of massage for helping workers stay healthy and productive. Massage can relieve muscular tension caused by prolonged sitting at workstations, and by repetitive tasks. It helps reduce the stresses of the work environment. Studies show that massage can increase mental clarity and alertness. It leaves workers feeling revitalized and ready to return to work.

The invention of a special massage chair in the 1980s has made massage more accessible to the workplace. With the special chair, massage can be given in small spaces to workers who are fully clothed.

In seated massage for the workplace, recipients are asked to take off their jackets, ties, jewelry, and other things that may interfere with the massage. Massage techniques that do not require oil are used, e.g., compression and kneading (petrissage), friction, tapotement, and other forms of bodywork such as amma, shiatsu, and polarity therapy. Areas massaged usually include neck and shoulders, head and scalp, upper back, forearms, wrists and hands.

Effective seated massage techniques include kneading the shoulders, direct pressure on either side of the spine, and arm and hand massage. Tension headaches are relieved by kneading the neck and shoulders, pressure to points along the trapezius and cervical muscles, and friction to the head and scalp. Light tapotement on the head is stimulating and increases alertness before getting back to work.

Seated massage is popular with both employers and employees since it has immediate positive effects, complements other heath practices, increases good feelings about the workplace, and improves worker productivity.

REFERENCES

No author (1996). Massage helps lower stress of working, taking final exams. In *Massage, 62* (July/August), p. 148.

Benjamin, P. J. (1994). *On-site therapeutic massage: Investment for a healthy business*. Information brochure. Rockford, IL: Hemingway Publications.

Field, T. M., Fox, N., Pickens, J., Ironsong, G., & Scafidi, F. (1993). Job stress survey. Unpublished manuscript, Touch Research Institute, University of Miami School of Medicine. Reported in *Touchpoints: Touch Research Abstracts, 1*(1).

Hodge, M., Robinson, C., Boehmer, J., & Klein, S. (2002). "Employee outcomes following work-site acupressure and massage." Chapter 9 in *Massage therapy: The evidence for practice*. New York: Mosby.

Palmer, D. (1995). The death of on-site massage? *Massage Therapy Journal, 34*(3), pp. 119–120.

WEB SITE

TouchPro Institute (*www.touchpro.org*)

ADDITIONAL RESOURCES

Videos

"Chair Massage with Connie Scholl." Riverside, CT: At Peace Media. (*www.atpeacemedia.com*)

"Japanese Chair Massage Video." (2002) By Shogo Mochizuki. Boulder, CO: Kotobuki Publications.

CHAPTER SIXTEEN

Infectious and Noninfectious Conditions

OBJECTIVES

- Discuss the risk factors for infectious diseases.
- Describe the most common pathogens infecting humans today.
- Explain how your immune system works to protect you and what factors may make it less effective.
- Explain the major emerging and resurgent diseases affecting humans; discuss why they are increasing in incidence and what actions are being taken to reduce risks.
- Discuss the various sexually transmitted infections, their means of transmission, and actions that can be taken to prevent their spread.
- Discuss human immunodeficiency virus and acquired immune deficiency syndrome, trends in infection and treatment, and the impact on special populations, such as women and members of the international community.
- Discuss the chronic lung diseases, common neurological disorders, diabetes and other digestion-related disorders, and the varied musculoskeletal diseases.

Every moment of every day, you are in contact with microscopic organisms that have the ability to cause illness or even death. These disease-causing agents, known as **pathogens,** are found in air and food and on nearly every object or person with whom you come in contact. Although new varieties of pathogens arise all the time, scientific evidence indicates that many have existed for as long as there has been life on the planet. Fossil evidence shows that infections, cancer, heart disease, and a host of other ailments afflicted the earliest human beings. At times, infectious diseases wiped out whole groups of people through epidemics such as the Black Death, or bubonic plague, which killed half the population of Europe in the 1300s. A pandemic, or global epidemic, of influenza killed more than 20 million people in 1918, while strains of tuberculosis and cholera continue to cause premature death throughout the world.

In spite of our best efforts to eradicate them, these diseases are a continuing menace to all of us. The news isn't all bad, however. Even though we are bombarded by potential pathogenic threats, our immune systems are remarkably adept at protecting us. *Endogenous microorganisms* are those that live in peaceful coexistence with their human host most of the time. For people in good health and whose immune systems are functioning properly, endogenous organisms are usually harmless. But in sick people or those with weakened immune systems, these normally harmless pathogenic organisms can cause serious health problems.

Exogenous microorganisms are organisms that do not normally inhabit the body. When they do, however, they are apt to produce an infection and/or illness. The more easily these pathogens can gain a foothold in the body and sustain themselves, the more **virulent,** or aggressive, they may be in causing disease. However, if your immune system is strong, you will often be able to fight off even the most virulent attacker. Several factors influence your susceptibility to disease.

ASSESSING YOUR DISEASE RISKS

Most diseases are **multifactorial diseases**—that is, they are caused by the interaction of several factors from inside and outside the person. For a disease to occur, the *host* must be *susceptible,* which means that the immune system must be in a weakened condition; an *agent* capable of transmitting a disease must be present; and the *environment* must be hospitable to the pathogen in terms of temperature, light, moisture, and other requirements. Other risk factors also apparently increase or decrease susceptibility. Figure 16.1 summarizes the body's defenses against invasion.

Risk Factors You Can't Control

Unfortunately, some risk factors are beyond our control. Here are some of the most common.

Heredity Perhaps the single greatest factor influencing longevity is the longevity of a person's parents. Being born into a family in which heart disease, cancer, or other illnesses are prevalent seems to increase risk. Still other diseases are caused by direct chromosomal inheritance. For example, **sickle-cell anemia,** an inherited blood disease that primarily affects African Americans, is often transmitted to the fetus if both parents carry the sickle-cell trait. It is often unclear whether hereditary diseases occur as a result of inherited chromosomal traits or inherited insufficiencies in the immune system.

Aging After age 40 we become more vulnerable to most of the chronic diseases. Moreover, as we age, our immune systems respond less efficiently to invading organisms, thus increasing risk for infection and illness. The same flu that produces an afternoon of nausea and diarrhea in a younger person may cause days of illness or even death in an older person. The very young are also at risk for many diseases, particularly if they are not vaccinated against them.

Environmental Conditions Unsanitary conditions and the presence of drugs, chemicals, and hazardous pollutants and wastes in food and water probably have a great effect on our immune systems. It is well documented that poor environmental conditions can weaken **immunological competence**—the body's ability to defend itself against pathogens.

Organism Resistance Some organisms, such as the food-borne organism **botulism,** are particularly virulent, and even tiny amounts may make the most hardy of us ill. Other organisms have mutated and are resistant to the body's defenses as well as to other conventional treatments designed to protect against them. Still other, newer pathogens pose unique challenges for our immune systems—ones that our bodily defenses are ill adapted to fight.

Risk Factors You Can Control

The good news is that we all have some degree of personal control over many risk factors for disease. Too much stress, inadequate nutrition, a low physical fitness level, lack of sleep, misuse or abuse of legal and illegal substances, poor personal hygiene, high-risk behaviors, and other variables significantly increase the risk for a number of diseases. Various chapters of this text discuss these variables. Several factors influence our individual susceptibility to various diseases. Those we have the most control over, via lifestyle decisions and behaviors, are noted on the following list with an asterisk (*):

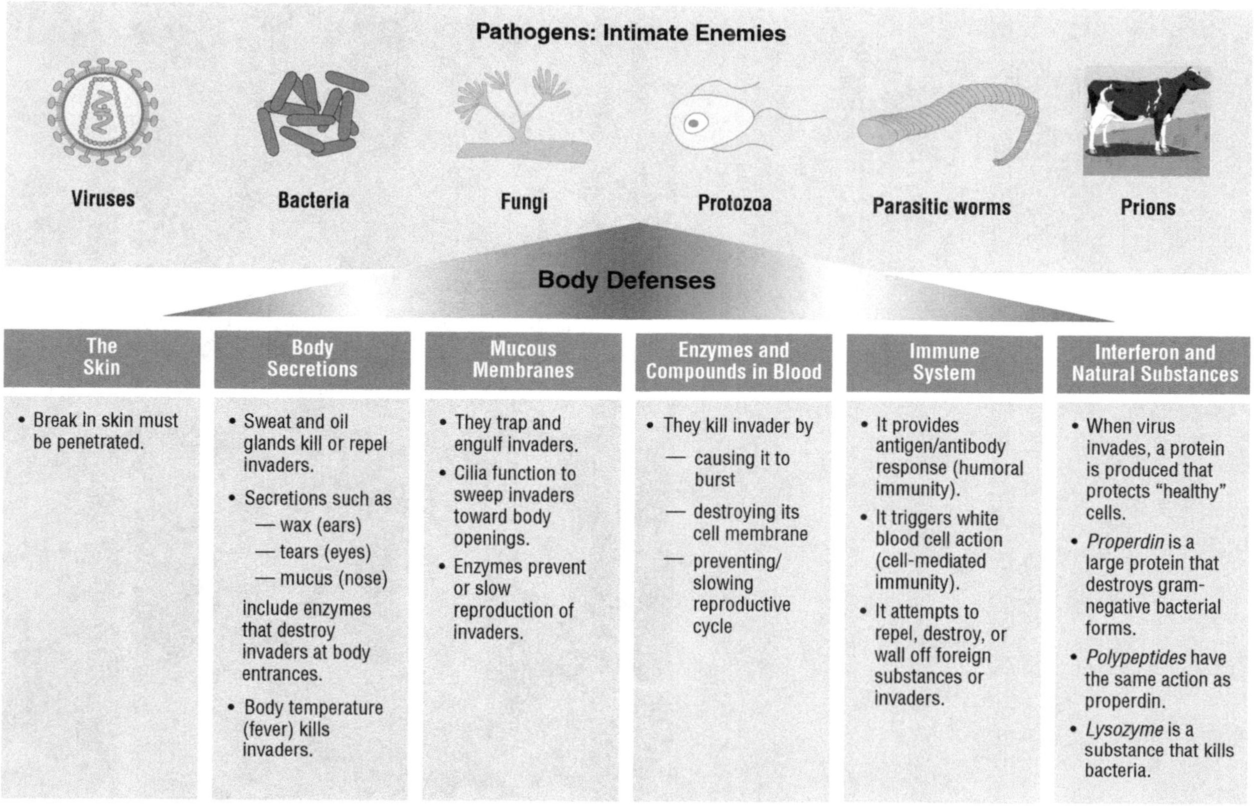

FIGURE 16.1. The Body's Defenses Against Disease-Causing Pathogens

- Dosage, virulence, and portal of entry of agent
- Age at time of infection
- Preexisting level of immunity*
- Nature and vigor of immune response*
- Genetic factors controlling immune response
- Nutritional status*
- Preexisting diseases*
- Personal habits: smoking, alcohol, exercise, drugs*
- Dual infection or superinfection with other agents
- Psychological factors (e.g., motivation, emotional status, and so on)*

Types of Pathogens and Routes of Transmission

Pathogens enter the body in several ways. They may be transmitted by *direct contact* between infected persons, such as during sexual relations, kissing, or touching, or by *indirect contact*, such as by touching an object the infected person has had contact with. The hands are probably the greatest source of infectious disease transmission. You may also **autoinoculate** yourself, or transmit a pathogen from one part of your body to another. For example, you may touch a sore on your lip that is teeming with viral herpes, then transmit the virus to your eye when you scratch your itchy eyelid.

Pathogens are also transmitted by *airborne contact*—you can breathe in air that carries a particular pathogen—or by *food-borne infection* if you eat something contaminated by microorganisms. Recent episodes of food poisoning from *Salmonella* bacteria found in certain foods and *E. coli* bacteria found in undercooked beef have raised concerns about the safety of the U.S. food supply. As a direct result of these concerns, food labels now caution consumers to cook meats thoroughly, wash utensils, and take other food-handling precautions.

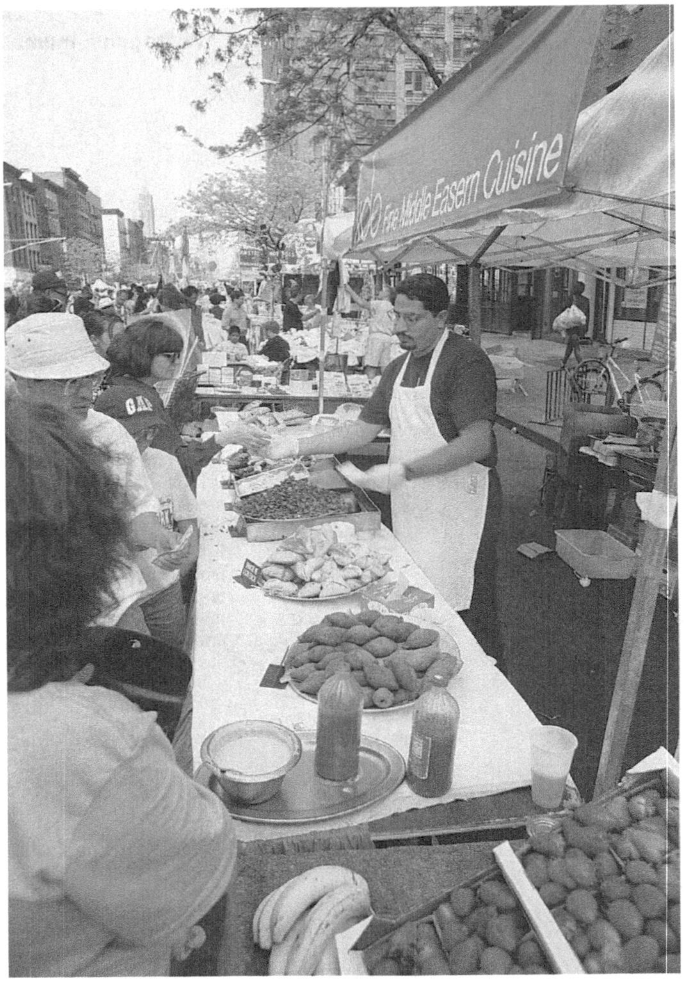

Airborne pathogens can be transmitted easily and unknowingly, so special precautions must be taken to ensure the health and safety of patrons of food markets and other public places.

Your best friend may be the source of *animal-borne pathogens*. Dogs, cats, livestock, and wild animals can spread numerous diseases through their bites or feces or by carrying infected insects into living areas and transmitting diseases either directly or indirectly. Although **interspecies transmission** of diseases (diseases passed from humans to animals and vice versa) is rare, it does occur. *Waterborne diseases* are transmitted directly from drinking water and indirectly from foods washed or sprayed with contaminated water. These pathogens can also invade your body if you wade or swim in contaminated streams, lakes, or reservoirs. Pathogens may also transmit *insect-borne diseases* via mosquitoes, ticks, and other hosts that spread disease through sucking or biting. Mothers may transmit diseases *perinatally* to an infant in the womb or as the baby passes through the vagina during birth.

We can categorize pathogens into six major types: bacteria, viruses, fungi, protozoa, parasitic worms, and prions.

Bacteria

Bacteria are single-celled organisms that are plantlike in nature but lack chlorophyll (the pigment that gives plants their green coloring). There are three major types of bacteria: cocci, bacilli, and spirilla. Bacteria can be viewed under a standard light microscope.

Although there are several thousand species of bacteria, only approximately 100 cause diseases in humans. In many cases, it is not the bacteria themselves that cause disease but rather the poisonous substances, called **toxins,** that they produce. The following are the most common bacterial infections.

Staphylococcal Infections **Staphylococci** are normally present on our skin at all times and usually cause few problems. But when there is a cut or break in the **epidermis,** or outer layer of the skin, staphylococci may enter and cause a localized infection. If you have ever suffered from acne, boils, styes (infections of the eyelids), or infected wounds, you have probably had a staph infection. Although most such infections are readily defeated by your immune system, resistant forms of staph bacteria are on the rise. These bacteria must be treated with heavy doses of antibiotics and pose serious risks to those infected.

At least one staph-caused disorder, **toxic shock syndrome,** is potentially fatal. Although most cases of toxic shock syndrome have occurred in menstruating women, the disease was first reported in 1978 in children and continues to be reported in people recovering from wounds, surgery, or other injury. To reduce the likelihood of toxic shock syndrome, take the following precautions: (1) avoid superabsorbent tampons except during the heaviest menstrual flow; (2) change tampons at least every four hours; and (3) use napkins at night instead of tampons.

Streptococcal Infections At least five types of the **streptococcus** microorganism are known to cause bacterial infections. Group A streptococcus causes the most common diseases, such as streptococcal pharyngitis (strep throat) and scarlet fever. Group B streptococcus can cause illness in newborn babies, pregnant women, the elderly, and adults with other illnesses such as diabetes or liver disease.

Pneumonia In the early twentieth century, **pneumonia** was one of the leading causes of death in the United States. This lung disease is characterized by chronic cough, chest pain, chills, high fever, fluid accumulation, and eventual respiratory failure. One of the most common forms of pneumonia is caused by bacterial infection and responds readily to antibiotic treatment in the early stages. Other forms are caused by viruses, chemicals, or other substances in the lungs and are more difficult to treat. Although medical advances have reduced the overall incidence of pneumonia, it continues to be a major threat in the United States and throughout the world. Vulnerable populations include the poor, the elderly, and those already suffering from other illnesses.

Legionnaires' Disease This bacterial disorder gained widespread publicity in 1976, when several Legionnaires at the American Legion convention in Philadelphia contracted the disease and died before the invading organism was isolated and effective treatment devised. Although it is not well known, the water-borne nature of Legionnaires' Disease has led to several recent outbreaks in the United States. The symptoms are similar to those of pneumonia, which sometimes makes identification difficult. In people whose resistance is lowered, particularly the elderly, delayed identification can have serious consequences.

Tuberculosis A major killer in the United States during the early twentieth century, **tuberculosis (TB)** was largely controlled in America by 1950 due to improved sanitation, isolation of infected persons, and treatment with drugs such as *rifampin* or *isoniazid.* But though many health professionals assumed that TB had been conquered, that appears not to be the case. During the past 20 years, several factors have led to an epidemic rise in the disease: deteriorating social conditions, including overcrowding and poor sanitation; failure to isolate active cases of TB; a weakening of public health infrastructure, which has led to less funding for screening; and migration of TB to the United States through international travel. In 2002, there were more than 15,075 active cases of TB in the United States. More than one-half of all TB cases in the U.S. in 2002 occurred in foreign-born individuals. Newer strains of multiple drug-resistant TB make this epidemic potentially more devastating than previous outbreaks.

Although increases in the incidence of TB in the United States are troubling, U.S. statistics pale by comparison to the staggering TB burden in the global population. Assuming no significant improvements in prevention and control between now and 2020, the World Health Organization (WHO) estimates that 1 billion people will acquire new TB infection, 200 million will develop active disease, and 70 million will die.

TB is caused by bacterial infiltration of the respiratory system that results in a chronic inflammatory reaction in the lungs. Airborne transmission via the respiratory tract is the primary and most efficient mode of transmitting TB. People with active cases can transmit the disease while talking, coughing, sneezing, or singing. Fortunately, TB is fairly difficult to catch, and prolonged exposure, rather than single exposure, is the typical mode of infection. Only about 20 to 30 percent of people exposed to an active case will become infected. Symptoms include persistent coughing, weight loss, fever, and spitting up blood. A simple skin test will indicate infection, and treatments are effective for most nonresistant cases. Many people have a form of latent TB in which the bacteria are present in the body but the person is symptom-free and not infectious. Most of these people never develop active TB, unless their immune system becomes compromised.

Periodontal Diseases Diseases of the tissue around the teeth, called **periodontal diseases,** affect three out of four adults over age 35. Improper tooth care, including lack of flossing and poor brushing habits, and the failure to obtain professional dental care lead to increased bacterial growth, caries (tooth decay), and gum infections. If left untreated, permanent tooth loss may result.

What do you think?

Why do you think we are experiencing global increases in diseases such as TB? • Should we be concerned about diseases in other countries? • Do we have an obligation to help the world's population in their struggle against these diseases? • What policies, programs, and services might help?

Viruses

Viruses are the smallest pathogens, approximately 1/500th the size of bacteria. Because of their tiny size, they are visible only under an electron microscope and were not identified until the twentieth century. More than 150 viruses are known to cause diseases in humans, although their role in various cancers and chronic diseases is still unclear.

Essentially, a virus consists of a protein structure that contains either *ribonucleic acid (RNA)* or *deoxyribonucleic acid (DNA)*. Incapable of carrying out the normal cell functions of respiration and metabolism, a virus cannot reproduce on its own and can exist only in a parasitic relationship with the cell it invades.

Viral diseases can be difficult to treat because many viruses can withstand heat, formaldehyde, and large doses of radiation with little effect on their structure. Drug treatment for viral infections is also limited. Drugs powerful enough to kill viruses generally kill the host cells too, although some medications block stages in viral reproduction without damaging host cells.

When exposed to certain viruses, the body produces a protein substance known as **interferon.** Interferon does not destroy the invading microorganisms but sets up a protective mechanism to aid healthy cells in their struggle against the invaders. Although interferon research is promising, it should be noted that not all viruses stimulate interferon production.

The Common Cold Colds are responsible for more days lost from work and more uncomfortable days spent at work than any other ailment. Caused by any number of viruses (some experts claim there may be more than 200 different viruses responsible for the common cold), colds are **endemic** (always present to some degree) among people throughout the world. In the course of a year, Americans suffer more than 1 billion colds. Otherwise healthy people carry cold viruses in their noses and throats most of the time. These viruses are held in check until the host's resistance is lowered. It is possible to "catch" a cold—from the airborne droplets of another person's sneeze or from skin-to-skin or mucous membrane contact—though recent studies indicate that the hands are the greatest avenue for transmitting colds and other viruses. Although many people believe that a cold results from exposure to cold weather or from getting chilled or overheated, experts believe that such things have little or no effect on cold development. Stress, allergy disorders that affect the nasal passages, and menstrual cycles do, however, appear to increase susceptibility.

REALITY CHECK

Body Piercing and Tattooing: Risks to Health

A look around almost any college campus reveals many examples of the widespread trend of body piercing and tattooing, also referred to as "body art." People are getting their ears and bodies pierced in record numbers, in such places as the eyebrows, tongues, lips, noses, navels, nipples, genitals, and just about any place possible. Many view the trend as a fulfillment of a desire for self-expression, as this University of Wisconsin–Madison student points out: "The nipple [ring] was one of those things that I did as a kind of empowerment, claiming my body as my own and refuting the stereotypes that people have about me. . . . The tattoo was kind of a lark and came along the same lines and I like it too. . . . [T]hey both give me a secret smile." Whatever the reason, tattoo artists are doing a booming business in both tattooing and the "art" of body piercing.

However, health professionals cite several concerns over health risks. The most common health-related problems associated with tattoos and body piercing include skin reactions, infections, and scarring. The average healing times for piercings depend on the size of the insert, location, and the person's overall health. Facial and tongue piercings tend to heal more quickly than areas not commonly exposed to open air or light and which are often teeming with bacteria, such as the genitals. Because the hands are great germ transmitters, "fingering" pierced areas poses a significant risk for infection.

Of even greater concern is the potential transmission of dangerous pathogens that any puncture of the human body exacerbates. The use of unsterile needles—which can cause serious infections and can transmit HIV, hepatitis B (HBV) and hepatitis C (HCV), tetanus, and a host of other diseases—poses a very real risk. (Actress Pamela Anderson claims to have contracted HCV from sharing a tattoo needle with her ex-husband Tommy Lee.) Body piercing and tattooing are performed by unlicensed "professionals" who generally have learned their trade from other body artists. Laws and policies regulating body piercing and tattooing vary greatly by state. While some states don't allow tattoo and body-piercing parlors, others may regulate them carefully, and still others provide few regulations and standards by which parlors have to abide. Standards for safety usually include minimum age of use, standards of sanitation, use of aseptic techniques, sterilization of equipment, informed risks, instructions for skin care, record keeping, and recommendations for dealing with adverse reactions. Because of the lack of standards regulating this business and the potential for transmission of dangerous pathogens, anyone who receives a tattoo, body piercing, or permanent makeup tattoo cannot donate blood for one year.

If you opt for tattooing or body piercing, remember the following points:

- Look for clean, well-lit work areas, and ask about sterilization procedures.
- Before having the work done, watch the artist at work. Tattoo removal is expensive and often impossible. Make sure the tattoo is one you can live with for years.
- Immediately before piercing or tattooing, the body area should be carefully sterilized. The artist should put on new latex gloves and touch nothing else while working.
- Packaged, sterilized needles should be used only once and then discarded. A piercing gun should not be used because it cannot be sterilized properly.
- Only jewelry made of noncorrosive metal, such as surgical stainless steel, niobium, or solid 14-karat gold, is safe for new piercing.
- Leftover tattoo ink should be discarded after each procedure. Do not allow the artist to reuse ink that has been used for other customers.
- If any signs of pus, swelling, redness, or discoloration persist, remove the piercing object and contact a physician.

Sources: U.S. Food and Drug Administration, Center for Food Safety and Applied Nutrition, "Tattoos and Permanent Makeup," Office of Cosmetics and Colors Fact Sheet, 2000, www.cfsan.fda.gov/ ~dms/cos-204.html; M. L. Armstrong and K. P. Murphy, "Adolescent Tattooing and Body Piercing," *The Prevention Researcher* (Integrated Research Services, Eugene, Oregon) 5, no. 3 (1998): 5.

The best rule of thumb is to keep your resistance level high. Sound nutrition, adequate rest, stress reduction, and regular exercise appear to be the best bets in helping fight off infection. Avoid people with newly developed colds (colds appear to be most contagious during the first 24 hours of onset). If you contract a cold, bed rest, plenty of fluids, and aspirin to relieve pain and discomfort are the tried-and-true remedies for adults. Children should not take aspirin for colds or the flu because this could lead to *Reye's syndrome*, a potentially fatal disease.

Influenza In otherwise healthy people, **influenza,** or flu, is usually not serious. Symptoms, including headaches, fatigue, aches and pains, fever, and coldlike ailments, generally pass quickly. However, in combination with other disorders or among the elderly, those with respiratory or heart disease, or children under age five, the flu can be very serious. Contrary to common belief, the flu is primarily a respiratory disease. You cannot have a "stomach flu." Nausea, vomiting, and diarrhea are extremely rare with the flu, except in small children. The period of November through March is the typical flu season.

To date, three major varieties of flu virus have been discovered, with many different strains existing within each variety. The "A" form of the virus is generally the most virulent, followed by the "B" and "C" varieties. If you contract one form of flu you may develop immunity to it, but you will not necessarily be immune to other forms of the disease. Little can be done to treat flu patients once the infection has become established. Some vaccines have proved effective against certain strains of flu virus, but they are totally ineffective against others. In spite of minor risks, it is recommended that people over age 65, pregnant women, people with heart or lung disease, and those with certain other illnesses be vaccinated. In fall of 2003, an inhaled vaccine called FluMist was released for use with healthy, nonpregnant adults up to age 49. Because the vaccine contains a weakened version of the live virus, people who receive the vaccine may pose a risk to anyone with a weakened immune system who is around them. More investigation into the risks are needed.

Infectious Mononucleosis Initial symptoms of mononucleosis, or mono, include sore throat, fever, headache, nausea, chills, and pervasive weakness/fatigue. As the disease progresses, lymph nodes may enlarge, and jaundice, spleen enlargement, aching joints, and body rashes may occur.

Caused by the *Epstein-Barr virus,* mono is readily detected through a *monospot test,* a blood test that measures the percentage of specific forms of white blood cells. Because many viruses are caused by transmission of body fluids, many people once believed that young people contracted mono through kissing (hence its nickname, "the kissing disease"). Although this is still considered a possible cause, mono is not believed to be highly contagious. It does not appear to be easily spread through normal, everyday personal contact.

Treatment of mono is often a lengthy process that involves bed rest, balanced nutrition, and medications. Gradually, the body develops immunity to the disease, and the person returns to normal activity.

Hepatitis One of the most highly publicized viral diseases is **hepatitis,** a virally caused inflammation of the liver. Hepatitis symptoms include fever, headache, nausea, loss of appetite, skin rashes, pain in the upper right abdomen, dark yellow (with brownish tinge) urine, and jaundice (yellowing of the whites of the eyes and the skin). In some regions of the United States and among certain segments of the population, hepatitis has reached epidemic proportions. Internationally, viral hepatitis is a major contributor to acute and chronic liver disease and accounts for high morbidity and mortality. Currently, there are seven known forms, with the following three indicating the highest rate of incidence (see the Centers for Disease Control and Prevention [CDC] website for further information on the types not discussed here).

- *Hepatitis A (HAV).* HAV is contracted from eating food or drinking water contaminated with human excrement. Each year, more than 150,000 people in the United States are infected, typically through something in the household, sexual contact, day care attendance, or international travel. Fortunately, people with HAV do not become chronic carriers.
- *Hepatitis B (HBV).* This disease, spread primarily through body fluids, particularly during unprotected sex, can lead to chronic liver disease or liver cancer. However, it can also be contracted via sharing needles when injecting drugs, or passed by an infected mother to her baby during birth. One of the fastest growing sexually transmitted infections (STIs) in the United States, with more than 300,000 new cases per year, HBV infection is more prevalent than human immunodeficiency virus (HIV). More than 1.2 million people are chronic carriers. Most people recover within six months, although some become chronic carriers.
- *Hepatitis C (HCV).* HCV infections are on an epidemic rise in many regions of the world, as resistant forms are emerging. Currently, it is estimated that there are 150,000 new cases of HCV in the United States each year, with more than 4 million people infected. More than 85 percent of those infected develop chronic infections; if the infection is left untreated, the person may develop cirrhosis of the liver, liver cancer, or liver failure. Liver failure due to chronic HCV is the leading cause of liver transplants in the United States. Some cases can be traced to blood transfusions or organ transplants.

In the United States, hepatitis continues to be a major threat in spite of a safe blood supply and massive efforts at education about hand washing (HAV) and safer sex (primarily HBV). Treatment of all forms of viral hepatitis is somewhat limited.

Measles **Measles** is a viral disorder that often affects young children. Symptoms, appearing about ten days after exposure, include an itchy rash and a high fever. **German measles (rubella)** is a milder viral infection that is believed to be transmitted by inhalation, after which it multiplies in the upper respiratory tract and passes into the bloodstream. It causes a rash, especially on the upper extremities. It is not generally a serious health threat and usually runs its course in three to four days. The major exceptions to this rule are newborns and pregnant women. Rubella can damage a fetus, particularly during the first trimester, by creating a condition known as congenital rubella in which the infant may be born blind, deaf, cognitively impaired, or with heart defects. Immunization has reduced the incidence of both measles and German measles. Infections in children not immunized against measles can lead to fever-induced problems such as rheumatic heart disease, kidney damage, and neurological disorders.

Other Pathogens

Fungi Hundreds of species of fungi, multicellular or unicellular primitive plants, inhabit our environment. Many fungi are useful, providing such foodstuffs as edible mushrooms and some cheeses. But some species of fungi can produce infections. Candidiasis (a vaginal yeast infection), athlete's foot, ringworm, and jock itch are examples of fungal diseases. Keeping the affected area clean and dry plus treatment with appropriate medications will generally bring prompt relief.

Protozoa **Protozoa** are microscopic, single-celled organisms that are generally associated with tropical diseases such as African sleeping sickness and malaria. Although these pathogens are prevalent in nonindustrialized countries, they are largely controlled in the United States. The most common protozoal disease in the United States is *trichomoniasis*, which we will discuss later in this chapter's section on STIs. A common water-borne protozoan disease in many regions of the country is *giardiasis*. People who drink or are exposed to the *Giardia* pathogen may suffer intestinal pain and discomfort weeks after infection. Protection of water supplies is the key to prevention.

Parasitic Worms **Parasitic worms** are the largest of the pathogens. Ranging in size from the small pinworms typically found in children to the relatively large tapeworms found in all warm-blooded animals, most parasitic worms are more a nuisance than a threat. Of special note today are the worm infestations associated with eating raw fish in Japanese sushi restaurants. Cooking fish and other foods to temperatures sufficient to kill the worms and their eggs can prevent this.

Prions A **prion,** or unconventional virus, is a self-replicating, protein-based *agent* that can infect humans and other animals. Believed to be the underlying cause of spongiform diseases such as "mad cow disease," this agent systematically destroys brain cells. We will say more about prion-based diseases later in this chapter.

YOUR BODY'S DEFENSES: KEEPING YOU WELL

Although all the pathogens just described pose a threat if they take hold in your body, the chances that they will do so are actually quite small. First, they must overcome a number of effective barriers, many of which were established in your body before you were born.

Physical and Chemical Defenses

Perhaps our most critical early defense system is the skin. Layered to provide an intricate web of barriers, the skin allows few pathogens to enter. **Enzymes,** complex proteins manufactured by the body that appear in body secretions such as sweat, provide additional protection; they destroy microorganisms on skin surfaces by producing inhospitable pH levels. Microorganisms that flourish at a selected pH will be weakened or destroyed as these changes occur. A third protection is our frequent slight elevations in body temperature, which create an inhospitable environment for many pathogens. Only when cracks or breaks occur in the skin can pathogens gain easy access to the body.

The linings of the body provide yet another protection. Mucous membranes in the respiratory tract and other linings of the body trap and engulf invading organisms. *Cilia,* hairlike projections in the lungs and respiratory tract, sweep invaders toward body openings, where they are expelled. Tears, nasal secretions, earwax, and other secretions found at body entrances contain enzymes designed to destroy or neutralize pathogens. Finally, any organism that manages to breach such initial lines of defense faces a formidable specialized network of defenses thrown up by the immune system.

The Immune System: Your Body Fights Back

Immunity is a condition of being able to resist a particular disease by counteracting the substance that produces the disease. Any substance capable of triggering an immune response is called an **antigen.** An antigen can be a virus, a bacterium, a fungus, a parasite, or a tissue or cell from another individual. When invaded by an antigen, the body responds by forming substances called **antibodies** that are matched to the specific antigen much as a key is matched to a lock. Antibodies belong to a mass of large molecules known as *immunoglobulins,* a group of nine chemically distinct protein substances, each of which plays a role in neutralizing, setting up for destruction, or actually destroying antigens.

Once an antigen breaches the body's initial defenses, the body begins a process of antigen analysis. It considers the size and shape of the invader, verifies that the antigen is not part of the body itself, and then produces a specific antibody to destroy or weaken the antigen. This process, which is much more complex than described here, is part of a system called *humoral immune responses.* Humoral immunity is the body's major defense against many bacteria and bacterial toxins.

Cell-mediated immunity is characterized by the formation of a population of lymphocytes that can attack and destroy the foreign invader. These lymphocytes constitute the body's main defense against viruses, fungi, parasites, and some bacteria. Key players in this immune response are specialized groups of white blood cells known as *macrophages* (a type of phagocytic, or cell-eating, cell) and *lymphocytes,* other white blood cells in the blood, lymph nodes, bone marrow, and certain glands.

Two forms of lymphocytes in particular, the *B-lymphocytes* (B-cells) and *T-lymphocytes* (T-cells), are involved in the immune response. There are different types of B-cells, named according to the area of the body in which they develop. Most are manufactured in the soft tissue of the hollow shafts of the long bones. T-cells, in contrast, develop and multiply in the thymus, a multilobed organ that lies behind the breastbone. T-cells assist the immune system in several ways. *Regulatory T-cells* help direct the activities of the immune system and assist other cells, particularly B-cells, to produce antibodies. Dubbed "helper T's," these cells are essential for activating B-cells, other T-cells, and macrophages. Another form of T-cell, known as the "killer T" or "cytotoxic T," directly attacks infected or malignant cells. Killer T-cells enable the body to rid itself of cells that have been infected by viruses or transformed by cancer; they are also responsible for the rejection of tissue and organ grafts. The third type of T-cell, "suppressor T," turns off or suppresses the activity of B-cells, killer T-cells, and macrophages. Suppressor T-cells circulate in the bloodstream and lymphatic system where they neutralize or destroy antigens, thus enhancing the effects of the immune response and helping to return the activated immune system to normal levels. After a successful attack on a pathogen, some of the attacker T- and B-cells are preserved as *memory T-* and *B-cells* that enable the body to quickly recognize and respond to subsequent attacks by the same kind of organism at a later time. Thus, macrophages, T- and B-cells, and antibodies are the key factors in mounting an immune response.

Once people have survived infectious diseases, they become immune to those diseases, which means that in all probability they will not develop them again. Upon subsequent attack by the disease-causing microorganism, their memory T- and B-cells are quickly activated to come to their defense.

Autoimmune Diseases Although white blood cells and the antigen–antibody response generally work in our favor by neutralizing or destroying harmful antigens, the body sometimes makes a mistake and targets its own tissue as the enemy, builds up antibodies against that tissue, and attempts to destroy it. This is known as *autoimmune disease* (*auto* means "self"). Common autoimmune disorders are rheumatoid arthritis, systemic lupus erythematosus (SLE), and myasthenia gravis.

In some cases, the antigen–antibody response completely fails to function. The result is a form of *immune deficiency syndrome*. Perhaps the most dramatic case of this syndrome was the "bubble boy," a youngster who died in 1984 after living his short life inside a sealed-off environment designed to protect him from all antigens. A much more common immune system disorder is *acquired immune deficiency syndrome (AIDS)*, which we will discuss later in this chapter.

Fever

If an infection is localized, pus formation, redness, swelling, and irritation often occur. These symptoms indicate that the invading organisms are being fought systematically. Another indication is the development of a fever, or a rise in body temperature above the norm of 98.6°F. Fever is frequently caused by toxins secreted by pathogens that interfere with the control of body temperature. Although this elevated temperature is often harmful to the body, it is also believed to act as a form of protection. Raising body temperature by even one or two degrees provides an environment that destroys some disease-causing organisms. A fever also stimulates the body to produce more white blood cells, which destroy more invaders.

Pain

Although we do not usually think of pain as a defense mechanism, it is a response to injury, and it plays a valuable role in the body's response to invasion. Pain may be either *direct pain*, caused by the stimulation of nerve endings in an affected area, or **referred pain,** meaning that it is present in one place although the source is elsewhere. Most pain responses are accompanied by inflammation. Pain tends to be the earliest sign that an injury has occurred and often causes the person to slow down or stop the activity that was aggravating the injury, thereby protecting against further damage. Because it is often one of the first warnings of disease, persistent pain should not be overlooked or masked with short-term pain relievers.

Vaccines: Bolstering Your Immunity

Recall that once people have been exposed to a specific pathogen, subsequent attacks will activate their memory T- and B-cells, thus giving them immunity. This is the principle on which **vaccination** is based.

A vaccine consists of killed or attenuated (weakened) versions of a disease-causing microorganism, or an antigen that is similar to but less dangerous than the disease antigen. It is administered to stimulate the person's immune system to produce antibodies against future attacks—without actually causing the disease. Vaccines are given orally or by injection, and this form of artificial immunity is termed **acquired immunity,** in contrast to **natural immunity,** which a mother passes to her fetus via their shared blood supply.

Depending on the virulence of the organism, vaccines containing live, attenuated, or dead organisms are given for a variety of diseases. In some instances, if a person is already weakened by other health problems, vaccination may provoke an actual mild case of the disease. Figure 16.2 on page 252 shows the recommended schedule for childhood vaccinations.

EMERGING AND RESURGENT DISEASES

Although our immune systems are remarkably adept at responding to many challenges, they are threatened by an army of microbes that is so diverse, virulent, and insidious that the invaders appear to be gaining ground. According to the WHO's *World Health Report* issued in 2002, trends such as the aging

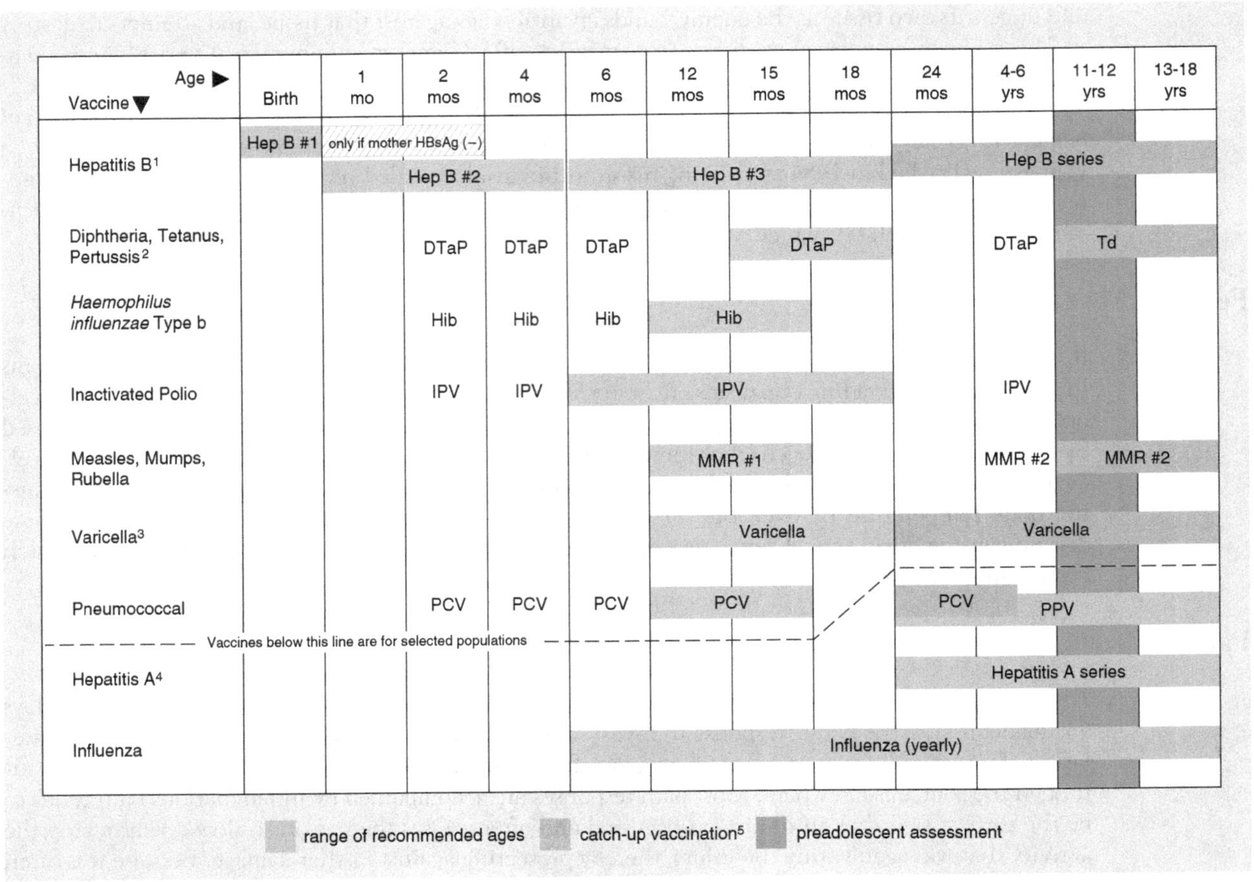

FIGURE 16.2. Recommended Childhood and Adolescent Immunization Schedule, 2003

1. Mothers who have tested positive for hepatitis B (HBV) should consult their doctors about their infant's vaccinations.
2. Tetanus and diphtheria toxoids (Td) are recommended at age 11–12 years if at least 5 years have elapsed since the last dose of tetanus and diphtheria vaccines. Subsequent routine Td boosters are recommended every 10 years.
3. Varicella is recommended at any visit or after age 12 months for children who lack a reliable history of chicken pox. Susceptible persons over 13 years should receive 2 doses, given at least 4 weeks apart.
4. Hepatitis A (HAV) vaccine is recommended for use in selected states and regions and for certain high-risk groups; consult your physician.
5. "Catch-up vaccination" indicates age groups that warrant special effort to administer any missed vaccines.

Source: Centers for Disease Control and Prevention, "Recommended Childhood and Adolescent Immunization Schedule," *Morbidity and Mortality Report* 52, no. 4 (2003): Q1–Q4.

of the population (the young and old are particularly vulnerable), the urbanization of developing countries, poverty, environmental pollution, globalization of the food supply, and crumbling health care systems bode very badly for the future. As international travel increases (more than 1 million people per day cross international boundaries), with germs transported from remote regions of developing countries to huge urban centers within a matter of hours, the likelihood of infection by microbes previously unknown on U.S. soil increases. Table 16.1 identifies major contributors to the emergence and resurgence of infectious diseases.

Tiny Microbes: Lethal Threats

Today's arsenal of antibiotics appears to be increasingly ineffective. Penicillin-resistant strains of diseases are on the rise as microbes become able to outlast and outsmart even the best of our antibiotic weapons. Old scourges are back, and new ones are emerging.

Table 16.1. FACTORS CONTRIBUTING TO EMERGENT/RESURGENT DISEASE SPREAD AND POSSIBLE SOLUTIONS

Contributing Factors	***Possible Solutions***
Hardier bugs: tiny size, adaptability, resistant strains, misuse of antibiotics	Increased pharmaceutical efforts, new drug development, selective use of new drugs; improved vaccination rates; funding of new research
Failure to prioritize public health initiatives on national level	Increased government funding; improved efforts aimed at prevention and intervention (Less than 1 percent of the federal budget goes to prevention programs.)
Explosive population growth: resource degradation, overcrowding, land use atrocities, increased urbanization	Population control, wise use of natural resources, environmental controls, reduced deforestation, and increased pollution prevention efforts
International travel	Education or risk reduction; restrictions related to unvaccinated populations; improved air quality and venting on commercial airlines
Human behaviors, particularly intravenous (IV) drug use and risky sexual behavior	Education about risky behaviors; incentives for improved behaviors; increased personal motivation
Vector management failures: widespread overuse/misuse of pesticides and antimicrobial agents that hasten resistance	Management of pesticide use; focus on pollution prevention; regulation; enforcement of laws
Food and water contamination; globalization of food supply and centralized processing	Control of population growth; animal controls; food controls; improved environmental legislation; food safety; pollution prevention
Complacency and apathy	Education—develop "we" mentality rather than "me" mentality
Poverty	Government support; international aid for vaccination programs, early diagnosis, and treatment; care for disadvantaged
War and mass refugee migration, famine, disasters	Government intervention; international aid
Aging of population	Support for prevention/intervention against controllable age-related health problems
Irrigation, deforestation, and reforestation projects that alter habitats of disease-carrying insects and animals	Improved techniques for conservation; responsible use of resources; policies and programs that protect environment
Increased human contact with tropical rainforests and other wilderness habitats that are reservoirs for insects and animals that harbor unknown infectious agents	Increased regulation to reduce human impact; more research to improve interactions between humans and environment

Sources: Author, plus information from U.S. Department of Health and Human Services, Centers for Disease Control and Prevention, "Emerging Infectious Diseases: A Strategy for the 21st Century," 2001. www.cdc.gov/ncidod/emergplan

"Mad Cow Disease" The American beef industry has been the subject of a great amount of media attention, with the first confirmed case of *bovine spongiform encephalitis* (BSE, or "mad cow disease") being detected in December 2003. BSE may be linked to a disease in humans known as *new variant Creutzfeldt-Jakob disease* (NvCJD). Both disorders are invariably fatal brain diseases with unusually long incubation periods measured in years, and both are caused by unconventional transmittable agents known as *prions*.

BSE is thought to have been transmitted when cows were fed a protein-based substance (slaughterhouse leftovers from sheep and other cows) to help them put on weight and grow faster. Failure to treat this protein by-product sufficiently to kill the BSE organism allowed it to infect the cows. The disease is believed to be transmitted to humans through the meat of these slaughtered cows. The resultant variant of BSE in humans, known as NvCJD disease and characterized by progressively worsening neurological damage and possible death, was noted in ten people in England and linked by some studies to the BSE-diseased cows. It should be noted that this link has not yet been scientifically verified.

A related prion-caused disease, *chronic wasting disease,* has been found in deer and is similar to BSE. Studies are underway investigating the implications of this disease for human health.

Dengue and Dengue Hemorrhagic Fever Transmitted by mosquitoes, **dengue** viruses are the most widespread insect-borne viruses in the world. Today, dengue is found on most continents, and more than one half of all United Nations member states are threatened. Dengue symptoms include flulike nausea, aches, and chronic fatigue and weakness. As urban areas become increasingly infected with mosquitoes, nearly 1.5 billion people, including about 600 million children, are at risk. Each year, it is estimated that more than 100 million people are infected, and more than 8,000 die. A more serious form of the disease, **dengue hemorrhagic fever,** can kill children in 6 to 12 hours, as the virus causes capillaries to leak and spill fluid and blood into surrounding tissue. Dengue is on the rise in the United States, largely because of increased international travel.

Ebola Hemorrhagic Fever (Ebola HF) Another emerging disease, Ebola HF is a severe, often fatal disease in humans and nonhuman primates (monkeys, gorillas, and chimpanzees). Although much about Ebola HF is unknown, researchers believe that the virus is animal-borne and normally occurs in animal hosts that are native to the African continent. The virus is spread via direct contact with blood and/or secretions, and possibly through the air. With an incubation period of 2 to 21 days, the course of the disease is quick and characterized by fever, headache, joint and muscle aches, sore throat, and weakness, followed by diarrhea, vomiting, stomach pain, and internal and external bleeding. Although there have been no known cases of human transmission in the United States, several outbreaks have occurred in various regions of Africa. In 1995, an Ebola HF outbreak in Zaire killed 245 of the 316 people infected, thus forcing strict government-enforced quarantine of the entire region. Subsequent infections in other regions of the world have caused increasing concern. Fortunately, Ebola HF is not as prevalent worldwide as dengue fever.

Cryptosporidium In 1993, the intestinal parasite *Cryptosporidium,* or crypto, infected the municipal water supply of Milwaukee, Wisconsin. The result was the largest water-borne protozoan disease outbreak ever recognized in this country; it caused many deaths and sickened hundreds of thousands of people with acute diarrhea. Exactly how the water supply became infected remains in question; however, the fact that humans, birds, and animals can carry the infective agent and be highly contagious suggests many possible routes. Today crypto is one of the most common waterborne diseases in the United States.

Escherichia coli O157:H7 *Escherichia coli O157:H7* is one of more than 170 types of *E. coli* bacteria that can infect humans. Commonly called *E. coli 0157:H7,* it produces a lethal toxin and can cause severe illness or death. Eating ground beef that is rare or undercooked is a common way of becoming infected. Drinking unpasteurized milk or juices and drinking or swimming in sewage-contaminated water or public pools can also cause infection via ingestion of feces that contain *E. coli.* In 2003, several children were infected at a fair in Oregon when they petted infected farm animals and did not wash their hands. Recent findings indicate that simple changes in the way cattle are fed prior to slaughter may reduce the growth of *E. coli* in cattle stomachs.

Cholera Cholera, an infectious disease transmitted through fecal contamination of food or water supplies, has been rare in the United States since the early 1900s. Recent epidemic outbreaks in the Western Hemisphere (more than 900,000 cases), however, have started to affect the United States. Efforts to control cholera may be increasingly difficult as international travel and trade increase.

Hantavirus Transmitted via rodent feces, this virus was responsible for many deaths in the southwestern United States in 1994 before experts were able to identify the culprit. Victims were believed to have come into contact with this organism through breathing the virus-laden dust in rodent-infested homes. Within hours, victims showed serious symptoms as their lungs filled with fluid; they subsequently experienced respiratory collapse and died. Today, cases of hantavirus have been noted in more than 20 states, and vaccines are being developed to counteract it.

Bioterrorism: The New Global Threat The idea of using infectious microorganisms as weapons is not new. In fact, in the English wars with Native Americans, blankets impregnated with scabs from patients with smallpox were traded to Native Americans in hopes of causing disease. The threat of deliberate spreading of deadly microorganisms is a topic of much discussion among today's world leaders, particularly after the instances of anthrax delivered via the mail following the September 11, 2001, terrorist attacks. For more on those biological threats considered to pose the greatest risk.

SEXUALLY TRANSMITTED INFECTIONS

Sexually transmitted infections (STIs) have been with human beings since earliest recorded history. Today, there are more than 20 known types of STIs. Once referred to as venereal diseases and then as sexually transmitted diseases, the current terminology is more reflective of the number and types of these communicable diseases. More virulent strains and more antibiotic-resistant forms spell trouble for at-risk populations in the days ahead.

A report issued by the CDC in 2000 indicated that there were 16.2 million new occurrences of STIs in 1999, an increase of more than 3.5 million since 1988. Although exact numbers are not available for each STI, the number of cases did increase for several in 2001 after years of decline. Syphilis was among those showing the greatest increase. According to Felicia Stewart of the Kaiser Family Health Foundation, "[T]here is no indication that STIs are coming rapidly under control. . . . In fact, people vastly underestimate risks and fail to take precautions. A Kaiser survey found that just 14% of men and 8% of women felt at risk for STIs, even though at least one third will get one."

Early symptoms of an STI are often mild (Figure 16.3). Left untreated, some of these infections can have grave consequences, such as sterility, blindness, central nervous system destruction, disfigurement, and even death. Infants born to mothers carrying the organisms for these infections are at risk

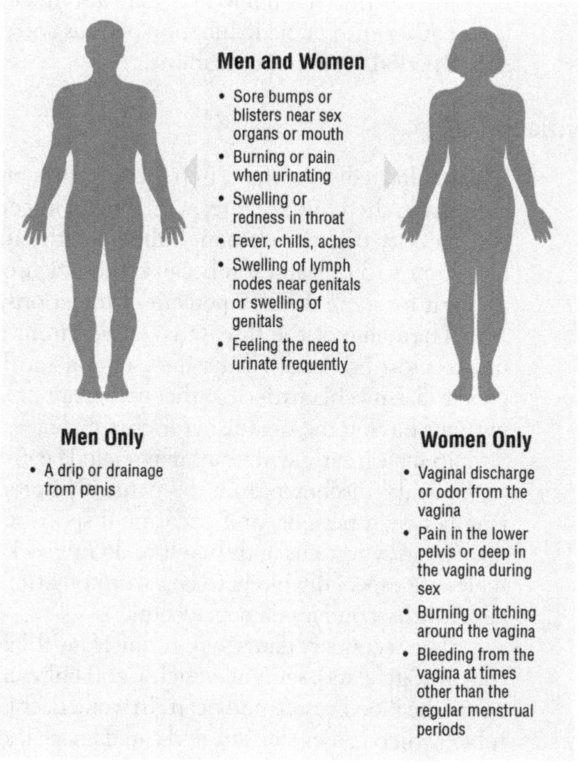

FIGURE 16.3. Signs or Symptoms of an STI

for a variety of health problems. As with many communicable diseases, much of the pain, suffering, and anguish associated with STIs can be eliminated through education, responsible action, simple preventive strategies, and prompt treatment.

Possible Causes: Why Me?

Several reasons have been proposed to explain the present high rates of STIs. The first relates to the moral and social stigma associated with these infections. Shame and embarrassment often keep infected people from seeking treatment. Unfortunately, they usually continue to be sexually active, thereby infecting unsuspecting partners. People who are uncomfortable discussing sexual issues may also be less likely to use and ask their partners to use condoms to protect against STIs and pregnancy.

Another reason proposed for the STI epidemic is our culture's casual attitude about sex. Bombarded by media hype that glamorizes easy sex, many people take sexual partners without considering the consequences. Others are pressured into sexual relationships they don't really want. Generally, the more sexual partners a person has, the greater the risk for contracting an STI. Evaluate your own attitude about STIs by completing the Assess Yourself box on page 258.

Ignorance—about the infections, their symptoms, and the fact that someone can be asymptomatic (symptom-free) but still infected—is also a factor. A person who is infected but asymptomatic can unknowingly spread an STI to an unsuspecting partner, who may, in turn, ignore or misinterpret any symptoms. By the time either partner seeks medical help, he or she may have infected several others.

Modes of Transmission

STIs are generally spread through some form of intimate sexual contact. Sexual intercourse, oral–genital contact, hand–genital contact, and anal intercourse are the most common modes of transmission. More rarely, pathogens for STIs are transmitted from mouth to mouth or through contact with fluids from body sores. Although each STI is a different infection caused by a different pathogen, all STI pathogens prefer dark, moist places, especially the mucous membranes lining the reproductive organs. Most of them are susceptible to light, excess heat, cold, and dryness, and many die quickly on exposure to air. (A toilet seat is not a likely breeding ground for most bacterial or viral STIs!) Although most STIs are passed on by sexual contact, other kinds of close contact, such as sleeping on sheets used by someone who has pubic lice, may also infect you. Like other communicable infections, STIs have both pathogen-specific incubation periods and periods of time during which transmission is most likely, called periods of communicability.

Chlamydia

Chlamydia, a disease that often presents no symptoms, tops the list of the most commonly reported infections in the United States. Chlamydia infects about 800,000 people annually in the United States, the majority of them women. Public health officials believe that the actual number of cases is probably closer to 3 or 4 million because these figures represent only those cases reported. College students account for more than 10 percent of infections, and these numbers seem to be increasing yearly.

The name of the disease is derived from the Greek verb *chlamys*, meaning "to cloak," because, unlike most bacteria, *Chlamydia* bacteria can live and grow only inside other cells. Although many people classify chlamydia as either *nonspecific* or *nongonococcal urethritis (NGU)*, a person may have NGU without having the organism for chlamydia.

In males, early symptoms may include painful and difficult urination, frequent urination, and a watery, puslike discharge from the penis. Symptoms in females may include a yellowish discharge, spotting between periods, and occasional spotting after intercourse. However, many chlamydia victims display no symptoms and therefore do not seek help until the disease has done secondary damage. Females are especially likely to be asymptomatic; more than 70 percent do not realize they have the disease until secondary damage occurs.

The secondary damage resulting from chlamydia is serious in both sexes. Men can suffer damage to the prostate gland, seminal vesicles, and bulbourethral glands as well as arthritislike symptoms and damage to the blood vessels and heart. In women, chlamydia-related infection can injure the cervix or fallopian tubes, which causes sterility, and can damage the inner pelvic structure, which leads to pelvic inflammatory disease (PID). If an infected woman becomes pregnant, she has a high risk for miscarriage and stillbirth. *Chlamydia* may also be responsible for one type of **conjunctivitis,** an eye infection that affects not only adults but also infants, who can contract the disease from an infected mother during delivery. Untreated conjunctivitis can cause blindness. If detected early, chlamydia is easily treatable with antibiotics.

What do you think?

Even though many college students have heard about the risks of STIs and AIDS, why do so many fail to use condoms and take other precautions? • What actions could be taken to make more of your friends heed the warnings about STIs?

Pelvic Inflammatory Disease

Pelvic inflammatory disease (PID) is a term used to describe a number of infections of the uterus, fallopian tubes, and ovaries. Although PID often results from an untreated STI, especially chlamydia or gonorrhea, it is not actually an STI. Several nonsexual factors increase the risk of PID, particularly excessive vaginal douching, cigarette smoking, and substance abuse.

In the United States, PID affects 11 percent of women of reproductive age. Approximately 1 million women experience PID each year, and 20 percent require hospitalization for treatment. Symptoms vary but generally include acute inflammation of the pelvic cavity, severe pain in the lower abdomen, menstrual irregularities, fever, nausea, painful intercourse, tubal pregnancies, and severe depression. Major consequences of untreated PID are infertility, ectopic pregnancy, chronic pelvic pain, and recurrent upper genital infections. Risk factors include young age at first sexual intercourse, multiple sex partners, high frequency of sexual intercourse, and change of sexual partners within the past 30 days. Regular gynecological examinations and early treatment for STI symptoms reduce risk.

Gonorrhea

One of the most common STIs in the United States, **gonorrhea** is surpassed only by chlamydia in number of cases. The Institute of Medicine estimates that there are more than 800,000 cases per year and that large numbers go unreported. Health economists estimate that the annual cost of gonorrhea and its complications is more than $1.1 billion. Caused by the bacterial pathogen *Neisseria gonorrhoeae,* this infection primarily infects the linings of the urethra, genital tract, pharynx, and rectum. It may spread to the eyes or other body regions via the hands or body fluids, typically during vaginal, oral, or anal sex. Most victims are males between the ages of 20 and 24; sexually active females between the ages of 15 and 19 are also at high risk.

In males, a typical symptom is a white milky discharge from the penis accompanied by painful, burning urination two to nine days after contact. This is usually enough to send most men to the physician for treatment. However, about 20 percent of all males with gonorrhea are asymptomatic.

In females, the situation is just the opposite: only 20 percent experience any discharge, and few develop a burning sensation upon urinating until much later in the course of the infection (if ever). The organism can remain in the woman's vagina, cervix, uterus, or fallopian tubes for long periods with no apparent symptoms other than an occasional slight fever. Thus, a woman can be unaware that she has been infected and is infecting her sexual partners.

If the infection is detected early, antibiotic treatment is generally effective within a short period of time. If the infection goes undetected in a woman, it can spread throughout the genital–urinary tract to the fallopian tubes and ovaries, thus causing sterility or, at the very least, severe inflammation and PID. The bacteria can also spread up the reproductive tract or, more rarely, can spread through the blood and infect the joints, heart valves, or brain. If an infected woman becomes pregnant, the infection can cause conjunctivitis in her infant. To prevent this, physicians routinely administer silver nitrate or penicillin preparations to the eyes of newborn babies.

Untreated gonorrhea may spread to the prostate, testicles, urinary tract, kidney, and bladder. Blockage of the vasa deferentia due to scar tissue may cause sterility. In some cases, the penis develops a painful curvature during erection.

ASSESS YOURSELF

Sexually Transmitted Infections: Attitude and Belief Scale

The following quiz will help you evaluate whether your beliefs and attitudes about STIs lead you to take risks that increase your risk of infection.

DIRECTIONS

Indicate that you believe the following items are true or false by circling the T or the F. Then consult the answer key that follows.

1. You can usually tell whether someone is infected with an STI, especially HIV infection.	T	F
2. Chances are that if you haven't caught an STI by now, you probably have a natural immunity and won't get infected in the future.	T	F
3. A person who is successfully treated for an STI needn't worry about getting it again.	T	F
4. So long as you keep yourself fit and healthy, you needn't worry about STIs.	T	F
5. The best way for sexually active people to protect themselves from STIs is to practice safer sex.	T	F
6. The only way to catch an STI is to have sex with someone who has one.	T	F
7. Talking about STIs with a partner is so embarrassing that it's better not to raise the subject and instead hope the other person will.	T	F
8. STIs are mostly a problem for people who have numerous sex partners.	T	F
9. You don't need to worry about contracting an STI as long as you wash yourself thoroughly with soap and hot water immediately after sex.	T	F
10. You don't need to worry about contracting AIDS if no one you know has ever come down with it.	T	F
11. When it comes to STIs, it's all in the cards. Either you're lucky, or you're not.	T	F
12. The time to worry about STIs is when you come down with one.	T	F
13. As long as you avoid risky sexual practices, such as anal intercourse, you're pretty safe from STIs.	T	F
14. The time to talk about safer sex is before any sexual contact occurs.	T	F
15. A person needn't be concerned about an STI if the symptoms clear up on their own in a few weeks.	T	F

ASSESS YOURSELF (continued)

ANSWER KEY

1. False. While some STIs have telltale signs, such as the appearance of sores or blisters on the genitals or disagreeable genital odors, others do not. Several STIs, such as chlamydia, gonorrhea (especially in women), internal genital warts, and even HIV infection in its early stages cause few if any obvious signs or symptoms. You often cannot tell whether your partner is infected with an STI. Many of the nicest-looking and best-groomed people carry STIs, often unknowingly. The only way to know whether a person is infected with HIV is by means of an HIV-antibody test.
2. False. If you practice unprotected sex and have not contracted an STI to this point, count your blessings. The thing about good luck is that it eventually runs out.
3. False. Sorry. Successful treatment does not render immunity against reinfection. You still need to take precautions to avoid reinfection, even if you have had an STI in the past and were successfully treated. If you answered true to this item, you're not alone. About one in five college students polled in a recent survey of more than 5,500 college students across Canada believed that a person who gets an STI cannot get it again.
4. False. Even people in prime physical condition can be felled by the tiniest of microbes that cause STIs. Physical fitness is no protection against these microscopic invaders.
5. True. If you are sexually active, practicing safer sex is the best protection against contracting an STI.
6. False. STIs can also be transmitted through nonsexual means, such as by sharing contaminated needles or, in some cases, through contact with disease-causing organisms on towels and bed sheets or even toilet seats.
7. False. Because of the social stigma attached to STIs, it's understandable that you may feel embarrassed about raising the subject with your partner. But don't let embarrassment prevent you from taking steps to protect your own and your partner's welfare.
8. False. It stands to reason that people who are sexually active with numerous partners stand a greater chance that one of their sexual partners will carry an STI. Nevertheless, all it takes is one infected partner to pass along an STI to you, even if he or she is the only partner you've had, or even if the two of you had sex only once. STIs are a potential problem for anyone who is sexually active.
9. False. While washing your genitals immediately after sex may have some limited protective value, it is no substitute for practicing safer sex.
10. False. You can never know whether you may be the first among your friends and acquaintances to become infected. Moreover, symptoms of HIV infection may not appear for years after initial infection with the virus, so you may have sexual contacts with people who are infected but don't know it and who are capable of passing along the virus to you. You, in turn, may then pass it along to others, whether or not you are aware of any symptoms.
11. False. Nonsense. While luck may play a part in determining whether you have a sexual contact with an infected partner, you can significantly reduce your risk of contracting an STI.
12. False. The time to start thinking about STIs (thinking helps, but worrying only makes you more anxious than you need be) is now, not after you have contracted an infection. Some STIs, like herpes and AIDS, cannot be cured. The only real protection you have against them is prevention.
13. False. Any sexual contact between the genitals, or between the genitals and the anus, or between the mouth and genitals, is risky if one of the partners is infected with an STI.
14. True. Unfortunately, too many couples wait until they have commenced sexual relations to have "a talk." By then it may already be too late to prevent the transmission of an STI. The time to talk is before any intimate sexual contact occurs.
15. False. Several STIs, notably syphilis, HIV infection, and herpes, may produce initial symptoms that clear up in a few weeks. But while the early symptoms may subside, the infection is still at work within the body and requires medical attention. Also, as noted previously, the infected person is capable of passing along the infection to others, regardless of whether noticeable symptoms were ever present.

INTERPRETING YOUR SCORE

First, add up the number of items you got right. The higher your score, the lower your risk. The lower your score, the greater your risk. A score of 13 correct or better may indicate that your attitudes toward STIs would probably decrease your risk of contracting them. Yet, even one wrong response on this test may increase your risk of contracting an STI. You should also recognize that attitudes have little effect on behavior unless they are carried into action. Knowledge alone isn't sufficient to protect yourself from STIs. You need to ask yourself how you are going to put knowledge into action by changing your behavior to reduce your chances of contracting an STI.

Source: Jeffrey S. Nevid with Fern Gotfried, *Choices: Sex in the Age of STDs* (Boston: Allyn and Bacon, 1995), 10–13.

Syphilis

Syphilis is also caused by a bacterial organism, the *spirochete* known as *Treponema pallidum*. Because it is extremely delicate and dies readily upon exposure to air, dryness, or cold, the organism is generally transferred only through direct sexual contact. Typically, this means contact between sexual organs during intercourse, but in rare instances, the organism enters the body through a break in the skin, through deep kissing, or through some other transmission of body fluids.

Syphilis is called the "great imitator" because its symptoms resemble those of several other infections. Left untreated, syphilis generally progresses through distinct stages. It should be noted, however, that some people experience no symptoms at all.

Primary Syphilis The first stage of syphilis, particularly for males, is often characterized by the development of a **chancre** (pronounced "shank-er"), a sore at the site of initial infection. This dime-sized chancre is painless, but it oozes with bacteria, ready to infect an unsuspecting partner. Usually the chancre appears three to four weeks after contact.

In males, the site of the chancre tends to be the penis or scrotum because this is the site where the organism first enters the body. But if the infection was contracted through oral sex, the sore can appear in the mouth, throat, or other "first contact" area. In females, the site of infection is often internal, on the vaginal wall or high on the cervix. Because the chancre is not readily apparent, the likelihood of detection is not great. In both males and females, the chancre will completely disappear in three to six weeks.

Secondary Syphilis From a month to a year after the chancre disappears, secondary symptoms may appear, including a rash or white patches on the skin or on the mucous membranes of the mouth, throat, or genitals. Hair loss may occur, lymph nodes may enlarge, and the victim may develop a slight fever or a headache. In rare cases, sores develop around the mouth or genitals. As during the active chancre phase, these sores contain infectious bacteria, and contact with them can spread the infection. In a few cases, there may be arthritic pain in the joints. Because symptoms vary so much and appear so much later than the sexual contact that caused them, the victim seldom connects the two. The infection thus often goes undetected even at this second stage. Symptoms may persist for a few weeks or months and then disappear, thus leaving the victim thinking that all is well.

Latent Syphilis After the secondary stage, the syphilis spirochetes begin to invade body organs. Symptoms, including infectious lesions, may reappear periodically for two to four years after the secondary period. After this period, the infection is rarely transmitted to others, except during pregnancy, when it can be passed to the fetus. The child will then be born with *congenital syphilis*, which can cause death or severe birth defects such as blindness, deafness, or disfigurement. Because in most cases the fetus does not become infected until after the first trimester, treatment of the mother during this period will usually prevent infection of the fetus.

In some instances, a child born to an infected mother will show no apparent signs of the infection at birth but within several weeks will develop body rashes, a runny nose, and symptoms of paralysis. Congenital syphilis is usually detected before it progresses much further. But sometimes the child's immune system will ward off the invading organism, and further symptoms may not surface until the teenage years. Fortunately, most states protect against congenital syphilis by requiring prospective marriage partners to be tested for syphilis prior to obtaining a marriage license.

If untreated, latent syphilis will progress and infect more and more organs.

Late Syphilis Years after syphilis has entered the body, its effects become all too evident. Late-stage syphilis indications include heart damage, central nervous system damage, blindness, deafness, paralysis, premature senility, and, ultimately, insanity.

Treatment for Syphilis Because the organism is bacterial, it is treated with antibiotics. The major obstacle to treatment is misdiagnosis of this "imitator" infection.

Pubic Lice

Pubic lice, often called "crabs," are small parasites that are usually transmitted during sexual contact. More annoying than dangerous, they move easily from partner to partner during sex. They have an affinity for pubic hair and attach themselves to the base of these hairs, where they deposit their eggs (nits). One to two weeks later, these nits develop into adults that lay eggs and migrate to other body parts, thus perpetuating the cycle.

Treatment includes washing clothing, furniture, and linens that may harbor the eggs. It usually takes two to three weeks to kill all larval forms. Although sexual contact is the most common mode of transmission, you can "catch" pubic lice from lying on sheets that an infected person has slept on. Sleeping in hotel and dormitory rooms in which sheets are not washed regularly, or sitting on toilet seats where the nits or larvae have been dropped and lie in wait for a new carrier, will put you at risk.

Genital HPV

Genital warts (also known as venereal warts or condylomas) are caused by a small group of viruses known as **human papillomaviruses (HPVs).** A person becomes infected when an HPV penetrates the skin and mucous membranes of the genitals or anus through sexual contact. HPV is among the most common forms of STI. The virus appears to be relatively easy to catch. The typical incubation period is from six to eight weeks after contact. Many people have no symptoms, particularly if the warts are located inside the reproductive tract. Others may develop a series of itchy bumps on the genitals that range in size from small pinheads to large cauliflowerlike growths. On dry skin (such as the shaft of the penis), the warts are commonly small, hard, and yellowish-gray, resembling warts that appear on other parts of the body. Genital warts are of two different types: (1) *full-blown genital warts* that are noticeable as tiny bumps or growths, and (2) the much more prevalent *flat warts* that are not usually visible to the naked eye.

Risks and Treatments of Genital Warts Many genital warts eventually disappear on their own. Others grow and generate unsightly flaps of irregular flesh on the external genitalia. If they grow large enough to obstruct urinary flow or become irritated by clothing or sexual intercourse, they can cause significant problems.

The greatest threat from genital warts lies in the apparent relationship between them and a tendency for *dysplasia,* or changes in cells that may lead to a precancerous condition. It is known that within five years after infection, 30 percent of all HPV cases progress to the precancerous stage. If precancerous cases are left untreated, 70 percent of them will result in actual cancer. New research also implicates HPV as a possible risk factor for coronary artery disease, possibly because it causes an inflammatory response in artery walls. In addition, venereal warts pose a threat to a pregnant woman's fetus if it is exposed to the virus during birth. Cesarean deliveries may be considered in serious cases.

Genital warts can be treated with topical medications or removed by being frozen with liquid nitrogen. Large warts may require surgical removal.

Candidiasis *(Moniliasis)*

Unlike many STIs, which are caused by pathogens that come from outside the body, the yeastlike fungus caused by the *Candida albicans* organism normally inhabits the vaginal tract in most women. Only under certain conditions, in which the normal chemical balance of the vagina is disturbed, will these organisms multiply and cause problems.

The likelihood of **candidiasis** (also known as moniliasis or a *yeast infection*) increases if a woman has diabetes; if her immune system is overtaxed or malfunctioning; if she is taking birth control pills, other hormones, or broad-spectrum antibiotics; or if she uses douches or spermicides. All of these factors decrease the acidity of the vagina and create favorable conditions for a yeastlike infection.

Symptoms of candidiasis include severe itching and burning of the vagina and vulva, swelling of the vulva, and a white, cheesy vaginal discharge. These symptoms are collectively called **vaginitis,** or inflammation of the vagina. When this microbe infects the mouth, whitish patches form, and the condition is referred to as *thrush.* This monilial infection also occurs in males and is easily transmitted between sexual partners.

Candidiasis strikes at least half a million American women a year. Antifungal drugs applied on the surface or by suppository usually cure it in just a few days. For approximately one out of ten women, however, nothing seems to work, and the infection returns again and again. Symptoms can be aggravated by contact of the vagina with soaps, douches, perfumed toilet paper, chlorinated water, and spermicides. Tight-fitting jeans and pantyhose can provide the combination of moisture and irritant the organism thrives on.

Trichomoniasis

Unlike many STIs, **trichomoniasis** is caused by a protozoan. Although as many as half of the men and women in the United States may carry this organism, most remain free of symptoms until their bodily defenses are weakened. Both men and women may transmit the infection, but women are the more likely candidates for infection. Symptoms include a foamy, yellowish, unpleasant-smelling discharge accompanied by a burning sensation, itching, and painful urination. These symptoms are most likely to occur during or shortly after menstruation, but they can appear at any time or be absent altogether. Although usually transmitted by sexual contact, the "trich" organism can also be spread by toilet seats, wet towels, or other items that have discharged fluids on them. You can also contract trichomoniasis by sitting naked on the locker room bench at your local gym. Treatment includes oral metronidazole, usually given to both sexual partners to avoid the possible "ping-pong" effect of repeated cross-infection so typical of STIs.

General Urinary Tract Infections

Although *general urinary tract infections (UTIs)* can be caused by various factors, some forms are sexually transmitted. Anytime invading organisms enter the genital area, they can travel up the urethra and enter the bladder. Similarly, organisms normally living in the rectum, urethra, or bladder may travel to the sexual organs and eventually be transmitted to another person.

You can also get a UTI through autoinoculation, often during the simple task of wiping yourself after defecating. Wiping from the anus forward can transmit organisms found in feces to the vaginal opening or the urethra. Contact between the hands and the urethra and between the urethra and other objects are also common means of autoinoculation. Women, with their shorter urethras, are more likely to contract UTIs. Hand washing with soap and water prior to sexual intimacy, foreplay, and so on, is recommended. Treatment depends on the nature and type of pathogen.

Herpes

Herpes is a general term for a family of infections characterized by sores or eruptions on the skin. Herpes infections range from mildly uncomfortable to extremely serious. **Genital herpes** is an infection caused by the herpes simplex virus (HSV).

There are two types of HSV. Historically, the herpes simplex type 2 virus was considered the primary culprit in genital herpes, and herpes simplex virus type 1 was thought to affect the area of the lips and other body areas. We now know that both type 1 and type 2 can infect any area of the body and produce lesions (sores) in and around the vaginal area, on the penis, around the anal opening, on the buttocks or thighs, and occasionally on other parts of the body. HSV remains in certain nerve cells for life and can flare up, or cause symptoms, when the body's ability to maintain itself is weakened.

The prodromal (precursor) phase of the infection is characterized by a burning sensation and redness at the site of infection. During this time, prescription medicines will often keep the disease from spreading. However, this phase of the disease is quickly followed by the second phase, in which a blister filled with a clear fluid containing the virus forms. If you pick at this blister or otherwise touch the site and spread this fluid with fingers, lipstick, lip balm, or other products, you can autoinoculate other body parts. Particularly dangerous is the possibility of spreading the infection to your eyes, for a herpes lesion on the eye can cause blindness.

Over a period of days, the unsightly blister will dry up and disappear, and the virus will travel to the base of an affected nerve supplying the area and become dormant. Only when the victim becomes overly stressed, when diet and sleep are inadequate, when the immune system is overworked, or when excessive exposure to sunlight or other stressors occurs will the virus become reactivated (at the same site every time) and begin the blistering cycle all over again. These sores cast off (shed) viruses that can be highly infectious. However, it is important to note that a herpes site can shed the virus even when no overt sore is present, particularly during the prodromal stages (the interval between the earliest symptoms and blistering). People may get genital herpes by having sexual contact with others who don't know they are infected or who are having outbreaks of herpes without any sores. A person with genital herpes can also infect a sexual partner during oral sex. The virus is spread only rarely, if at all, by touching objects such as a toilet seat or hot tub seat.

Genital herpes is especially serious in pregnant women because the baby could be infected as it passes through the vagina during birth. Many physicians recommend cesarean deliveries for infected women. Additionally, women who have a history of genital herpes appear to have a greater risk of cervical cancer.

Although there is no cure for herpes at present, certain drugs can reduce symptoms. Unfortunately, they seem to work only if the infection is confirmed during the first few hours after contact. As you may guess, this is rather rare. The effectiveness of other treatments, such as L-lysine, is largely unsubstantiated. Newer over-the-counter medications seem to be moderately effective in reducing the severity of symptoms. Although lip balms and cold-sore medications may provide temporary relief, remember that rubbing anything on a herpes blister can spread herpes-laden fluids to other body parts.

Preventing Herpes You can take precautions to reduce your risk of herpes.

- Avoid any form of kissing if you notice a sore or blister on your partner's mouth. Kiss no one, not even a peck on the cheek, if you know that you have a herpes lesion. Allow time after the sores go away before you start kissing again.
- Be extremely cautious if you have casual sexual affairs. Not every partner will feel obligated to tell you that he or she has a problem. It's up to you to protect yourself.
- Wash your hands immediately with soap and water after any form of sexual contact.
- If you have questionable sores or lesions, seek medical help at once. Do not be afraid to name your contacts.
- If you have herpes, be responsible in your sexual contacts with others. If you have any suspicious lesions that might put your partner at risk, say so. Find an appropriate time and place, and hold a candid discussion.
- Reduce your risk of herpes outbreaks by avoiding excessive stress, sunlight, or whatever else appears to trigger an episode.

HIV/AIDS

Acquired immune deficiency syndrome (AIDS) is a significant global health threat. Since 1981, when AIDS was first recognized, more than 60 million people in the world have become infected with human immunodeficiency virus (HIV), the virus that causes AIDS. Today, more than 42 million people are estimated to be living with HIV or AIDS, and an estimated 5 million new cases were diagnosed worldwide in 2002. Women are becoming increasingly affected by the virus and account for approximately 50 percent of cases. In the United States, as of 2002, more than 886,575 men, women, and children with AIDS have been reported to the CDC, and at least 501,669 have died. The CDC estimates that at least 40,000 new infections occur each year in the United States. See the Health in a Diverse World box on page 264 for more on the global impact of HIV/AIDS.

A Shifting Epidemic

Under old definitions, people with HIV were diagnosed as having AIDS only when they developed blood infections, the cancer known as Kaposi's sarcoma, or any of 21 other indicator diseases, most of which were common in males. The CDC has expanded the indicator list to include pulmonary tuberculosis, recurrent pneumonia, and invasive cervical cancer. Perhaps the most significant new indicator is a drop in the level of the body's master immune cells, called CD4s, to 200 per cubic millimeter (one-fifth the level in a healthy person).

AIDS cases have been reported state by state throughout the United States since the early 1980s as a means of tracking the disease. While the numbers of actual reported cases have always been suspect, im-

HEALTH IN A DIVERSE WORLD

The Staggering Toll of HIV/AIDS in the Global Community

Although the rates of HIV/AIDS may be slowing in the United States, the disease has had an increasingly devastating impact on other regions of the world. By the year 2003, an estimated 34 to 46 million people from all regions of the world were infected with HIV, which translates to nearly 1 out of every 100 men, women, and children. Every day in 2003, an estimated 14,000 people were newly infected with HIV. Here are some facts about this global epidemic.

AFRICA

- In southern Africa, one in every five people is now infected. Almost 39% of the population in Botswana and Swaziland is living with HIV.
- About 30% of people living with HIV worldwide live in southern Africa, an area that is home to just 2% of the world's population.
- South Africa is home to an estimated 5.3 million people with HIV, more than any other country in the world.

LATIN AMERICA AND THE CARIBBEAN

- In 2003, an estimated 2 million people in this region were living with the HIV virus. The epidemic was mainly spread through heterosexual intercourse, injecting drug use, and men who have sex with men.
- Haiti was worst hit, with 6% of adults infected.

EASTERN EUROPE AND CENTRAL ASIA

- In eastern Europe and central Asia combined, an estimated 1.5 million people were living with the AIDS virus at the end of 2003.
- Rates of infection are increasing among drug users sharing needles in eastern Europe and Russia.

ASIA

- An estimated 7.4 million people in the region were living with the AIDS virus in 2003.
- Thailand has an infection rate of 2%. This country and Cambodia seem to have controlled the once-rampant spread of HIV by promoting condom use, especially among sex workers.
- An estimated 3.82 to 4.58 million people in India live with the virus, the second highest national total behind South Africa, with an infection rate of 0.7%.

Source: Joint United Nations Programme on HIV/AIDS (UNAIDS), "AIDS Epidemic Update 2003," December 2003. www.unaids.org/wad/ 2003/press/epiupdate.html

proved reporting and surveillance methods have helped increase accuracy. Today, the CDC recommends that all states report HIV infections as well as AIDS. Because of medical advances in treatment and increasing numbers of HIV-infected persons who do not progress to AIDS, it is believed that AIDS incidence statistics may not provide a true picture of the epidemic, the long-term costs of treating HIV-infected individuals, and other key information. HIV incidence data also provide a better picture of infection trends. Currently, most states mandate that those who test positive for the HIV antibody be reported.

What do you think?

Do you favor mandatory reporting of HIV and AIDS cases? • If you knew that your name and vital statistics would be "on file" if you tested positive for HIV, would you be less likely to take the HIV test? • On the other hand, do people who carry this contagious fatal disease have a responsibility to inform the general public and the health professionals who will provide their care? Explain your answer.

Women and AIDS

HIV is an equal-opportunity pathogen that can attack anyone who engages in high-risk behaviors. This is true regardless of race, gender, sexual orientation, or socioeconomic status. Consider the following facts:

- Women are four to ten times more likely than men to contract HIV through unprotected sexual intercourse with an infected partner.

- By 2002, women accounted for more than 50 percent of all AIDS cases in the United States.
- HIV/AIDS due to heterosexual sexual transmission is increasing faster in rural America than in any other part of the country. Women most at risk are ethnic minorities and the economically disadvantaged. Among sexually active heterosexual teenagers, college students, and health care workers, nearly 60 percent of HIV cases are women.
- Most women with AIDS were infected through heterosexual exposure to HIV, followed by injection drug use (sharing needles).
- Women of color are disproportionately affected by HIV; African American and Hispanic women together account for 76 percent of AIDS cases among women in the United States, though they comprise less than 25 percent of all U.S. women.
- Of all AIDS cases among women, 61 percent were reported from five states: New York (26 percent), Florida (13 percent), New Jersey (10 percent), California (7 percent), and Texas (5 percent).
- AIDS is the leading cause of death among African American women age 25 to 44, and the fourth leading cause of death among all American women in this age group.
- AIDS is one of the top ten causes of death for people age 15 to 64 in the United States.

Compounding the problems are serious deficiencies in our health and social service systems, including inadequate treatment for women addicts and lack of access to child care, health care, and social services for families headed by single women. Women with HIV/AIDS are of special interest because they are the major source of infection in infants. Virtually all new HIV infections among children in the United States are attributable to perinatal transmission of HIV.

Although contracting HIV is a serious problem for both males and females, women often have an even more difficult time protecting themselves from infection and taking care of themselves once they become ill. Irrefutable evidence indicates that HIV/AIDS disproportionately affects women. This discrepancy can be traced to biological and socioeconomic factors.

Biological factors include:

- HIV can enter through mucous membrane surfaces of the genital tract; the vagina has a greater exposed mucous membrane than does the urethra of the penis.
- The vaginal area is more likely to incur micro-tears during sexual intercourse, which facilitates entry of HIV.
- During intercourse, a woman is exposed to more semen than is the male to vaginal fluids.
- Semen is more likely to enter the vagina with force, whereas vaginal fluids do not enter the penis with force.
- Women who have STIs are more likely to be asymptomatic and therefore unaware they have an STI; STIs increase the risk of HIV transmission.

Socioeconomic factors include:

- There are more HIV-infected men than HIV-infected women in the United States; thus, it is more likely for a woman to have an HIV-infected male partner.
- Women have been underrepresented in clinical trials for HIV treatment and prevention.
- Many cultural norms place women in subordination to men, especially in developing nations. This reduces women's decision-making power and ability to negotiate safer sex.
- Women are more vulnerable to sexual abuse from their male partners.
- Women are more likely to be economically dependent on men.
- Women may be less likely to seek medical treatment because of lack of money, caregiving burdens, and transportation problems.
- In the United States, HIV-positive women are more likely than are HIV-positive men to be younger and less educated.

What do you think?

Why do you think HIV/AIDS is increasing among women and minority groups in America? • Why are some women particularly vulnerable? • What actions can we take as a nation to reduce the spread of HIV/AIDS among women and among minority groups? • Should Americans be concerned about the global HIV/AIDS epidemic? Why or why not?

How HIV Is Transmitted

HIV typically enters one person's body when another person's infected body fluids (semen, vaginal secretions, blood, etc.) gain entry through a breach in body defenses. Mucous membranes of the genital organs and the anus provide the easiest route of entry. If there is a break in the mucous membranes (as can occur during sexual intercourse, particularly anal intercourse), the virus enters and begins to multiply. After initial infection, HIV multiplies rapidly, invading the bloodstream and cerebrospinal fluid. It progressively destroys helper T-lymphocytes, thus weakening the body's resistance to disease. The virus also changes the genetic structure of the cells it attacks. In response to this invasion, the body quickly begins to produce antibodies.

Despite some myths, HIV is not a highly contagious virus. Studies of people living in households with a person with HIV/AIDS have turned up no documented cases of HIV infection due to casual contact. Other investigations provide overwhelming evidence that insect bites do not transmit HIV.

Engaging in High-Risk Behaviors AIDS is not a disease of gay people or minority groups. If you engage in high-risk behaviors, you increase your risk for the disease. If you do not practice these behaviors, your risk is minimal. Anyone who engages in unprotected sex is at risk, especially sex with a partner who has engaged in other high-risk behaviors. Sex with multiple partners is the greatest threat.

Exchange of Body Fluids The greatest risk factor is the exchange of HIV-infected body fluids during vaginal and anal intercourse. Substantial research evidence indicates that blood, semen, and vaginal secretions are the major fluids of concern. Most health officials state that saliva is not a high-risk body fluid unless blood is present. But the fact that the virus has been found in isolated samples of saliva does provide a good rationale for using caution when engaging in deep, wet kissing.

Initially, public health officials also included breast milk in the list of high-risk fluids because a few infants apparently contracted HIV while breast-feeding. Subsequent research has indicated that HIV transmission could have been caused by bleeding nipples as well as by actual consumption of breast milk and other fluids. Infection through contact with feces and urine is believed to be highly unlikely though technically possible.

Receiving a Blood Transfusion Prior to 1985 A small group of people became infected with HIV after receiving blood transfusions. In 1985, the Red Cross and other blood donation programs implemented a stringent testing program for all donated blood. Today, because of these massive screening efforts, the risk of receiving HIV-infected blood is almost nonexistent.

Injecting Drugs A significant percentage of AIDS cases in the United States are believed to result from sharing or using HIV-contaminated needles and syringes. Though users of illegal drugs are commonly considered the only members of this category, others may also share needles—for example, people with diabetes who inject insulin or athletes who inject steroids. People who share needles and also engage in sexual activities with members of high-risk groups, such as those who exchange sex for drugs, increase their risks dramatically.

Mother-to-Infant Transmission (Perinatal) Approximately one in three of the children who has contracted AIDS received the virus from an infected mother while in the womb or while passing through the vaginal tract during delivery.

Symptoms of HIV Disease

A person may go for months or years after infection by HIV before any significant symptoms appear. The incubation time varies greatly from person to person. Children have shorter incubation periods than do adults. Newborns and infants are particularly vulnerable to AIDS because human beings do not become fully immunocompetent (that is, their immune system is not fully developed) until they are 6 to 15 months old. New information suggests that some very young children show the "adult" progression of AIDS.

For adults who receive no medical treatment, it takes an average of eight to ten years for the virus to cause the slow, degenerative changes in the immune system that are characteristic of AIDS. During

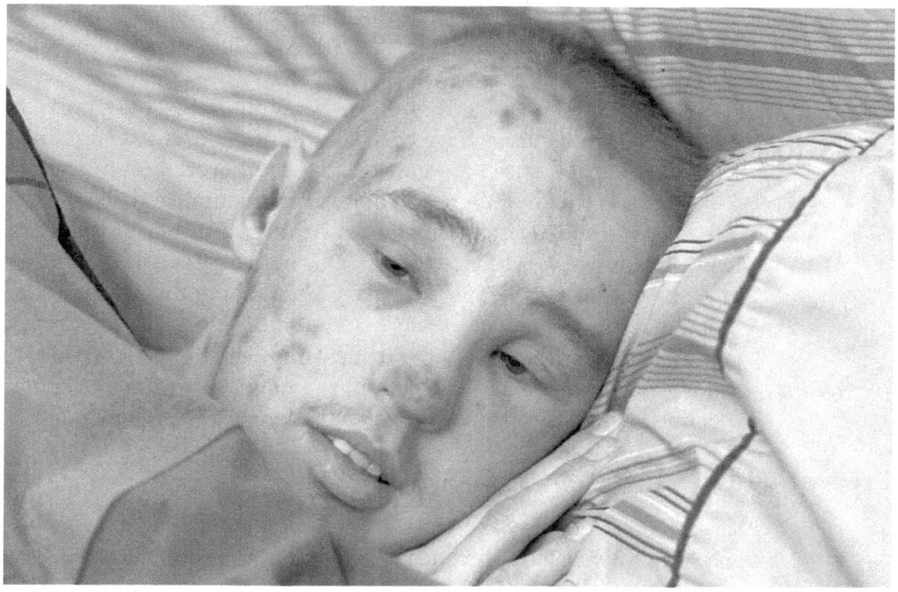

The effects of HIV/AIDS can be seen here in the form of Kaposi's sarcoma and wasting syndrome.

this time, the person may experience a large number of opportunistic infections (infections that gain a foothold when the immune system is not functioning effectively). Colds, sore throats, fever, tiredness, nausea, night sweats, and other generally non–life-threatening conditions commonly appear, and are described as pre-AIDS symptoms.

Testing for HIV Antibodies

Once antibodies have formed in reaction to HIV, a blood test known as the **ELISA** test may detect their presence. If sufficient antibodies are present, the ELISA test will be positive. When a person who previously tested *negative* (no HIV antibodies present) has a subsequent test that is *positive,* seroconversion is said to have occurred. In such a situation, the person would typically take another ELISA test, followed by a more expensive, precise test known as the **Western blot,** to confirm the presence of HIV antibodies.

It should be noted that these tests are not AIDS tests per se. Rather, they detect antibodies for the disease that would indicate the presence of HIV in the person's body. Whether the person will develop AIDS depends to some extent on the strength of the immune system. However, the vast majority of all infected people develop some form of the disease.

As testing for HIV antibodies has been perfected, scientists have explored various ways of making it easier for individuals to be tested. Health officials distinguish between *reported* and *actual* cases of HIV infection because it is believed that many HIV-positive people avoid being tested. One reason may be fear of knowing the truth. Another is the fear of discrimination from employers, insurance companies, and medical staff if a positive test becomes known to others. However, early detection and reporting are important, because immediate treatment for someone in the early stages of HIV disease is critical.

New Hope and Treatments

New drugs have slowed the progression from HIV to AIDS and have prolonged life expectancies for many AIDS patients. While these new therapies offered the promise of life for many, they may have inadvertently led to increases in risky behaviors. This may have led to a noteworthy rise in cases by 2 percent in 2002. Although the death rate from AIDS has declined each year since 1995, many fear that we are taking steps backward. Advocates for AIDS patients believe the medications still cost too much money and cause too many side effects. Multidrug treatment for AIDS for one person now exceeds $20,000 per year.

Current treatments combine selected drugs, especially protease inhibitors and reverse transcriptase inhibitors. Protease inhibitors (for example, Amprenavir, Ritonavir, and Saquinavir) resemble pieces of the protein chain that the HIV protease normally cuts. They block the HIV protease enzyme from cutting the protein chains needed to produce new viruses. Older AIDS drugs work by preventing the virus from infecting new cells.

Although protease inhibitors show promise, they have proved difficult to manufacture, and some have failed while others have been successful. Side effects vary, and getting the right dose is critical for effectiveness. All of the protease drugs seem to work best in combination with other therapies. These combination treatments are still quite experimental, and no combination has proved to be absolute for all people as yet. Also, as with other antiviral treatments, resistance to the drugs can develop. Individuals who already show resistance to AZT may not be able to use a protease-AZT combination. This can pose a problem for many people who have been taking the common drugs and then find their options for combination therapy limited.

Although these drugs provide new hope and longer survival for people living with HIV, we are still a long way from a cure. In addition, the number of people becoming HIV-infected each year has not declined which means that we are still a long way from beating this disease.

Preventing HIV Infection

Although scientists have been searching for an HIV vaccine since 1983, they have had no success so far. The only way to prevent HIV infection is to avoid risky behaviors. HIV infection and AIDS are not uncontrollable conditions. You can reduce your risk by the choices you make in sexual behaviors and by taking responsibility for your health and the health of your loved ones. The Skills for Behavior Change box on page 269 presents ways to reduce your risk for contracting HIV.

NONINFECTIOUS DISEASES

Typically, when we think of major noninfectious ailments, we think of "killer" diseases such as cancer and heart disease. Clearly, these diseases make up the major portion of life-threatening diseases—accounting for nearly two-thirds of all deaths. Yet, although these diseases capture much media attention, other chronic conditions can also cause pain, suffering, and disability. Fortunately, most of them can be prevented or their symptoms relieved.

Generally, noninfectious diseases are not transmitted by a pathogen or by any form of personal contact. Lifestyle and personal health habits are often implicated as underlying causes. Healthy changes in lifestyle and public health efforts aimed at research, prevention, and control can minimize the effects of these diseases.

CHRONIC LUNG DISEASE

Chronic lung diseases pose a serious and significant threat to Americans today. Collectively, they have become the fourth leading cause of death, with most sufferers living with a condition known as chronic **dyspnea,** or chronic breathlessness. Depending on the situation, dyspnea may limit the ability to climb stairs, walk unassisted, or even sleep. Chronic lung disease can result in major disability and lack of function as the lungs fill with mucous, become susceptible to bacterial or viral infections, or cause acute stress on the heart as they struggle to get valuable oxygen. Chronic cough, excessive phlegm, wheezing, or coughing up blood are frequent symptoms. Over time, many of these underlying conditions lead to hospitalization and possible death.

Among the more deadly chronic lung diseases are the **chronic obstructive pulmonary diseases (COPDs):** asthma, emphysema, and chronic bronchitis. Other chronic lung diseases also cause significant health risks, the most common of which are allergy-induced problems and hay fever. Each of these may exacerbate or contribute to the development of COPD.

Allergy-Induced Respiratory Problems

An **allergy** occurs as a part of the body's attempt to defend itself against a specific *antigen* or *allergen* by producing specific *antibodies*. When foreign pathogens such as bacteria or viruses invade the body, the

SKILLS FOR BEHAVIOR CHANGE

Staying Safe in an Unsafe Sexual World

HIV transmission depends on specific behaviors; this is true of other STIs as well. The following will help you protect yourself and reduce your risk.

- Avoid casual sexual partners. Ideally, have sex only if you are in a long-term, mutually monogamous relationship with someone who is equally committed to the relationship and whose HIV status is negative.
- Avoid unprotected sexual activity involving the exchange of blood, semen, or vaginal secretions with people whose present or past behaviors put them at risk for infection. Do not be afraid to ask intimate questions about your partner's sexual past. Remember, whenever you choose to have sexual relations, you expose yourself to your partner's history. Postpone sexual involvement until you are assured that he or she is not infected.
- All sexually active adults who are not in a lifelong monogamous relationship should practice safer sex by using latex condoms. Remember, however, that condoms still do not provide 100% safety.
- Never share injecting needles with anyone for any reason.
- Never share any devices through which the exchange of blood could occur, including needles, razors, tattoo instruments, body-piercing instruments, and any other sharp objects.
- Avoid injury to body tissue during sexual activity. HIV can enter the bloodstream through microscopic tears in anal or vaginal tissues.
- Avoid unprotected oral sex or any sexual activity in which semen, blood, or vaginal secretions could penetrate mucous membranes through breaks in the membrane. Always use a condom or a dental dam during oral sex.
- Avoid using drugs that may dull your senses and affect your ability to make decisions about responsible precautions with potential sex partners.
- Wash your hands before and after sexual encounters. Urinate after sexual relations and, if possible, wash your genitals.
- Although total abstinence is the only absolute means of preventing the sexual transmission of HIV, abstinence can be a difficult choice to make. If you have any doubt about the potential risks of having sex, consider other means of intimacy, at least until you can assure your safety. Try massage, dry kissing, hugging, holding and touching, and masturbation (alone or with a partner).
- Be sure medical professionals take appropriate precautions to prevent potential transmission, including washing their hands and wearing gloves and masks. All equipment used for treatment should be properly sterilized.
- If you are worried about your own HIV status, have yourself tested. Don't risk infecting others inadvertently.
- If you are a woman and HIV positive, you should take the steps necessary to ensure that you do not become pregnant.
- If you suspect that you may be infected or if you test positive for HIV antibodies, do not donate blood, semen, or body organs.

At no time in your life is it more important to communicate openly than when you are considering an intimate relationship. Ask questions, so you can then make an informed decision about whether to get involved. Remember that you can't tell if someone has an STI. Anyone who has ever had sex with anyone else or has injected drugs is at risk, and they may not even know it. The following will help you to communicate about potential risks.

- Remember that you have a responsibility to your partner to disclose your own status. You also have a responsibility to yourself to stay healthy. Ask about your partner's HIV status. Suggest going through the testing together as a means of sharing something important.
- Be direct, honest, and determined in talking about sex before you become involved. Do not act silly or evasive. Get to the point, ask clear questions, and do not be put off in receiving a response. A person who does not care enough to talk about sex probably does not care enough to take responsibility for his or her actions.
- Discuss the issues without sounding defensive or accusatory. Develop a personal comfort level with the subject prior to raising the issue with your partner. Be prepared with complete information, and articulate your feelings clearly. Reassure your partner that your reasons for desiring abstinence or safer sex arise from respect and not distrust. Sharing feelings is easier in a calm, suspicion-free environment in which both people feel comfortable.
- Encourage your partner to be honest and to share feelings. This will not happen overnight. If you have never had a serious conversation with this person before you get into an intimate situation, you cannot expect honesty and openness when the lights go out.
- Analyze your own beliefs and values ahead of time. Know where you will draw the line on certain actions, and be very clear with your partner about what you expect. If you believe that using a condom is necessary, make sure you communicate this.
- Decide what you will do if your partner does not agree with you. Anticipate potential objections or excuses, and prepare your responses accordingly.
- Ask about your partner's history. Although it may seem as though you are prying into another person's business, your own health future depends upon knowing basic information about your partner's past sexual practices and use of injectable drugs.
- Discuss the significance of monogamy in your partner's relationships. Ask, "How important is a committed relationship to you?" Decide early how important this relationship is to you and how much you are willing to work at arriving at an acceptable compromise on lifestyle.

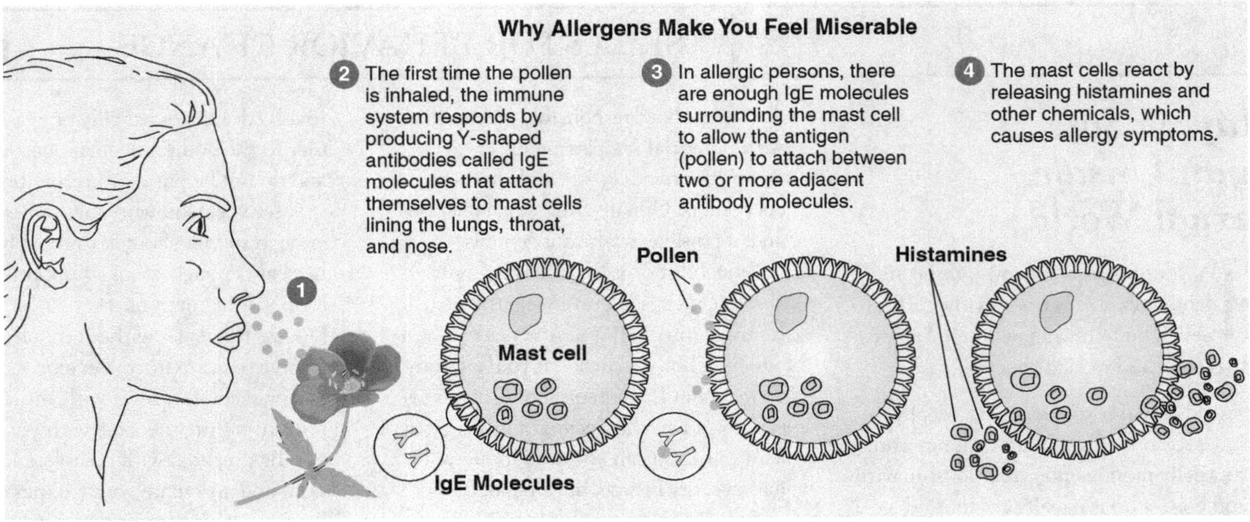

FIGURE 16.4. Steps of an Allergy Response

body responds by producing antibodies to destroy these invading antigens. Under normal conditions, the production of antibodies is a positive element in the body's defense system. However, for unknown reasons, in some people the body overreacts by developing an overly elaborate protective mechanism against relatively harmless substances. The resultant *hypersensitivity reaction* to specific allergens or antigens in the environment is fairly common, as anyone who has awakened with a runny nose or itchy eyes will testify. Most commonly, these hypersensitivity, or allergic, responses occur as a reaction to environmental antigens such as molds, animal dander (hair and dead skin), pollen, ragweed, or dust. Once excessive antibodies to these antigens are produced, they trigger the release of **histamines,** chemical substances that dilate blood vessels, increase mucous secretions, cause tissues to swell, and produce other allergy-like symptoms, particularly in the respiratory system (Figure 16.4).

Although many people think of allergies as childhood diseases, in reality allergies tend to become progressively worse with time and with increased exposure to allergens. In these circumstances, allergic responses become chronic in nature, and treatment becomes difficult. Many people take allergy shots to reduce the severity of their symptoms, with some success. In most cases, once the offending antigen has disappeared, allergy-prone people suffer few symptoms. Although allergies can cause numerous problems, one of the most significant effects is on the immune system.

Hay Fever

Perhaps the best example of a chronic respiratory disease is **hay fever.** Usually considered a seasonally related disease (most prevalent when ragweed and flowers are blooming), hay fever is common throughout the world. Hay fever attacks, which are characterized by sneezing and itchy, watery eyes and nose, make countless people miserable. The disorder appears to run in families, and research indicates that lifestyle is not as great a factor in developing hay fever as it is in other chronic diseases. Instead, an overzealous immune system and exposure to environmental allergens including pet dander, dust, pollen from various plants, and other substances appear to be the critical factors that determine vulnerability. For those people who are unable to get away from the cause of their hay fever response, medical assistance in the form of injections or antihistamines may provide the only relief.

Asthma

Unfortunately, for many persons who suffer from allergies such as hay fever, their condition often becomes complicated by the development of one of the major COPDs: asthma, emphysema, or bronchitis. **Asthma** is a long-term, chronic inflammatory disorder that blocks air flow in and out of the lungs. Asthma causes tiny airways in the lung to overreact with spasms in response to certain triggers. Symptoms include wheezing, difficulty breathing, shortness of breath, and coughing spasms. Although most

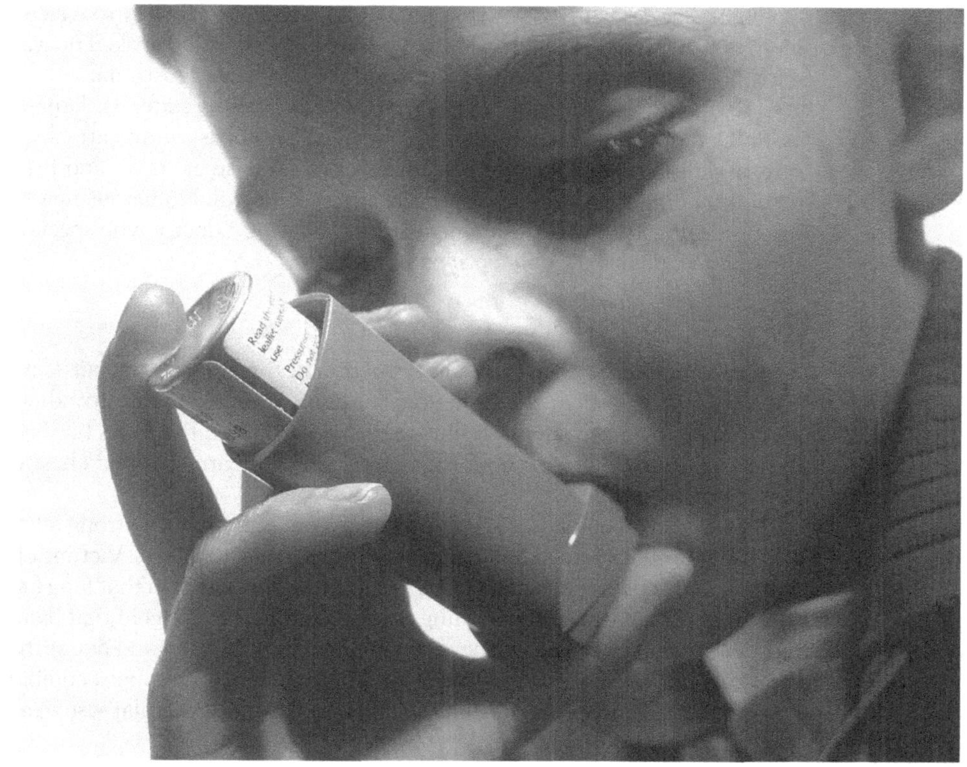

Although a number of new medications are available to relieve the symptoms of asthma, the marked increase of this problem among young children concerns health officials.

asthma attacks are mild and non–life-threatening, they can trigger bronchospasms (contractions of the bronchial tubes in the lungs) that are so severe that without rapid treatment, death may occur. Between attacks, most people have few symptoms.

A number of things can trigger an asthma attack, including air pollutants; particulate matter, such as wood dust; indoor air pollutants, such as sidestream smoke from tobacco; and allergens, such as dust mites, cockroach saliva, and pet dander. Stress is also believed to trigger attacks in some individuals.

Asthma can occur at any age, but it is most likely in children between infancy and age 5 and in adults before age 40. In childhood, asthma strikes more boys than girls; in adulthood, it strikes more women than men. Also, the asthma rate is 50 percent higher among African Americans than whites, and four times as many African Americans die of asthma than do whites. Midwesterners appear to be more prone to asthma than people from other areas of the country. In recent years, concern over the rise in incidence of asthma has grown considerably. Consider these points:

- Asthma has become the most common chronic disease of childhood and accounts for one-fourth of all school absences.
- Asthma is the number one cause of hospitalization and absenteeism.
- Asthma affects more than 17 million Americans, including 5 million children; 13 percent of all students age 5 to 19 have it.
- The number of asthma sufferers has increased by more than 65 percent since the 1980s; one in ten new asthma cases is diagnosed in people over age 65.
- The death toll from asthma has nearly doubled since 1980 to more than 5,000 persons per year.

People with asthma have one of two distinctly different types. The most common type, known as *extrinsic* (or *slow onset*) *asthma*, is most commonly associated with allergic triggers. This form tends to run in families and begins to develop in childhood. Often, by adulthood, a person has few episodes, or the disorder completely goes away. *Intrinsic asthma* also may have allergic triggers, but the main difference is that any unpleasant event or stimulant may trigger an attack. A common form of extrinsic asthma is *exercise-induced asthma (EIA)*, which may or may not have an allergic connection. Some athletes have no allergies yet live with asthma. Cold, dry air is believed to exacerbate EIA; thus, keeping the lungs moist and warming up prior to working out may reduce risk. The warm, moist air around a swimming pool is one of the best environments for people with asthma.

Relaxation techniques appear to help some asthma sufferers. Drugs may be necessary for serious cases. Determining whether a specific allergen provokes asthma attacks, taking steps to reduce exposure, avoiding triggers such as certain types of exercise or stress, and finding the most effective medications are big steps in asthma prevention and control. Numerous new drugs are available that cause fewer side effects than do older medications. Finding a doctor who specializes in asthma treatment and stays up-to-date on possible options is critical.

Emphysema

Emphysema involves the gradual destruction of the **alveoli** (tiny air sacs) of the lungs. As the alveoli are destroyed, the affected person finds it more and more difficult to exhale. The victim typically struggles to take in a fresh supply of air before the air held in the lungs has been expended. The chest cavity gradually begins to expand, thus producing the barrel-shaped chest characteristic of the chronic emphysema victim.

The cause of emphysema is uncertain. There is, however, a strong relationship between emphysema and long-term cigarette smoking and exposure to air pollution. Victims of emphysema often suffer discomfort over a period of many years. In fact, studies have shown that lung function decline may begin well before age 50 and the early morning "smoker's cough" may signal that damage has already begun. What most of us take for granted—the easy, rhythmic flow of air in and out of the lungs—becomes a continuous struggle for people with emphysema. Inadequate oxygen supply, combined with the stress of overexertion on the heart, eventually takes its toll on the cardiovascular system and leads to premature death.

Bronchitis

Bronchitis refers to an inflammation of the lining of the bronchial tubes. These tubes, the bronchi, connect the windpipe with the lungs. When the bronchi become inflamed or infected, less air is able to flow from the lungs, and heavy mucous begins to form. *Acute bronchitis* is the most common of the bronchial diseases and results in millions of visits to the doctor every year at a cost of more than $300 million per year. More than 95 percent of these acute cases are caused by viruses; however, they are often misdiagnosed and treated with antibiotics, even though little evidence supports this treatment. Typically, misdiagnosis occurs when a cluster of symptoms is labeled as bronchitis, despite the fact that there is no true laboratory diagnosis. *Chronic bronchitis*, in contrast, is defined by the presence of a productive (mucous-laden) cough most days of the month, more than three months of a year for two successive years without underlying disease to explain the cough. Typically, cigarette smoking causes chronic bronchitis, and once bronchitis begins, secondary bacterial or viral infections often make the condition worse. Air pollution and industrial dusts and fumes are also risk factors.

Sleep Apnea

Sleep apnea, although not as life threatening as asthma and other COPDs, affects about 5 percent of the general population. This condition is characterized by periodic episodes when breathing stops completely for ten seconds or longer. Each time it occurs, the sleeper awakens and breathing resumes, but the pattern causes a restless night's sleep. Over time, sleep apnea can lead to high blood pressure and subsequent risk of CVD. Reducing alcohol use, changing sleeping position and schedules, and other medical interventions are common treatments.

What do you think?

Which of the respiratory diseases described in this section do you or your family have problems with? • How many of your college friends have these COPDs? • What difficulties do they have in controlling their diseases? • Why do you think the incidence of COPDs, as a group, is increasing? • What actions can you or your community take to reduce risks and problems from these diseases?

NEUROLOGICAL DISORDERS

Headaches

Almost all of us have experienced at least one major headache. In fact, more than 80 percent of women and 65 percent of men experience headaches on a regular basis. Common types of headaches and their treatments are described below.

Tension Headache Tension headaches, also referred to as muscular contraction headaches, are generally caused by muscle contractions or tension in the neck or head. This tension may be caused by actual strain placed on neck or head muscles due to overuse, static positions held for long periods of time, or tension triggered by stress. Recent research indicates that tension headaches may be a product of a more "generic mechanism" in which chemicals deep inside the brain may cause the muscular tension, pain, and suffering often associated with an attack. Possible triggers include red wine, lack of sleep, fasting, menstruation, or other factors, and the same symptoms (sensitivity to light and sound, nausea, and/or throbbing pain) may characterize different types of headaches. Relaxation, hot water treatment, and massage have surfaced as the new holistic treatments, while aspirin, Tylenol, Aleve, and Advil remain the old standby forms of pain relief. Although such painkillers may bring temporary relief of symptoms, it is believed that, over time, the drugs may dull the brain's own pain-killing weapons and result in more rather than fewer headaches.

Migraine Headache **Migraine** is not just a name for an unusually bad headache; it is a specific diagnosis, involving pain that begins on one side of the head, often accompanied by nausea and sensitivity to light and sounds. Many migraine sufferers experience the sensation of an "aura" in their visual field, typically some form of disturbance such as flashing lights or blind spots, along with numbness or weakness on one side of the body or slurred speech, all signals of an ensuing bad headache. Most people report pain behind or around one eye and always on the same side of the head—a pain that can last for hours or days and then disappear. A migraine can strike at any time, although the hormonal changes around menstruation and ovulation often seem to set off migraines in women, who are three times more likely to get them than men.

Patients report that migraines can be triggered by emotional stress, weather, certain foods, lack of sleep, and a litany of other causes. When tested under laboratory settings, however, much of this evidence is inconclusive. What is known is that migraines occur when blood vessels dilate in the membrane that surrounds the brain. Historically, treatments have centered on reversing or preventing this dilation, with the most common treatment derived from the rye fungus *ergot*. Today, many fast-acting ergot compounds are available by nasal spray, thus vastly increasing the speed of relief. However, ergot drugs have many side effects, the least of which may be that they are habit forming, which causes users to wake up with "rebound" headaches each morning after use.

Critics of the blood vessel dilation theory question why only blood vessels of the head dilate in these situations. Furthermore, why aren't people who exercise or take hot baths more prone to migraine attacks? They suggest that migraines originate in the cortex of the brain, where certain pain sensors are stimulated.

When true migraines occur, relaxation is only minimally effective. Often, strong pain-relieving drugs prescribed by a physician are necessary. Imitrex, a drug tailor-made for migraines, works for about 80 percent of those who try it. Recently, treatment with lidocaine has also shown promising results, and newer drugs called triptans, such as Zomig, Amerge, and Maxalt, are now available.

Secondary Headaches Secondary headaches arise as a result of some other underlying condition. Hypertension, blocked sinuses, allergies, low blood sugar, diseases of the spine, the common cold, poorly fitted dentures, problems with eyesight, and other problems can trigger this condition. Relaxation and pain relievers such as aspirin are of little help in treating secondary headaches. Rather, medications or other therapies designed to relieve the underlying organic cause of the headache must be included in the treatment regimen.

Seizure Disorders

The word **epilepsy** is derived from the Greek *epilepsia*, meaning "seizure." Approximately 1 percent of all Americans suffer from some form of seizure-related disorder. These disorders are generally caused by abnormal electrical activity in the brain and are characterized by loss of control of muscular activity and unconsciousness. Symptoms vary widely from person to person. Common forms of epilepsy include the following.

- *Grand mal, or major motor seizure*. These seizures are often preceded by a shrill cry or a seizure aura (body sensations such as ringing in the ears or a specific smell or taste). Convulsions and loss of consciousness generally occur and may last from 30 seconds to several minutes or more. Keeping track of the length of time elapsed is one aspect of first aid.
- *Petit mal, or minor seizure*. These seizures involve no convulsions. Rather, a minor loss of consciousness that may go unnoticed occurs. Minor twitching of muscles may take place, usually for a shorter time than for grand mal convulsions.
- *Psychomotor seizure*. These seizures involve both mental processes and muscular activity. Symptoms may include mental confusion and a listless state characterized by activities such as lip smacking, chewing, and repetitive movements.
- *Jacksonian seizure*. This is a progressive seizure that often begins in one part of the body, such as the fingers, and moves to other parts, such as the hand or arm. Usually only one side of the body is affected.

In most cases, people afflicted with seizure disorders can lead normal, seizure-free lives when under medical supervision. Public ignorance about these disorders is one of the most serious obstacles confronting them. Improvements in medication and surgical intervention to reduce some causes of seizures are among the most promising treatments today.

What do you think?

Do you suffer from recurrent headaches or other neurological problems? • What might cause your problems? • What actions could you take to reduce your risks and symptoms?

Other Neurological Disorders

Parkinson's disease and multiple sclerosis are two other conditions related to the nervous system. Parkinson's has come to public attention due to actor Michael J. Fox's announcement that he suffers from it. **Parkinson's disease** is a chronic, slowly progressive condition that typically strikes after age 50. The symptom most commonly associated with the disease is a tremor. These tremors can become so severe that simple daily tasks can become difficult or impossible. The most common theories for the causes of the disease are familial disposition, acceleration of age-related changes, and exposure to environmental toxins. Although the disease is progressive and incurable, drug therapies can keep the symptoms under control, possibly for years.

Multiple sclerosis (MS) is a degenerative disease in which myelin, a material composed of fats that serves as an insulator and conduit for transmission of nerve impulses, breaks down and causes nerve malfunction. MS typically appears between ages 15 and 50 and is characterized by a periods of relapse, when symptoms flare up, and remissions, when symptoms are not present. Symptoms can range in severity from fatigue and episodic numbness to severe weakness. Most MS patients have few flare ups and can lead fairly normal lives. Theories for the cause of MS are inconclusive.

GENDER-RELATED DISORDERS

Menstrual Problems

Premenstrual syndrome (PMS) comprises the mood changes and physical symptoms that occur in some women a week to ten days preceding the menstrual period. Symptoms include depression, tension, irritability, headaches, tender breasts, bloated abdomen, backache, abdominal cramps, acne, fluid retention, diarrhea, and fatigue. About 80 percent of all women have some negative symptoms associated with their menstrual cycle; about 3 to 5 percent have more severe symptoms, which are known collectively as **premenstrual dysphoric disorder (PMDD).** Unlike PMS, PMDD symptoms are severe and difficult to manage. They include severe mood disturbances in addition to the physical symptoms associated with PMS.

Strategies for managing PMS include decreasing caffeine and salt intake, increasing intake of complex carbohydrates, practicing stress reduction techniques, and getting exercise. These strategies can also help PMDD. The use of SSRI antidepressants has shown significant promise in the treatment of the mood disturbances associated with PMDD.

Dysmenorrhea, a condition that causes pain in the lower abdomen just before or after menstruation, and toxic shock syndrome (discussed elsewhere in this chapter) are other problems associated with menstruation.

Endometriosis

Whether the incidence of **endometriosis** is on the rise in the United States or whether the disorder is simply attracting more attention is difficult to determine. Victims of endometriosis tend to be women between the ages of 20 and 40. Symptoms include severe cramping during and between menstrual cycles, irregular periods, unusually heavy or light menstrual flow, abdominal bloating, fatigue, painful bowel movements with periods, painful intercourse, constipation, diarrhea, menstrual pain, infertility, and low back pain.

Endometriosis is characterized by the abnormal growth and development of endometrial tissue (the tissue lining the uterus) in regions of the body other than the uterus. Among the most widely accepted theories concerning its causes are the transmission of endometrial tissue to other body regions during surgery or birth; backward flow of menstrual fluid through the fallopian tubes during menstruation; and abnormal cell migration through the movement of body fluids. Women with cycles shorter than 27 days and those with flows lasting over a week are at increased risk. The more aerobic exercise a woman engages in and the earlier she starts it, the less likely she is to develop endometriosis.

Treatment ranges from bed rest and stress reduction to **hysterectomy** (the removal of the uterus) and/or the removal of one or both ovaries and fallopian tubes. Recently, physicians have been criticized by some segments of the public for being too quick to select hysterectomy as the treatment of choice. More conservative treatments that involve dilation and curettage, surgically scraping endometrial tissue off the fallopian tubes and other reproductive organs, and combinations of hormone therapy have become more acceptable. Hormonal treatments include gonadotropin-releasing hormone (GnRH) analogs, various synthetic progesterone-like drugs (Provera), and oral contraceptives.

DIGESTION-RELATED DISORDERS

Diabetes

Diabetes is a serious, widespread, and costly chronic disease, affecting not just the more than 18 million Americans who must live with it, but their families and communities. Between 1990 and 2000, diagnosed diabetes increased 49 percent among U.S. adults, which gives it the dubious distinction of being the fastest growing chronic disease in American history. A recent CDC study indicated that diabetes seems to be increasing even more dramatically among younger adults—up by almost 70 percent among those in their thirties. More than 2,200 people are diagnosed with diabetes each day in America, and more than 200,000 die each year of related complications, thus making diabetes the sixth leading cause of death in America today.

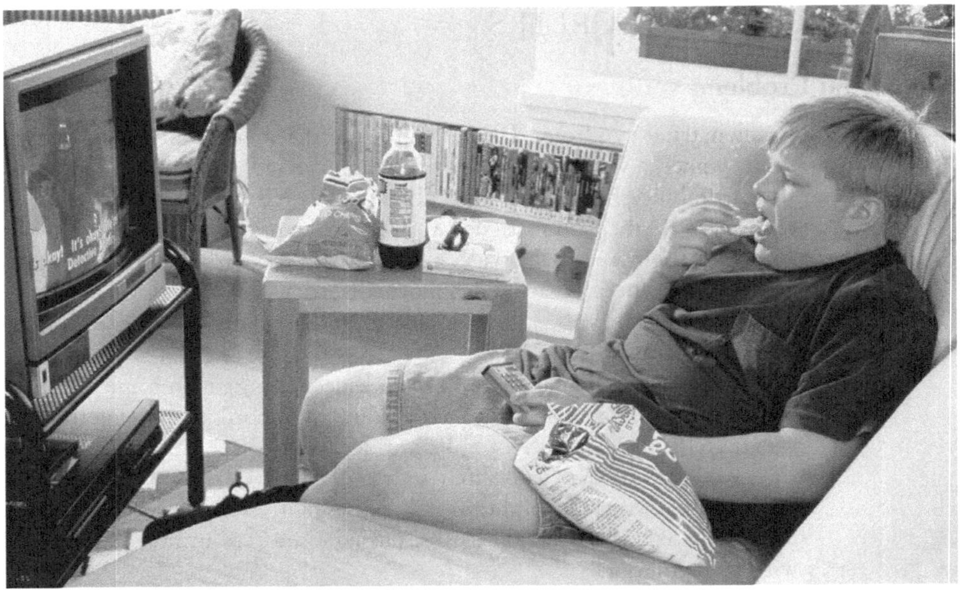

Unhealthy eating habits and a sedentary lifestyle can lead to type 2 diabetes even among children.

What causes this serious disease? In healthy people, the *pancreas*, a powerful enzyme-producing organ, secretes the hormone **insulin** in sufficient quantities to allow the body to use or store glucose (blood sugar). When the pancreas fails to produce enough insulin to regulate sugar metabolism or when the body fails to use insulin effectively, a disease known as **diabetes mellitus** occurs. Diabetics exhibit **hyperglycemia,** or elevated blood sugar levels, and high glucose levels in their urine. Other symptoms include excessive thirst, frequent urination, hunger, tendency to tire easily, wounds that heal slowly, numbness or tingling in the extremities, changes in vision, skin eruptions, and, in women, a tendency toward vaginal yeast infections.

The most serious form, known as type 1 (insulin-dependent) diabetes, is an autoimmune disease in which the immune system destroys the insulin-making beta cells. Type 1 diabetics typically must depend on insulin injections or oral medications for the rest of their lives because insulin is not present in their bodies. Type 2 (non–insulin-dependent) diabetes, in which insulin production is deficient or the body resists or is unable to utilize available insulin, tends to develop in later life. People with Type 2 diabetes can often control their symptoms with a healthy diet, weight control, and regular exercise. They may be able to avoid oral medications or insulin indefinitely. A third type of diabetes, *gestational diabetes*, can develop in a woman during pregnancy. The condition usually disappears after childbirth, but it does leave the woman at greater risk of developing type 2 diabetes at some point.

Understanding Risk Factors Diabetes tends to run in families. Being overweight, coupled with inactivity, dramatically increases the risk of type 2 diabetes. Older persons and mothers of babies weighing more than 9 pounds also run an increased risk. Approximately 80 percent of all type 2 patients are overweight at the time of diagnosis. Weight loss and exercise are important factors in lowering blood sugar and improving the efficiency of cellular use of insulin. Both can help to prevent overwork of the pancreas and the development of diabetes. In fact, recent findings show that modest, consistent physical activity and a healthy diet can cut a person's risk of developing type 2 diabetes by nearly 60 percent. African Americans, Hispanics, and Native Americans have the highest rates of type 2 diabetes in the world—much higher than that of Caucasians. The reasons for this increased risk are not clear.

Controlling Diabetes Most physicians attempt to control diabetes with a variety of insulin-related drugs. Most of these drugs are taken orally, although self-administered hypodermic injections are prescribed when other treatments are inadequate. Recent breakthroughs in individual monitoring and implantable insulin monitors and insulin infusion pumps that regulate insulin intake "on demand" have provided many diabetics with the opportunity to lead normal lives. Newer forms of insulin that last longer in the body and have fewer side effects are now available. An insulin inhaler is being tested and may soon be available.

Lactose Intolerance

As many as 50 million Americans are unable to eat dairy products such as milk, cheese, ice cream, and other foods that the rest of us take for granted. These people suffer from **lactose intolerance,** which means that they have lost the ability to produce the digestive enzyme lactase, which is necessary for the body to convert milk sugar (lactose) into glucose. That glass of milk becomes a source of stomach cramping, diarrhea, nausea, gas, and related symptoms. Once diagnosed, however, lactose intolerance can be treated by introducing low-lactose or lactose-free foods into the diet. Through trial and error, people usually find that they can tolerate one type of low-lactose food better than others. As an alternative to eating foods without lactose, some purchase special products that contain the missing lactase and thus eat dairy foods without serious side effects. Most large grocery chains, food cooperatives, and drug stores have these products available in liquid or tablet form. It should be noted, however, that these products do not work for everyone. Someone who is lactose intolerant may need to experiment before settling into a diet that works.

Colitis and Irritable Bowel Syndrome

Ulcerative colitis is a disease of the large intestine in which the mucous membranes of the intestinal walls become inflamed. Victims with severe cases may have as many as 20 bouts of bloody diarrhea a day. Colitis can also produce severe stomach cramps, weight loss, nausea, sweating, and fever. Although some experts believe that colitis occurs more frequently in people with high stress levels, this theory is controversial. Hypersensitivity reactions, particularly to milk and certain foods, have also been considered as a cause. It is difficult to determine the cause of colitis because the disease goes into unexplained remission and then recurs without apparent reason. This pattern often continues over periods of years and may be related to the later development of colorectal cancer. Since the cause of colitis remains unknown, treatment focuses on relieving the symptoms. Increasing fiber intake and taking anti-inflammatory drugs, steroids, and other medications designed to reduce inflammation and soothe irritated intestinal walls can relieve symptoms.

Many people develop a related condition known as **irritable bowel syndrome (IBS),** characterized by nausea, pain, gas, diarrhea attacks, or cramps that occur after eating certain foods or when a person is under unusual stress. IBS symptoms commonly begin in early adulthood. Symptoms may vary from week to week and can fade for long periods of time, only to return. The cause is unknown, but researchers suspect that people with IBS have digestive systems that are overly sensitive to food and drink, stress, and certain hormonal changes. They may also be more sensitive to pain signals from the stomach. Stress management, relaxation techniques, regular activity, and diet can bring IBS under control in the vast majority of cases. Problems with diarrhea can be reduced by cutting down on fat and avoiding caffeine and excessive amounts of sorbitol, a sweetener found in dietetic foods and chewing gum.

Peptic Ulcers

An ulcer is a lesion or wound that forms in body tissue as a result of some irritant. A **peptic ulcer** is a chronic ulcer that occurs in the lining of the stomach or the section of the small intestine known as the *duodenum*. The lining of these organs becomes irritated, the protective covering of mucous is reduced, and the gastric acid begins to digest the dying tissue, just as it would a piece of food. Typically, this irritation causes pain that disappears when the person eats, but it returns about an hour later.

Research indicates that most peptic ulcers result from infection by a common bacterium, *Helicobacter pylori*. The disorder, which affects more than 4 million Americans every year, generally responds to antibiotics. Peptic ulcers caused by excess stomach acid or overuse of stomach-irritating drugs such as aspirin and ibuprofen can be treated with acid-reducing medications.

What do you think?

What role can a healthy diet play in reducing risks for and symptoms of the diseases discussed here? • *Are you or any of your family members at risk for these problems?* • *What actions can you take today that will cut your risk?*

MUSCULOSKELETAL DISEASES

Arthritis

Called the "nation's primary crippler," **arthritis** strikes one in seven Americans, or more than 38 million people. Symptoms range from the occasional tendinitis of the weekend athlete to the severe pain of rheumatoid arthritis. There are more than 100 types of arthritis diagnosed today. Together, they cost the U.S. economy over $65 billion per year in lost wages and productivity and untold amounts in hospital and nursing home services, prescriptions, and over-the-counter pain relief.

Osteoarthritis, also known as degenerative joint disease, is a progressive deterioration of bones and joints that has been associated with the wear-and-tear theory of aging. More recent research indicates that as joints are used, they release enzymes that digest cartilage while other cells in the cartilage try to repair the damage. When the enzymatic breakdown overpowers cellular repair, the cartilage is destroyed, thus causing bones to rub against each other. Weather extremes, excessive strain, and injury often lead to osteoarthritis flare-ups, but a specific precipitating event does not seem to be necessary. Obesity, joint trauma, and repetitive joint usage all contribute to increased risk, and thus are important targets for prevention.

Of the 20.7 million Americans with osteoarthritis, the majority of them are women. Although age and injury are undoubtedly factors, heredity, abnormal use of the joint, diet, abnormalities in joint structure, and impaired blood supply to the joint may also contribute. Joint replacement and bone fusion are common surgical repair techniques. For most people, anti-inflammatory drugs and pain relievers such as aspirin and cortisone-related agents ease discomfort. Heat, mild exercise, and massage may also relieve the pain.

Rheumatoid arthritis is an autoimmune disease involving chronic inflammation that can appear at any age, but most commonly between ages 20 and 45. Rheumatoid arthritis is three times more common among women than among men during early adulthood but equally common among men and women in the over-70 age group. Symptoms include stiffness, pain, and swelling of multiple joints, often including the joints of the hands and wrists; they can be gradually progressive or sporadic, with occasional unexplained remissions.

Treatment for rheumatoid arthritis is similar to that for osteoarthritis. Emphasis is placed on pain relief and attempts to improve the functional mobility of the patient. Sometimes immunosuppressant drugs can reduce the inflammatory response.

Fibromyalgia

Fibromyalgia is a chronic, painful, rheumatoidlike disorder that affects as many as 5 to 6 percent of the general population. Persons with fibromyalgia experience an array of symptoms, including headaches, dizziness, numbness and tingling, itching, fluid retention, chronic joint pain, abdominal or pelvic pain, and even occasional diarrhea. Suspected causes include sleep disturbances, stress, emotional distress, viruses, and autoimmune disorders; however, none has been proved in clinical trials. Because of fibromyalgia's multiple symptoms, it is usually diagnosed only after myriad tests have ruled out other disorders. The American College of Rheumatology identifies these major diagnostic criteria:

- History of widespread pain of at least three months' duration in the axial skeleton as well as in all four quadrants of the body
- Pain in at least 11 of 18 paired tender points on digital palpation of about 4 kilograms of pressure

Fibromyalgia primarily affects women in their 30s and 40s. It can be extremely debilitating, causing feelings of unrelieved pain, bloating or swelling, and fatigue. Many people with fibromyalgia also become depressed and report chronic fatigue-like symptoms. Treatment varies based on the severity of symptoms. Typically, adequate rest, stress management, relaxation techniques, dietary supplements and selected herbal remedies, and pain medications are prescribed.

Systemic Lupus Erythematosus

Systemic lupus erythematosus (SLE), or **lupus,** is an autoimmune disease in which antibodies destroy or injure organs such as the kidneys, brain, and heart. The symptoms vary from mild to severe and may disappear for periods of time. A butterfly-shaped rash covering the bridge of the nose and both cheeks is common. Nearly all SLE sufferers have aching joints and muscles, and 60 percent of them develop redness and swelling that move from joint to joint. The disease affects 1 in 700 Caucasians but 1 in 250 African Americans; 90 percent of all victims are females. Extensive research has not yet found a cure for this sometimes fatal disease.

Low Back Pain

Approximately 80 percent of all Americans will experience low back pain (LBP) at some point. Some LBP episodes result from muscular damage and may be short-lived and acute. Other episodes may involve dislocations, fractures, or other problems with spinal vertebrae or discs, thus resulting in chronic pain or requiring surgery. Low back pain is epidemic throughout the world. It is the major cause of disability for people age 20 to 45 in the United States, who suffer more frequently and severely from this problem than older people do. LBP causes more lost work time in the United States than any other illness except upper respiratory infections. In fact, costs associated with back injury exceeded those associated with all other industrial injuries combined.

Almost 90 percent of all back problems occur in the lumbar spine region (lower back). You can avoid many problems by consciously maintaining good posture. Other preventive hints include:

- Purchase a firm mattress, and avoid sleeping on your stomach.
- Avoid high-heeled shoes, which often tilt the pelvis forward.
- Control your weight.
- Lift objects with your legs, not your back.
- Buy a good chair for doing your work, preferably one with lumbar support.
- Move your car seat forward so your knees are elevated slightly.
- Warm up before exercising.
- Engage in regular exercise, particularly exercises that strengthen the abdominal muscles and stretch the back muscles.

OTHER MALADIES

During the past 20 years, several afflictions have surfaced that seem to be products of our time. Some of these health problems relate to specific groups of people; some are due to technological advances; and others have not been explained (Table 16.2).

Chronic Fatigue Syndrome

Fatigue is a subjective condition in which people feel tired before they begin activities, lack the energy to accomplish tasks that require sustained effort and attention, or become abnormally exhausted after normal activities. In the late 1980s, several U.S. clinics noted a characteristic set of symptoms including chronic fatigue, headaches, fever, sore throat, enlarged lymph nodes, depression, poor memory, general weakness, nausea, and symptoms remarkably similar to mononucleosis.

Despite extensive testing, No viral cause has been found. In the absence of a known pathogen, many researchers believe that the illness, commonly referred to as *chronic fatigue syndrome (CFS)*, may have strong psychosocial roots. Our heightened awareness of health makes some of us scrutinize our bodies so carefully that the slightest deviation becomes amplified. In addition, people who suffer from depression seem to be good candidates for CFS. Experts worry, however, that too many people approach CFS as something that is "in the person's head" and that such an attitude may prevent scientists from doing the serious research needed to find a cure.

The diagnosis of CFS depends on two major criteria and eight or more minor criteria. The major criteria are debilitating fatigue that persists for at least six months and the absence of other illnesses that could cause the symptoms. Minor criteria include headaches, fever, sore throat, painful lymph nodes, weakness, fatigue after exercise, sleep problems, and rapid onset of these symptoms. Treatment focuses on improved nutrition, rest, counseling for depression, judicious exercise, and development of a strong support network.

Table 16.2. OTHER MODERN AFFLICTIONS		
Disease	***Description***	***Treatment***
Cystic fibrosis	Inherited disease occurring in 1 out of every 1,600 births. Characterized by pooling of large amounts of mucus in lungs, digestive disturbances, and excessive sodium excretion. Results in premature death.	Most treatments are geared toward relief of symptoms. Antibiotics are administered for infection. Recent strides in genetic research suggest better treatments and potential cure in the near future.
Sickle-cell anemia	Inherited disease affecting 8–10% of all African Americans. Disease affects hemoglobin, forming sickle-shaped red blood cells that interfere with oxygenation. Results in severe pain, anemia, and premature death.	Reduce stress, and attend to minor infections immediately. Seek genetic counseling.
Cerebral palsy	Disorder characterized by the loss of voluntary control over motor functioning. Believed to be caused by a lack of oxygen to the brain at birth, brain disorders or an accident before or after birth, poisoning, or brain infections.	Follow preventive actions to reduce accident risks; improved neonatal and birthing techniques show promise.
Graves' disease	A thyroid disorder characterized by swelling of the eyes, staring gaze, and retraction of the eyelid. Can result in loss of sight. The cause is unknown, and the disease can occur at any age.	Medication may help control symptoms. Radioactive iodine supplements also may be administered.

Repetitive Stress Injuries

The Bureau of Labor Statistics estimates that 25 percent of all injuries in the labor force that result in lost work time are due to a **repetitive stress injury (RSI).** These are injuries to nerves, soft tissue, or joints that result from the physical stress of repeated motions. They are estimated to cost employers more than $22 billion a year in workers' compensation and an additional $85 billion in related costs, such as absenteeism.

One of the most common RSIs is **carpal tunnel syndrome.** Hours spent typing at the computer, flipping groceries through computerized scanners, or other jobs made simpler by technology can irritate the median nerve in the wrist, thus causing numbness, tingling, and pain in the fingers and hands. Although carpal tunnel syndrome risk can be reduced by proper placement of the keyboard, mouse, wrist pads, and other techniques, RSIs are often overlooked until significant damage has been done. Better education and ergonomic workplace designs can eliminate many injuries of this nature.

TAKING CHARGE

Make It Happen!

Assessment: The Assess Yourself box on page 376 gave you the chance to consider your beliefs and attitudes about STIs, and possible risks you may be facing. Now that you have considered these results, you can begin to take steps toward changing certain behaviors that may be putting you at risk.

Making a Change: In order to change your behavior, you need to develop a plan. Follow these steps.

1. Evaluate your behavior, and identify patterns and specific things you are doing. What can you change now? What can you change in the near future?
2. Select one pattern of behavior that you want to change.
3. Fill out a Behavior Change Contract. It should include your long-term goal for change, your short-term goals, the rewards you'll give yourself for reaching these goals, potential obstacles along the way, and strategies for overcoming these obstacles. For each goal, list the small steps and specific actions that you will take.

4. Chart your progress in a journal. At the end of a week, consider how successful you were in following your plan. What helped you be successful? What made change more difficult? What will you do differently next week?
5. Revise your plan as needed. Are the short-term goals attainable? Are the rewards satisfying?

Example: Carlos had never thought that he was at risk for an STI. He only dated one woman at a time, and he had never had an STI himself. After he reviewed his answers to the self-assessment, however, he saw that there were several ways in which he was putting himself at risk.

He had thought that he would be able to tell whether someone was infected with an STI but the answer to question #1 described how, especially among women, there are few if any obvious signs or symptoms of some STIs. Carlos also believed that he was not at risk because he dated only one woman at a time, but the answer to question #8 pointed out that a person can pass on an STI that he or she contracted from a previous sex partner. Carlos decided it was time to take responsibility for his sexual activity. He had been on three dates with Sherry, and felt things were progressing to a more intimate stage soon. He wanted to be sure that they took the time to discuss STIs before they put themselves at risk.

Carlos was nervous when he thought about talking to Sherry about STIs, so he wrote out a few ideas of ways to bring up the subject. This made him more confident that he would be able to talk honestly with Sherry before they became more intimate. He also made sure that he had a supply of condoms, so there wouldn't be any reason not to practice safe sex. At the end of their next date, Carlos asked Sherry if they could have a serious conversation about the next step. When he told her that he wanted to talk about STIs, she told him that she was relieved that he had brought up the subject. She knew that she was healthy, and hadn't been sure how to find out his status. Carlos was relieved that Sherry was as concerned about the issue as he was, and they were both glad that embarrassment had not prevented them from having this conversation.

SUMMARY

- The major uncontrollable risk factors for contracting infectious diseases are heredity, age, environmental conditions, and organism resistance. The major controllable risk factors are stress, nutrition, fitness level, sleep, hygiene, avoidance of high-risk behaviors, and drug use.
- The major pathogens are bacteria, viruses, fungi, protozoa, prions, and parasitic worms. Bacterial infections include staphylococcal infections, streptococcal infections, pneumonia, Legionnaire's disease, tuberculosis, and periodontal diseases. Major viruses include the common cold, influenza, mononucleosis, hepatitis, and measles.
- Your body uses a number of defense systems to keep pathogens from invading. The skin is the body's major protection, helped by enzymes. The immune system creates antibodies to destroy antigens. In addition, fever and pain play a role in defending the body. Vaccines bolster the body's immune system against specific diseases.
- Emerging and resurgent diseases pose significant threats for future generations. Many factors contribute to these risks. Possible solutions focus on a public health approach to prevention.
- Sexually transmitted infections (STIs) are spread through intercourse, oral sex, anal sex, hand–genital contact, and sometimes through mouth-to-mouth contact. Major STIs include chlamydia, pelvic inflammatory disease (PID), gonorrhea, syphilis, pubic lice, genital warts, candidiasis, trichomoniasis, and herpes. Sexual transmission may also be involved in some general urinary tract infections.
- Acquired immune deficiency syndrome (AIDS) is caused by the human immunodeficiency virus (HIV). HIV is not confined to certain high-risk groups. Globally, HIV/AIDS has become a major threat to the world's population. Anyone can get HIV by engaging in high-risk sexual activities that include exchange of body fluids, by having received a blood transfusion before 1985, and by injecting drugs (or having sex with someone who does). Women appear to be particularly susceptible to infection. You can cut your risk for AIDS by deciding not to engage in risky sexual activities.
- Chronic lung diseases include allergies, hay fever, asthma, emphysema, and chronic bronchitis. Allergies are part of the body's natural defense system. Chronic obstructive pulmonary diseases are the fifth leading cause of death in the United States.

- Neurological conditions include headaches, seizure disorders, Parkinson's disease, and multiple sclerosis. Headaches may be caused by a variety of factors, the most common of which are tension, dilation and/or rapid contraction of blood vessels in the brain, chemical influences on muscles and vessels that cause inflammation and pain, and underlying physiological and psychological disorders.
- Premenstrual syndrome (PMS) and premenstrual dysphoric disorder (PMDD) are conditions related to the menstrual cycle. Endometriosis is the buildup of endometrial tissue in regions of the body other than the uterus.
- Diabetes occurs when the pancreas fails to produce enough insulin to regulate sugar metabolism. Other conditions, such as colitis, irritable bowel syndrome (IBS), and peptic ulcers, are the direct result of functional problems in various digestion-related organs or systems.
- Musculoskeletal diseases such as arthritis, lower back pain, repetitive stress injuries, and other problems cause significant pain and disability in millions of people. Chronic fatigue syndrome (CFS) and repetitive stress injuries (RSIs, such as carpal tunnel syndrome) have emerged in the past decade as major chronic maladies. CFS is associated with depression. Repetitive stress injuries are preventable by proper equipment placement and usage.

QUESTIONS FOR DISCUSSION AND REFLECTION

1. What are the major controllable risk factors for contracting infectious diseases? Using this knowledge, how would you change your current lifestyle to prevent such infection?
2. What is a pathogen? What are the similarities and differences between pathogens and antigens? Discuss uncontrollable and controllable risk factors that can threaten your health.
3. What are the six types of pathogens? What are the various means by which they can be transmitted? How have social conditions among the poor and homeless increased the risks for certain diseases, such as tuberculosis, influenza, and hepatitis? Why are these conditions a challenge to the efforts of public health officials?
4. Identify possible reasons for the spread of emerging and resurgent diseases. Indicate public policies and programs that might reduce this trend.
5. Identify five STIs. What are their symptoms? How do they develop? What are their potential long-term effects?
6. Should Americans be concerned about soaring HIV/AIDS rates elsewhere in the world? Explain your answer.
7. What are some of the major noninfectious chronic diseases affecting Americans today? Do you think there is a pattern in the types of diseases that we get? What are the common risk factors?
8. List common respiratory diseases affecting Americans. Which of these diseases has a genetic basis? An environmental basis? An individual basis? What, if anything, is being done to prevent, treat, and control each of these conditions?
9. Describe the symptoms and treatment of diabetes. What is the difference between type 1 diabetes and type 2 diabetes?
10. What are the major disorders of the musculoskeletal system? Why do you think there aren't any cures? Describe the difference between osteoarthritis and rheumatoid arthritis.

ACCESSING YOUR HEALTH ON THE INTERNET

Visit the following Internet sites to explore further topics and issues related to personal health. To visit an organization's website, go to the Companion Website for *Health: The Basics, Sixth Edition* at www.aw-bc.com/donatelle, click on the book image, and select "Accessing Your Health on the Internet" from the navigation menu on the left.

1. *American Academy of Allergy, Asthma, and Immunology*. Provides an overview of asthma and allergies. Offers interactive quizzes to test your knowledge and an "ask an expert" section.

2. *American Diabetes Association*. Excellent resource for diabetes information.
3. *Centers for Disease Control and Prevention (CDC)*. Home page for the government agency dedicated to disease intervention and prevention, with links to all the latest data and publications put out by the CDC, including the *Morbidity and Mortality Weekly Report, HIV/AIDS Surveillance Report,* and the *Journal of Emerging Infectious Diseases*, and access to the CDC research database, Wonder.
4. *National Center for Chronic Disease Prevention and Health Promotion*. Provides access to a wide range of information from this CDC-affiliated organization dedicated to chronic diseases and health promotion.
5. *World Health Organization (WHO)*. Provides access to the latest information on world health issues, including infectious disease, as put out by WHO. Provides direct access to publications and fact sheets, with keywords to help users find topics of interest.

FURTHER READING

Champeau, D., and R. Donatelle. *AIDS and STIS: A Global Perspective*. Englewood Cliffs, NJ: Prentice Hall, 2002. *An overview of issues, trends, and ethics surrounding the global pandemic of HIV/AIDS and STIs.*

Chin, J., ed. *Control of Communicable Diseases Manual, 17th ed.* Washington, D.C.: American Public Health Association, 2003. *Outstanding pocket reference for information on infectious diseases. Updated every three to five years to cover emerging diseases.*

National Center for Health Statistics. *Monthly Vital Statistics Report and Advance Data from Vital and Health Statistics*. Hyattsville, MD: Public Health Service. *Detailed government reports, usually published monthly, concerning mortality and morbidity data for the United States. Includes changes occurring in the rates of particular diseases and in health practices so patterns and trends can be analyzed.*

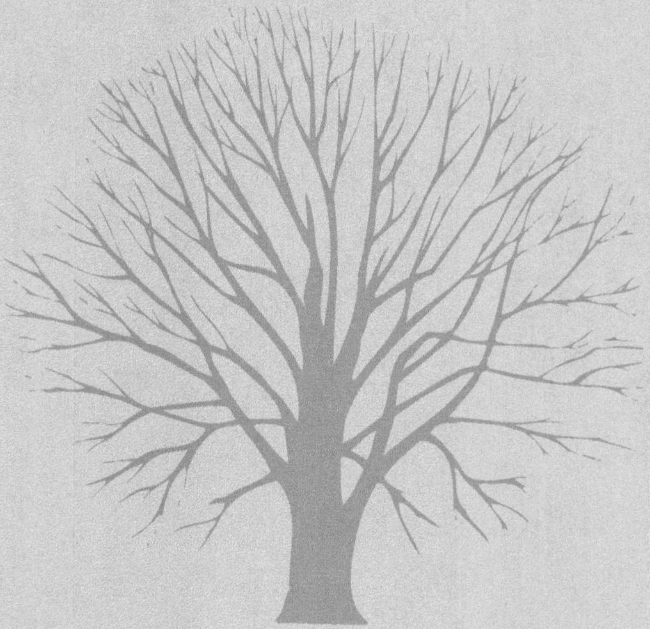

III

Study Guide

CHAPTER ONE

Healing Massage—A Wellness Perspective

STUDY GUIDE

LEARNING OUTCOMES

Use the learning outcomes at the beginning of the chapter as a guide to your studies. Perform the task given in each outcome, either in writing or verbally into a tape recorder or to a study partner. This may start as an "open book" exercise, and then later from memory.

KEY TERMS/CONCEPTS

To study key words and concepts listed at the beginning of this chapter, choose one or more of the following exercises. Writing or talking about ideas helps you remember them better, and explaining them to someone else helps deepen your understanding.

1. Write a one or two sentence explanation of each key word and concept.
2. Make study cards by writing the explanation from problem 1 on one side of a 3 × 5 card, and the key word or concept on the other. Shuffle the cards and read one side, trying to recite either the explanation or word on the other side.
3. Pick out two or three key words or concepts and explain how they are related.
4. With a study partner, take turns explaining key words and concepts verbally.
5. Make up sentences using one or more key words or concepts.
6. Read your sentences from problem 5 to a study partner, who will ask you to clarify your meaning.

STUDY OUTLINE

The following questions test your memory of the main concepts in this chapter. Locate the answers in the text using the page number given for each question.

Natural Healing Art

1. Along with other therapies that use the healing gifts of nature, massage is considered a ____________. (p. 4)
2. The natural healing philosophy includes these tenets: (1) ________________, (2) ________________, (3) ________________________________. (p. 4)
3. Massage is considered manual therapy because it is performed ______________________. (p. 4)
4. The term *healing* means ____. (p. 4)
5. In contrast to the term *healing*, the term *curing* implies ________________________________. (p. 4)
6. The term *holistic* includes a person's (1) ________, (2) ________, (3) ________, and (4) ________ (p. 4)

Massage Definition

1. *Massage* is the ____________________ and ________________ manipulation of the ______ ____________ of the body to enhance health and healing. (p. 5)
2. The ________ and ________ of the practitioner constitute the massage technique. (p. 5)
3. The aim that guides the action is called its ________. (p. 5)
4. The words ________ and ________ are often used together to describe the broad scope of the occupational field of massage therapy. (p. 5)

Massage and Bodywork Traditions

1. A *tradition* is an element of culture that is passed down from ____________________________. (p. 5)
2. Four major world traditions of massage and bodywork are (1) ________, (2) ________, (3) ________, (4) ________. (p. 5)
3. The system of soft tissue manipulation that evolved out of the work of Ling and Mezger in the 19th century is known as ____________________. (p. 6)
4. Match the classic Western massage techniques listed below with the descriptions on the right: (p. 7)

_____ effleurage	a. percussion
_____ petrissage	b. rubbing surfaces together
_____ tapotement	c. sliding or gliding
_____ friction	d. oscillating
_____ vibration	e. kneading or pressing

5. Two additional techniques commonly performed in Western massage are ____________ and ____________. (p. 7)
6. Lymphatic massage, trigger points, and reflexology are categorized as __________________ Western massage and bodywork systems. (p. 7)
7. Practitioners who incorporate techniques from two or more traditions or systems of massage and bodywork are said to be ________________________. (p. 7)

Massage and Western Medicine

1. When massage is considered an either/or option outside of mainstream medicine, it is referred to as ____________. (p. 7)
2. When massage is used to contribute to a patient's recovery, but as secondary to a treatment by mainstream medicine, it is referred to as ____________. (p. 7).
3. CAM is an acronym for C ________ & A ________ M ________. (p. 7)
4. In ________ health care systems, different therapies exist on an equal footing and are chosen for the greatest benefit of the patient. (p. 7)

Wellness Perspective

1. A wellness perspective goes beyond the old idea of health as the absence of disease to one of achieving ________________. (p. 9)
2. The diagram by Travis that shows the scope of the wellness model from premature death to high level wellness is called the ________________. (p. 9)
3. The goal of treatment is to bring a person to the ________________ point on the illness/wellness continuum. (p. 9)

4. Since it addresses many different aspects of a person's life, the idea of high level wellness is _____ _____________ at its core. (p. 9)

5. The wellness massage pyramid is a tool for understanding the ______________________________ ________ on the journey to high level wellness. (p. 11)

6. The levels of the wellness massage pyramid from the foundation up to high level wellness are (1) ________________, (2) ________________, (3) ________________________, (4) neutral zone, (5) ________________, (6) ________________, and (7) ________________ (Figure 1–4)

7. Which of the following statements are true according to a wellness perspective? (pp. 9–12)

   _____ a. Treatment for a medical condition is an aspect of wellness.

   _____ b. A person with a chronic illness cannot achieve high level wellness.

   _____ c. Health care professionals are responsible for their patients achieving high level wellness.

   _____ d. Freedom from illness or injury is a neutral point in terms of wellness.

   _____ e. Once high level wellness is achieved, it remains for life.

Wellness and the Health Professions

1. The professions that include massage in their scope of practice are ______________________________ ________________________. (p. 12)

2. A method of treating a pathology is called a ________________. (p. 12)

3. Rather than calling systems of massage bodywork *modalities*, it is recommended that they be called ________________ or ________________. (p. 12)

4. True or False. Physical therapists only perform treatment applications of massage and other therapeutic modalities. Explain. (p. 12)

5. True or False. Massage therapists only perform massage for personal growth and pleasure. Explain. (p. 12)

4. Nurses sometimes include massage as part of ________________ care of patients in hospitals and nursing homes. (p. 12)

5. Although different health professions use massage somewhat differently, they share a common bond, that is, the ________________ themselves. (p. 12)

Clarifying Terminology

1. Someone trained in massage and who uses massage in the practice of his or her profession is called a ________________. (p. 13)

2. A ________________ refers to the period of time in which massage is performed. (p. 13)

3. The word ________________ is reserved for descriptions of medical applications of massage. (pp. 12–13)

FOR GREATER UNDERSTANDING

The following exercises are designed to take you from the realm of theory into the real world. They will help give you a deeper understanding of the subjects covered in this chapter. Action words are *underlined* to emphasize the variety of activities presented to address different learning styles, and to encourage deeper thinking.

1. Visit two or more places where massage is offered, for example, a spa, health club, rehabilitation clinic, or integrative medicine facility. Compare and contrast the settings, clientele, and types of massage offered. Get a massage at one or more places for a more personal experience.

2. Interview someone who receives regular massage to find out how they think massage has benefited them over a period of time. Ask them to be specific. Analyze their responses using the wellness massage pyramid.

3. Interview two or more people as in problem 2, and compare their responses.

4. Receive a massage from a trained practitioner. After the massage, interview the practitioner about their choice of techniques and their intention(s) in applying the techniques during the session. Write a report of your experience.

5. Interview someone who performs massage in his or her occupation and analyze their work according to the wellness massage perspective. Note their

occupational field or profession, the setting, clientele, goals of massage sessions, and types of massage and bodywork provided.

6. Think about how you might use massage for your own health and healing, looking at benefits for body, mind, emotions, and spirit. Discuss your thoughts in class or a study group, and compare with others.

7. Using Table 1–2, write a short story about a client or patient using wellness or treatment terminology as appropriate. For example: (Wellness) Jane went to the spa for a massage session after planting her vegetable garden and experiencing sore and stiff back and legs. The massage therapist took a health history, assessed the situation, developed a session strategy, and performed Western massage focusing on circulation and muscle relaxation in the back and legs. (Treatment) John's doctor referred him for massage to help in recovery from a repetitive strain injury in the shoulder. The therapist took a medical history, noting that John was taking muscle relaxants and pain medication. Using clinical reasoning skills, the therapist developed a treatment plan, and performed Western massage with trigger point therapy on the affected region.

8. Look through a massage and bodywork magazine or journal, and make a list of the types of massage and bodywork written about or advertised. Categorize the types into the four world traditions. Explain your decisions.

9. Read the White House Commission Report on Complementary and Alternative Medicine Policy, and in class or with a study group, discuss the implications of the report for the future of massage therapy. (*www.whccamp.hhs.gov*).

10. Visit the Web sites listed throughout this chapter for further information about a particular topic.

CHAPTER TWO

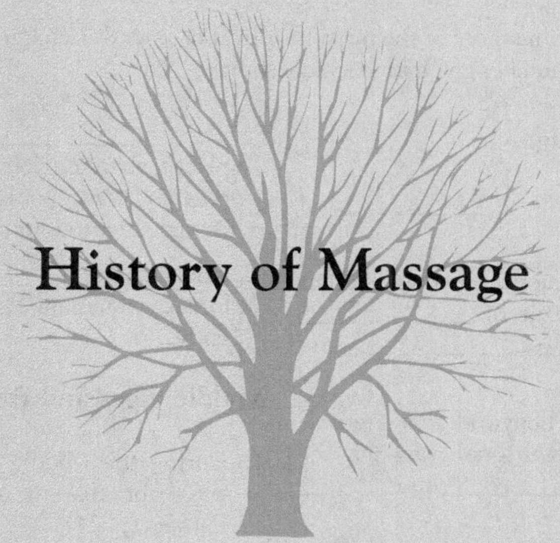

History of Massage

STUDY GUIDE

LEARNING OUTCOMES

Use the learning outcomes at the beginning of the chapter as a guide to your studies. Perform the task given in each outcome, either in writing or verbally into a tape recorder or to a study partner. This may start as an "open book" exercise, and then later from memory.

KEY HISTORICAL PEOPLE, KEY TERMS/CONCEPTS

To study key historical people, places, events, and forms of massage listed at the beginning of this chapter, choose one or more of the following exercises. Writing or talking about these stories will help you remember them better, and deepen your understanding of their significance.

1. Summarize the contributions of a key person in the development of massage at a particular period of time. Try to capture their contributions in one or two concise statements.
2. Make study cards by writing the name of a key historical person, place or event on one side of a 3 × 5 card, and details about them on the other. Shuffle the cards and read one side, trying to recite information from the other side.
3. Match key historical people to places and events or other people related to them in some way, and explain how they are related.
4. With a study partner(s), take turns telling the stories of key people, places or events in the history of massage. Telling the stories verbally to someone else can help you remember them, and help clarify details in your mind.
5. After each story in problem 4, ask each other questions to clarify the significance of the person, place, or event in the history of massage.

STUDY OUTLINE

The following questions test your memory of the main historical facts in this chapter. Locate the answers in the text using the page number given for each question.

Ancient and Global Heritage

1. The history of massage is both ____________ and ____________. (p. 17)
2. The exchange of ideas and practices among different cultures happens as the result of ____________, ____________, ____________, ____________, and ____________. (p. 17)
3. Some of forms of massage and bodywork that continue to be performed in their traditional ways may be considered both __________________ and ____________________. (p. 17)

Native and Folk Traditions

1. An example of wellness massage practiced by people of the South Sea Islands for centuries is __________________. (p. 18)
2. Hispanic healers called __________________ use massage in their tradition of folk medicine developed in the 15th century when Catholic Spaniards came in contact with the __________________ civilization in Mexico. (p. 18)

Ancient Civilizations

1. One of the oldest records describing rubbing for medicinal purposes was found on clay tablets written in _______________ in 2100 BCE. (pp. 18–19)
2. Written over 2,500 years ago, __________________ __________________ is often cited as the first book written on Chinese medicine. (p. 19)
3. Traditional Japanese massage called ____________ developed in Japan in the 6th century BCE when Chinese health and healing practices reached the islands. (p. 19)
4. Shiatsu is a modern form of Japanese bodywork developed in the ______________ by __________________. (p. 19)
5. The traditional healing practices of India, called _________________, can be traced back to the 5th century CE, and included forms of massage. (p. 20)
6. The ancient Greek medical writings of ____________ mentioned massage used to treat sprains and dislocations. (p. 20)
7. Massage given to athletes in the Greek ___________ used a lot of oil, and was given before and after exercises. (p. 20)
8. The __________________ were communal gathering places where citizens of the Roman empire enjoyed cool and warm pools of water, steam rooms, and received a rigorous form of bodywork. (pp. 20–21)
9. The modern __________________ is a legacy of the Greek gymnasium, Roman baths, and ____________ baths. (p. 21)

Middle Ages and Renaissance Europe

1. During the Middle Ages, the practice of massage was kept alive in the __________________ of Europe. (p. 21)
2. Classic Greek and Roman writings about the use of massage in medicine were preserved during the Dark Ages by the ____________, and by the __________________. (p. 21)
3. A book called the __________________, translated from Arabic into Latin in the 11th century, is evidence of the early development of the philosophy of natural health and healing. (p. 21)
4. Classic Greek and Roman writings were brought back to Europe during the period called the __________________. (pp. 21–22)

Western Massage

1. Western massage is a synthesis of techniques developed by __________________ of Sweden and __________________ of Amsterdam in the 1800s. (p. 22)
2. Pehr Ling developed a system of medical gymnastics to treat chronic ailments called the __________________ __________________ in the United States. (p. 22)
3. Ling's school in Stockholm, called the ______________________, was founded in __________. (p. 23)
4. Johann Mezger categorized the many soft tissue techniques, calling them by the French terms ____________, ____________, ____________, and ____________. These, plus the technique of ____________, make up the categories of Western massage. (p. 23)
5. Ling's medical gymnastics was brought to the United States by ____________________ of New York in ____________. (p. 24)

Conventional and Natural Healing

1. Words used to describe massage technique in early conventional medical practice were ____________, ____________, and ____________. (p. 24)
2. Massage and bodywork was called the ____________ art by Walter Johnson in an 1866 book on the history of soft tissue manipulation. (p. 24)
3. Lucas-Championnière of France (c. 1880) advocated the use of soft tissue manipulation in the treatment of ____________. (p. 24)
4. The Reconstruction Department of the United States Army was established in 1918 to help in the rehabilitation of soldiers wounded in (war) ____________. Women trained to use massage, movements, and hydrotherapy in this effort were called ____________. (p. 25)
5. ____________________ was a prominent figure in the history of physical therapy who trained Reconstruction Aides at the Walter Reed Clinic during World War I. She wrote *Massage and Therapeutic Exercise* while director of physiotherapy at ____________ in the 1920s. (p. 25)
6. The director of the Battle Creek Sanitarium in Michigan in the late 1800s, and a famous advocate of natural healing, was ________________________. His book ______________ was published in 1895. (p. 26)
7. A man named __________________ popularized natural health practices in the late 19th and early 20th centuries through his resorts, *Physical Culture Magazine*, and radio shows. (p. 26)
8. The heyday of Swedish massage was from about ____________ to ____________. (p. 26)
9. Swedish massage practice consisted of Western massage, the Swedish movements, various forms of ____________________, ____________________, ____________________, reducing massage, and ____________________ irrigation. (p. 26)
10. Many Swedish massage practitioners in the early 20th century worked as natural healers, and with non-conventional doctors of __________________ and __________________. (p. 26)

Sports and Fitness

1. The ______________________ was a simple form of massage given to athletes in the late 1800s and early 1900s. (p. 27)
2. A book written in 1916 by H. J. Fay called __________________ describes massage for recovery after athletic events. (p. 27)
3. Sports massage was revived by __________________ in the (year) __________________, and is now a popular specialty within the field. (p. 27)
4. Massage has been part of the health services at the __________________, an American health and fitness institution, since the early 1900s. (p. 28)

Decline and Revival in the 20th Century

1. The ______________ (decade) was a period of decline in the practice of massage in the United States. (p. 28)
2. Massage __________________ were used as a cover for prostitution, ruining the image of legitimate massage practitioners. (p. 28)
3. A simplified version of Western massage developed in the 1970s that emphasized long flowing strokes and the sensual experience of scented oils, relaxing music, and incense was called ____________________ (p. 29)
4. Two important social movements in the development of the form of massage described in problem 3 were ________________ and the ______________. (p. 28)
5. A movement of the 1970s that had a major impact on health professions, including massage therapy, and that developed within the field of health, physical education, and recreation was the ______________. (p. 29)

Milestones at the Turn of the 21st Century

1. A national organization whose mission is to advance massage therapy research is the ______________________, incorporated in ___________ (year). (p. 30)
2. The first center in the world devoted to research on the use of touch in human health was the __________________ at the University of Miami. It was founded in ____________ (year), and its first director was __________________. (p. 30)
3. The U.S. National Institutes of Health (NIH) established the ___________________________ in 1992 to explore unconventional medical practices. This was elevated to a center at NIH in 1998 called the ______________________________________. (p. 30)
4. The first National Certification Examination for Therapeutic Massage and Bodywork was given in ______________ (year). (p. 30)
5. The Commission on Massage Therapy Accreditation received U.S. Department of Education recognition in ______________ (year). (p. 31)

FOR GREATER UNDERSTANDING

The following exercises are designed to make history come alive by connecting it to the real world of human experience. The exercises will introduce you to primary sources for learning more about history, and help you gain a deeper understanding of the historical subjects covered in this chapter.

1. Choose one or two major figures introduced in this chapter, and research their lives and contributions to the development of massage therapy. Try to locate their original writings to read about their work in their own words.

2. Locate an old Turkish bath or spa in your community that is still in operation. Research its history, and visit the place, looking at its architecture and floor space. Receive a massage there if still available, or enjoy the baths. See if they have old photos or an archive. This is also a good vacation adventure.

3. Look through old newspapers, magazines, or playbills for advertisements related to the history of massage, e.g., Turkish baths, reducing salons, health clubs, massage parlors. From the 1890s to 1930s are good times to explore.

4. Visit an antique shop and look for things related to the history of massage, such as advertisements mentioned in problem 3, old books, electrical vibrators, or lotion and oil bottles that might have been used with massage.

5. Interview someone who remembers the 1950s and how massage was perceived at that time. Ask them how their view of massage has changed over the years, and what has influenced that change. Share your interview with a study partner or group.

6. Interview someone who learned Esalen massage in the 1970s or early 1980s. Where did they learn it and what was their experience of it? How was it different from massage therapy today? Share your interview with a study partner or group.

7. Interview someone from a different culture who is familiar with massage as passed down within their family. How far back in time and where has it been practiced? Who did they learn it from? What was it like? How is it different or similar to Western massage?

8. Interview a nurse or physical therapist who was working in the 1950s, 1960s, or another period from the past. Ask them about how massage was used in health care at that time, and how it changed over the years. Report your findings.

9. Be alert to references about massage in old movies, especially from the 1930–1940s. Some movies set in historical periods also show massage as given at that time.

10. Visit the website of the World of Massage Museum (*www.worldofmassagemuseum.com*). Look at its mission and the content of its collection.

CHAPTER THREE

Effects and Benefits of Massage

STUDY GUIDE

LEARNING OUTCOMES

Use the learning outcomes at the beginning of the chapter as a guide to your studies. Perform the task given in each outcome, either in writing or verbally into a tape recorder or to a study partner. This may start as an "open book" exercise, and then later from memory.

KEY TERMS/CONCEPTS

To study key words and concepts listed at the beginning of this chapter, choose one or more of the following exercises. Writing or talking about ideas helps you remember them better, and explaining helps deepen your understanding.

1. Write a one- or two-sentence explanation of each key word and concept.
2. Make study cards by writing the explanation from problem 1 on one side of a 3 × 5 card, and the key word or concept on the other. Shuffle the cards and read one side, trying to recite either the explanation or word on the other side.
3. Pick out two or three key words or concepts and explain how they are related.
4. With a study partner, take turns explaining key words and concepts verbally.
5. Make up sentences using one or more key words or concepts.
6. Read your sentences from problem 5 to a study partner, who will ask you to clarify your meaning.

STUDY OUTLINE

The following questions test your memory of the main concepts in this chapter. Locate the answers in the text using the page number given for each question.

Effects of Massage

1. Changes in the body, mind, and emotions of the recipient as a result of soft tissue manipulation and related techniques are called ____________________. (p. 35)
2. Practitioners who know how to apply massage techniques to obtain specific effects will be more successful in achieving ____________________. (p. 35)

Tissue Level Effects

1. Massage promotes the overall health of tissues, primarily through increased blood and lymph ____________________. (p. 35)
2. Massage is ____________________ during the inflammation phase of tissue repair. (p. 37)
3. During the regeneration phase of tissue repair, massage removes ____________________, and transports ____________________ to the affected area. (p. 37)
4. During the remodeling phase of tissue repair, massage helps in healthy ________________ formation. (p. 37)
5. A study showed that wounds heal more slowly in people suffering from ____________________. (p. 37)
6. The property of connective tissue whereby it become more pliable when it is mobile is called ____________________. (p. 37)
7. The type of connective tissue that surrounds all muscles, bones, and organs, and gives them their shape is called ____________________. (p. 37)
8. When fascial tissues stick together, ____________________ are formed. (p. 37)

Organ System Level Effects

Integumentary System

1. Benefits of stimulating the sensory receptors in the skin with massage include ____. (p. 38)
2. Friction that occurs with massage helps keep ____________________ free from blockage. (p. 38)
3. Oil and lotion applied with massage ____________________ the skin. (p. 38)

Skeletal System

1. Movement of the joints stimulates production of ____________________. (p. 38)
2. Optimal range of motion is achieved when the bones are in ____________________. and the tissues surrounding the joints are ____________________. (p. 38)

Muscular System

1. Muscular *under-activity* caused by illness or injury results in ____. (p. 39)
2. Massage techniques that simulate ____________________ can alleviate negative effects of muscular *under-activity*. (p. 39)
3. Muscular *over-activity* such as from strenuous exercise can cause ____. (p. 39)
4. Massage techniques that increase blood flow, for example ________________ and ________________, can alleviate negative effects of *over-activity*. (p. 39)
5. General muscle relaxation may be elicited by massage through activation of the ____________________ nervous system, by conscious release of ____________________, or by increased sensory ____________________. (p. 39)
6. Muscles that are tense and in a state of partial contraction are said to be ________________. (p. 39)
7. The muscle relaxation technique in which the practitioner slowly and forcibly draws the muscle attachments together is called ________________. (p. 40)
8. The muscle relaxation technique in which cross-fiber and with-fiber friction is performed on the attachments of the targeted muscle is called ________________. (p. 40)
9. Movement at joints is restricted by ____. (p. 40)
10. Proper body alignment is commonly called ____________________. (p. 40)
11. Massage and joint movements can improve posture by ________________ and ________________ shortened muscles, lengthening muscle groups with ____________________, and unsticking fascial ____________________ that are contributing to posture distortion. (p. 40)

Nervous and Endocrine Systems

1. An example of a massage and joint movement technique that utilizes the nervous system to effect desired results is ____. (p. 41)
2. The ____________________ occurs with activation of the parasympathetic nervous system, which has ef-

fects on skeletal muscles as well as several other organ systems. (p. 41)

Cardiovascular System

1. Superficial friction massage can cause release of a chemical called ________________. that leads to capillary vessel dilation and ________________ ________________ in skin and underlying connective tissue. (p. 41)
2. Increase in the amount of blood in an area is referred to as ________________. (p. 41)
3. A condition in which normal blood flow in the veins is slowed or halted is called ______________. (p. 42)
4. Venous return is facilitated by the mechanical action of these massage techniques: ________________ ________________. (pp. 41–42)
5. The dictum in classic Western massage that deep effleurage should always be ________________ reflects the thought that valves in the larger veins would be damaged if blood flow were forced backwards against them. (p. 42)
6. Blood pressure may be temporarily decreased during massage. This is thought to be the result of ________________________________. (p. 42)
7. The number of circulating red blood cells may be (choose one: increased or decreased) with massage. (p. 42)

Lymphatic System and Immunity

1. Movement of lymph through the lymph vessel system depends on outside sources such as ____________ ________________. (p. 42)
2. Resistance to injuries and disease caused by foreign substances is called ____________________. (p. 42)
3. Massage improves immunity through these effects: ____ ____________________. (pp. 42–43)

Respiratory System

1. Respiratory system function is enhanced by massage through improved ______________________ to the lungs, encouraging deep ________________ breathing, and relieving tension and shortening in ________________ involved in respiration. (p. 43)
2. By facilitating good posture, massage and bodywork helps clients achieve the ____________________ and ______________________ needed for optimal vital capacity. (p. 43)

Digestive System

1. Activation of the parasympathetic nervous system in relaxation massage (choose one: increases or decreases) digestive activity. (p. 43)
2. The stimulation of bowel movement through abdominal massage is useful for normal digestion function as well as treatment for ________________. (p. 43)
3. Bowel movements stimulated through massage are the result of direct ____________ effects, as well as reflex stimulation of ________________ movement of the large intestine. (p. 43)

Urinary System

1. The kidney function enhanced by increased circulation is ____________________ of the blood. (p. 43)
2. Parasympathetic nervous system activation (choose one: increases or decreases) urinary output and bladder tension. (p. 43)

Reproductive System

1. Male and female genitals are not ____________ ____________ for therapeutic massage. (p. 43)
2. There is evidence that chronic stress (choose one: improves or impairs) sexual function. (p. 43)
3. Breast massage is a specialized skill that promotes well-breast health. Breast massage requires ____________ ________ from the client, and may be beyond the ____________________________ of some practitioners. (pp. 43–44)

Organism Level Effects

1. Stimulation of the ______________________ in the skin and muscle tissue is essential for proper growth and development of infants. (p. 44)
2. Lack of blood supply to an area is called ______________________. (p. 44)
3. Massage can provide increased sensory input that blocks slower pain-transmitting nerve impulses. This is called the ____________________________ mechanism. (p. 44)
4. Myofascial trigger points can be deactivated by massage techniques such as ______________________ ________ and ______________________. (p. 45)
5. Pain may also be modulated by the release of neurochemicals called ______________ and ________

________________ that induce relaxation and feelings of wellbeing. (p. 45)

6. Relaxation massage is known to elicit the ________________________ Response by activating the parasympathetic nervous system. (p. 45)

7. Psychological effects of massage include improved mental ______________, ______________ anxiety, emotional ________________, and increased feeling of wellbeing. (p. 46)

Mechanisms of Massage

1. Effects of massage that are the result of physical forces such as compression, stretching, and vibration of body tissues are called __________________ effects. (p. 48)

2. Functional changes mediated by the ______________ system are called reflex effects. (p. 48)

3. Effects of massage involving organic processes at the cellular, tissue and organ system level are called ________________ effects. (p. 48)

4. Body-mind effects acknowledge the interplay of ________________, ________________, and ________________ in health and disease. (p. 49)

5. Theories of energy effects of bodywork are currently outside of purview of ________________; however, they have persisted over time and have been found useful by many people. (p. 49)

A Holistic View

1. A ________________ view of massage appreciates that we live as whole beings, and the separate effects of massage interact in complex ways to produce an overall effect that may be greater than the sum of its parts. (p. 49)

2. The connection of mind and body can be traced to our beginnings as embryos, when the outer layer of cells or ectoderm eventually develops into the ________________, ________________ and ________________ system. (p. 49)

3. Research on infant massage demonstrates the need for touch for proper ______________ and ______________. (p. 50)

4. The limbic system is group of structures in the brain related to the experience of ______________, and in the formation of ______________ memories. (p. 50)

5. Character ________________ is a concept used to explain muscular tension caused by suppressed emotions. (p. 50)

6. Massage is considered a ________________ therapy since it works primarily through touch and movement of the body to produce holistic effects in the recipient. (p. 50)

Benefits for Everyone

1. Effects of massage that support general health and wellbeing are ________________ by definition. (p. 51)

2. Massage provides health touch, which is a basic ________________. (p. 51)

Benefits for Special Populations

1. People with special needs that can benefit from massage include ________________________________. (p. 51)

2. Even if massage is not an appropriate ________________ for a certain medical condition, it may provide other health ________________ that improve the lives of those living with the condition. This is the essence of the wellness perspective. (p. 52)

FOR GREATER UNDERSTANDING

The following exercises are designed to take you from the realm of theory into the real world. They will help give you a deeper understanding of the subjects covered in this chapter. Action words are underlined to emphasize the variety of activities presented to address different learning styles, and to encourage deeper thinking.

1. <u>Write</u> a brief personal health history for the past 1 or 2 years. Using the information in this chapter, <u>identify</u> any areas that might have benefited (or did benefit) from receiving massage. <u>Discuss</u> your conclusions with a study partner or group.

2. <u>Interview</u> a family member or friend, and complete problem 1 for their case.

3. Choose a special population to study. <u>List</u> their special needs that result from their unique situation. If possible, <u>interview</u> someone from that population. Using the information in this chapter, <u>identify</u> any areas that might have benefited (or did benefit) from receiving massage.

4. For the special population studied in problem 3, <u>identify</u> a nonprofit organization that offers support. <u>Read</u>

their brochures or check out their Web sites for information on their mission and services. Do they recommend massage as being beneficial for the population? Write a letter to the organization providing evidence of the benefits of massage for the population and encouraging their recommendation. The letter may actually be sent or just written as a learning exercise.

5. Choose one particular effect of massage to study in more depth. Search several sources for further information including anatomy and physiology textbooks, and the AMTA Foundation research database. Discuss your findings with a study partner or group.

CHAPTER FOUR

Clinical Applications of Massage

STUDY GUIDE

LEARNING OUTCOMES

Use the learning outcomes at the beginning of the chapter as a guide to your studies. Perform the task given in each outcome, either in writing or verbally into a tape recorder or to a study partner. This may start as an "open book" exercise, and then later from memory.

KEY TERMS/CONCEPTS

To study key words and concepts listed at the beginning of this chapter, choose one or more of the following exercises. Writing or talking about ideas helps you remember them better, and explaining helps deepen your understanding.

1. Write a one- or two-sentence explanation of each key word and concept.
2. Make study cards by writing the explanation from problem 1 on one side of a 3 × 5 card, and the key word or concept on the other. Shuffle the cards and read one side, trying to recite either the explanation or word on the other side.
3. Pick out two or three key words or concepts and explain how they are related.
4. With a study partner, take turns explaining key words and concepts verbally.

STUDY OUTLINE

The following questions test your memory of the main concepts in this chapter. Locate the answers in the text using the page number given for each question.

Value of Research

1. Applications of massage for the treatment of pathologies are called ____________________ massage therapy. (p. 56)
2. Therapies for which there is supportive scientific research are called ____________________ - based. (p. 56).
3. In recipe-based therapy, every patient receives the ____________________. (p. 57)
4. In principle-based therapy, appropriate treatment techniques are ____________________, ____________________, and ____________________ as necessary to achieve specific effects. (p. 57)
5. Research is most useful when it adds to our understanding of the effectiveness of certain massage applications, and not as a means of developing ____________________ for treatment. (p. 57)
6. Research literacy includes understanding the ____________________ method, locating ____________________, and reading, analyzing and evaluating ____________________. (p. 57)

Clinical Approach

1. Massage is considered ____________________ to a primary treatment to enhance its effectiveness and create a more favorable environment for healing. (p. 57)
2. Massage is considered ____________________ care when it reduces discomforts related to a disease or its treatment. (p. 57)
3. Massage has ____________________ effects for treating a number of pathologies. (p. 57)

Musculo-Skeletal Pathologies

1. Direct therapeutic effects related to musculo-skeletal pathologies include ____________________, ____________________, ____________________, and ____________________. (p. 58)
2. Deep transverse friction is used effectively in treatment of ____________________ strain injuries. (p. 58)
3. Massage is an effective treatment for hypertonic muscles, e.g., in ____________________ and ____________________. (p. 58)
4. Symptoms of fibromyalgia relieved with massage include ____. (p. 58)

Cardiovascular and Lymphatic Pathologies

1. Cardiovascular pathologies for which massage is beneficial include ____________________ and ____________________. (p. 58)
2. Hospitalized heart patients experienced reduced ____________________ with massage. (p. 58)
3. Edema, the condition of excess ____________________ in the tissues, can be relieved with massage. (p. 58)
4. Massage may be contraindicated in cases of edema due to chronic ____________________, ____________________, or ____________________ problems. (p. 59)

Immune Function

1. Massage is thought to be of benefit to clients who are HIV positive because of its ____________________ effects. (p. 59)
2. Massage can be an important ____________________ measure for health problems that result from compromised immune function. (p. 59)

Respiratory Pathologies

1. Respiratory conditions for which massage is a good complementary therapy include ____________________, ____________________, and ____________________. (p. 59)
2. Massage and bodywork techniques studied for their effectiveness in treating respiratory conditions include ____________________, ____________________, and ____________________. (p. 59)
3. ____________________ techniques on the back and chest, and rib cage ____________________ techniques are effective in helping to produce productive coughs. (p. 59)

Anxiety Reduction in Hospitalized Patients

1. Nursing studies have found massage to be an effective complement to treatment for hospitalized patients, particularly its ____________________ and ____________________ effects. (pp. 59–60)
2. Massage holds potential for reducing the ____________________ effects of institutional care. (p. 60)

Massage for Cancer Patients

1. General effects of massage especially beneficial for cancer patients include __________, __________, __________, __________, and __________. (p. 60)
2. Massage can reduce some of the negative side effects of cancer treatments, such as __________ and __________. (p. 60)
3. The benefits of massage after cancer surgery include __________. (p. 60)
4. Emotional benefits of massage for cancer patients may include __________, __________, __________, __________, and __________. (p. 60)
5. __________ massage benefits women who have had breast cancer by enhancing post-mastectomy wound healing, and healthy scar formation. (p. 60)
6. Lymphatic massage helps reduce __________ that often accompanies mastectomy. (p. 60)

Pediatric Care

1. Tactile stimulation of preterm infants through massage enhances __________, __________, __________, and __________ (pp. 60–61)
2. Massage has been found to be an effective complementary treatment for children with a variety of medical conditions including __________, __________, __________, and __________. (p. 61)

Psychological Aspects of Treatment

1. Massage can be a valuable complement to treatment for people with diseases induced by or aggravated by __________. (p. 61)
2. The effects of massage that can benefit psychiatric patients include __________, __________, __________, and receiving pleasurable non-sexual __________. (p. 62)

Therapeutic Touch

1. Therapeutic Touch is an __________ approach to manual therapy developed by a nurse, Dolores Krieger, in the 1970s. (p. 62)
2. Theories about the mechanisms of Therapeutic Touch range from the physiological (e.g., __________), to those beyond the realm of science (e.g., __________ the patient's energy field). (p. 62)

Complement to Chiropractic

1. Massage can help __________ a person for a chiropractic adjustment, relieve tension and pain in soft tissues as a __________ to chiropractic treatment, and help __________ future musculo-skeletal misaligment. (pp. 62–63)

FOR GREATER UNDERSTANDING

The following exercises are designed to take you from the realm of theory into the real world. They will help give you a deeper understanding of the subjects covered in this chapter. Action words are underlined to emphasize the variety of activities presented to address different learning styles, and to encourage deeper thinking.

1. Choose a specific pathology to study. Locate research studies about the effectiveness of massage in treating that pathology. Write a review of the research that you find.
2. Choose one research study to read, analyze and evaluate. Present your findings and conclusions to a study partner or group.
3. Choose a specific pathology to study. Locate information about contraindications and cautions related to the pathology. Identify implications for giving massage to a person with the pathology studied. Discuss with a study partner or group.
4. Interview someone who is receiving massage as treatment for a particular pathology. Ask them to identify the benefits they feel from receiving massage. Compare this with conventional wisdom and available research.
5. Interview a massage practitioner who specializes in clinical applications, or the director of a clinical massage setting. Ask them about the types of pathologies they see in their practices and the benefits patients receive from massage. Report to a study partner or group.
6. Develop plans for a research study related to a specific pathology.

CHAPTER FIVE

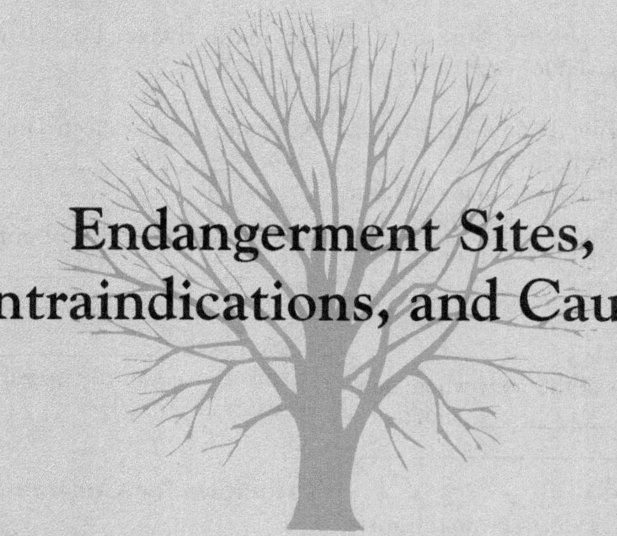

Endangerment Sites, Contraindications, and Cautions

STUDY GUIDE

LEARNING OUTCOMES

Use the learning outcomes at the beginning of the chapter as a guide to your studies. Perform the task given in each outcome, either in writing or verbally into a tape recorder or to a study partner. This may start as an "open book" exercise, and then later from memory.

KEY TERMS/CONCEPTS

To study key words and concepts listed at the beginning of this chapter, choose one or more of the following exercises. Writing or talking about ideas helps you remember them better, and explaining them helps deepen your understanding.

1. Write a one- or two-sentence explanation of each key word and concept.
2. With a study partner, take turns explaining key words and concepts verbally.
3. Make up sentences using one or more key words or concepts.
4. Read your sentences to a study partner, who will ask you to clarify your meaning.

STUDY OUTLINE

The following questions test your memory of the main concepts in this chapter. Locate the answers in the text using the page number given for each question.

1. One of most basic rules of giving therapeutic massage is to ________________ harm. (p. 67)
2. An endangerment site or contraindication in one form of massage and bodywork may be considered ________________ for a different form. (p. 67)

Endangerment Sites

1. Endangerment sites are areas of the body where delicate structures are ________________ and, therefore, may be more easily ________________ when receiving massage. (p. 67)
2. Endangerment sites for Western massage on the anterior part of the body include ________________ ________________. (pp. 67–69)
3. Endangerment sites for Western massage on the posterior part of the body include ________________ ________________. (pp. 67–69)
4. Deep effleurage or stroking should always move from ________________ to ________________ to avoid damage to the valves in the large veins. (p. 69)

General Principles of Safety around Endangerment Sites

1. Always adjust the pressure you use to match the ________________, the ________________, and the ________________ you are working on. (p. 69)
2. Avoid ________________ pressure over nerves, blood vessels, and lymph vessels close to the body surface. (p. 69)
3. Move off of the spot if you feel a ________________, or if the client reports ________________ sensations indicating pressure on a nerve. (p. 69)
4. Proceed with ________________ around abnormal structures. (p. 69)
5. Always work with ________________, and do not take a chance that may lead to ________________. (p. 69)

Contraindications

1. Contraindications are conditions or situations that make receiving massage inadvisable because of the ________________. (p. 69)
2. Avoid massage altogether for ________________ contraindications. (p. 69)
3. Avoid the area affected for ________________ or ________________ contraindications. (p. 69)
4. Cautions are areas of potential danger that require ________________ and possible modifications of ________________. (p. 69)
5. A client ________________ should be taken to identify possible contraindications and cautions. (p. 69)

Principles for Contraindications

1. Severe distress is a general contraindication for massage, for example, ________________, ________________, ________________, and ________________. (p. 70)
2. Acute inflammation is a general or local contraindication for massage, e.g., any condition that ends in "________________." (p. 70)
3. Loss of structural integrity occurs with surgery, ________________, ________________, and ________________. (p. 70)
4. Avoid massage near a ________________ skin condition, or when massage would make a skin condition worse. (p. 70)
5. ________________ may prevent a client from giving accurate feedback regarding pressure, so use care in amount of pressure used during massage. (p. 70)
6. ________________ to touch calls for massage only to recipient's tolerance level. (p. 71)
7. Avoid massage when there is pathology that might spread through blood or lymph ________________ ________________. (p. 71)
8. Bruising is a ________________ contraindication. (p. 71)
9. In cases of edema from infection, deep vein thrombosis, and general edema from cardiac, liver, or kidney disease ________________. (p. 71)
10. A client's compromised immunity calls for extra care in personal and environmental ________________. (p. 71)
11. Avoid ________________ on clients with diagnosed osteoporosis, or frail clients in high-risk categories. (p. 71)

Medications

1. A client's medications may affect the ______________ and ______________________ of massage sessions, techniques used, their method of application, and client ________________________. (p. 72)
2. Types of medications that require caution include those that __________________, __________________, __________________, and __________________. (p. 72 ; Table 5–1)
3. Clients under the influence of recreational drug or alcohol should not receive massage since these drugs ______________________, ___________ ________________________. (p. 72)

Person-Centered Massage

1. From a wellness perspective, massage can be thought of as ______________________- centered rather than *pathology-centered*. (p. 73)
2. Light massage that adds care, comfort and stress reduction may be appropriate even for someone for whom more vigorous massage is ____________ ____________________. (p. 73)

Resources

1. Resources for information on pathologies and conditions can be found ______________________, ____________________, ____________________. (p. 73; Table 4–1)
2. Every massage practitioner should have a personal ______________________ for looking up information related to contraindications and cautions. (p. 73)
3. The client himself or herself may be one of the best sources of information about their condition and relevant ______________________ when they are receiving massage. (p. 73)

FOR GREATER UNDERSTANDING

The following exercises are designed to take you from the realm of theory into the real world. They will help give you a deeper understanding of the subjects covered in this chapter. Action words are underlined to emphasize the variety of activities presented to address different learning styles, and to encourage deeper thinking.

1. On yourself, or working with a study partner, <u>explore the surface anatomy</u> of the major endangerment sites. Carefully and safely <u>feel</u> the structure of the area and visualize the tissues, and anatomical structures underneath the skin. <u>Imagine</u> how deep specific structures are to the surface and how exposed to pressure. Use an anatomy book or atlas as an aid to visualization.
2. Choose a specific pathology to study. <u>Locate information</u> about contraindications and cautions related to the pathology. <u>Identify implications</u> for giving massage to a person with the pathology studied. <u>Discuss</u> with a study partner or group.
3. <u>Interview</u> someone who receives massage regularly and who has the pathology studied in problem 2. Ask them to identify any restrictions related to massage that they are aware of related to their pathology. <u>Compare</u> this with information you have located. <u>Explain</u> to them what you found out related to contraindications and cautions.
4. <u>Interview</u> a massage practitioner who specializes in clinical applications, or the director of a clinical massage setting. Ask them about the types of pathologies they see in their practices and the cautions they take in working with those clients. Report to a study partner or group.
5. <u>Interview</u> a person taking one or more medications. List the medications they take and the related pathology that they are being treated for. <u>Identify modifications</u> you would make in a massage session with this person. <u>Discuss</u> your session plan with a study partner or group.

C H A P T E R   S I X

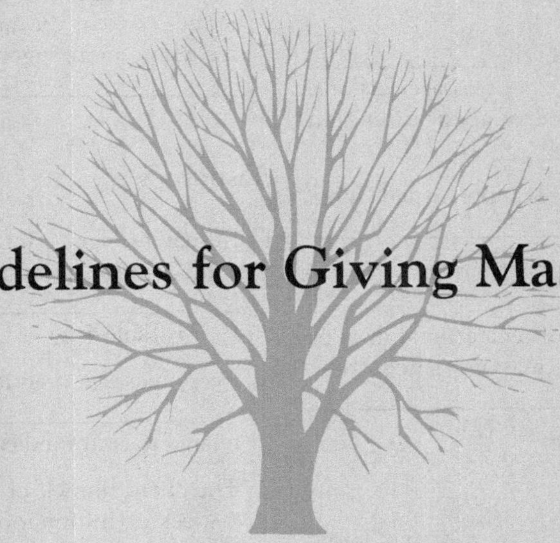

Guidelines for Giving Massage

S T U D Y   G U I D E

LEARNING OUTCOMES

The learning outcomes for this chapter list skills developed by successful massage practitioners. For each outcome, discuss the guidelines and key points to remember when developing the skill listed. This can be in writing, or discussed with a study partner or group.

KEY TERMS/CONCEPTS

To study key words and concepts listed at the beginning of this chapter, choose one or more of the following exercises. Writing or talking about ideas helps you remember them better, and explaining them helps deepen your understanding.

1. Write a one- or two-sentence explanation of each key word and concept.
2. Find key words or concepts that are related in some way. Explain the relationship. For example: "*Liniments*, *lotions*, and *oils* are all topical substances used in massage." Or "Guidelines for the *therapeutic relationship* are outlined in *standards of practice*."
3. Repeat problem 2 for groups of 3–5 words or concepts.
4. Pair each key word with one of the learning outcomes. For example: "Air quality is a part of 10: Create an ideal physical environment for massage." Go on to explain the guidelines related to the word; for example, "The air in the massage space should be fresh . . ."

STUDY OUTLINE

The following questions test your memory of the main concepts in this chapter. Locate the answers in the text using the page number given for each question.

The Therapeutic Relationship

1. The ______________ involves an implicit agreement regarding the roles of the massage practitioner and the client. (p. 76)
2. Clarity about roles is maintained by keeping ______________. (p. 76)
3. A ______________ relationship is any relationship other than the primary one of practitioner and client. (p. 76)
4. When clients unconsciously bring unresolved feelings from their past into the practitioner–client relationship, it is called ______________. (p. 77)
5. When practitioners unconsciously bring unresolved feelings from their past into the practitioner–client relationship, it is called ______________. (p. 77)

Professional Demeanor

1. The practitioner's appearance and behavior help establish a good therapeutic relationship by ______________ ______________. (p. 77)
2. Professional clothing is ______________, ______________, and ______________. (p. 77)
3. Offensive odors such as ______________, ______________, and ______________ should be eliminated. (p. 77)
4. The practitioner's language should avoid ______________, as well as unduly ______________ language and jargon; and speak to the ______________ level of the client. (p. 77)
5. The relationship between giver and receiver should be understanding and sympathetic, but never ______________ ______________. (p. 77)

Touching Another Person

1. Human beings have an innate touch ______________ ______________. (p. 77)
2. To touch means ______________ ______________. (p. 77)
3. From the holistic perspective, what seems to be simple physical touch often has profound effects on the ______________, ______________, and ______________ of the receiver. (p. 77)
4. Touch can communicate ______________, ______________, ______________, and ______________. (p. 78)
5. Examples of self-care for preventing absorption of a client's negative "vibes" are ______________, ______________, and ______________. (p. 78)
6. Comfort levels with touch vary among clients because ______________ ______________. (p. 78)
7. ______________ touch is never appropriate in a professional setting. (p. 78)

Permission to Touch

1. Informed consent is a process initiated when ______________. (p. 78)
2. Informed consent includes ______________, ______________, ______________, and ______________. (Table 6–1)
3. For informed consent the client should clearly have the option of ______________ to the proposed action. (pp. 78–79)

Gender Considerations

1. In cross-gender and same-gender massage, be clear about the ______________ nature of massage therapy, and establish clear ______________. (p. 79)
2. Many people, especially women, have been victims of ______________ and ______________, and have special needs for clear ______________. (p. 79)

Intervention Model

1. The intervention model is used when ______________ ______________. (p. 80)
2. The steps in the seven-step intervention model are (a) ______________, (b) ______________, (c) ______________, (d) ______________, (e) ______________, (f) ______________, (g) ______________. (Table 6–2)

Talking and Feedback

1. The degree of verbal interaction that goes on during a massage session depends on ____________ and ____________. (p. 80)
2. When relaxation is the goal, talking should be ____________. (p. 80)
3. Verbal and non-verbal communication that gives the practitioner information from the receiver about the massage performance is called ____________. (p. 80)
4. Emotional release is the result of ____________ ____________. (p. 81)
5. During emotional release, the practitioner's reaction is to ____________, and *not* to ____________. (p. 81)
6. An exception to the "minimal talk during massage" guideline might be ____________ ____________. (p. 81)
7. A good way to avoid letting your own life come into the talk during massage is to ____________ ____________. (p. 81)

Confidentiality

1. Confidentiality is an ethical principle in the professional relationship based on the client's right to ____________. (p. 81)
2. Confidential information about the client or patient includes ____________, ____________, and ____________. (p. 81)
3. Exceptions to the general rule of confidentiality are ____________ and ____________. (p. 81)
4. It is considered unethical to give out information about a client without ____________ ____________. (p. 81)
5. The National Certification Board for Therapeutic Massage and Bodywork has adopted a document called ____________ that gives detailed guidelines about professional ethical behavior. (p. 81)

HIPAA Privacy Rule

1. HIPAA stands for the ____________ ____________ act. (p. 81)
2. HIPAA was designed to protect the ____________ of individuals. (p. 81)
3. Clients should be able to see their ____________, and ask for ____________ if they find mistakes. (p. 82)
4. According to HIPAA, client records must be kept in ____________ file cabinets, preferably in ____________ records rooms. (p. 82)
5. Clients must give ____________ consent for use and disclosure of information for ____________, ____________, and ____________. (p. 82)

The Physical Environment

1. Essential features of a massage table are adjustable ____________ and ____________. (p. 82)
2. The type of massage table you choose depends on ____________ and the ____________. (p. 82)
3. A typical massage chair consists of a ____________, ____________, ____________, ____________, and ____________. (p. 83)
4. A comfortable temperature for a massage room is approximately ____________ degrees. (p. 83)
5. A ____________ can help remove dust, mold, and other allergens from a room. (p. 84)
6. Lighting for massage should be ____________ and ____________. (p. 84)
7. Sound, including music, can help create a ____________ and ____________ environment, or a ____________ one. (p. 84)
8. When clients are ____________ or ____________, it is appropriate to help them disrobe and get onto the table. (p. 84)
9. Used sheets and towels should be kept ____________ ____________. (p. 84)

Topical Substances

1. Ingredients commonly found in liniments include ____________, ____________, ____________, ____________, ____________, and ____________. (p. 84)
2. Liniments are usually applied (choose one: before, during, after) a massage. (p. 84)
3. Vegetable oils commonly used for massage include ____________, ____________, ____________, and ____________. (p. 84)

4. Practitioners choose the oils the use for their ____________________, ____________________, and ____________________. (p. 85)
5. Lotions are absorbed into ______________, unlike oils, which tend to stay on __________. (p. 85)

Safety and Comfort of the Receiver

1. The purpose of positioning the receiver is ____________________, and ____________________. (p. 85)
2. In the supine (i.e., face-__________) position, bolsters are placed under the ______________, and ________________. (Figure 6–3)
3. In the prone (i.e., face-__________) position, a bolster is placed under ______________ to take pressure off of the ______________. (Figure 6–4)
4. In the side-lying position support is provided for ____________________, ____________________, and ____________________. (Figure 6–6)
5. Draping during massage serves to ____________________, ____________________, and ____________________. (p. 86)
6. Body areas to be draped at all times include ______________ and ______________. (p. 86)
7. A technique to use when the receiver is turning from prone to supine is called ______________. (p. 89)

Physical Self-Care for the Practitioner

1. Practitioners can protect themselves from hand, arm, and back injuries by ____________________, ____________________, ____________________, and ____________________. (p. 92)
2. A protective technique in which pressure is applied through a straight line of joints is called ______________ the ______________. (p. 92)
3. Avoid pressure with the thumb (choose one: abducted or adducted). (p. 92)
4. When applying compression with the palms, avoid ____________________ of the wrist. (p. 92)
5. When reinforcing one hand with the other during compression, the top hand should be placed over the ____________________. (p. 92)
6. Bend your ____________________ to lower your body when performing massage. (p. 93)
7. When facing the head or the foot of the table, use a ____________________ stance. (p. 93)
8. Pressure is applied by ____________________, not by using the arms. (p. 93)
9. The maximum number of one-hour massage sessions that can be done safely in a week is ________. (p. 94)

Emotional Self-Care

1. Emotional self-care is important to prevent ______________ and ______________. (p. 97)
2. Strategies for emotional self-care include ____________________. (p. 97)

Performance Elements

1. The length of a massage session is determined by ____________________. (p. 98)
2. Use the least amount of lubricant needed to ____________________. (p. 99)
3. Too much lubricant can ______________. (p. 99)
4. Deep specific techniques should be preceded and followed by ____________________ ____________________ ones. (p. 100)
5. Sequences of techniques performed in almost the same way each time are called ______________. (p. 100)
6. The direction of technique application is expressed in general anatomical terms, for example, proximal, ____________________, ____________________, and ____________________. (p. 100)
7. Massage practitioners are working with ____________________ if they focus their techniques on a particular anatomical structure. (p. 100)
8. A ____________________, ____________________, ____________________ rhythm helps evoke relaxation. (p. 100)
9. It is the skillful blending of performance techniques that comprise the ____________________ of massage. (p. 100)

FOR GREATER UNDERSTANDING

The following exercises are practical applications of the guidelines presented in this chapter. Action words are underlined to emphasize the variety of activities presented, and to encourage advanced skill development. These exercises can be done with a study partner or group, or in class.

1. Analyze a professional relationship you have with a doctor, lawyer, psychotherapist, religious leader, or teacher. Is it similar to the therapeutic relationship described in this chapter? Do they have a professional demeanor? How is it similar or different from a massage practitioner? Discuss your observations.
2. Receive a massage from a professional practitioner. Notice how they establish a therapeutic relationship and maintain professional boundaries. Was there anything that seemed unprofessional to you? Discuss your observations.
3. Receive a massage from a professional practitioner. Afterwards, analyze the amount and content of talking that occurred in the session. Did their communication enhance or detract from the experience for you? Write down your observations giving specific examples. Discuss with a study partner or group.
4. Look through a magazine written for massage practitioners (e.g., Massage Therapy Journal (AMTA), Massage & Bodywork (ABMP), Massage magazine). Critique photographs of massage practitioners, pointing out examples of professional and unprofessional images. Present and discuss your findings.
5. Interview two people with cultural backgrounds different from yourself. Ask them about touch in their cultures. For example: How do people greet each other? How much do they touch when they talk? Walk together? Other occasions? Are there restrictions related to touch between men and women, two adults of the same gender, or between people of different ages? Compare and contrast the cultures. How might a client's touch background affect his/her openness to massage, and how would this affect your behavior as the massage practitioner? Present and discuss your findings.
6. Role play a situation that calls for informed consent. Have observers critique your performance. Repeat the situation using their suggestions.
7. Role play a situation that calls for the intervention model. Have observers critique your performance. Repeat the situation using their suggestions.
8. Visit the Web sites of two different table manufacturers. Create a comparison chart of the features of their most basic massage table, and of options available.
9. Repeat problem 8 for a massage chair.
10. Envision your massage practice over the next five years. Describe your ideal massage table in detail. Visit Web sites, showrooms, or consult brochures. Determine which table is best for you and its approximate cost.
11. Visit a facility that offers massage (e.g., private office, spa, health club, beauty salon, rehabilitation clinic, hospital, nursing home). Describe in detail the elements of the space such as temperature, air quality, lighting, sound, dressing arrangements, and cleanliness. How is it conducive to massage? How could it be made better? Discuss your findings in a group or class, and compare experiences.
12. Each person in a group or class brings a different liniment, oil or lotion used for massage. Compare ingredients of these products. Perform massage techniques with the substances, noting how they feel and how they enhance the massage technique. Choose your favorite and discuss your choice with the group.
13. Practice placing a study partner in different positions, (e.g., supine, prone, side-lying, and reclining) using bolsters and other props as needed. Adjust the face-cradle when they are prone. Using their feedback, rearrange the position or use of bolsters for maximum comfort. Practice on different size people and different body types. Identify factors to consider with different people.
14. Practice sheet draping with a recipient in different positions (e.g., supine, prone, side-lying, and reclining). Uncover and recover different body parts. Practice draping women's breasts. Get feedback from the recipient on how they feel. Do you seem confident? Do they feel safe and their modesty preserved?
15. Videotape yourself performing massage for about 10 minutes. Analyze your performance for good hand and wrist care, and general body mechanics. Get feedback from observers. Re-tape your performance, making corrections.
16. Practice performing massage with the table at different heights. Identify the height at which you can best maintain good body mechanics. Get feedback from observers.

17. Practice different massage techniques with different amounts of lubricant. Determine the right amount for each technique performed. Identify factors that had an impact on your judgment, e.g., your intent, the type of lubricant, or skin condition of the recipient. Discuss your findings with a group.

18. Perform a sequence of massage techniques varying the pressure, rhythm, and pacing. Get feedback from the recipient regarding how the variations felt and their effect.

CHAPTER SEVEN

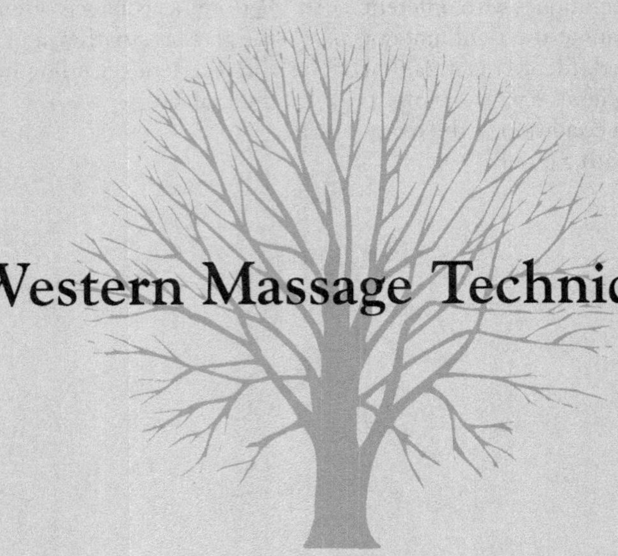

Western Massage Techniques

STUDY GUIDE

LEARNING OUTCOMES

Use the learning outcomes at the beginning of the chapter as a guide to your studies. Perform the task given in each outcome using the information in the chapter. This may start as an "open book" exercise, and then later from memory.

KEY TERMS/CONCEPTS

To study key techniques listed at the beginning of this chapter, choose one or more of the following exercises. Writing or talking about ideas helps you remember them better, and explaining helps deepen your understanding. Some exercises are designed to sharpen your focus on the details of performing the techniques.

1. Write a description of the six technique categories presented in this chapter. Describe how they differ from each other.
2. Demonstrate technique variations while explaining them verbally to a study partner.
3. Describe how each technique might be used in a massage session, e.g., for warming tissues, as a transition technique, or for ending a session.
4. Explain the physiological/psychological effects of each soft tissue technique variation.

STUDY OUTLINE

The following questions test your memory of the main concepts in this chapter. Locate the answers in the text using the page number given for each question.

Western Massage

1. Western massage is the basis of most massage therapy performed in ________________ and ________________ today. (p. 106)
2. Today's Western massage traces its origin to the work of ________________ of Sweden and ________________ of Amsterdam in the 19th century. (p. 106)
3. The effects, benefits and indications of Western massage are explained in terms of Western ________________ and ________________, and Western notions of ________________ and ________________. (p. 106)
4. The seven technique categories of Western massage include the five classic massage categories of ________________, ________________, ________________, ________________, and ________________, plus ________________ and ________________. (p. 106)
5. The number of technique variations within each category are ________________. (p. 106)

Effleurage

1. Effleurage techniques ________________ or ________________ over the skin with a smooth continuous motion. (p. 106)
2. Effleurage has many uses in a massage session, including to ________________, ________________, ________________, or ________________. (p. 106)
3. The effects of effleurage depend on the manner of application, but may include ________________, ________________, or ________________ (p. 107)

Petrissage

1. Petrissage techniques ________________, ________________, or ________________ soft tissues in a kneading motion, or ________________ or ________________ the tissues under or between the hands. (p. 112)
2. Petrissage is used to "milk" muscles of ________________, increase local ________________, relax ________________, and broaden or separate ________________. (p. 112)
3. Pressure used during petrissage should vary according to the condition of ________________, and should avoid ________________ or ________________. (p. 112)
4. Kneading or lifting types of petrissage include basic ________________, ________________, ________________, ________________, and ________________. (pp. 112–114)
5. Pressing petrissage techniques include ________________, and ________________. (pp. 114–115)

Friction

1. Friction is performed by rubbing one surface over ________________ repeatedly. (p. 115)
2. ________________ friction generates heat on the skin by brisk rubbing over the skin surface, and is done best with little or no lubricant. (p. 115)
3. Superficial friction variations are created by varying the part of the hand used, for example ________________, or by using a back and forth ________________ motion with the ulnar side of the hand. (p. 116)
4. Deep friction creates movement between ________________ tissues and helps to keep them from ________________ to each other. (p. 116)
5. Deep friction is performed either in ________________ fiber, ________________ fiber, or ________________ motion. (p. 117)
6. Deep friction is used for specific attention to small areas, and areas around ________________ and on ________________. (p. 117)
7. Tissues should be warmed thoroughly before performing deep friction, and pressure should be monitored carefully to avoid ________________. (p. 117)
8. ________________ friction is a specific type of cross-fiber friction applied directly to the site of a lesion, and is used to aid healthy ________________ formation, and in healing of ________________. (p. 118)
9. ________________ is a specific application of deep transverse friction used in rehabilitation. (p. 118)

Tapotement

1. Tapotement consists of a series of brisk ______________ movements following each other in light, rapid, rhythmic, alternating fashion. (p. 119)
2. Hands should ______________ the surface of the body providing pleasant stimulation, and avoid ______________ that feels uncomfortable. (p. 119)
3. Tapotement is used when finishing ______________ or ______________ of the body, or to ______________ the session, or when ______________ rather than sedation is desired. (p. 120)
4. Variations of tapotement are achieved by altering ______________ and include hacking, rapping, cupping, clapping, slapping, tapping, pincement, quacking, and squishes. (p. 120)

Vibration

1. Vibration may be described as an ______________, ______________, or ______________ motion, or movement back and forth or up and down performed ______________ and ______________. (p. 122)
2. Vibration can be ______________, ______________, or ______________ depending on how it is performed. (p. 122)
3. Fine vibration or trembling motion is imparted by the fingertips, but generated by ______________. (p. 123)
4. Various types of ______________ vibrators may be used for fine vibration. (p. 122)
5. ______________ is coarse vibration of an individual muscle or muscle group, and used for relaxation. (p. 124)
6. ______________ is a variation of shaking with movement back and forth from hand to hand, usually of a limb. It causes movement in related joints. (p. 124)

Touch Without Movement

1. Touch without movement is a unique massage technique category. It is not casual or social touch, but ______________ with ______________. (p. 125)
2. ______________ is simply laying the fingers, one hand, or both hands lightly on the body. It may impart ______________, have a ______________ effect, or help balance ______________. (p. 125)
3. When applying direct pressure, there is no ______________ after the initial compression of tissues. (p. 125)
4. Ischematic compression is a form of direct pressure applied with enough pressure to cause ______________ of tissues. After pressure is released, local ______________ is increased. (p. 125)
5. Direct pressure has a variety of uses including relieving ______________, diminishing ______________, and helping muscles ______________. (p. 125)
6. Different types of "point" therapy that involve direct pressure include ______________, ______________, ______________, ______________, and ______________. (p. 127)

FOR GREATER UNDERSTANDING

The following exercises are designed to take you from the realm of theory into practical applications. They will help give you a deeper understanding of the techniques covered in this chapter. Action words are underlined to emphasize the variety of activities presented to address different learning styles, and to encourage deeper thinking.

1. One person <u>performs</u> a key massage technique variation, while another observes. The observer <u>verbally describes</u> the hand and body position of the person performing the technique.
2. <u>Evaluate</u> how closely their performance matches the written descriptions and illustrations in the book and CD video. Instruct the giver on how to alter their performance to more closely resemble the technique as illustrated.
3. After completing problems 1 and 2, <u>experiment with variations</u> on the technique.
4. <u>Videotape</u> your performance of each of the technique variations. <u>Watching</u> the video, <u>analyze</u> your hand and body mechanics. <u>Perform</u> the techniques again, correcting mechanics. (You may substitute an observer for the videotape).
5. <u>Watching a video</u> of a full-body Western massage (or portion of a session), identify the techniques as you

observe them. Identify broad technique categories, and any specific variations you see. (You may substitute a live performance for the video.)

6. Watching a video of a full-body Western massage (or portion of a session), identify how the techniques are being used in the session, e.g., warming, transition, ending, and for their different effects, e.g., circulatory, muscle relaxation, general relaxation. (You may substitute a live performance for the video.)

7. Watching a video of a full-body Western massage (or portion of a session), become aware of the richness of techniques used, i.e., how many variations and combinations of techniques the practitioner applies. Watch two or more sessions and compare them.

8. Receive a massage and pay attention to the feel of the different techniques, naming them in your mind as they are applied. Notice how they are used by the practitioner.

CHAPTER EIGHT

Joint Movements

STUDY GUIDE

LEARNING OUTCOMES

Use the learning outcomes at the beginning of the chapter as a guide to your studies. Perform the task given in each outcome using the information in the chapter. This may start as an "open book" exercise, and then later from memory.

KEY TERMS/CONCEPTS

To study the key concept and terminology listed at the beginning of this chapter, choose one or more of the following exercises. Writing or talking about ideas helps you remember them better, and explaining them helps deepen your understanding. Some exercises are designed to sharpen your focus on the details of performing the techniques.

1. Write a one-sentence explanation of the different categories of joint movements: active, passive, assisted, resisted. Demonstrate and explain them to a study partner or group.
2. Explain the difference between mobilizing techniques and stretches. Demonstrate the difference on one or two joints.
3. Perform a specific stretch using static, contract-relax-stretch, and reciprocal inhibition. Explain the details of the three stretching approaches to a study partner or group.
4. Demonstrate mobilizing techniques for major joints in the body. With a study partner lying clothed on a massage table, start at the head and move clockwise around the body. Name and describe the movements as you perform them.
5. Repeat problem 4 for stretches of major joints.

STUDY OUTLINE

The following questions test your memory of the main concepts in this chapter. Locate the answers in the text using the page number given for each question.

Joint Movements

1. Joint movements are categorized into ____________ (i.e., without practitioner assistance), and ________________________ (i.e., initiated and controller by practitioner) movements. (p. 131)
2. In ________________________ movements, the client initiates the movement, while the practitioner helps in completion of the movement. (p. 131)
3. In ______________________ movements, the practitioner provides resistance to the active movement of the client. (p. 131)
4. Mobilizing techniques or joint mobilizations, in the context of massage therapy, are passive movements performed within ________________________ of joint movement. (p. 131)
5. ______________________ is a type of passive joint movement that is performed to the limit of range of motion, and used to elongate muscles and tendons. (p. 131)
6. Three different approaches to stretching a joint include ____________________________ stretch, contract- ________________________- stretch, and ________________________. (p. 132)
7. Joint movements are used to stretch ______________, increase range of ____________________, enhance ______________ awareness, stimulate ___________ relaxation, build muscle __________________, and improve _______________. (p. 131)
8. Some contemporary forms of bodywork use joint movement to affect the ______________________ system, i.e., re-educate muscles and integrate function (e.g., Trager Psychophyscial Integration). (p. 131)
9. Joint ________________ or __________________ intended to realign a misaligned joint by sudden thrusting movements, and characterized by "popping" or "cracking" at the joints, are <u>not</u> within the ____________________ of massage therapy. (p. 131)

General Principles of Joint Movements

1. Stay within the ________________________ range of motion of the joint when performing joint movement techniques. (p. 131)
2. Mobilizing techniques can be characterized as smooth, _______________, and _______________. (p. 132)
3. Warm surrounding __________________________ before stretching. (p. 132)
4. Use breathing to enhance a stretch, ______________________ holding the breath, and time the stretch to the client's (choose one: inhalation or exhalation). (p. 132)
5. Stay with the ________________________ range of the recipient during joint movements. (p. 132)
6. Be aware of ________________________ of joint structure and adapt movements accordingly. (p. 132)

JOINT MOVEMENTS

Neck

1. The neck is a general term for the region between the head and the trunk, which includes the seven ________________________ vertebrae and surrounding ________________________. (p. 132)
2. Mobilizing techniques of the neck are performed best with the recipient (choose one: prone or supine, or side-lying). (p. 132)
3. Simple mobilizing techniques of the neck may be performed by lifting the head slightly off the table, and moving the neck through its full _______________. (p. 133)
4. Finger push-ups may be used to produce a gentle movement between the ______________________. (p.133)
5. The melt-down is a variation of the finger push-up used primarily in the ______________________ region. (p. 133)
6. A ________________________ movement can be created in the neck by applying deep effleurage on both sides at the same time, traveling from the base of the neck to the suboccipital space. (p. 133)
7. Neck stretches include lateral __________________, __________________, forward __________________, and cross- __________________ stretch. (pp. 133–134)

Shoulder Girdle

1. The shoulder girdle is a complex structure and the most mobile area of the body. It includes the gleno-______________, acromio-______________, and scapulo-______________ joints. (p. 134)
2. Mobilizing techniques for the shoulder girdle may be performed with the recipient in the ______________, ______________, ______________, or ______________ position. (p. 134)
3. Mobilizing the joints of the shoulder may be accomplished indirectly by movement of the ______________ or by movement of the ______________. (p. 134)
4. Mobilizing techniques for the shoulder when the recipient is prone include ______________, ______________, direct mobilizing, and ______________ mobilizing. (p. 134)
5. Stretches to the shoulder in supine include horizontal ______________, and the over ______________ stretch. (p. 136)

Elbow

1. Movements of the elbow are limited to ______________, ______________, ______________, and ______________. (p. 136)
2. Mobilizing the elbow may be performed by ______________ and ______________ of the hand, or ______________ the forearm with upper arm immobilized. (p. 137)
3. Stretches of muscles that cross the elbow are accomplished largely by stretching the whole arm, as in the ______________ stretch for the shoulder. (p. 137)

Wrist

1. Movements of the wrist include flexion, extension, ______________ extension, radial and ulnar ______________, and ______________. (p. 138)
2. Mobilizing movements of the wrist include (choose one: passive or resisted) movement of the wrist through its *full range of motion*, and waving. (p. 138)
3. Flexion and ______________ are the most common stretches of the wrist. (p. 138)

Hand

1. Movements of the hand distal to the wrist involve movements of the fingers, i.e., flexion, extension, ______________, ______________; movements between the meta ______________; and the more complex movements of the ______________. (p. 138)
2. Mobilizing techniques for the hand include passive movements of all joints; ______________ at the knuckles; ______________ between metacarpals. (pp. 138–139)
3. Stretches of the hand involve ______________ at the knuckles ______________ and ______________ at the wrist. (p. 139)

Chest

1. The chest is a general term for the front and sides of the ______________, *generally* defined by the ______________, ______________, and ______________. (p. 140)
2. Mobilizing the rib cage is performed in supine by gentle ______________ from side to side. (p. 140)
3. Stretch of the arm muscles that attach to the chest may be accomplished by the ______________ stretch. (p. 140)

Hip

1. The large muscles of the hip are located on the upper ______________ and ______________. (p. 140)
2. Movements possible at the hip joint itself include flexion, ______________, hyper ______________, ab ______________, ad ______________, diagonal ______________ and ______________, outward and inward ______________, and ______________. (p. 140)
3. Rhythmic ______________ of the straight leg with recipient in supine position is a mobilizing technique of the hip joint. (p. 140)
4. The hip joint can be taken through its full range of motion using ______________ movement. (p. 142)
5. Some useful stretches of the hip joint with recipient in supine include knee to ______________ flexion, straight ______________ flexion, diagonal ______________ with knee flexed. (p. 142)

Knee

1. The knee is a hinge joint, and its movements are largely limited to __________ and __________. (p. 142)
2. The knee is best mobilized with the recipient in the __________ position. Simple mobilizing techniques include the __________ toss, __________ the lower leg at the knee. (p. 142)
3. Some stretches of the __________ leg also stretch the muscles that cross the knee. (p. 144)
4. Bringing the heel of the foot towards the buttocks (flexion) will stretch the __________ muscles of the thigh. (p. 144)

Ankle

1. The ankle is a hinge joint, and its movements include __________ flexion (flexion), __________ flexion (extension), __________ (eversion/abduction), and __________ (inversion/adduction). (p. 144)
2. Mobilizing techniques at the ankle include thumb pressure to bottom of foot while __________ flexing the ankle (prone); __________ movement of the ankle through full range of motion (prone); side to side mobilizing of the ankle using __________ (supine). (pp. 144–145)
3. Stretches at the ankle primarily involve __________ and __________ flexion. (p. 145)

Foot

1. The foot itself is a complex structure with two types of joints (i.e., __________ and __________) and two arches (i.e., __________ and __________). Movement can occur at the articulation of any of the (number) __________ bones. (p. 145)
2. Mobilizing techniques for the foot are similar to those for the hands, and are applied easiest with the recipient in __________ position. These include figure __________ with the toes; __________ between metatarsals; and straightening toes with __________ along the underside of phalanges. (p. 146)
3. Stretches for the foot include __________ flexion; __________ of the toes; foot widening at the __________; and interlocking __________ (giver) and __________ (receiver). (p. 147)

FOR GREATER UNDERSTANDING

The following exercises are designed to take you from the realm of theory into practical applications. They will help give you a deeper understanding of the techniques covered in this chapter. Action words are underlined to emphasize the variety of activities presented to address different learning styles, and to encourage deeper thinking.

1. For each of the stretches covered in the chapter, name muscles involved, and locate their attachments on a skeleton. If possible, perform the joint movements on the skeleton and observe how the bones move in relation to each other.
2. One person performs mobilizing techniques on a joint, while another observes. The observer verbally describes the hand and body position of the person performing the technique.
3. For problem 2, the observer evaluates the giver's body mechanics, and offers suggestions on how they might be improved.
4. In a group of three, one person talks another through performing a particular stretch to a receiver lying on the massage table. He or she describes step by step how the technique is performed. Include static, contract-relax-stretch, and reciprocal inhibition.
5. Videotape your performance of mobilizing techniques. Watching the video, analyze your body mechanics. Perform the technique again, correcting body mechanics.
6. Perform *active* versions of the passive movements (mobilizing techniques and stretches) covered in this chapter. Include static, contract-relax-stretch, and reciprocal inhibition techniques.

CHAPTER NINE

Full-Body Western Massage

STUDY GUIDE

LEARNING OUTCOMES

Use the learning outcomes at the beginning of the chapter as a guide to your studies. Perform the task given in each outcome, either in writing or verbally into a tape recorder or to a study partner. This may start as an "open book" exercise, and then later from memory.

KEY TERMS/CONCEPTS

To study key words and concepts listed at the beginning of this chapter, choose one or more of the following exercises. Writing or talking about ideas helps you remember them better, and explaining them helps deepen your understanding.

1. Write a one- or two-sentence explanation of each key word and concept.
2. Make study cards by writing the explanation from problem 1 on one side of a 3 × 5 card, and the key word or concept on the other. Shuffle the cards and read one side, trying to recite either the explanation or word on the other side.
3. Pick out two or three key words or concepts and explain how they are related.
4. With a study partner, take turns explaining key words and concepts verbally.
5. Make up sentences using one or more key words or concepts.
6. Read your sentences to a study partner, who will ask you to clarify your meaning.

STUDY OUTLINE

The following questions test your memory of the main concepts in this chapter. Locate the answers in the text using the page number given for each question.

Guidelines for Full-Body Western Massage

1. From a wellness perspective, a full-body Western massage focuses on general ____________, as well as meeting the ____________ needs of the recipient. (p. 150)
2. Goals for general health promotion include to ____________, ____________, ____________, ____________, ____________, and create a general sense of ____________. (p. 150)
3. A full-body massage typically lasts from ________ minutes to ________ minutes. (p. 150)
4. Full-body includes massage of the general body regions of the back, legs, ________, ________, ________, and ________. (p. 151)
5. The practitioner blends the ____________ techniques into logical sequence or routine. (p. 150)
6. The recipient is typically ____________ with a sheet for modesty. (p. 151)
7. 7. Oil or lotion is used to enhance ____________ over the skin and to prevent ____________. (p. 150)

Draping

1. Recipients should be draped with a sheet or ____________, and body parts skillfully uncovered and ____________ as needed. (p. 151)
2. Genitals should be ____________ at all times. (p. 151)
3. Women's breasts are always ____________, except when breast massage is performed by a practitioner with ____________ and then only with ____________ from the recipient. (p. 151)

Sequence of Body Regions

1. A massage sequence has a ____________ point, a ____________, and an ____________ point. (p. 151)
2. If the session starts in prone position, an effective sequence is back, ____________, ____________, turn to supine, and proceed with legs, ____________, ____________, ____________, ____________, and ending with head and ____________. (p. 151)
3. If the session starts in supine position, an effective sequence is head and face, ____________, shoulders and ____________, chest and ____________, legs and ____________, turn to prone, and proceed to legs, buttocks, and ending on the ____________. (p. 151)
4. Advantages of starting prone are that it often feels ____________ to those new to massage, starting on the back seems to lead to ____________ sooner, and ending supine helps the client be more ____________ at the end of the session. (p. 151)
5. An advantage of starting supine is that beginning with massage of the head, face, and neck is relaxing for many who work at ____________. (p. 151)

Order of Techniques

1. Massage of each region of the body begins with ____________ techniques such as ____________ and ____________. (p. 152)
2. ____________ of techniques are then applied for their general health promotion and specific ____________ effects. (p. 152)
3. Work on a particular area is concluded with ____________ techniques to reconnect, smooth out, and gradually lighten touch. (p. 152)
4. Common finishing techniques include light ____________, ____________, or ____________. (p. 152)
5. ____________ techniques serve to provide continuity and flow from one section to another. (p. 152)

Continuity and Flow

1. Establishment or removal of touch should never be ____________. (p. 152)
2. A sense of flow is achieved through an orderly ____________, and ____________ transitions from one region of the body to the next. (p. 152)

Rhythm, Pacing, and Specificity

1. Full-body Western massage is usually performed with a ________________ rhythm at ________________ pace. (p. 152)
2. The shorter the session (e.g., 30 minutes), the less ________________ is possible on any one region. (p. 152)
3. The more need for specific attention to a particular body region, the less specificity is possible ________________. (p. 152)

Full-Body Western Massage Routine

1. Practitioners develop their own ________________ and ________________ ways of performing a massage session. These routines typically change with further ________________ and ________________. (p. 152)
2. Routines are modified to meet the ________________ of the recipient on the table. (p. 152)
3. Today's ________________ practitioners often use Western massage as a starting point and integrate other forms of massage and bodywork as desired to meet the goals of the session. (p. 152)
4. Practitioners use routines as a general ________________, but vary actual techniques according to the needs and goals of the client at the time of the massage. (p. 152)

FOR GREATER UNDERSTANDING

The following exercises are designed to take you from the realm of theory into the real world. They will help give you a deeper understanding of the subjects covered in this chapter. Action words are underlined to emphasize the variety of activities presented to address different learning styles, and to encourage deeper thinking. Keeping a journal of your experiences can help make the lessons more valuable and accessible for review later.

1. Receive professional full-body massages from two different practitioners. Compare and contrast the two experiences. Notice the sequence used, the techniques chosen, and other elements of a session.
2. Receive two professional massages from the same person. Compare and contrast the two experiences. Did you notice a routine way of working, favorite techniques, and other similarities? Were there differences in the two sessions? If yes, what were they and why do you think there were differences?
3. Receive a 60-minute full-body massage and, at a later time, a 30-minute full-body massage from the same practitioner. Analyze how the practitioner shortened the second session. How did the two experiences compare?
4. Write out an ideal 60-minute full-body massage routine noting sequence, and techniques to be used on each region of the body. Plan how much time to spend on each region of the body, opening techniques, finishing techniques and other elements of a session. Perform your routine. Analyze your experience. Did you stick to the plan? Why or why not?
5. Videotape the first 15 minutes of a full-body routine. Watch the videotape and analyze the elements of the routine with particular attention to the techniques chosen, and the continuity and flow. Discuss with a study partner or group.
6. Repeat problem 5 for the last 15 minutes of a routine.

CHAPTER TEN

Regional Applications

STUDY GUIDE

LEARNING OUTCOMES

Use the learning outcomes at the beginning of the chapter as a guide to your studies. Perform the task given in each outcome, either in writing or verbally into a tape recorder or to a study partner. This may start as an "open book" exercise, and then later from memory.

KEY TERMS/CONCEPTS

To study key words and concepts listed at the beginning of this chapter, choose one or more of the following exercises. Writing or talking about ideas helps you remember them better, and explaining them helps deepen your understanding.

1. Write a one- or two-sentence explanation of each key word and concept.
2. With a study partner, take turns explaining key words and concepts verbally.

STUDY OUTLINE

The following questions test your memory of the main concepts in this chapter. Locate the answers in the text using the page number given for each question.

Wholeness and Meaning

1. Practitioners may want to focus more time and attention on a particular part of the body as the result of ________________, ________________, ________________, or ________________. (p. 166)
2. Even though the body is massaged region by region during a session, its ________________ should always be kept in mind. (p. 166)
3. The human meaning of a particular body region is determined by ________________, ________________, ________________. (p. 166)
4. As you interact with a client, be aware that you are not just touching a body, you are touching a ________________. (p. 166)

Head and Face

1. The head is the center for ________________ and ________________. (p. 166)
2. Tension in the head and face may be caused by ________________, and ________________. (p. 166)
3. Worry and anxiety can lead to tension in the ________________ and ________________. (p. 166)
4. Pathologies that affect the face include ________________ and ________________. (p. 166)
5. The musculature of the head and face is complex and includes muscles of ________________, ________________, and ________________ (p. 167)
6. Always ask a client if they are wearing ________________ to avoid damage to the eyes. (p. 167)
7. Two types of muscles in the face are ________________ and ________________. (p. 167)
8. Squeeze to the tissues along the eyebrow feels good to people who ________________, ________________, or ________________. (p. 167)
9. When performing effluerage over the eyelids, keep pressure ________________. (p. 168)
10. Muscles that perform mastication (chewing) are ________________, ________________, and ________________. (p. 169)
11. The ears are massaged between the ________________, and the ________________. (p. 169)
12. The scalp is massaged using ________________ techniques. (p. 169)
13. A technique similar to the self-comforting gesture of holding your face in your hands is ________________. (p. 170)

Neck

1. The neck is a ________________ region that links the head with the torso, and facilitates movement of the head for ________________, ________________, ________________ and ________________. (p. 170)
2. Massage can help relieve tension in the neck caused by ________________, ________________, or long periods of ________________. (p. 171)
3. ________________ headaches can be relieved with massage. (p. 171)
4. A useful technique for specific massage of the neck is ________________. (p. 172)

Back

1. The back is the core area for maintaining ________________, and a place of attachment for muscles that ________________. (p. 174)
2. Soothing back massage is associated with the qualities of ________________, ________________, and ________________. (p. 174)
3. Tension in the upper trapezius can refer pain to the ________________. (p. 174)
4. It is important for practitioners to develop a ________________ dimensional concept of the back. (p. 175)
5. A technique in which superficial tissues are lifted from the underlying muscles is called ________________. (p. 175)
6. Warming friction for the back can be performed with ________________. (p. 175)
7. Effleurage between the ribs affects the ________________ muscles. (p. 175)

8. Back massage for relaxation avoids causing ____________ and includes long flowing ____________ with oil performed with full firm contact with the palms. (p. 177)

9. Sedating effleurage of the back is performed with the fingertips lightly stroking the skin from ____________ to ____________. Hands alternate stroking for a ____________ movement. (p. 177)

Buttocks

1. The large muscles of the buttocks region help support ____________ and provide power for ____________. (p. 178)

2. Positive associations with this region include ________. (p. 178)

3. Negative associations with this region include ____________. (p. 178)

4. Take great care in this region to create a feeling of ____________ and ____________. (p. 178)

5. Populations that can benefit greatly from massage of this region include ____________, ____________, and ____________. (p. 178)

6. Use of the ____________, ____________ and ____________ to apply techniques can help with massage of the large muscles of this region. (p. 179)

Lower Extremities

1. The lower extremities are the principal means of ____________ for bipedal human beings. (p. 208)

2. Massage of the feet is especially appreciated by those who ____________ for long periods of time. (p. 180)

3. The lower extremities are generally massaged in three sections, i.e., ____________, ____________, and ____________. (p. 180)

4. Caution is in order when massaging the legs of people with ____________ veins. (p. 181)

Upper Extremities

1. Upper extremities are used for everyday activities, as well as ____________, ____________, and ____________. (p. 185)

2. Tennis and golf elbow are categorized as ____________ (RSI). (p. 186)

3. Loss of shoulder mobility may be caused by ____________, ____________, ____________, or ____________. (p. 186)

4. For the purposes of massage, the upper extremities may be thought of in four sections: ____________, ____________, ____________, ____________. (p. 186)

Chest and Abdomen

1. Expansion and contraction of the chest for ____________ is evidence of life itself. (p. 190)

2. Women's chests and breasts are associated with ____________, while well developed chests in men signify ____________ and ____________. (p. 190)

3. In the United States, women's breasts are kept ____________ in public and should therefore be draped to maintain ____________ and proper ____________. (p. 190)

4. Breast massage for wellness and clinical applications is becoming more accepted in the United States and may be performed after special ____________ and with ____________. (p. 190)

5. The abdomen is associated with deep feeling and ____________, and is ____________ for many people. (p. 190)

6. Massage and stretching of the muscles of the chest and abdomen can help correct poor ____________. (p. 190)

FOR GREATER UNDERSTANDING

The following exercises are designed to take you from the realm of theory into the real world. They will help give you a deeper understanding of the subjects covered in this chapter. Action words are underlined to emphasize the variety of activities presented to address different learning styles, and to encourage deeper thinking.

1. Write a description of the human meaning of your own body and body regions. Explain the meaning of regions with special significance, and how that might affect how you experience touch and massage there. Report verbally to a study partner or group.
2. Sketch your body on a piece of paper using different colors to represent different regions and their significance to you. Explain your drawing to a study partner or group.
3. Interview someone else about the meaning of their body regions as described in problems 1 and 2. Discuss findings with a study partner or group.
4. Interview someone who has received massage recently. Ask if massage of any particular body region was uncomfortable for them, and if so, ask them to explain why. Report your findings to a study partner or group, and discuss.
5. Interview two or more people who have received massage recently. Ask them to identify their favorite part of the massage, and explain their choice. Report your findings to a study partner or group, noting similarities and differences.
6. Receive a massage from a professional practitioner. Ask for special attention to a particular body region. Note how they address the request, and their approach to massage of the region. Report on their performance to a study partner or group.
7. Perform the therapeutic sequences in Tables 10–1 to 10–5 exactly as written. Then create variations identifying warming, therapeutic combinations, and finishing and transition techniques. Develop a routine way of approaching each body region that is well thought out.
8. Choose one of the following body regions for your focus: arm, leg, foot, back, head and face. Create a 30-minute massage for the region including warming, therapeutic combinations, and finishing and transition techniques. Perform your sequence, noting how you achieved specificity, avoided monotony, and made transitions.

CHAPTER ELEVEN

Hydrotherapy/Thermal Therapies

STUDY GUIDE

LEARNING OUTCOMES

Use the learning outcomes at the beginning of the chapter as a guide to your studies. Perform the task given in each outcome using the information in the chapter. This may start as an "open book" exercise, and then later from memory.

KEY TERMS/CONCEPTS

To study the key concept and terminology listed at the beginning of this chapter, choose one or more of the following exercises. Writing or talking about ideas helps you remember them better, and explaining them helps deepen your understanding.

1. Match historical people, places, and modalities that are related in some way. Explain your choices and their relationship to a study partner or group.
2. Research the biography of an important person in the history of hydrotherapy. Write a report or make a verbal report to a study group.
3. Write out the definition of key terms and concepts.
4. With a study partner, take turns defining key terms and concepts verbally from memory.
5. Group key terms and concepts that are related in some way. Explain your choices and their relationship to a study partner or group.
6. Explain your choices and their relationship to a study partner or group.

STUDY OUTLINE

The following questions test your memory of the main concepts in this chapter. Locate the answers in the text using the page number given for each question.

1. Hydrotherapy is the use of ____________________ in health and healing practices. (p. 197)
2. Therapeutic use of local hot and cold applications is called ____________________ therapy. (p. 197)

History of Hydrotherapy

1. Native Americans visited ____________________ and ____________________ springs for their healing effects for centuries. (p. 197)
2. Resorts were later built at the sites of mineral springs in places like ____________________ Springs, NY; ____________________ Spring, Arkansas, and ____________________, CA. (p. 197)
3. Archeologists studying ancient ______________ and ______________ civilizations have found the ruins of ______________ throughout Central America. (p. 197)
4. The sauna was developed in ____________________. (p. 197)
5. A tradition of bathhouses is found all over the world, i.e., the ancient Greek ____________________, ______________ and ______________ baths, and in ancient India, China, ______________ and ________________. (p. 197)
6. The Greek physician ______________ (c. 460 BCE) used compresses, sponging, and bathing to treat disease. (p. 197)
7. Vincent ____________________ of the Austro-Hungarian Empire developed an entire system of hot and cold water therapy (c. 1840). (p. 197)
8. Sebastian ____________________ from Bavaria further developed therapeutic use of water adding his knowledge of herbs (c. 1880). (p. 198)
9. European spas adopted the methods of Kneipp in places like Baden-____________________, Germany; Montecatini, Italy; and Evian-les-______________, France. (p. 198)
10. At the natural healing resort, the ______________ Creek Sanitarium in Michigan, ______________ offered hydrotherapy and wrote two books on the subject (c.1900). (p. 198)
11. ________________ hospitals controlled by physicians were opened in England in the 1700–1800s at Bath, Harrogate, Droitwich, and Buxton. (p. 198)
12. By the early 20th century, the old water therapies were largely the province of naturopaths, ______________, and ________________ practitioners. (p. 199)
13. Injured soldiers in World War I (1914–1918) were treated with hydrotherapy, massage, and related therapies, thus beginning the evolution of today's profession of ____________________. (p. 199)

Healing Properties of Water

1. Therapeutic use of water taken ______________ is outside the scope of massage therapy except for encouraging clients to drink plenty of clean pure water. (p. 199)
2. ____________________ applications of water, and ____________________ in water have been associated with massage since ancient times. (p. 199)
3. Hydro- and thermal therapies can be roughly divided into temperature ranges called ________________- (above body temperature), ________________- (at body temperature), and ________________- (below body temperature). (p. 199)
4. Healing properties of water are related to its uses in ______________ the body, and its effects for raising or lowering core ____________________ and the temperature of specific ________________. (p. 199)
5. Water ____________ acts as a form of massage. (p. 199)

Whirlpool Baths, Showers, Steam Room, Sauna

1. Temperatures for hydrotherapy and thermal therapy methods range from ______________ cold to hot ____________ and ____________ heat. (Table 11–1)
2. Massage practitioners should know something about hydrotherapy facilities to be able to give their clients ____________________, and to suggest their ____________________ and ____________________ use in relation to massage. (p. 200)
3. Benefits of warm/hot hydrotherapy include ____________________ the body temperature, causing ____________, cleansing ____________, increase in ____________________ circulation, and general relaxation. They are best taken (choose one: before or after) massage. (p. 200)

4. Benefits of cool/cold hydrotherapy include __________ body temperature, __________ pores, __________ superficial circulation, and general stimulation. They are best taken (choose one: before or after) massage. (p. 200)

5. Thermo- or heat therapy (choose one: increases or decreases) body temperature, pulse rate, and respiratory rate; (choose one: increases or decreases) blood pressure and muscle tone; and has a (choose one: sedating or invigorating) effect. (Table 11–3)

6. Cryo- or cold therapy (choose one: increases or decreases) body temperature, pulse rate, and respiratory rate; (choose one: increases or decreases) blood pressure and muscle tone; and has a (choose one: sedating or invigorating) effect. (Table 11–3)

7. The __________ bath consists of a water tub with air or water jets that cause water movement or churning. Healing effects are from water __________ and the pressure from __________ as a massage. (p. 200)

8. __________ showers are relaxing and increase superficial circulation. (p. 200)

9. __________ showers are stimulating and reduce overall body temperature. (p. 200)

10. __________ showers surround the bather from head to toe. (p. 200)

11. __________ showers are taken lying down on a table, and may include a salt or shampoo scrub. (p. 200)

12. Steam rooms provide __________ heat from 105° to 130°F (41° to 54°C) with 100% humidity. (p. 201)

13. Steam __________ apply steam to the body, but not the head. (p. 201)

14. __________ steam devices are used in skin care and to improve respiration. (p. 201)

15. Steam can help clear sinuses and __________ congestion, (choose one: raise or lower) body temperature, and induce sweating. (p. 201)

16. __________ provide dry heat from 160° to 180°F (71° to 82°C) with 6 to 8% humidity. (p. 201)

17. A cold shower or plunge into a pool following a sauna helps return __________ to normal. (p. 201)

18. General __________ for thermo- (hot) hydrotherapy include circulatory diseases, pregnancy, some systemic diseases, seizures, multiple sclerosis, skins rashes, certain allergies, contagious conditions. (p. 201)

19. __________ that alter skin sensation, how blood vessels react to heat, or the body's temperature control mechanisms are contraindications for hot and cold hydrotherapies. (Table 11–4)

Hot Applications—Thermo-Therapy

Healing Effects of Heat

1. Heat applied locally feels good, helps muscles __________, increases __________ circulation, makes connective tissue more __________, and __________ core body temperature slightly. (p. 203)

2. Raising temperature of tissues to 104° to 113°F (40° to 45°C) increases cell __________ and __________ flow for certain therapeutic effects. (p. 203)

3. General contraindications for __________-hydrotherapy may also apply to hot applications. (p. 203)

4. Local __________ for heat applications include burns, wounds, swelling, and skin conditions that could be made worse with heat. (p. 203)

Hot Packs and Massage

1. Hot packs applied prior to massage can begin muscle __________, increase circulation __________, and prepare area for __________ massage techniques. (p. 203)

2. Moist hot packs come in various shapes and sizes, and are heated in electrical units called __________. (p. 203)

3. __________ are placed between the hot pack and the client's skin to prevent burns. (p. 204)

Cold Applications—Cryotherapy

Healing Effects of Cold

1. Cold applied locally causes vasoconstriction; and (choose one: increased or decreased) local circulation, cell metabolism, __________ conduction velocity, pain, muscle spindle activity, and spasm. It can also act to (choose one: raise or lower) core body temperature slightly. (p. 204)

2. Cold applied for over __________ minutes may induce vasodilation. (p. 204)

3. Cold applied to tissues after trauma or injury can (choose one: increase or decrease) secondary cell or tissue damage, and prevent further __________. (p. 204)

4. Cold applications are part of first aid for trauma to limbs, i.e., R.I.C.E.S. (____________________, ____________________, ____________________, ____________________, ____________________). (p. 204)

5. Contraindications to local cold applications include ____________________ and heart problems, allergy to ____________________ cold hypersensitivity, chilling, multiple ____________________, asthma, arthritis, infection, depression, and pregnancy. (Table 11–7)

6. Medications that alter skin ____________________, how blood vessels react to ____________________, or the body's ____________________ control mechanisms are contraindications for hot and cold hydrotherapy. (Table 11–7)

Cold Packs, Ice, Ice Massage

1. Cold packs are commercially available, or may be made from ____________________ or ____________________ in plastic bags. (p. 205)

2. Cold or ice packs may be used as adjunct to massage to reduce muscle ____________________, muscle ____________________, or tissue ____________________. (p. 205)

3. Cold may be applied for up to ____________________ hour at a time. (p. 205)

4. ____________________ involves rubbing ice directly on a small area in a circular motion using an ice cube or ice cup. (p. 205)

5. Ice massage is performed for 5 to 10 minutes until the area is ____________________. It is sometimes used with ____________________ friction to an injury site. (p. 205)

6. Stages of sensation when applying ice are (1) ____________________, (2) ____________________, (3) ____________________, (4) ____________________. (p. 205)

FOR GREATER UNDERSTANDING

The following exercises are designed to take you from the realm of theory into practical applications. They will help give you a deeper understanding of the information covered in this chapter. Action words are underlined to emphasize the variety of activities presented to address different learning styles, and to encourage deeper thinking. *Do not do any exercise if it is a contraindication for you or your practice partner.*

1. Visit a spa or health club with hydrotherapy facilities. Experience as many facilities or treatments as you can. Write about which ones you enjoyed or didn't enjoy, and which were beneficial and why you think so. Report your findings to a study partner or group.

2. Visit a spa or health club with hydrotherapy facilities. Observe how other people use the facilities. Was there anything you thought they needed instruction about, for example, contraindications or how best to enjoy the experience? Were there any signs or people to instruct patrons on how to use the facilities? Report your observations to a study partner or group.

3. Practice applying hot packs to a study partner. Observe all of the guidelines in Table 11–6.

4. Repeat problem 3, applying hot packs to the back. Apply moist heat for 10 minutes. Remove the hot packs and perform a 10-minute back massage. Note the effects of the heat on the massage. Discuss your observations with the practice partner.

5. Practice applying cold or ice packs to a study partner. Observe all of the guidelines in Table 11–8.

6. Immerse your foot or hand into a bucket of ice water. Notice the phases of sensation you experience. Say them out loud to a study partner as you experience them. (Variation: Apply cold pack instead.)

7. Practice ice massage on yourself or a practice partner. Discuss the effects you see and feel with a study partner.

8. Visit a training room with a certified athletic trainer. Observe how they use hydro- and thermal therapy in treatment of athletes. Report your observations to a study partner or group.

CHAPTER TWELVE

Mother and Child

STUDY GUIDE

LEARNING OUTCOMES

Use the learning outcomes at the beginning of the chapter as a guide to your studies. Perform the task given in each outcome, either in writing or verbally into a tape recorder or to a study partner. This may start as an "open book" exercise, and then later from memory.

KEY TERMS/CONCEPTS

To study key words and concepts listed at the beginning of this chapter, choose one or more of the following exercises. Writing or talking about ideas helps you remember them better, and explaining them helps deepen your understanding.

1. Write a one- or two-sentence explanation of each key word and concept.
2. With a study partner, take turns explaining key words and concepts verbally.
3. Make up sentences using one or more key words or concepts.

STUDY OUTLINE

The following questions test your memory of the main concepts in this chapter. Locate the answers in the text using the page number given for each question.

Benefits of Pregnancy Massage

1. Deviations from the nonpregnant state that cause discomforts that can be relieved by massage include ______________, ______________, and ______________ deviations. (p. 208)
2. Typical pregnancy posture may be described as head ______________, chest ______________, belly ______________, hips tilted ______________, ______________ knees, and feet turned ______________. (p. 208)
3. Massage can help relieve strain on the ______________ and ______________ caused by pregnancy posture. (p. 208)
4. Pressure from the additional weight carried during pregnancy often causes ______________ of the hands, legs, and feet. (p. 208)
5. Softening of ______________ tissue during pregnancy causes joint instability and pain. (p. 208)

Contraindications and Cautions

1. Massage is ______________ in most cases of pregnancy, but it is best to check with the mother's physician for any special ______________ or ______________. (p. 208)
2. Massage of the abdomen is ______________ for pregnant women. (p. 208)
3. Massage should be avoided if the mother is experiencing ______________, ______________, ______________, or any unusual ______________, ______________ or ______________. (p. 208)
4. Chinese medicine dictates that heavy pressure over the ______________ channel, and (choose one: yin or yang) meridians on inside of the lower legs, and ______________ to LI4 and Sp6 should be avoided on pregnant women. (p. 208)

Positioning and Environment

1. The room temperature is kept a little ______________ than usual for pregnancy massage. (p. 208)
2. Air should be ______________ and ______________. (p. 208)
3. Atmosphere and music should be ______________. (p. 209)
4. A ______________ should be accessible since pregnant women have to urinate frequently. (p. 209)
5. The massage table may be adjusted (choose one: higher or lower) than usual. (p. 209)
6. A ______________ may be useful for the recipient to get onto the table. (p. 209)
7. In the first few weeks of pregnancy, women may lie ______________ or ______________. (p. 209)
8. As the belly gets larger, switch to the ______________ or ______________ positions. (p. 209)
9. Some doctors caution against pregnant women lying on their (choose one: right or left) side. (p. 210)
10. In side-lying position, pillows are placed under the client's ______________, ______________, and ______________. (p. 210)
11. Use ______________ to support the body comfortably. (p. 210)

Pregnancy Massage Session

1. The characteristics of pregnancy massage can be described as ______________ and ______________. (p. 211)
2. Traditional Western massage, ______________, and ______________ are types of bodywork found to address pregnant women's needs. (p. 211)
3. Focus of the pregnancy massage sessions is on these parts of the body: ______________, ______________, ______________, and ______________. (p. 211)
4. A goal of pregnancy massage is general ______________. (p. 211)
5. Massage may be performed during ______________ to help reduce anxiety and ease labor pain. (p. 212)

Massage After Delivery

1. Massage may be received during the weeks after birth to help ______________ areas stressed during delivery. (p. 212)

2. Women who receive ______________________ may also benefit from massage during recovery and from techniques that help form healthy ______________________ tissue. (p. 212)

3. Women with infants and small children may benefit from taking time for ______________________ and receiving ______________________ massage as part of their regular self-care. (p. 212)

4. Breast massage has been found useful for relieving the discomforts of mothers ________ their infants. (p. 212)

Infant Massage

1. Massage given to newborns by parents, grandparents, and other caregivers is an excellent way to provide the ________________ and ________________ stimulation essential for healthy growth and development of infants. (p. 213)

2. Research has shown infant massage to be beneficial not only for healthy babies, but also for promoting recovery of ________________, ________________, ______________________, and other high risk infants. (p. 213)

3. Other benefits for infants include releasing ____________, learning to ________________, ______________________ with parents, aiding ______________________ and elimination, improving ______________________, easing ______________________ pains, and helping calm ______________________ babies. (p. 213)

4. Infant massage techniques include gentle ________________, ________________, ________________, and ________________. (p. 213)

5. Caregivers should maintain ________________ contact during massage when the infant is supine. (p. 217)

FOR GREATER UNDERSTANDING

The following exercises are designed to take you from the realm of theory into the real world. They will help give you a deeper understanding of the subjects covered in this chapter. Action words are underlined to emphasize the variety of activities presented to address different learning styles, and to encourage deeper thinking.

1. Interview a pregnant woman, and ask what changes she has noticed in her body and emotions as her pregnancy progresses. Observe her posture, how she moves, and other physical challenges. Write a report of your findings, and in it, discuss how massage might meet the needs of this particular woman.

2. Analyze a massage practice space in a private office, health club, or spa to determine how conducive it is for pregnancy massage. Draw the space and note its proximity to a bathroom. Evaluate other aspects of the environment and the equipment available for pregnancy massage. Write a report and share with a study partner or group.

3. Observe massage of a pregnant woman in the side-lying or reclining position. How did the massage practitioner position the woman? How was draping handled? What areas did the practitioner concentrate on? What specific techniques were used? Write a report of your observations and share it with a study partner or group. (Alternative: Watch a video of massage given to a pregnant woman.)

4. Observe infant massage given by a caregiver trained by a certified practitioner. Write a report describing how techniques were applied, how they were adapted for the individual infant, and the reaction of the infant and the caregiver. Interview the caregiver regarding the benefits they have observed from infant massage.

5. Take a training in infant massage, and practice techniques on a doll. How are they similar and different from massage of an adult?

6. Visit the Web sites mentioned in Additional Resources. What organizations exist for infant massage? What are their missions? What resources do they have available? What training and certifications? Report your findings to a study partner or group.

CHAPTER THIRTEEN

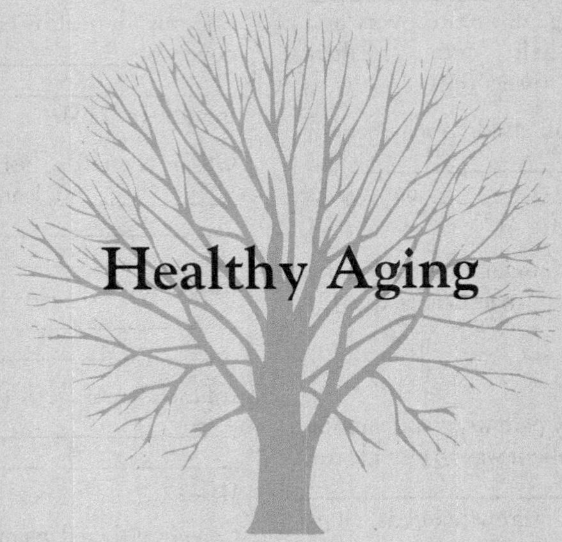

Healthy Aging

STUDY GUIDE

LEARNING OUTCOMES

Use the learning outcomes at the beginning of the chapter as a guide to your studies. Perform the task given in each outcome, either in writing or verbally into a tape recorder or to a study partner. This may start as an "open book" exercise, and then later from memory.

KEY TERMS/CONCEPTS

To study key words and concepts listed at the beginning of this chapter, choose one or more of the following exercises. Writing or talking about ideas helps you remember them better, and explaining them helps deepen your understanding.

1. Write a one- or two-sentence explanation of each key word and concept.
2. Make study cards by writing the explanation from problem 1 on one side of a 3 × 5 card, and the key word or concept on the other. Shuffle the cards and read one side, trying to recite either the explanation or word on the other side.
3. With a study partner, take turns explaining key words and concepts verbally.

STUDY OUTLINE

The following questions test your memory of the main concepts in this chapter. Locate the answers in the text using the page number given for each question.

1. Massage can be an important part of life-long ______________________, and an aid to caring for elders in ______________________ settings. (p. 221)

Effects of Aging and Benefits of Aging

1. The physical effects of aging begin around age ______________________ and include decrease in general mobility, slower ______________________ conduction, less ______________________ circulation, less ______________________ elasticity, ______________________ and ______________________ skin, loss of bone ______________________, decreased sensory function, and a less ______________________ immune system. (p. 221)
2. Regular massage can help retard some of the decreases in function and condition that are part of the normal aging process. For example, massage promotes ______________________ skin, improves general blood ______________________ and lymph ______________________, helps keep fascia and muscles more ______________________, improves joint ______________________, and ______________________ immune system function. (p. 221)
3. Massage also reduces the physical and mental effects of ______________________ that may accelerate the ______________________ process. (p. 221)

Benefits for Elders

1. Massage is especially beneficial for elders of __________ years or older. (p. 221)
2. Massage helps elders maintain mobility and ______________________ longer, and helps ease the emotional pain of loss and ______________________ experienced in later years. (p. 221)
3. Massage may alleviate some common physical problems of the elderly such as ______________________, ______________________, ______________________, physical discomfort, and ______________________. (p. 221)
4. Massage may also alleviate some common emotional problems such as ______________________, ______________________, ______________________, feeling alone, and ______________________. (p. 221)
5. Massage offers regular caring ______________________, ______________________, and ______________________ interaction to homebound elders and those in ______________________. (p. 221)
6. Benefits of massage for elders in hospitals include relaxation, improved ______________________, and reducing the ______________________ effects of institutional care. (pp. 221–222)
7. Massage has been found to reduce negative behavior in some ______________________ elderly in nursing homes. (p. 222)

Working with the Elderly

1. It is useful to think of older adults in terms of ______________________ age rather than ______________________ age. (p. 223)
2. ______________________ elders show few outward signs of impaired health. (p. 223)
3. ______________________ elders show typical signs of aging. (p. 223)
4. ______________________ elders look and feel fragile to touch. (p. 223)
5. After the massage, leave the room only when you are sure that the recipient is not ______________________ and can get off of the table ______________________. (p. 223)
6. Be gentle in lifting ______________________ elders. ______________________ their bodies to help them change position. (p. 223)

Massage for Elders

1. Limit the prone position of elders to ______________ minutes. (p. 223)
2. Use bolsters to relieve stress on ______________________. (p. 223)
3. There are no special massage techniques that ______________________ the aging process. (p. 225)
4. Elements to include in massage sessions for older people. (p. 225)
    a. ______________________ enhancing massage, e.g., effleurage.
    b. Petrissage for ______________________ and ______________________ connective tissue.
    c. Joint movements to improve ______________________ and ______________________.

d. Joint movements in upper extremities to improve ____________________ functions.

e. Passive movement of cervical muscles to improve ____________________ rotation.

f. Techniques to improve upright __________.

g. ________________ massage for improved digestion and elimination.

Cautions

1. Common conditions of the elderly that may be contraindications, or for which special cautions apply, include use of prescribed ____________________, thinning ________________, ________________ growths, cancer, circulatory problems such as ________________ veins and ________________, and joint disease such as ____________________. (p. 225)
2. Observe limitations around ____________________ replacements. (p. 225)
3. Avoid ________________ and ________________ with hip replacements. (p. 225)
4. Avoid massage of the ____________________ neck. (p. 225)
5. Pressure used to apply techniques should be light to moderate to avoid ____________________. (p. 225)
6. Tell the client of any skin growths that you suspect may be ______________________. (p. 225)

FOR GREATER UNDERSTANDING

The following exercises are designed to take you from the realm of theory into the real world. They will help give you a deeper understanding of the subjects covered in this chapter. Action words are underlined to emphasize the variety of activities presented to address different learning styles, and to encourage deeper thinking.

1. <u>Observe</u> people of a variety of ages in a public place like a park or shopping mall. <u>Note differences</u> in the way they move, their posture, and other visible characteristics. Compare and contrast children, young adults, older adults, and the elderly. <u>Summarize</u> your findings in writing and report to a study partner or group.
2. <u>Observe</u> a number of different elderly people. <u>Categorize</u> them as robust, age appropriate, or frail. <u>Explain</u> the basis for your decisions. <u>Summarize</u> your findings in writing and report to a study partner or group.
3. <u>Visit a nursing home</u> or extended care facility for the elderly. <u>Observe</u> the patients' mobility, activity, and limitations. <u>Describe</u> your observations and how massage could add to their health and wellbeing. <u>Report</u> to a study partner or group.
4. <u>Interview</u> an older adult (50–65 years old) and ask them what changes they have noticed in themselves as they age. <u>Describe</u> what specific effects of massage may apply directly to improving their lives. Plan a massage session including approaches to address their unique needs.
5. <u>Give a massage</u> to an older adult or elder. How does it differ from massage of a younger person? <u>Note</u> contraindications and cautions, medications, skin condition, quality of tissues, flexibility, past injuries, and other factors related to age. <u>Report</u> your experience.
6. <u>Volunteer</u> to give seated massage (head, shoulders, hands or feet) to the elderly in a senior center, nursing home, or other facility. How did you modify the massage for each person? What was their reaction to you and the massage? What benefit do you think they got from the experience? What benefit did you get from the experience? <u>Report</u> your experience.
7. <u>Visit the Web sites</u> of organizations for the elderly listed as additional resources at the end of the chapter. What are their missions, and in what way do they benefit older people? Do they have anything of value to offer massage therapists? <u>Report</u> your findings.
8. <u>Take a training</u> specifically for massage of the elderly. How is massage modified to address the needs of this special population?

CHAPTER FOURTEEN

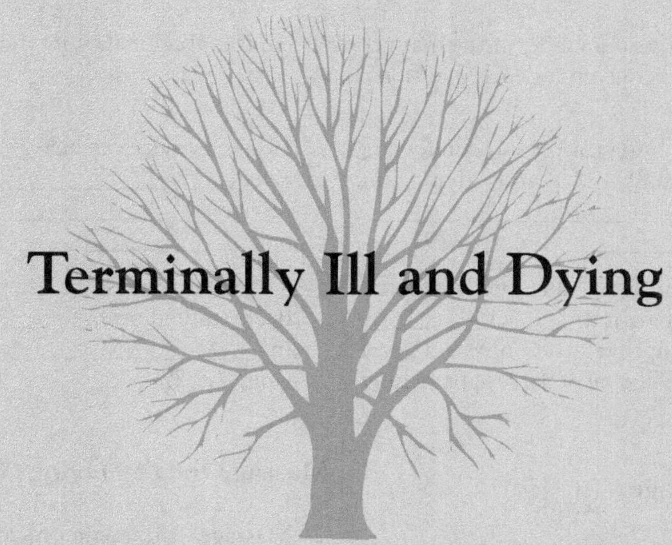

Terminally Ill and Dying

STUDY GUIDE

LEARNING OUTCOMES

Use the learning outcomes at the beginning of the chapter as a guide to your studies. Perform the task given in each outcome, either in writing or verbally into a tape recorder or to a study partner. This may start as an "open book" exercise, and then later from memory.

KEY TERMS/CONCEPTS

To study key words and concepts listed at the beginning of this chapter, choose one or more of the following exercises. Writing or talking about ideas helps you remember them better, and explaining them helps deepen your understanding.

1. Write a one- or two-sentence explanation of each key word and concept.
2. Pick out two or three key words or concepts and explain how they are related.
3. With a study partner, take turns explaining key words and concepts verbally.
4. Make up sentences using one or more key words or concepts.

STUDY OUTLINE

The following questions test your memory of the main concepts in this chapter. Locate the answers in the text using the page number given for each question.

1. Massage may be used to bring caring and comforting touch to the terminally ill and dying in ______________, ______________, and ______________ care. (p. 229)
2. Simple massage techniques may be used by health practitioners and taught to ______________ caregivers to help improve the physical and ______________ wellbeing of those approaching the end of life. (p. 229)

Caring Touch of Massage

1. From the ______________ perspective, even those with terminal illness or nearing death continue to strive for optimal ______________ in their life circumstances. (p. 229)
2. Although massage will not ______________ or save someone from imminent ______________, it can help improve physical function and ease some of the pain and ______________ felt. (p. 229)
3. Massage can address some of the special problems of those who have been physically ______________ or ______________ for a long period of time. (p. 229)
4. These people often suffer from poor ______________, ______________, ______________ and ______________, difficulty ______________, and skin ______________. (p. 229)
5. Massage can help prevent bed ______________. (p. 229)
6. Relaxing massage can help alleviate emotional distress from feelings of ______________, ______________, ______________, ______________, ______________, and touch ______________. (p. 229)
7. Massage can provide a sense of ______________, and generate feelings of general ______________. (p. 229)

Hospice and Palliative Care

1. Hospice and palliative care programs provide ______________ care at the end of life, and typically involve a ______________-oriented approach. (p. 229)
2. Hospice services include ______________ care, ______________ care, ______________ services, ______________ visits, ______________, and ______________ services. (p. 229)
3. The value of massage as a palliative care method has been studied and ______________ in ______________ medical settings. (p. 229)

Massage for the Dying

1. Massage can communicate caring and love in a ______________ way. (p. 229)
2. TLP (Tender Loving ______________) is a program in New Zealand for the dying that provides short-term ______________ to ease the transition from life to death. (p. 229)
3. Therapeutic Touch has been used to help the dying experience a feeling of ______________ and deep ______________. (pp. 229–230)
4. Massage offered by caregivers in hospice settings provides a means of ______________, even for patients unable to speak. (p. 230)

Knowledge and Skills

1. A medical profile of the terminally ill person is essential for ______________ a massage session, and ______________ both the recipient and the practitioner. (p. 230)
2. Specific technique is less important when working with the terminally ill than qualities such as ______________ and ______________. (p. 230)
3. Other useful skills include active ______________, listening and ______________, ______________, guided ______________, shared ______________. (p. 230)
4. In general, massage sessions with the dying are ______________, ______________, and ______________. (p. 230)
5. Massage sessions with the dying last about ______________ minutes. (p. 230)

6. The recipient may be lying on a massage table, sitting in a regular chair or ______________ chair, or lying in a ______________ or ______________ bed. (p. 230)

7. The key to massage for the dying is to be ______________, ______________, and ______________. (p. 230)

Self-Care

1. Working with the terminally ill and dying calls for a strategy of ______________ self-care on the part of the massage practitioner. (p. 230)

2. Practitioners should maintain good ______________ while working with recipients in chairs and lying in bed. (p. 230)

3. Proper ______________ should be observed when recipients have communicable diseases. (p. 231)

4. Maintaining ______________ wellness when working with the dying may involve confronting your own issues about illness and dying, and discussing those feelings with a ______________, ______________ or ______________. (p. 231)

5. Eventual ______________ of your client is to be expected and ongoing professional supervision may be helpful in your own process of ______________ and ______________. (p. 231)

FOR GREATER UNDERSTANDING

The following exercises are designed to take you from the realm of theory into the real world. They will help give you a deeper understanding of the subjects covered in this chapter. Action words are underlined to emphasize the variety of activities presented to address different learning styles, and to encourage deeper thinking.

1. <u>Interview</u> a health professional who is working or who has worked with the terminally ill or dying. Ask them about the type of setting, and their personal challenges working in that environment. What were their patients' greatest needs? Inquire about the role of massage, if any, where they worked, and the potential benefits of massage for this special population. Discuss your findings with a study partner or group.

2. <u>Repeat Problem 1</u> with a massage therapist who is working or who has worked with the terminally ill or dying.

3. <u>Visit</u> a hospice or palliative care facility. What is the approach to providing care at the end of life? What types of services do they offer, and what types of health professionals do they employ? <u>Report</u> your findings to a study partner, and <u>compare</u> with others who also completed the assignment.

4. <u>Visit the Web sites</u> given as additional resources at the end of the chapter, and any others you find related to hospice and palliative care programs. What is the mission of the organization? Services offered? Any mention of massage? <u>Report</u> your findings to a study partner or group.

5. <u>Volunteer</u> to give massage at a hospice or in a palliative care program. <u>Take training</u> offered to orient you to the setting. <u>Keep a journal</u> of your experience.

CHAPTER FIFTEEN

Seated Massage in the Workplace

STUDY GUIDE

LEARNING OUTCOMES

Use the learning outcomes at the beginning of the chapter as a guide to your studies. Perform the task given in each outcome, either in writing or verbally into a tape recorder or to a study partner. This may start as an "open book" exercise, and then later from memory.

KEY TERMS/CONCEPTS

To study key words and concepts listed at the beginning of this chapter, choose one or more of the following exercises. Writing or talking about ideas helps you remember them better, and explaining them helps deepen your understanding.

1. Write a one- or two-sentence explanation of each key word and concept.
2. Pick out two or three key words or concepts and explain how they are related.
3. With a study partner, take turns explaining key words and concepts verbally.
4. Make up sentences using one or more key words or concepts.

STUDY OUTLINE

The following questions test your memory of the main concepts in this chapter. Locate the answers in the text using the page number given for each question.

1. Massage is an increasingly popular workplace ____________ offering. (p. 234)
2. Seated massage is popular with businesses exploring ways to reduce ____________ on the job, and to minimize job-related ____________. (p. 234)

History of Workplace Massage

1. In the late 19th and early 20th centuries, massage and physiotherapy were offered by many businesses as part of their employee ____________. These in-house wellness programs largely ____________ by mid-20th century. (p. 234)
2. Workplace wellness programs were revived in ____________ as an offshoot of the larger ____________ movement. (p. 234)
3. The invention of the ____________ in the 1980s by David Palmer made massage at the workplace more convenient. (p. 234)
4. The term ____________ massage was coined to describe offering massage in massage chairs in public places like parks, stores, and the workplace. (p. 234)
5. Massage chairs can be easily ____________, use less ____________ than a massage table, and allow people to receive massage in a seated position with their ____________ on. (p. 234)

Benefits of Massage in the Workplace

1. Massage in the workplace may help minimize ____________ injuries (RSI), and reduces ____________ among employees. (p. 234)
2. Massage has been found to increase ____________ clarity and ____________ that can only enhance worker productivity. (p. 234)
3. Massage can help reduce the adverse effects of ____________ for long periods of time. (p. 235)
4. Massage can address problems such as ____________ headaches and ____________ and ____________ muscles. (p. 235)
5. Massage improves ____________ function for more healthy employees. (p. 235)
6. Massage leaves employees feeling ____________ and ready for ____________. (p. 235)

Seated Massage for Office Workers

1. Seated massage in the workplace typically lasts ____________ minutes. (p. 236)
2. Sessions mainly focus on the ____________ body. (p. 237)
3. Techniques that work well without ____________ are emphasized. (p. 237)
4. Seated massage techniques include ____________, ____________, ____________, ____________, light ____________, and ____________ movements. (p. 237)
5. Shiatsu and other forms of ____________ bodywork are particularly adaptable for seated massage. (p. 237)
6. A technique combination to alleviate tension headache includes ____________ of the neck and shoulders, ____________ on either side of the spine, and ____________ of the head and scalp. (p. 237)

Popularity of Workplace Massage

1. Workplace massage is popular because it has immediate ____________ effects, addresses aches and pains related to ____________, requires no ____________ on the part of the recipient, and complements other health practices like ____________ reduction. (p. 237)
2. Workplace massage promotes loyalty, and boosts ____________. (p. 238)

FOR GREATER UNDERSTANDING

The following exercises are designed to take you from the realm of theory into the real world. They will help give you a deeper understanding of the subjects covered in this chapter. Action words are underlined to emphasize the variety of activities presented to address different learning styles, and to encourage deeper thinking.

1. Interview a massage practitioner who specializes in seated massage. Ask them about the goals of their sessions, the approach and techniques used, and what type of clients they have. How do they market their practices? Report your findings to a study partner or group.
2. Receive a seated massage offered in a public place like a shopping mall, airport, or street fair. How did the practitioner prepare you for the session? Adjust the chair? What techniques were used? How long did it last? How did you feel afterwards? Report your experience to a study partner or group.
3. Interview someone who receives massage at their workplace. Ask them to describe the seated massage sessions. What benefits do they experience personally? Report your findings to a study partner or group.
4. Observe workplace seated massage sessions. Notice the physical space and environment for massage. Watch how the practitioner greets and prepares the recipient for seated massage. Observe the body mechanics and techniques used. Observe how the recipients respond during and after the session. Report your observations to a study partner or group.
5. Take a training in seated massage. Note the differences in body mechanics and techniques used compared to regular table massage.

APPENDIX A

25 Forms of Therapeutic Massage and Bodywork

The therapeutic massage and bodywork forms described below are some of the major systems practiced today. Descriptions include a summary of their origins and history, techniques and applications, the theory on which they are based, and some resources for further information. Noncommercial Web sites are listed when available, and books for forms that do not have relevant Web sites (e.g., Ayurvedic massage) are also cited. Readers are encouraged to check the Internet for Web sites appearing after publication of this text.

Many of the forms of massage and bodywork listed are root systems from which other forms or spin-offs have been derived. Because the field of massage therapy is an emerging profession with a large entrepreneurial component, there are several trademarked forms, e.g., Rolfing®. Spin-offs of originals may also be trademarked, or there may be generic spin-offs without trademarks.

For further explanations of these and other forms of massage and bodywork see *Discovering the Body's Wisdom* by Mirka Knaster (New York: Bantam Books, 1996).

1. Alexander Technique

   Origin: Alexander Technique was developed by an Australian named Frederick Matthias Alexander (1869–1955), who practiced in London in the early 1900s. Alexander, a Shakespearean actor, cured himself of loss of voice through correction of faulty posture in the head and neck. He later worked with other actors and public speakers using the same method to improve their vocal abilities.

   Technique: Alexander Technique is a form of contemporary bodywork in which a teacher guides the student through various movements like sitting, walking, and bending. The emphasis is on achieving balance in the head-neck relationship, called Primary Control. Poor habitual patterns are replaced by light, easy, simple, and integrated movement.

   Theory: Proper body alignment and movement patterns are achieved by heightened kinesthetic awareness, and conscious movement.

   Web Sites: Alexander Technique (www.alexandertechnique.com)
   Alexander Technique International (www.ati-net.com)
   American Society for the Alexander Technique (www.alexandertech.org)

2. Aromatherapy Massage

   Origin: The use of natural plant essences for health and therapeutic effects is ancient. The modern term "aromatherapie" was coined by a French chemist named Rene Maurice Gattefosse (1881–1950) as he studied the use of fragrant oils for their healing

properties in the 1920–1930s. Later, Madame Marguerite Maury (1895–1968) started prescribing essential oils for her patients, and is credited with the modern use of essential oils for massage. She wrote an important aromatherapy guide in French in 1961 that was translated into English in 1964.
Technique: Aromatherapy massage involves the use of essential oils in massage oil blends for their therapeutic effects. Techniques of Western massage, Ayurvedic massage, and other systems of soft tissue manipulation may be used in the application of aromatherapy massage oils.
Theory: Essential oils are highly concentrated aromatic extracts that are cold-pressed or steam distilled from plants such as grasses, leaves, flowers, fruit peels, wood, and roots. Each essential oil has a specific therapeutic effect such as relaxing, boosting immune system, relieving congestion, or soothing muscular aches and pains. Common massage blends contain essential oils such as peppermint, lavender, citrus, tea tree, and rosemary.
Web Site: National Association for Holistic Aromatherapy (www.naha.org)

3. Ayurvedic Massage
   Origin: Ayurvedic massage is one of the healing practices of ancient India. Vedic scriptures of India dating back to 3000 BCE describe healing practices including massage with oil.
   Technique: Ayurvedic massage techniques include rubbing, kneading, squeezing, tapping, and pulling or shaking the body. Emphasis is given to massage of the head and feet. Sessions are invigorating and the recipient changes position several times. Pressure is applied to *marmas*, or pressure points on the body.
   Theory: Ayurvedic massage is based in traditional Ayurvedic medicine of India. Massage is thought to remove obstructions to the flow of *vayu* (wind) through *siras* or wind-carrying vessels to reduce pain, relieve tension, and encourage more natural breathing patterns. Massage oils are chosen according to body type, the atmosphere and the season.
   Reference: *Ayurvedic Massage: Traditional Indian Techniques for Balancing Body and Mind* by Harish Johari (Rochester, VT: Healing Arts Press, 1996).
4. Clinical Massage Therapy
   See Medical Massage
5. Craniosacral Therapy (CST)
   Origin: Craniosacral therapy stems from the work of an osteopath named Dr. William Garner Sutherland (1873–1954) in the early 1900s. Dr. Sutherland developed the basic theory of CST, including cranial suture movement, rhythmic motion of cerebrospinal fluid (i.e., Breath of Life), and the relationship between craniosacral rhythm and health. John E. Upledger, D.O., has continued development of this work, and added the concept of SomatoEmotional Release (SER) of negative emotions stored in traumatized tissues. The Upledger Foundation was established in 1987 to study CST.
   Technique: Craniosacral therapy is a form of contemporary bodywork that uses gentle compression to realign the skull bones and stretch related membranes to balance the craniosacral rhythm (CSR), and improve function of the nervous system.
   Theory: CST is based in Western anatomy and physiology, and osteopathic science. The craniosacral system (i.e., cranium, spine, and sacrum) is connected by a fascial membrane called the dura mater that houses the brain and central nervous system. Cerebralspinal fluid is pumped throughout the system, creating a pulse or craniosacral rhythm (CSR). CST techniques aim to balance the CSR so that cerebralspinal fluid flows freely through the system. Once this is achieved, the body's own healing mechanism can function properly.
   Web Sites: The Upledger Institute (www.upledger.com)
   Craniosacral Therapy Association of North America (www.craniosacraltherapy.org)
6. Esalen Massage
   Origin: Esalen massage was developed at the Esalen Institute in Big Sur, California in the 1970s. Its development grew out of the Human Potential Movement and counterculture of the 1960s. Esalen massage was popularized in the classic *The Massage Book* by George Downing, published in 1972.

Technique: Esalen massage is a form of Western massage loosely based in Swedish massage. It emphasizes the sensual qualities of massage, and is associated with scented oils, incense, and New Age music. It initially was performed without draping, but accepted draping standards are now observed in most settings.
Theory: Esalen massage is applied to help the recipient get in touch with their senses, and their inner self, and is considered a meditative and personal growth experience. General health benefits of Swedish massage apply to Esalen massage.
Reference: *The Massage Book* by George Downing (New York: Random House Trade Paperbacks, 1998) (1st edition, 1972).
Web Site: Esalen Institute (www.esalen.org)

7. Feldenkrais Method®
Origin: The Feldenkrais Method was developed by Moshe Feldenkrais (1904–1984), who was an engineer, physicist, judo master, and mathematician. In efforts to heal himself of a knee injury, Feldenkrais developed a system of movement re-education. The Feldenkrais Method came to light during the human potential movement of the 1970–1980s.
Technique: Feldenkrais Method is a form of contemporary bodywork consisting of Functional Integration, i.e., hands-on table work in which the practitioner uses her hands to communicate new sensory movement patterns to the recipient through passive movements. In Awareness Through Movement, a teacher leads a group through structured movement experiences performed on the floor.
Theory: Feldenkrais Method is based in Western anatomy and physiology. Integrated movement patterns are established by re-educating the sensory-motor nervous system through repeated movements.
Web Sites: Feldenkrais Guild® of North America (www.feldenkrais. com)
International Feldenkrais Federation (www.feldenkrais-method.org)

8. Infant Massage
Origin: Massage has been given to infants from time immemorial by their mothers, grandmothers and other caregivers. Instances of infant massage are found among native tribes in Africa, South Sea Islands, and North America, in ancient and modern India, and folk cultures of Europe. Recent interest in infant massage was revived by Vimala Schneider in the 1980s, and by the research of Dr. Tiffany Fields at the University of Miami in the 1990s.
Technique: Infant massage is a specialty within Western massage and consists of simple techniques like stroking, kneading, twisting, and pressing performed with gentle pressure. Some passive joint movements are incorporated. Eye contact and communication with the infant are emphasized.
Theory: Infant massage is based in Western anatomy, physiology, and theories of child development. It aims to help the infant relax, improve circulation and other body functions, improve immune function, and promote neurological development. Research confirms the necessity of touch and movement for healthy human development, and the benefits of massage for premature infants.
Reference: *Infant Massage: A Handbook for Loving Parents* by Vimala Schneider McClure, revised edition (New York: Bantam Doubleday Dell, 2000).
Web Sites: International Institute of Infant Massage (www.infantmassageinstitute.com)
Loving Touch Foundation (www.lovingtouch.com) infant massage
Touch Research Institute (www.miami.edu/touch-research)

9. Lomi-Lomi
Origin: Lomi-lomi is a traditional massage of the natives of the Hawaiian Islands practiced from time immemorial. Different styles of lomi-lomi were developed within families. Typically a tutu, i.e., grandmother, or other respected family member was the keeper of the tradition. Its modern form was popularized by Aunty Margaret Machado of Kona, Hawaii in the 1970–1980s.
Technique: Lomi-lomi is a form of traditional native massage consisting of pressing and squeezing techniques performed with the fingers, palm and elbow. Kukui nut, macadamia, or coconut oil may be used. The recipient lies on a mat, or in modern

times, a massage table to receive lomi-lomi. Associated methods include baths, bone adjusting techniques, and prayer.
Theory: Lomi-lomi is based in traditional Hawaiian culture, and emphasizes letting go of stress, unconditional love, and opening the heart to harmony, acceptance, and healing.
Reference: *Hawaiian Lomi-Lomi: Big Island Massage* by Nancy S. Kahalewai (Hilo, HI: Island Massage Publishing, 2000).
Web Site: Aunty Margaret Homepage (www.hawaiian.net/~kea/aunty.html)

10. Lymphatic Drainage Massage
    Origin: Manual techniques applied to enhance lymphatic system function and treat lymphedema were developed as early as the 1880s. Emil and Astid Vodder developed their Manual Lymph Drainage (MLD), or Vodder Method, in the 1930s in France. In the 1970s, Hungarians Michael and Ethel Foldi combined Vodder's MLD with other modalities to create a treatment for lymphedema called Complete Decongestive Therapy (CDT).
    Technique: Lymphatic drainage massage is a specialized form of Western massage consisting of gentle techniques applied to the superficial skin layers to stretch the tissue and open the superficial lymphatic vessels so that lymph fluid can enter the vessels more easily. Classic Vodder techniques include stationary circles, scoop, pump, rotary, and light effleurage applied rhythmically and in specific directions.
    Theory: Lymphatic drainage massage is based on Western anatomy and physiology, and knowledge of the lymphatic system. Techniques are applied in such a way to enhance the movement of lymph fluid into superficial vessels and through the system. Lymphatic drainage massage improves immune function, reduces areas of edema, and aids injury healing.
    Web Sites: Academy of Lymphatic Studies (www.acols.com)
    Dr. Vodder School North America (www.vodderschool.com)
11. Medical Massage
    Origin: Massage has been used to treat ailments from time immemorial all over the globe. Historically in Western medicine, it has been called medical rubbing, frictions, massage, massotherapeutics, and physiotherapy. Medical massage is emerging in the 21st century as a specialty within the broader field of therapeutic massage and bodywork. It is sometimes called *clinical massage*.
    Technique: Medical massage is a specialty of Western massage in which soft tissue manipulation and related techniques are used in the treatment of pathological conditions. A subspecialty is the treatment of musculoskeletal dysfunction.
    Theory: Medical massage is based in Western anatomy, physiology, kinesiology, and pathology. Traditional and contemporary massage techniques are used as appropriate in treatment plans.
    References: *Basic Clinical Massage Therapy: Integrating Anatomy and Treatment* by James H. Clay and David M. Pounds (Philadelphia: Lippincott Williams & Wilkins, 2003) (Treating Musculoskeletal Dysfunction).
    Clinical Massage Therapy: Understanding, Assessing and Treating over 70 Conditions by Fiona Rattray and Linda Ludwig (Toronto, Canada: Talus Incorporated, 2000).
    Massage for Orthopedic Conditions by Thomas Hendrickson (Philadelphia: Lippincott Williams & Wilkins, 2003).
    Medical Massage by Ross Turchaninov and Connie Cox (Scottsdale, AZ: Stress Less Publishing, 1998).
12. Myofascial Massage
    Origin: Manual techniques that target the myofascial tissues were developed in the 1950s by Ida Rolf (1896–1979) in her system of Rolfing®, and by osteopath Robert Ward as myofascial release technique in the 1960s. Since then several systems of bodywork that treat myofascial tissues have been developed.
    Technique: Myofascial massage techniques apply traction to the skin and underlying tissues to slowly and gently push, pull, and stretch fascial tissues and break fascial adhesions. They are applied without oil so that restrictions can be palpated and techniques applied without slipping.

Theory: Myofascial massage is based in Western anatomy and physiology. It focuses on connective or myofascial tissues that surround muscles, nerves, blood vessels, and all organs of the body. Restrictions in fascial tissues can cause a variety of dysfunctions, including limited mobility, postural distortion, poor cellular nutrition, and pain. Myofascial massage produces a softening of tissues and freeing of fascial restrictions.
Reference: *The Myofascial Release Manual,* 3rd edition, by Carol J. Manheim (Thorofare, NJ: Slack, Inc., 2001)

13. Neuromuscular Therapy (NMT)

Origin: A precursor to today's NMT was developed by a natural healer named Stanley Lief in the 1920s. Trigger Point Therapy was brought to public attention through the work of Janet Travell, MD (1901–1997), an expert in myofascial pain, and her treatment of Presidents Kennedy and Johnson in the 1960s. Fitness expert Bonnie Prudden developed a popular system of NMT called Myotherapy® in the 1970s.
Technique: Neuromuscular Therapy is a form of contemporary Western massage in which trigger points, i.e., hyperirritable taut bands in the myofascial tissues, are located and deactivitated using ischematic compression. Pressure is applied to trigger points for about 30 seconds using the thumb, fingers, or small hand tool. A stretch of the affected muscle follows application of pressure on trigger points.
Theory: A trigger point is a taut band or irritable spot in myofascial tissue that causes muscle pain at the trigger point and in its referral zones. It also causes muscle shortening, and decreased strength. Under a microscope, trigger points appear to be bands of contracted muscle tissue.
References: Travell, J. G., & Simons, D. G. (1999). *Myofascial pain and dysfunction: The trigger point manual, Volume 1—Upper half of the body,* 2nd editon. Baltimore: Williams & Wilkins.
Travell, J. G., & Simons, D. G. (1992). *Myofascial pain and dysfunction: The trigger point manual, Volume 2—The lower extremities.* Baltimore: Williams & Wilkins.
Web Site: Bonnie Prudden Myotherapy (www.bonnieprudden.com)

14. Polarity Therapy

Origin: Polarity Therapy was developed by Randolph Stone (1890–1981) in the 1930–1950s. Stone combined Western knowledge with theories from Chinese and Ayurvedic medicine, particularly regarding energy balancing. Upon his retirement in 1973, Stone's successors taught Polarity Therapy throughout the United States. The American Polarity Therapy Association was founded in 1984.
Technique: Polarity Therapy is an eclectic form of energy bodywork. Most Polarity Therapy techniques consist of placing the hands in different positions on the body to affect the free flow of energy. Other techniques include pressing, gentle rocking, and brushing.
Theory: Polarity Therapy techniques aim to remove obstructions to the free flow of energy in the body. Stone developed his own esoteric theories of energy flow after studying Chinese and Ayurvedic medicine.
Web Site: American Polarity Therapy Association (www.polaritytherapy.org)

15. Reflexology

Origin: Modern reflexology was developed by Eunice Ingham Stopfel (1889–1974), who combined the theory of Zone Therapy with compression massage of the feet and hands. She mapped the feet for their corresponding zones of reference, and developed pressure techniques for stimulating points on the feet to affect specific organs and structures of the body. She started her work in the 1930s, and taught throughout the United States in the 1950–1960s.
Technique: Reflexology is performed primarily on the feet. Pressure is applied to areas of the feet to stimulate other parts of the body. Reflexology techniques include thumb walking, finger walking, hook and backup, along with Western massage and joint movements applied to the feet.
Theory: Reflexology is based in Zone Therapy, which postulates that 10 longitudinal zones of the body end in the feet and the hands. Pressure to a zone in the feet causes stimulation of the entire zone. Reflexology charts map out which specific organs or

body structures will be affected by pressure on specific areas of the feet. Reflexology is thought to normalize function, improve circulation, and promote relaxation. Knowledge of Western anatomy, physiology, and pathology are important in reflexology.
Web Sites: Home of Reflexology (www.reflexology.org)
International Institute of Reflexology (www.reflexology-usa.net)

16. Rolfing® Structural Integration
Origin: Rolfing was developed by Ida P. Rolf (1896–1979), and brought to public recognition during the 1970s within the human potential movement. The Rolf Institute® of Structural Integration was founded in 1971, and provides training and certification for Rolfing practitioners.
Technique: Rolfing is a form of contemporary Western bodywork, also called Structural Integration. It includes soft tissue manipulation and movement education. In Rolfing, myofascial tissues are manipulated so that they lengthen and glide, to balance the body around its vertical axis, achieving proper alignment or posture. In the process of working with deep myofascial tissues, past emotional trauma is also released.
Theory: Rolfing is based in Western anatomy and physiology, especially of fascial tissues, and psychology.
Web Site: The Rolf Institute for Structural Integration (www.rolf.org)

17. Shiatsu—Namikoshi
Origin: Shiatsu evolved from traditional Japanese massage called Amma. Tokujiro Namikoshi (1905–) developed a system of finger pressure to treat various ailments. He founded the first Shiatsu Institute of Therapy on Hokkaido in 1925, and the Japan Shiatsu Institute in Tokyo in 1940. His son, Toru Namikoshi (1931–), popularized Shiatsu in Japan and throughout the world in the 1950–1970s.
Technique: Shiatsu is a form of Asian Bodywork Therapy. Shiatsu literally means finger pressure (shi-atsu) in Japanese. Pressure is applied along energy (ki) meridians and to acupoints with the thumbs, fingers, or elbow. Recipient is either lying on a mat on the floor or on a bodywork table.
Theory: Shiatsu, as developed by Namikoshi, combines traditional Chinese medicine and Western anatomy and physiology. Important acupoints are pressed to elicit desired results.
Web Site: American Organization of Bodywork Therapies of Asia (www.aobta.org)

18. Sports Massage
Origin: Sports massage can be traced to ancient Greece and Rome where massage was given in the gymnasia and public baths. Massage prepared athletes for exercises, and helped in recovery from competition. In the late 19th century, rubbers and athletic masseurs used massage in the training of athletes. Sports massage was revived in the 1970s within the context of Western massage.
Technique: Sports massage is a specialty within Western massage. Western massage techniques are applied to enhance athletic performance, prevent injuries, prepare for and recover from competition, and in rehabilitation of injuries. Modern sports massage given at events emphasizes the technique of compression and other forms of petrissage. Individual practitioners may add other bodywork approaches to achieve the goals of the athlete.
Theory: Sports massage is based in Western anatomy, physiology, kinesiology, pathology, and sports science.
Reference: *Understanding Sports Massage* by Patricia J. Benjamin & Scott Lamp (Champaign, IL: Human Kinetics, 1996).

19. Stone Massage
Origin: Stones have been used in healing practices all over the world, including Asia. Healing or hot stone massage is a treatment that gained popularity in North American spas in the 1990–2000s.
Technique: Stone massage is a form of contemporary bodywork and spa treatment. Stones of various sizes, shapes and textures are used as massage tools, and as a form of thermal therapy. As massage tools, stones are used instead of the hands to apply pressure during techniques such as effleurage. As thermal therapy, stones may be heated and

placed on the body over certain anatomical structures or in patterns over energy centers and meridians; or cooled and used as cryotherapy to reduce swelling and cool tissues.
Theory: Stone massage is practiced as an eclectic form of bodywork incorporating Western anatomy and physiology with traditional Asian medicine. Geological properties of various kinds of stones are considered. Hot stones applied to the body impart weight and heat that promotes relaxation, normal body function, and energy balancing.
References: *Healing Stone Massage*. Video with Carollanne Crichton (Real Bodywork, 2001).
Japanese Hot Stone Massage by Mark Hess and Shogo Mochizuki (Kotobuki Publications, 2002).

20. Swedish Massage
Origin: Swedish massage and related techniques were developed in Europe in the early 1800s, and brought to North America in the 1860s. It can be traced historically to the work of two men, Pehr Henrick Ling (1776–1839) of Sweden, and Johann Mezger (1838–1909) of Amsterdam. The heyday of Swedish massage in the United States was the 1930–1950s, when it was offered in health clubs, salons, and as part of physiotherapy.
Technique: Swedish massage is a form of traditional Western massage. The five classic technique categories of Swedish massage soft tissue manipulation are effleurage (stroking, sliding), petrissage (kneading, compression), tapotement (percussion), friction, and vibration. Joint movements and hydrotherapy are also within the scope of Swedish massage.
Theory: Swedish massage is based in Western anatomy, physiology, and pathology. It is applied to support the normal function of the human body and its systems, as well as enhance its innate healing capacity.
See Western Massage.

21. Thai Massage
Origin: Nuad bo-Rarn means "ancient massage" in the language of Thailand. It has been practiced for over 2500 years. At the Temple of the Reclining Buddha in Bangkok, 200 year–old stone engravings illustrate the energy lines and points, and techniques of this ancient practice. Thai massage is passed down in families, and also taught at schools of Traditional Thai Medicine.
Technique: In Thai massage, the practitioner uses passive movement, yoga-like stretching, and pressure techniques to stimulate energy channels called *sen lines*, and release tension in the body. Application is gentle and rhythmic. Recipients lie on floor mats to receive Thai Massage.
Theory: Thai massage is based on Ayurvedic (India) and Chinese medicine, and was influenced by yoga, as it evolved in ancient Thailand. Techniques stimulate the free flow of energy through channels.
Web Site: Institute of Thai Massage (www.thai-massage.org)

22. Therapeutic Touch (TT)
Origin: Therapeutic Touch was developed by Delores Krieger, a professor of nursing, and her teacher, Dora Kunz in the 1960–1970s. It is a modification of the ancient practice of laying on of the hands.
Technique: Therapeutic Touch is a system of energy bodywork performed in five steps: (1) centering of the practitioner, (2) assessment of the energy field of the recipient with the palms of the hands, (3) clearing blockages, imbalances or congestion of energy with sweeping hand movements, (4) establishing harmony in the energy field using the mind, (5) smoothing out the energy field by sweeping the hands outward toward the periphery of the field.
Theory: Therapeutic Touch is based in theories of bioelectricity and electromagnetic energy fields. The sweeping hand movements of TT move energy to create balance and harmony in a person's energy field. Imbalances, blockages, and congestion in the energy field are thought to result in disease and dysfunction. TT is used in the treatment of many different ailments.
Web Sites: Nurse Healers–Professional Associates International (www.therapeutic touch.org)

23. Trager® Approach
    Origin: Trager Approach, also known as Psychophysical Integration, was developed by Milton Trager, MD (1908–1997). After earning a medical degree after World War II, Trager opened a practice in Hawaii in 1959, and gave a public demonstration of his work in 1973.
    Technique: The Trager Approach is a system of contemporary Western bodywork that combines tissue and joint mobilization, relaxation and movement re-education. The practitioner applies continuous rhythmic movement to different joints in the body with the recipient lying on a table. Recipients recreate the easy, light, free movements of the table work in a system of active exercise called Mentastics.
    Theory: Trager focuses on creating the sensations of lighter, easier, and freer movement through affecting neurological mechanisms of the body. It imparts an experience of deep relaxation, and greater joint mobility.
    Web Site: Trager International (www.trager.com)
24. Tuina
    Origin: The origin of Tuina, or Chinese medical massage, is clouded in the mists of time. It developed from the same roots as acupuncture in Chinese medicine. Tuina is written about in several ancient medical texts, and a Tuina department was set up in the Imperial Health Administration in the Tang Dynasty (618–907 CE). Tuina for infants and children became popular in the Qing Dynasty (1644–1911 CE)
    Technique: Tuina is a form of Chinese medical massage, i.e., Asian Bodywork Therapy. Techniques of Tuina include stroking, pushing, grasping, pressing, palm-rubbing, twisting, pinching, rubbing, rolling, tapping, stretching, kneading, lifting, and holding. Techniques are applied to stimulate acupoints and affect blood circulation. Tuina also includes joint manipulation, herbal remedies, and therapeutic exercise.
    Theory: Tuina is based in theory of Chinese medicine including *qi* or energy, energy channels, and yin-yang. Modern Tuina incorporates knowledge of Western anatomy, physiology, and pathology. Tuina is used to treat ailments recognized by Chinese medicine, as well as Western pathology.
    Reference: *Chinese Tuina Therapy* by Wang Fu (Bejing, China: Foreign Languages Press, 1994).
25. Western Massage
    Origin: Western massage can be traced to health and healing practices of ancient Greece and Rome. Techniques of soft tissue manipulation were further developed through the centuries in Europe and North America. Western massage today is an outgrowth of Swedish massage, massage used in Western medicine, and various contemporary systems of massage and bodywork.
    Description: Western massage techniques include classic Swedish massage techniques, plus various forms of contemporary massage, e.g., neuromuscular therapy, myofascial massage, lymphatic drainage massage, and other forms of massage therapy based in Western anatomy, physiology, and pathology. Western massage practitioners tend to be eclectic, incorporating various techniques, including energy approaches, with classic Swedish massage.
    Theory: Western massage is based in Western anatomy, physiology, and pathology. It aims to enhance the normal functioning of the body and its systems, including the innate healing power in each person.
    Web Sites: American Massage Therapy Association (www.amtamassage.org)
    Associated Bodywork & Massage Professionals (www.abmp.com)

Glossary

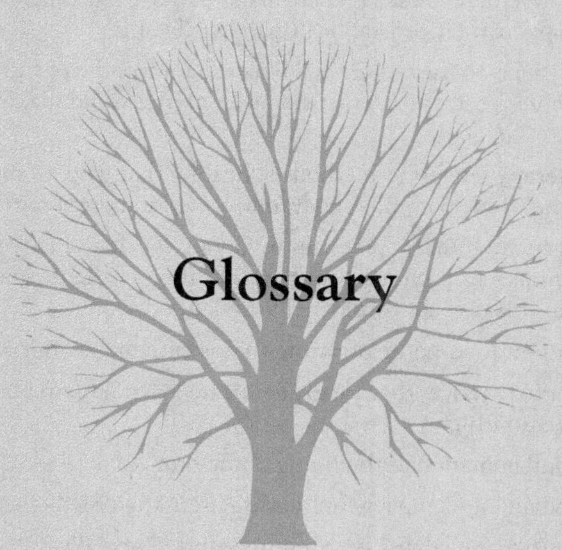

Acquired immune deficiency syndrome (AIDS) Extremely virulent sexually transmitted disease that renders the immune system inoperative.

Acquired immunity Immunity developed during life in response to disease, vaccination, or exposure.

Active movements are performed voluntarily by a person with no or some assistance from a practitioner. Types of active movements are free, assistive, and resistive.

Acupressure is a Western term for a form of Asian bodywork therapy based on Chinese meridian theory in which acupuncture points are pressed to stimulate the flow of energy or chi.

Allergy Hypersensitive reaction to a specific antigen or allergen in the environment in which the body produces excessive antibodies to that antigen or allergen.

Alternative therapy refers to methods or systems of healing outside of mainstream medicine.

Alveoli Tiny air sacs of the lungs.

Amma is a term for traditional Japanese massage.

Antibodies Substances produced by the body that are individually matched to specific antigens.

Antigen Substance capable of triggering an immune response.

Arthritis Painful inflammatory disease of the joints.

Asian bodywork therapies (ABT) are forms of massage and bodywork whose theoretical basis is Traditional Asian (Chinese) Medicine.

Assistive movement is a type of active movement in which the recipient initiates the movement, and the practitioner helps perform the movement. Also called **assisted movement**.

Asthma A chronic respiratory disease characterized by attacks of wheezing, shortness of breath, and coughing spasms.

Autoinoculation Transmission of a pathogen from one part of the body to another.

Ayurvedic massage is a system of soft tissue manipulation based in traditional theories of health and disease from India, i.e., Ayurvedic medicine.

Bacteria Single-celled organisms that may cause disease.

Benefits are positive outcomes. The benefits of massage are experienced by recipients when the effects of massage support their general health and wellbeing.

Body mechanics refers to the posture and biomechanics of the practitioner when performing massage. Good body mechanics protect the practitioner from injury and maximize the efficiency of technique applications.

Body-centered therapy refers to methods of healing that work primarily through the physical body, but which affect the whole person — body, mind, emotions, and spirit.

Bodywork is a general term for practices involving touch and movement in which the practitioner uses manual techniques to promote health and healing of the recipient. The healing massage techniques described in this text are considered forms of bodywork.

Botulism A resistant food-borne organism that is extremely virulent.

Boundaries refer to practices that clearly delineate and maintain practitioner and client roles within the therapeutic relationship.

Bronchitis An inflammation of the lining of the bronchial tubes.

CAM is an acronym for Complementary and Alternative Medicine.

Candidiasis Yeastlike fungal disease often transmitted sexually.

Chancre Sore often found at the site of syphilis infection.

Chlamydia Bacterially caused STI of the urogenital tract.

Chronic obstructive pulmonary diseases (COPDs) A collection of chronic lung diseases including asthma, emphysema, and chronic bronchitis.

Clinical massage therapy describes applications of massage for the treatment of pathologies. Also called medical massage.

Complementary therapy refers to healing methods that are used as secondary treatments to enhance the effectiveness of primary treatments, and that contribute to a patient's recovery.

Confidentiality is an ethical principle that upholds clients' right to privacy, and prohibits giving information about clients to others without the client's permission. See **HIPAA.**

Conjunctivitis Serious inflammation of the eye caused by any number of pathogens or irritants; can be caused by STDs such as chlamydia.

Contemporary massage and bodywork is a general category for systems of manual therapy that were developed in the 20th century, e.g., myofascial massage, neuromuscular therapy, polarity therapy.

Contraindications are conditions or situations that make receiving massage inadvisable because of the harm that it might do.

Counter-transference is a psychological phenomenon that occurs when a practitioner responds to a client as if they were relating to someone important in their, i.e., the practitioner's, past (e.g., mother), and transferring those positive or negative feelings onto the therapeutic relationship. See **transference.**

Cryotherapy is the application of cold (e.g., ice) for its therapeutic effects.

Deep friction is a type of friction in which the practitioner's fingers do not move over the skin, but instead, move the skin over tissues underneath. Cross-fiber and circular friction are types of deep friction.

Deep transverse friction is a specific type of deep friction used in rehabilitation to break adhesions, facilitate healthy scar formation, and treat muscle and tendon lesions. It is performed across the tissues, causing broadening and separation of fibers. Deep transverse friction was popularized by James Cyriax. Also called **Cyriax friction.**

Dengue A disease transmitted by mosquitoes, which causes flulike symptoms.

Dengue hemorrhagic fever A more serious form of dengue.

Diabetes mellitus A disease in which the pancreas fails to produce enough insulin or the body fails to use insulin effectively.

Direct pressure, or direct static pressure, is the application of force to compress tissues in a specific spot; it is applied with a thumb, finger, elbow, or knuckle. It can be considered a form of compression without movement and has also been called **static friction.**

Draping refers to the use of sheets, towels, or other materials to cover recipients of massage to preserve their privacy and modesty, to maintain professional boundaries, and for warmth.

Dyspnea Chronic breathlessness.

Eclectic practitioners combine two or more systems of massage and bodywork into their own unique approach to manual therapy.

Effectiveness of a massage performance refers to the degree to which intended goals are achieved and to which the recipient is satisfied.

Effects of massage refer to the basic physiological and psychological changes that occur to the recipient during a massage session.

Effleurage is a Western massage technique category that includes movements that slide or glide over the body with a smooth continuous motion.

ELISA Blood test that detects presence of antibodies to HIV virus.

Emphysema A respiratory disease in which the alveoli become distended or ruptured and are no longer functional.

Endangerment sites are areas of the body where delicate body structures are less protected and, therefore, may be more easily damaged when receiving massage.

Endemic Describing a disease that is always present to some degree.

Endometriosis Abnormal development of endometrial tissue outside the uterus; results in serious side effects.

Environment for massage includes the room, air quality, lighting, sound, dressing arrangements, equipment, and overall cleanliness and neatness of the space in which a session is given.

Enzymes Organic substances that cause bodily changes and destruction of microorganisms.

Epidermis The outermost layer of the skin.

Epilepsy A neurological disorder caused by abnormal electrical brain activity; can be accompanied by altered consciousness or convulsions.

Esalen massage is a genre of bodywork based on a simplified form of Swedish massage, whose main purpose is to enhance nonverbal connection with the inner self and with others. It emphasizes the sensual aspects of massage. It was developed at the Esalen Institute in Big Sur, California in the 1970s as part of the human potential movement.

Evidence-based therapy is founded on scientific research that provides verifiable evidence of the effectiveness of a specific treatment.

Fibromyalgia A chronic rheumatoidlike disorder that can be highly painful and difficult to diagnose.

Folk and native massage traditions are found all over the world among families, tribes, and villages. They are based on tradition and experience and often involve herbal remedies, ritual, and religious beliefs.

Foot reflexology See **reflexology.**

Free active movements or free exercises are performed entirely by a person with no assistance from a practitioner.

Friction is a Western massage technique category that includes movements that rub one surface over another repeatedly and includes superficial and deep friction.

Full-body Western massage refers to a massage session lasting from 30 to 90 minutes, in which traditional Western massage techniques are combined into a routine to address the whole body. These sessions are generally wellness oriented and aim to improve circulation, relax the muscles, improve joint mobility, induce general relaxation, promote healthy skin, and create a general sense of wellbeing.

Fungi A group of plants that lack chlorophyll and do not produce flowers or seeds; several microscopic varieties are pathogenic.

General contraindications are conditions or situations that make receiving any massage inadvisable because of the harm that it might do.

Genital herpes STI caused by the herpes simplex virus.

Genital warts Warts that appear in the genital area or the anus; caused by the human papillomaviruses (HPVs).

German measles (rubella) A milder form of measles that causes a rash and mild fever in children and may cause damage to a fetus or a newborn baby.

Gonorrhea Second most common STD in the United States; if untreated, may cause sterility.

Hay fever A chronic respiratory disorder that is most prevalent when ragweed and flowers bloom.

Healing means enhancing health and wellbeing. It is the process of regaining health or optimal functioning after an injury, disease, or other debilitating condition. "To heal" means to make healthy, whole, or sound; restore to health; or free from ailment.

Hepatitis A virally caused disease in which the liver becomes inflamed, which produces symptoms such as fever, headache, and jaundice.

HIPAA is an acronym for the Health Insurance Portability and Accountability Act of 1996.

HIPAA Privacy Rules specify how medical records must be secured, who may have access to medical records, and under what conditions records may be shared with others. See **confidentiality.**

Histamines Chemical substances that dilate blood vessels, increase mucous secretions, and produce other symptoms of allergies.

Holistic massage refers to forms of massage which take into account the wholeness of human beings, i.e., body, mind, emotions, and spirit.

Human immunodeficiency virus (HIV) The slow-acting virus that causes AIDS.

Human papillomaviruses (HPV) A small group of viruses that cause genital warts.

Human potential movement is an historical social movement in the 1960–1970s United States that advocated exploring the limits of human potential, and spawned many forms of massage and bodywork. See **Esalen massage.**

Hydrotherapy is the use of water in different forms for its therapeutic effects. See **thermal therapies.**

Hyperglycemia Elevated blood sugar levels.

Hysterectomy Surgical removal of the uterus.

Immunological competence Ability of the immune system to defend the body from pathogens.

Indication is used in the treatment model to mean that when a specific medical condition is present, a particular modality is indicated or advised to alleviate the condition. Massage is indicated as a treatment for a number of medical conditions.

Infant massage involves soft tissue manipulation and joint movements designed to enhance the growth and development of newborns and children.

Influenza A common viral disease of the respiratory tract.

Informed consent is a procedure used to ask for explicit permission from a client to touch a certain body area, or perform a specific technique.

Insulin A hormone produced by the pancreas; required by the body for the metabolism of carbohydrates.

Integrative health care is an approach to healing in which mainstream medicine and alternative healing methods are offered as equal options for treating patients.

Intention is the aim that guides the action, that is, what the practitioner hopes to accomplish.

Interferon A protein substance produced by the body that aids the immune system by protecting healthy cells.

Interspecies transmission Transmission of disease from humans to animals or from animals to humans.

Intervention model is a procedure used to clarify a possible misunderstanding of intention by a client (e.g., sexual intent), and to make a decision whether to stop or continue with a massage session.

Irritable bowel syndrome (IBS) Nausea, pain, gas, or diarrhea caused by certain foods or stress.

Jin Shin Do® is a modern synthesis of traditional Chinese acupressure/acupuncture theory and techniques, breathing exercises, Taoist philosophy, and modern psychology. It was developed by Iona Marsaa Teeguarden in the 1970s in the United States.

Joint manipulations, sometimes called adjustments or chiropractic adjustments, refer to techniques that take a joint beyond its normal range of motion and that are specific attempts to realign a misaligned joint, usually using a thrusting movement. Joint manipulations are not part of Western massage and are not within the scope of this text.

Joint movements are techniques that involve motion in the joints of the body, and include mobilizing techniques and stretching.

Lactose intolerance The inability to produce lactase, an enzyme needed to convert milk sugar into glucose.

Local contraindications are conditions or situations that make receiving massage on a particular part of the body inadvisable because of the harm that it might do. Also called **regional contraindications.**

Lubricants are topical substances used in some massage sessions to enhance the effects of techniques and to minimize skin friction. Common lubricants include vegetable and mineral oils, jojoba, lotions, and combinations of these substances.

Lupus A disease in which the immune system attacks the body and produces antibodies that destroy or injure organs such as the kidneys, brain, and heart.

Lymphatic drainage massage (LDM) is a form of contemporary massage designed to assist the function of the lymphatic system by the application of slow, light, and repetitive strokes that help move lymph fluid through the system of vessels and nodes (also **manual lymph drainage**).

Manual therapy refers to healing methods applied with the practioner's hands touching or moving the recipient's body.

Massage is the intentional and systematic manipulation of the soft tissues of the body to enhance health and healing. Joint movements and stretching are commonly performed as part of massage. The primary characteristics of massage are touch and movement.

Massage therapy is a general term for health and healing practices involving touch and movement, which are based in massage and related manual techniques. It is sometimes used synonymously with the term **bodywork.** The term massage therapy has been adopted by some massage practitioners to define their profession, which is a licensed profession in many states.

Measles A viral disease that produces symptoms including an itchy rash and a high fever.

Medical massage See **clinical massage.**

Migraine A condition characterized by localized headaches that possibly result from alternating dilation and constriction of blood vessels.

Mobilizing techniques Mobilizing techniques are free and loose non-specific joint movements within the normal range of joint motion.

Modality is a method of treating a medical condition. Massage is considered a modality in the tradition of physiotherapy, along with other modalities such as ice packs, hot packs, ultrasound, or whirlpool baths.

Multifactorial disease Disease caused by interactions of several factors.

Multiple sclerosis (MS) A degenerative neurological disease in which myelin, an insulator of nerves, breaks down.

Myofascial massage is a general term for techniques aimed at restoring mobility in the body's fascia and softening connective tissue that has become rigid. Also called **myofascial release** and **myofascial unwinding.**

Natural healing refers to a philosophy that shows preference for methods of healing derived from nature, the belief in an innate healing force, and a holistic view of human life.

Natural healing arts are methods of healing derived from nature, for example, nutritious food, herbs, water therapy, exercise, relaxation, fresh air, sunshine, and massage.

Natural immunity Immunity passed to a fetus by its mother.

Neuromuscular therapy (NMT) is a form of contemporary massage focused on deactivating myofascial trigger points. See **trigger points.**

Organization of a session refers to the overall structure of a massage session into beginning, middle, and end; the progression from one section of the body to another; and the ordering of techniques into sequences. Organization includes the use of opening techniques, transitions, and finishing techniques.

Osteoarthritis A progressive deterioration of bones and joints that has been associated with the "wear and tear" theory of aging.

Pacing refers to the speed of performing techniques, which may vary from very slow to very fast for different effects.

Palliative care refers to methods of reducing symptoms and discomfort associated with certain diseases or their treatment.

Parasitic worms The largest of the pathogens, most of which are more a nuisance than a threat.

Parkinson's disease A chronic, progressive neurological condition that causes tremors and other symptoms.

Passive movements are body movements initiated and controlled by the practitioner, while the recipient remains relaxed and receptive.

Passive touch is simply laying the fingers, one hand, or both hands on the body. Passive touch may impart heat to an area, have a calming influence, or help balance energy.

Pathogen A disease-causing agent.

Pelvic inflammatory disease (PID) Term used to describe various infections of the female reproductive tract.

Peptic ulcer Damage to the stomach or intestinal lining, usually caused by digestive juices.

Periodontal diseases Diseases of the tissue around the teeth.

Person-centered massage refers to maintaining awareness of the whole person during a session, as opposed to focusing strictly on the pathology, i.e., pathology centered.

Petrissage is a Western massage technique category that includes movements that lift, wring, or squeeze soft tissues in a kneading motion; or press or roll the soft tissues under or between the hands.

Pneumonia Disease of the lungs characterized by chronic cough, chest pain, chills, high fever, and fluid accumulation; may be caused by bacteria, viruses, chemicals, or other substances.

Polarity therapy is a form of bodywork that uses simple touch and gentle rocking movements with the intention to balance life energy and to encourage relaxation. It was developed by Randolph Stone in the mid-20th century.

Positioning the receiver refers to placing the recipient of massage in a position (e.g., supine, prone, side-lying, seated) to maximize his or her comfort and safety. Bolsters and other props may be used to support specific body areas.

Practitioner refers to someone trained in massage techniques and who uses massage in the practice of his or her profession.

Pregnancy massage refers to massage and bodywork adapted to meet the needs of pregnant women, and relieve some of the discomforts related to the pregnant state.

Premenstrual dysphoric disorder (PMDD) A group of symptoms similar to but more severe than PMS; especially involves mood disturbances.

Premenstrual syndrome (PMS) The mood changes and physical symptoms that occur in many women prior to menstruation.

Pressure is related to the force used in applying techniques and to the degree of compaction of tissues as techniques are applied. The amount of pressure used in massage will depend on the intended effect and the tolerance or desires of the recipient.

Principle-based massage utilizes a broad base of knowledge and skills to plan a unique session or treatment strategy, as opposed to relying on a set protocol or formula.

Prions A self-replicating protein-based agent that systematically destroys brain cells.

Professional demeanor refers to the appearance, language, and behavior of practitioners, which meets professional standards and inspires trust and respect.

Professional library includes the resources a practitioner has accessible within their own office, including some basic sources of information about conditions, pathologies, and special populations commonly encountered in their massage practice.

Protozoa Microscopic, single-celled organisms.

Pubic lice Parasites that can inhabit various body areas, especially the genitals; also called "crabs."

Referred pain Pain that is present at one point, but whose source is elsewhere.

Reflexology is a form of bodywork based on the theory of zone therapy, in which specific spots on the feet or hands are pressed to stimulate corresponding areas in other parts of the body.

Research literacy refers to knowledge and skills needed to understand and use scientific research. It includes an understanding of the scientific method, locating research articles, and reading, analyzing, and evaluating research studies.

Resistive movements are a type of active movement in which the practitioner offers resistance to the motion, thereby challenging the muscles used. Also called **resisted movements.**

Rheumatoid arthritis A serious inflammatory joint disease.

Rhythm refers to a recurring pattern of movement with a specific cadence, beat, or accent and may be described as smooth, flowing, or uneven.

Scope of practice describes the legally allowed, or professionally defined, methods used by a certain profession, as well as their intention in performing them. Different professions have different scopes of practice as defined by law or by the profession. Massage techniques fall within the scope of practice of several professions.

Seated massage refers to massage given with the recipient seated in an ordinary or a special massage chair. It is called **on-site massage** when the chair is taken to a public place such as an office or commercial establishment. Also called **chair massage.**

Session refers to a period of time in which massage is given to a recipient by a practitioner. Sessions have logical organization, have a wellness or a treatment purpose, and generally vary from 10 minutes to two hours.

Sexually transmitted infections (STIs) Infectious diseases transmitted via some form of intimate, usually sexual, contact.

Shiatsu is a general term for Japanese bodywork based on Chinese meridian theory and Western science, in which tsubo (i.e., acupoints) are pressed to balance the flow of energy or ki.

Sickle-cell anemia Genetic disease commonly found among African Americans; results in organ damage and premature death.

Sleep apnea Disorder in which a person has numerous episodes of breathing stoppage during a night's sleep.

Sports massage is the science and art of applying massage and related techniques to ensure the health and wellbeing of the athlete and to enhance athletic performance. The major applications of sports massage are recovery, remedial, rehabilitation, maintenance, and event (i.e., pre-, inter-, and post-event).

Standards of practice are documents developed by professional associations that outline acceptable ethical professional conduct.

Staphylococci Round, gram-positive bacteria, usually found in clusters.

Streptococci Round bacteria, usually found in chain formation.

Stretching is a passive movement performed to the limit of the range of motion of a joint. Stretching increases flexibility in a joint; lengthens the muscles and connective tissues that cross a joint; and helps relax muscles involved.

Superficial friction is a type of friction in which the hand rubs briskly back and forth over the skin to improve circulation in superficial tissues and to create heat.

Swedish massage is a genre of bodywork that includes traditional Western massage, Swedish movements, hydrotherapy, heat lamps, and other modalities. Swedish massage is a popular form of massage in health clubs, spas, and resorts.

Swedish Movement Cure refers to Pehr Ling's system of medical gymnastics that was developed in the early 1800s and which, along with Mezger's massage, is the forerunner of today's Western massage.

Syphilis One of the most widespread STDs; characterized by distinct phases and potentially serious results.

Tapotement is a Western massage technique category consisting of brisk percussive movements that are performed in rapid rhythmic fashion. Forms of tapotement include hacking, rapping, cupping, clapping, slapping, tapping, and pincement.

Technique refers to the technical aspects of the application of massage, or how the body moves while performing massage. The broader concept of the term technique also includes the intent.

Therapeutic relationship is a model for understanding the separate and unique roles of the practitioner and the client in the therapeutic setting.

Thermal therapies involve the application of hot and cold modalities for their therapeutic effects, e.g., hot packs, ice. See **hydrotherapy.**

Touch means "to come into contact with." Massage practitioners touch their clients or patients in many ways, but primarily with their hands. Touch may happen on a physical or an energetic level.

Touch without movement is a Western massage technique in which the practitioner comes in contact with the recipient either physically or energetically, but no perceptible movement occurs that fits into the five traditional classic Western massage categories. Two common types of touch without movement are passive touch and direct static pressure.

Toxic shock syndrome A potentially life-threatening bacterial infection that is most common in menstruating women who use tampons.

Toxins Poisonous substances produced by certain microorganisms that cause various diseases.

Traditional Asian Medicine (TAM) is a system of healing based on Chinese medicine, and includes concepts such as yin/yang, the five elements, energy (Qi), and energy channels.

Transference is a psychological phenomenon that occurs when clients respond to practitioners as if they were relating to someone important in their past (e.g., father), and transferring those positive or negative feelings onto the therapeutic relationship. See **counter-transference.**

Treatment refers to interventions aimed at alleviating a specific medical condition.

Treatment model is a concept that explains the intention of using specific interventions or modalities to alleviate medical conditions.

Trichomoniasis Protozoan infection characterized by foamy, yellowish discharge and unpleasant odor.

Trigger points are small, hyperirritable spots in muscle or related connective tissue that may cause local pain or pain in a distant referral zone. Trigger points may be relieved manually with ischemic compression techniques, deep friction, deep stripping, and stretching. See **neuromuscular therapy (NMT).**

Tuberculosis (TB) A disease caused by bacterial infiltration of the respiratory system.

Ulcerative colitis An inflammatory disorder that affects the mucous membranes of the large intestine, producing bloody diarrhea.

Vaccination Inoculation with killed or weakened pathogens or similar, less dangerous antigens in order to prevent or lessen the effects of some disease.

Vaginitis Set of symptoms characterized by vaginal itching, swelling, and burning.

Vibration is a Western massage technique category that includes oscillating, quivering, or trembling movements; or movement of soft tissues back and forth, or up and down, performed quickly and repeatedly. Vibration may be described as fine or coarse (e.g., shaking, jostling).

Virulent Strong enough to overcome host resistance and cause disease.

Viruses Minute parasitic microbes that live inside another cell.

Wellness refers to a condition of optimal physical, emotional, intellectual, spiritual, social, and vocational wellbeing.

Wellness massage is massage performed with the intention of promoting the receiver's general wellbeing. It goes beyond the treatment of specific conditions to help the receiver achieve high-level wellness.

Wellness Massage Pyramid is a model for understanding the possible contributions of massage therapy to high-level wellness. Pyramid levels from the base to the top are: treatment, recovery, prevention, neutral zone, health maintenance, personal growth, and life enjoyment.

Wellness model is a concept that explains good health and wellbeing as aimed at living a healthy, vibrant, and meaningful life. It goes beyond the idea of health as the absence of disease and emphasizes personal responsibility. Also called the **wellness perspective.**

Western blot A test more accurate than the ELISA to confirm presence of HIV antibodies.

Western massage is a form of soft tissue manipulation and related techniques developed in Europe and the United States over the past 200 years. The technique categories commonly used to describe Western massage are effleurage, petrissage, tapotement, friction, vibration, touch without movement, and joint movements. See Swedish massage.

Zen Shiatsu is a form of Asian Bodywork Therapy from Japan developed by Shizuto Masunaga.

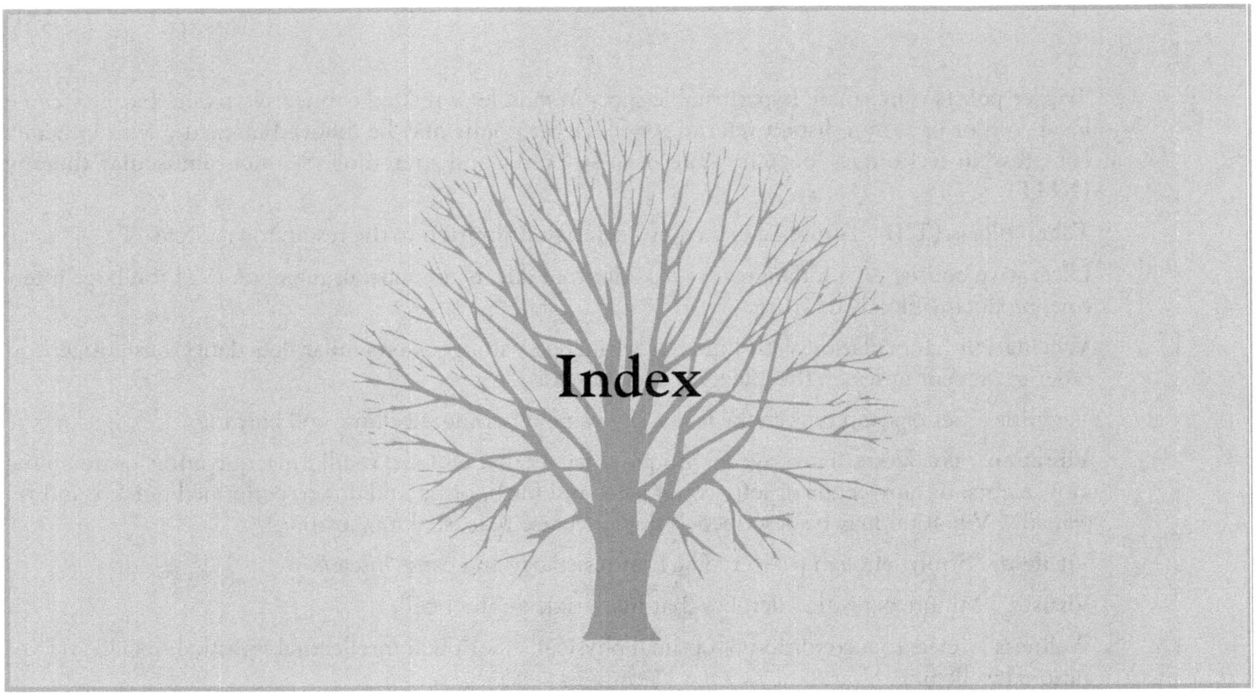

Index

A
Abdomen
  anatomy, 191
  full-body Western massage, 160–161
  massage, 194, 225
Acquired immune deficiency syndrome (AIDS), 263–268
Acquired immunity, 251
Acupressure points, 212
Adduction, diagonal (thigh), 142
Adhesions, 37
Adjustment, chiropractic, 62, 131
Aging
  as disease risk factor, 242
  physical effects of, 221
Airborne pathogens, 243
Air quality, 84
Alignment, body, 40
Allergy-induced respiratory problems, 268, 270
Alternating fingers-to-thumb petrissage, 113
Alternating one-handed kneading, 112
Alternative therapy, 7
Amma (Japanese massage), 19
AMTA Foundation, 30
Anatomy
  back, 175
  buttocks, 178
  chest and abdomen, 191
  face and head, 167
  lower extremities, 180–181
  neck, 171–172
  upper extremities, 186–187
Anatripic Art, 24
Animal-borne pathogens, 244
Ankle, movement techniques, 144–145
Anterior neck, 67
Antibodies, 250
HIV, 267
Antigens, 250
Anxiety
  reduced, 46
  reduction in hospitalized patients, 59–60
Arms
  anatomy, 187
  full-body Western massage, 158–160
Arrhythmias, cardiac, 71
Arthritis, 278
Asian bodywork therapy (ABT), 6
Asthma, 270–272
Asthmatic children, 61
Atherosclerosis, 71
Autistic children, 61
Autoimmune diseases, 250–251
Autoinoculate, 243
Avicenna, 22
Axilla, 68
Ayurvedic massage tradition, 6, 20

B
Back
  anatomy, 175
  applications of massage, 174
  full-body Western massage, 153
  low back pain, 279
  massage for relaxation, 177
  techniques, 175–178
Bacteria, 244–246
Basic sliding effleurage, 107
Basic two-handed kneading, 112

Baths
Maya sweat, 197
Roman, 20–21
Turkish, 21
whirlpool, 200
Battle Creek Sanitarium, 198
Behaviors, high-risk, 266
Bilateral tree stroking, 107
Bioterrorism, 255
Bleeding, 71
Blood circulation, 41
Blood pressure, 42
contraindications regarding, 71
Blood transfusion, and AIDS, 266
B-lymphocytes, 250
Body alignment, 40
Body awareness, 38
Body-centered therapy, 50
Body defenses
immune system, 250–251
physical and chemical, 249–250
vaccines, 251
Body fluids exchange, 266
Body mechanics, practitioner's, 92–94
Body–mind effects, 49
Body piercing, 247
Bodywork traditions, 5–7
Boundaries, 76
Bovine spongiform encephalitis, 253–254
Breasts
draping, 89
massage, 44, 191, 212
Bronchitis, 272
Bruising, 71
Buttocks
anatomy, 178
application of massage, 178
full-body Western massage, 153–156
techniques, 179

C
Cancer patients, 60
Candidiasis, 261–262
Cardiovascular system, 41–42
pathologies, 58–59
Carotid bruit, 71
Carpal tunnel syndrome, 280
Cautions, 69–72
Cell-mediated immunity, 250
Cellular level activity, of muscles, 39
Celsus, 20
Chairs, 82–83
Character armor, 50
Chemical defenses against disease, 249–250
Chest
anatomy, 191
applications of massage, 190–191
movement techniques, 140
techniques, 191–194
China, ancient, 19
Chiropractic, 62–63
Chlamydia, 256–257
Cholera, 254
Chronic fatigue syndrome (CFS), 279
Chronic lung disease, 268–272
Circling, lower leg, 144
Circular two-handed petrissage, 113
Circulatory massage, spreading disease by, 71
Clapping, 121
Cleanliness of massage space, 84
Clinical applications
anxiety reduction in hospitalized patients, 59–60
cardiovascular and lymphatic pathologies, 58–59
clinical approaches, 57
complement to chiropractic, 62–63
immune function, 59
massage for cancer patients, 60
musculoskeletal pathologies, 58
pediatric care, 60–61
psychological aspects of treatment, 61–62
respiratory pathologies, 59
therapeutic touch, 62
value of research, 56–57
Clinical massage therapy, 56
Cold
common, 246–247
healing effects of, 204–205
Colitis, 277
Combinations of techniques, 152
Commission on Massage Therapy Accreditation (COMTA), 31
Common cold, 246–247
Complementary and alternative medicine (CAM), 7
Complementary therapy, 7
Compression techniques, 114–115
ischemic, 125
Confidentiality, 81
Connective tissue, 37
Consumers of massage therapy, 31
Contact lenses, 71
Continuity, 152
Contract-relax-stretch (CRS), 132
Contraindications, 69–72
for massage in older adults, 225–226
for pregnancy massage, 208
for thermo-hydrotherapy, 201–202
Conventional medicine, massage in, 24–26
Counterculture, 28–29
Countertransference, 77
Crabs, 261
Cross-armed stretch, 134
Cross-gender massage, 79
Cryotherapy, 199, 204–205
Cryptosporidium, 254
Culture, and touch, 79
Cupping, 121
Curanderas, 18
Cycle of pain–spasm–pain, 44
Cyriax friction, 118–119

D
Deep friction, 116–118
Deep pressure, to suboccipitals, 172–173
Deep transverse friction, 118–119
Dengue, 254
Dengue hemorrhagic fever, 254
Depressed adolescent mothers, 61
Diabetes
  in children, 61
  risk factors, 276
  U.S. incidence of, 275
Digestive system, 43
  disorders related to, 275–279
Direct pressure, 125
  to buttocks, 179
  to cervical muscles, 172
Direct therapeutic effects, 57
Disease
  chronic fatigue syndrome, 279
  chronic lung disease, 268–272
  digestion-related, 275–277
  emerging and resurgent, 251–255
  gender-related disorders, 275
  HIV/AIDS, 263–268
  musculoskeletal, 278
  neurological disorders, 273–274
  noninfectious, 268
  repetitive stress injuries, 280
  risks for, 242–249
  sexually transmitted infections, 255–263
  spreading by circulation, 71
Distress, acute, 70
Do no harm, 67
Dorsiflexion, mobilizing with (ankle), 144
Dr. M. Roth, 23
Draping, 86–91, 151
Dressing arrangements, 84
Drugs
  for HIV, 267–268
  injecting, 266
Dual relationships, 76
Dying, massage for, 229–230

E
Ears, massaging, 169
Ebola hemorrhagic fever, 254
Edema, 58, 71
Effects of massage
  organism level, 44–46
  organ system level, 38–44
  psychological, 46–47
  tissue level, 35–37
Effleurage techniques, 7, 106–107
  light effleurage with vibration, 124
  over eyelids, 168
  between ribs, 175
  sedating effleurage of back, 177–178
  variations, 107–111
Elbow, 68
  direct pressure applied by, 179
  movement techniques, 136–137
Elderly
  cautions regarding massage, 225–226
  massage for, 221–222, 224–225
  working with, 223
Electric vibrators, 122
ELISA test, 267
Emerging and resurgent diseases, 251–255
Emotional release, 47, 81
Emotional self-care for practitioner, 97
Emphysema, 272
Endangerment sites, 67–69
  cervical region, 171–172
  popliteal fossa, 181
Endocrine system, 40–41
Endometriosis, 275
Endorphins, 45
Energetic effects, 49
Environment
  as disease risk factor, 242
  massage space, 83–84
  setting for pregnancy massage, 208–209
Enzymes, 249–250
Epidemic, HIV/AIDS, 263–264
Epilepsy, 274
Ergonomics, 234
Esalen massage (1970s), 28–30
Escherichia coli O157:H7, 254
Evidence-based therapies, 56
Eyebrows, squeeze to, 167–168
Eyelids, effleurage over, 168
Eyes, 69
  passive touch over, 170

F
Face
  anatomy, 167
  applications of massage, 166
  and head, 162
  techniques, 167–170
Facial steam, 201
Fascia, 37
Fever, 251
  dengue hemorrhagic, 254
  ebola hemorrhagic, 254
Fibromyalgia syndrome (FMS), 58, 278
Figure eights
  foot, 147
  hand, 139
Fine vibration, 123
Finger push-ups, neck, 133
Fingers, interlocking between toes, 147
Fingers-to-thumb petrissage, alternating, 113
Finishing techniques, 152
Finnish sauna, 197
Fist, direct pressure applied by, 179
Fitness, 28
Flexibility, joints, 40
Flow of techniques, 152
Folk traditions, 5–6, 17–18

Foot
  anatomy, 180–181
  massage, 181–182
  movement techniques, 145–147
Forearm
  direct pressure applied by, 179
  preventing strain of, 189–190
  pronation and supination, 137
Forward flexion, 133–134
Frail elders, 223
Friction, 115–119
  warming, 175
Full-body Western massage
  continuity and flow, 152
  draping, 151
  goals for health promotion, 150
  order of techniques, 151–152
  routines, 152–163
  sequence of body regions, 151
Fungi, 249

G
Galen, 20
Gender considerations, 79–80
  endometriosis, 275
  menstrual problems, 275
General UTIs, 262
Genital herpes, 262–263
Genital HPVs, 261
German measles, 249
Giving massage
  amount of lubricant, 99
  confidentiality, 81
  emotional self-care, 97
  gender considerations, 79–80
  HIPAA privacy rule, 81–82
  interventional model, 80
  length of session, 98
  permission to touch, 78–79
  physical environment, 82–84
  physical self-care for practitioner, 91–97
  positioning and draping, 85–91
  pressure, rhythm, and pacing, 100
  professional demeanor, 77
  sequence of techniques and routines, 100
  specificity and direction, 100
  talking and feedback, 80–81
  therapeutic relationship, 76–77
  topical substances, 84–85
  touching another person, 77–78
Gluteal attachments, 179
Gonorrhea, 257
Graham, Douglas, 24
Greece, ancient, 20
Groin, 69
Growth and development, 44
Gymnasia, Greek, 20, 197

H
Hacking, 120–121
Hands
  anatomy, 187
  practitioner: care of, 91–92
Hantavirus, 254–255
Hawaiian lomi-lomi, 18
Hay fever, 270
Head
  anatomy, 167
  applications of massage, 166
  face and, 162
  muscles on, 170
  techniques, 167–170
Headaches, 273
Health care, integrative, 7
Health history, 69
Health professions, wellness and, 12
Hearing aids, 71–72
Heat, healing effects of, 203
Hepatitis, 248–249
Heredity, 242
Herpes, 262–263
High-level wellness, 9–10
High-risk behaviors, 266
Hip
  massage, 183
  movement techniques, 140, 142
HIPAA privacy rule, 81–82
Hippocrates, 20
Histamines, 270
History of massage
  ancient and global heritage, 17
  native and folk traditions, 17–18
HIV/AIDS, 263–268
Holding, sides of head, 170
Holistic approach to health, 4–5
  body-centered therapy, 50
  character armor, 50
  indivisible body and mind, 49–50
  limbic system, 50
Horizontal flexion, 136
Horizontal stroking, 109–110
Hospice, 229
Hospitals, mineral water, 198
Hot packs, 203–204
Hot tub, 200
Human immunodeficiency virus (HIV), 263–268
Human papillomaviruses (HPVs), 261
Human potential movement, 28–29
Humoral immune responses, 250
Hydrocollator units, 203
Hydrotherapy
  in medicine, 198–199
  physical therapy, 199
  water-based, 197–198
Hyperemia, 41

Hyperextension
  hand, 139
  hip, 142
  at wrist, 138
Hypertonic muscles, 39

I
Ice massage, 205
Illness/wellness continuum, 9
Immune function, 59
Immune system, 250–251
Immunity, 42–43
  compromised, 71
Immunoglobulins, 250
India, ancient, 20
Indivisible body and mind, 49–50
Infant massage
  benefits, 213
  techniques, 213–217
Infectious mononucleosis, 248
Inflammation, 35–37
  acute, 70
Influenza, 247–248
Informed consent, 78–79
Inguinal area, 69
Insect-borne diseases, 244
Insulin, 276
Integumentary system, 38
Intention, 5
Interferon, 246
Interspecies transmission of disease, 244
Intervention model, 80
Irritable bowel syndrome (IBS), 277
Ischemia, 44
Ischemic compression, 125

J
Japan, ancient, 19
Jaw, massage around, 169
Joint movements, 7
  categories of, 131
  general principles of, 131–132
  techniques, 132–147
Joints, increased mobility and flexibility, 40
Jones, Sir Robert, 24–25
Jostling, 124

K
Kellogg, John Harvey, 26, 198
Kidney area, 68–69
Kneading, 112
Knee
  endangerment site, 181
  movement techniques, 142–144
Kneipp, Sebastian, 198
Knuckling, 111

L
Labor, massage during, 212
Lactose intolerance, 277
Latent syphilis, 260
Lateral flexion, neck, 133
Late syphilis, 260
Legionnaires' disease, 245
Leg toss, 144
Length of session, 98
Lice, pubic, 261
Lighting, 84
Limbic system, 50
Ling, Pehr Henrik, 22–23
Liniment, 84
Lomi-lomi, 18
Lotions, 85
Lower back, therapeutic sequence for, 175–177
Lower extremities
  anatomy, 180–181
  applications of massage, 180
  techniques, 181–185
Lower leg
  anatomy, 180
  general massage, 185
Lower limbs
  prone position, 153–156
  supine position, 156–158
Lubricant, amount of, 99
Lucas-Championnière, Marie Marcellin, 24
Lymphatic system, 42–43
Lymphedema, 59
Lymph fluid movement, 42

M
Macfadden, Bernarr, 26
Mad cow disease, 253–254
Manual therapy, 4
Massage. *See also* Giving massage
  effects of. *See* Effects of massage
  hot packs and, 203–204
  regional applications of, 165–195
  seated: in workplace, 233–239
  space, 83–84
  tables and chairs, 82–83
  techniques of, 5
  Western. *See* Western massage
  workplace. *See* Workplace massage
Maya sweat baths, 197
McMillan, Mary, 25
Measles, 249
Mechanical effects, 48
Mechanisms of massage, 47–49
Medications, massage and, 72
Medicine
  conventional: massage in, 24–26
  hydrotherapy in, 198–199
  Western: massage and, 7–9
Melt-down, neck, 133
Mennell's superficial stroking, 110
Menstrual problems, 275
Mental clarity, 46

Mezger, Johann Georg, 23
Microbes, 252–255
Middle Ages, 21–22
Migraine, 273
Mineral and hot springs, 197
Misalignment, 62
Mobility
  in lower extremities, 183
  shoulder girdle, 187–189
Mobilizing techniques
  ankle, 144–145
  buttocks, 179
  chest, 140
  elbow, 137
  foot, 146
  hip, 140, 142
  knee, 142–144
  neck, 132
  scalp, 169
  shoulder girdle, 134
  wrist, 138
Moniliasis, 261–262
Mononucleosis, infectious, 248
Mouth, massage around, 169
Multifactorial diseases, 242
Multiple sclerosis, 274
Muscles
  cellular level activity, 39
  cervical, 172, 225
  on head, 170
  hypertonic, 39
  relaxation, 39–40
Muscular system
  cellular level activity, 39
  health of, 38
  joint mobility and flexibility, 40
  muscle relaxation, 39–40
  posture, 40
Musculoskeletal diseases, 278–279
Musculoskeletal pathologies, 58

N
National Center for Complementary and Alternative Medicine (NCCAM), 30
Native traditions, 5–6, 17–18
Natural healing art, 4–5, 26
Natural immunity, 251
Neck
  anatomy, 171–172
  anterior, 67
  applications of massage, 171
  full-body Western massage, 161–162
  massage in prone position, 174
  movement techniques, 132–134
  protective responses, 170–171
  techniques, 172–174
Nerve strokes, 110
Nervous system, 40–41
Neural-gating mechanism, 44–45
Neurological disorders, 273–274
Neutro-therapy, 199
Noninfectious diseases, 268
Normal range of motion, 131
Nose, sliding of thumb along, 168
Nurturing touch, 229
NvCJD disease, 253–254

O
Oils, 84–85
One-handed kneading, 112
On-site massage, 234
Opening technique, 152
Order of techniques, 151–152
Organism level effects
  growth and development, 44
  pain reduction, 44–45
  stress reduction, 45–46
Organism resistance, 242
Organ system level effects
  cardiovascular system, 41–42
  digestive system, 43
  integumentary system, 38
  lymphatic system and immunity, 42–43
  muscular system, 38–40
  nervous and endocrine systems, 40–41
  reproductive system, 43–44
  respiratory system, 43
  skeletal system, 38
  urinary system, 43
Osteoarthritis, 278
Osteoporosis, 71
Overhead stretch, 136–137

P
Pacing, 100
  full-body massage, 152
Pain
  as defense mechanism, 251
  low back, 279
  reduction, 44–45
Palliative care, 57, 229
Parasitic worms, 249
Pare, Ambrose, 22
Parkinson's disease, 274
Passive shoulder roll, 134
Passive touch, 125
  over eyes, 170
Pathogens, 241
  routes of transmission, 243–244
Pediatric care, 60–61
Pelvic inflammatory disease (PID), 257
Peptic ulcers, 277
Perinatal transmission of AIDS, 266
Periodontal diseases, 246
Person-centered massage, 73
Petrissage techniques, 7, 35
  for healthy aging, 225
  variations, 112–115

Physical defenses against disease, 249–250
Physical environment
  massage space, 83–84
  massage tables and chairs, 82–83
Physical self-care, for practitioner, 91–97
Physical therapy, with water, 199
Physiological effects, 48
Pincement, 121
Plantar flexion, 145
Pneumonia, 245
Popliteal fossa, 69
Positioning, 85–86
  options for pregnancy massage, 209–210
Posttraumatic stress disorder, children with, 61
Posture, 40
  pregnancy, 208
  techniques for healthy aging, 225
Practitioners
  amount of lubricant, 99
  avoiding strain, 94
  eclectic, 7
  emotional self-care, 97
  good body mechanics, 92–94
  hand and wrist care, 91–92
  length of session, 98
  pressure, rhythm, and pacing, 100
  sequence of techniques and routines, 100
  specificity and direction, 100
Pregnancy massage
  contraindications, 208
  labor, delivery, and recovery, 212
  positioning options, 209–210
  session, 211–212
  setting the environment, 208–209
Premenstrual dysphoric disorder (PMDD), 275
Premenstrual syndrome (PMS), 275
Pressure, 100
  along zygomatic arch, 168
  to cervical muscles, 172
  on sides of head, 170
  to thoracic attachments, 173–174
Priessnitz, Vincent, 197
Primary syphilis, 260
Principle-based therapy, 57
Prions, 249
Productivity, worker, 234
Professional demeanor, 77
Pronation, forearm, 137
Prone position, 85
  full-body Western massage, 153–156
  neck massage in, 174
  upper extremity massage, 188
Protozoa, 249
Psychological effects, 61–62
  emotional release, 47
  feelings of general well-being, 47
  mental clarity, 46
  reduced anxiety, 46
Pubic lice, 261
Public policy, 30

Q
Quacking, 121

R
Range of motion
  full (hip), 142
  normal, 131
Rapping, 121
Reciprocal inhibition, 132
Reclining, for pregnancy massage, 210
Reconstruction aides, 25
Red blood cells, 42
Referred pain, 251
Reflex effects, 48
Rehabilitation, friction used in, 118–119
Relaxation
  back massage for, 177
  muscle, 39–40
  response, 45–46
Renaissance Europe, 21–22
Repair, tissue, 35–37
Repetitive strain injuries, 234
Repetitive stress injuries (RSI), 280
Reproductive system, 43–44
Research
  literacy, 57
  value of, 56–57
Resistance, organism, 242
Resources, 73
Respiration, enhancing, 192–194
Respiratory system, 43
  pathologies, 59
Rheumatoid arthritis, 278
Rhythm, 100
  full-body massage, 152
Ribs, effleurage between, 175
Risk factors for disease, 242–243
  diabetes, 276
Robust elders, 223
Rocking
  leg, 140
  rib cage, 140
Rolling, 115. *See also* Skin rolling
Rome, ancient, 20–21
Room temperature, 83
Rounded shoulders, 191–192
Routines, 100
  full-body Western massage, 152–163
Rubbing, medical, 24
Rubdown, 27
Rubella, 249

S
Safety, around endangerment sites, 69
Same-gender massage, 79
Sauna
  dry heat, 201
  Finnish, 197
Sawing, 116

Scalp, mobilizing, 169
Scapula, mobilizing, 134
Scissoring, 139, 146
Seated massage in workplace, 233–239
Secondary headache, 273
Secondary syphilis, 260
Sedating effleurage, of back, 177–178
Seizure disorders, 274
Self-care
  emotional, 97
  physical, 91–97
  when working with terminally ill, 230–231
Sensation, decreased, 70–71
Sensory input, 39
Sequence of body regions, 151
Session length, 98
Sexually transmitted infections (STIs), 255–263
Shaking
  form of vibration, 124
  shoulder mobilizing technique, 134
Shiatsu, 19
Shingles effleurage, 107
Shoulder girdle
  enhancing mobility of, 187–189
  movement techniques, 134–136
Shoulders
  anatomy, 187
  arms and, 158–160
  neck and, 161–162
  rounded, 191–192
Showers, 200–201
Side-lying position, 86
  for pregnancy massage, 210
Simple mobilizing movements, neck, 133
Skeletal system, 38
Skills, in working with terminally ill, 230
Skin conditions, contraindications, 70
Skin rolling, 114
  back, 175
Slapping, 121
Sleep apnea, 272
Sliding effleurage, basic, 107
Sliding of thumb along nose, 168
Socioeconomic factors and AIDS, 265
Sound, 84
South Sea Islands, 18
Spa
  European, 198
  medical, 9
Special populations, 51
Specificity
  and direction, 100
  of full-body massage, 152
Sports massage, 27
Squeeze, to eyebrows, 167–168
Squishes, 122
Standards and credentials, 30–31
Staphylococcal infections, 245
Static stretches, 132
Steam cabinet, 201
Steam rooms, 201
Sternocleidomastoid, 67
Strain, avoiding, 94
Streptococcal infections, 245
Stress reduction, 45–46
Stretches
  ankle, 145
  cervical muscles, 225
  chest, 140
  elbow, 137
  foot, 147
  hip, 142
  neck, 133–134
  shoulder girdle, 136
  wrist, 138
Stretching, buttocks, 179
Stripping effleurage technique, 107
Stroke, 71
Structural integrity, loss of, 70
Structure and movement
  ankle, 144
  chest, 140
  elbow, 136–137
  foot, 145–146
  hip, 140
  knee, 142
  neck, 132
  shoulder girdle, 134
  wrist, 138
Subluxations, 62
Sumer, 18
Superficial warming friction, 116
Supination, forearm, 137
Supine position, 85
  direct pressure to thoracic attachments, 173–174
  full-body Western massage, 156–163
  upper extremity massage, 189
Swedish massage, 26
Swedish movement cure, 23
Swiss shower, 200
Symptoms of HIV, 266–267
Syphilis, 260
Systemic lupus erythematosus (SLE), 278–279

T

Tables, 82–83
Talking and feedback, 80–81
Tapotement, 7, 119–122
Tapping, 121
Tattooing, 247
Taylor, Dr. George, 24
Tension headache, 273
Terminally ill, 228–231
Terminology, health professions, 12–13
Therapeutic relationship, 76–77
Therapeutic sequence, for lower back, 175–177
Therapeutic touch, 62
Thermal therapy, 196–206
Thermo-therapy, 199, 203–204

Thigh
  anatomy, 180
  deep effleurage, 183
  diagonal adduction, 142
Thixotropy, 37
Thoracic attachments, direct pressure to, 173–174
Thoracic cage, 67
Three-count stroking of trapezius, 107, 109
Tissue level effects
  connective tissue, 37
  tissue repair, 35–37
T-lymphocytes, 250
Toes, mobilized into extension, 146
Topical substances, 84–85
Touch
  deprivation of, 229
  increased sensitivity to, 71
  passive, 125, 170
  permission to, 78–79
  therapeutic, 62
  and therapeutic relationship, 78
Touching another person, 77–78
Touch Research Institute, 30, 60–61
Touch without movement, 7
  direct pressure, 125, 127
  passive touch, 125
Toxic shock syndrome, 245
Trager Psychophysical Integration, 59
Transference, 77
Transition techniques, 152
Transmission
  of AIDS, 266
  of STIs, 256
Trapezius, three-count stroking of, 109
Trichomoniasis, 262
Tuberculosis, 245–246
Turkey, ancient, 21
Turning over, 156
Two-handed kneading, basic, 112

U
Ulcer, peptic, 277
Umbilicus, 68
United States
  diabetes incidence, 275
  Swedish movement cure in, 23
Upper extremities, 185–190
  anatomy, 186–187
  applications of massage, 186
  techniques, 187–190
Urinary system, 43
Urinary tract infections (UTIs), 262

V
Vaccines, 251
Veins
  carotid and jugular, 171–172
  in extremities, 69
  varicose, 71
Venostasis, 42
Venous return, 41–42
Vertebral column, 67
Vibration, 7, 122–124
Vichy shower, 200–201
Viruses, 246–249

W
Wagging, 134, 137, 142
Warming friction
  of back, 175
  superficial, 116
Warming technique, 152
Warts, genital, 261
Water, healing properties of, 199
Water-based therapies, 197–198
Wavelike movement, neck, 133
Waving, 138
Well-being, feelings of, 47
Wellness, high-level, 9–10
Wellness massage pyramid, 10–12
Western blot, 267
Western massage
  full-body, 149–164
  healthy aging, 220–226
  hydrotherapy/thermal therapies, 196–206
  Johann Georg Mezger, 23
  joint movements, 129–148
  mother and child, 207–218
  overview of, 6
  Pehr Henrik Ling, 22–23
  regional applications, 165–195
  Swedish movement cure in U.S., 23–24
  of terminally ill and dying, 228–231
  in workplace, 233–239
Western massage techniques
  effleurage, 7, 106–111
  friction, 115–119
  petrissage, 7, 35, 112–115
  tapotement, 7, 119–122
  touch without movement, 7, 125–127
  vibration, 7, 122–124
Western medicine, massage and, 7–9
Whirlpool baths, 200
Wholeness and meaning, 167
Widening, foot, 147
Women and AIDS, 264–265
Workplace massage
  benefits of, 234–235
  history of, 234
  popularity of, 237–238
  seated massage for office workers, 236–237
Work-site acupressure massage, 235
Wrist
  movement techniques, 138
  practitioner: care of, 91–92

Y
Yellow Emperor's Classic of Internal Medicine, 19

Z
Zygomatic arch, direct pressure along, 168

Pearson Education, Inc.

YOU SHOULD CAREFULLY READ THE TERMS AND CONDITIONS BEFORE USING THE CD-ROM PACKAGE. USING THIS CD-ROM PACKAGE INDICATES YOUR ACCEPTANCE OF THESE TERMS AND CONDITIONS.

Pearson Education, Inc. provides this program and licenses its use. You assume responsibility for the selection of the program to achieve your intended results, and for the installation, use, and results obtained from the program. This license extends only to use of the program in the United States or countries in which the program is marketed by authorized distributors.

LICENSE GRANT

You hereby accept a nonexclusive, nontransferable, permanent license to install and use the program ON A SINGLE COMPUTER at any given time. You may copy the program solely for backup or archival purposes in support of your use of the program on the single computer. You may not modify, translate, disassemble, decompile, or reverse engineer the program, in whole or in part.

TERM

The License is effective until terminated. Pearson Education, Inc. reserves the right to terminate this License automatically if any provision of the License is violated. You may terminate the License at any time. To terminate this License, you must return the program, including documentation, along with a written warranty stating that all copies in your possession have been returned or destroyed.

LIMITED WARRANTY

THE PROGRAM IS PROVIDED "AS IS" WITHOUT WARRANTY OF ANY KIND, EITHER EXPRESSED OR IMPLIED, INCLUDING, BUT NOT LIMITED TO, THE IMPLIED WARRANTIES OR MERCHANTABILITY AND FITNESS FOR A PARTICULAR PURPOSE. THE ENTIRE RISK AS TO THE QUALITY AND PERFORMANCE OF THE PROGRAM IS WITH YOU. SHOULD THE PROGRAM PROVE DEFECTIVE, YOU (AND NOT PRENTICE HALL, INC. OR ANY AUTHORIZED DEALER) ASSUME THE ENTIRE COST OF ALL NECESSARY SERVICING, REPAIR, OR CORRECTION. NO ORAL OR WRITTEN INFORMATION OR ADVICE GIVEN BY PRENTICE HALL, INC., ITS DEALERS, DISTRIBUTORS, OR AGENTS SHALL CREATE A WARRANTY OR INCREASE THE SCOPE OF THIS WARRANTY.

SOME STATES DO NOT ALLOW THE EXCLUSION OF IMPLIED WARRANTIES, SO THE ABOVE EXCLUSION MAY NOT APPLY TO YOU. THIS WARRANTY GIVES YOU SPECIFIC LEGAL RIGHTS AND YOU MAY ALSO HAVE OTHER LEGAL RIGHTS THAT VARY FROM STATE TO STATE.

Pearson Education, Inc. does not warrant that the functions contained in the program will meet your requirements or that the operation of the program will be uninterrupted or error-free.

However, Pearson Education, Inc. warrants the diskette(s) or CD-ROM(s) on which the program is furnished to be free from defects in material and workmanship under normal use for a period of ninety (90) days from the date of delivery to you as evidenced by a copy of your receipt.

The program should not be relied on as the sole basis to solve a problem whose incorrect solution could result in injury to person or property. If the program is employed in such a manner, it is at the user's own risk and Pearson Education, Inc. explicitly disclaims all liability for such misuse.

LIMITATION OF REMEDIES

Pearson Education, Inc.'s entire liability and your exclusive remedy shall be:

1. the replacement of any diskette(s) or CD-ROM(s) not meeting Pearson Education, Inc.'s "LIMITED WARRANTY" and that is returned to Pearson Education, or
2. if Pearson Education is unable to deliver a replacement diskette(s) or CD-ROM(s) that is free of defects in materials or workmanship, you may terminate this agreement by returning the program.

IN NO EVENT WILL PRENTICE HALL, INC. BE LIABLE TO YOU FOR ANY DAMAGES, INCLUDING ANY LOST PROFITS, LOST SAVINGS, OR OTHER INCIDENTAL OR CONSEQUENTIAL DAMAGES ARISING OUT OF THE USE OR INABILITY TO USE SUCH PROGRAM EVEN IF PRENTICE HALL, INC. OR AN AUTHORIZED DISTRIBUTOR HAS BEEN ADVISED OF THE POSSIBILITY OF SUCH DAMAGES, OR FOR ANY CLAIM BY ANY OTHER PARTY.

SOME STATES DO NOT ALLOW FOR THE LIMITATION OR EXCLUSION OF LIABILITY FOR INCIDENTAL OR CONSEQUENTIAL DAMAGES, SO THE ABOVE LIMITATION OR EXCLUSION MAY NOT APPLY TO YOU.

GENERAL

You may not sublicense, assign, or transfer the license of the program. Any attempt to sublicense, assign or transfer any of the rights, duties, or obligations hereunder is void.

This Agreement will be governed by the laws of the State of New York.

Should you have any questions concerning this Agreement, you may contact Pearson Education, Inc. by writing to:

Director of New Media
Higher Education Division
Pearson Education, Inc.
One Lake Street
Upper Saddle River, NJ 07458

Should you have any questions concerning technical support, you may write to:

New Media Production
Higher Education Division
Pearson Education, Inc.
One Lake Street
Upper Saddle River, NJ 07458
1-800-677-6337 Monday–Friday, between 8:00 a.m. and5:00 p.m. CST.

You can also get support by filling out the web form located at http://247.pearsoned.com/mediaform

YOU ACKNOWLEDGE THAT YOU HAVE READ THIS AGREEMENT, UNDERSTAND IT, AND AGREE TO BE BOUND BY ITS TERMS AND CONDITIONS. YOU FURTHER AGREE THAT IT IS THE COMPLETE AND EXCLUSIVE STATEMENT OF THE AGREEMENT BETWEEN US THAT SUPERSEDES ANY PROPOSAL OR PRIOR AGREEMENT, ORAL OR WRITTEN, AND ANY OTHER COMMUNICATIONS BETWEEN US RELATING TO THE SUBJECT MATTER OF THIS AGREEMENT.

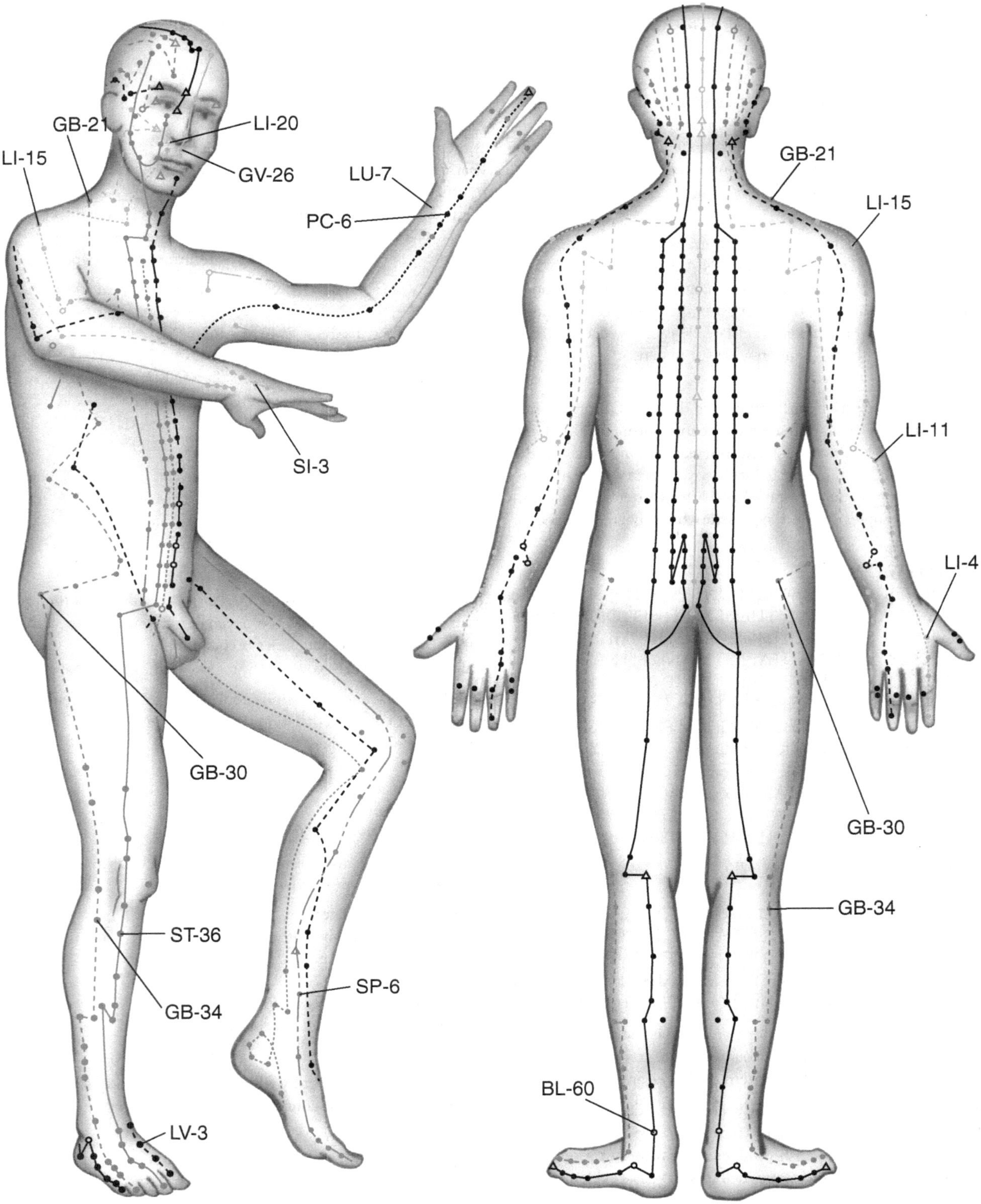
GB-21
LI-15
LI-20
GV-26
LU-7
PC-6
SI-3
GB-30
ST-36
GB-34
SP-6
LV-3
GB-21
LI-15
LI-11
LI-4
GB-30
GB-34
BL-60

Yes! I am interested in finding out how I can have a rewarding career in Health Care.

Please contact me now.

Name ______________________ Address ______________________
City __________________________ State ______ Zip ____________
Phone (______) ___________________ E-Mail __________________
High School __________________________ Year Grad. ____________

Also, please send a brochure to this friend.

Name ______________________ Address ______________________
City __________________________ State ______ Zip ____________
Phone (______) ___________________ E-Mail __________________

HERITAGE COLLEGE
Careers for lifelong fulfillment

Mail this card today! Or, call us at 800-887-8556.

NO POSTAGE
NECESSARY
IF MAILED
IN THE
UNITED STATES

BUSINESS REPLY MAIL

FIRST-CLASS MAIL PERMIT NO. 1347 DENVER CO

POSTAGE WILL BE PAID BY ADDRESSEE

HERITAGE COLLEGE
4704 HARLAN ST STE 100
DENVER CO 80212-9803

NO POSTAGE
NECESSARY
IF MAILED
IN THE
UNITED STATES

BUSINESS REPLY MAIL

FIRST-CLASS MAIL PERMIT NO. 1347 DENVER CO

POSTAGE WILL BE PAID BY ADDRESSEE

HERITAGE COLLEGE
4704 HARLAN ST STE 100
DENVER CO 80212-9803